Algorithms in
Infertility and Reproductive Medicine

Algorithms in Infertility and Reproductive Medicine

Editors

Kamini A Rao
MBBS DGO MCh FRCOG FNAMS FICOG PGDMLE
Medical Director
Milann Fertility Center
Bengaluru, Karnataka, India

Harpreet Kaur
MBBS MD DNB FNB (Rep Med) MRCOG (UK)
Associate Professor
Department of Obstetrics and Gynecology
All India Institute of Medical Sciences
Bilaspur, Himachal Pradesh, India

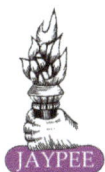

JAYPEE BROTHERS MEDICAL PUBLISHERS
The Health Sciences Publisher
New Delhi | London

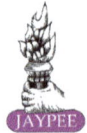 **Jaypee Brothers Medical Publishers (P) Ltd**

Headquarters
Jaypee Brothers Medical Publishers (P) Ltd
EMCA House, 23/23-B
Ansari Road, Daryaganj
New Delhi 110 002, India
Landline: +91-11-23272143, +91-11-23272703
+91-11-23282021, +91-11-23245672
Email: jaypee@jaypeebrothers.com

Corporate Office
Jaypee Brothers Medical Publishers (P) Ltd
4838/24, Ansari Road, Daryaganj
New Delhi 110 002, India
Phone: +91-11-43574357
Fax: +91-11-43574314
Email: jaypee@jaypeebrothers.com

Overseas Office
JP Medical Ltd
83 Victoria Street, London
SW1H 0HW (UK)
Phone: +44 20 3170 8910
Fax: +44 (0)20 3008 6180
Email: info@jpmedpub.com

Website: www.jaypeebrothers.com
Website: www.jaypeedigital.com

© 2024, Jaypee Brothers Medical Publishers

The views and opinions expressed in this book are solely those of the original contributor(s)/author(s) and do not necessarily represent those of editor(s) or publisher of the book.

All rights reserved. No part of this publication may be reproduced, stored or transmitted in any form or by any means, electronic, mechanical, photocopying, recording or otherwise, without the prior permission in writing of the publishers.

All brand names and product names used in this book are trade names, service marks, trademarks or registered trademarks of their respective owners. The publisher is not associated with any product or vendor mentioned in this book.

Medical knowledge and practice change constantly. This book is designed to provide accurate, authoritative information about the subject matter in question. However, readers are advised to check the most current information available on procedures included and check information from the manufacturer of each product to be administered, to verify the recommended dose, formula, method and duration of administration, adverse effects and contraindications. It is the responsibility of the practitioner to take all appropriate safety precautions. Neither the publisher nor the author(s)/editor(s) assume any liability for any injury and/or damage to persons or property arising from or related to use of material in this book.

This book is sold on the understanding that the publisher is not engaged in providing professional medical services. If such advice or services are required, the services of a competent medical professional should be sought.

Every effort has been made where necessary to contact holders of copyright to obtain permission to reproduce copyright material. If any have been inadvertently overlooked, the publisher will be pleased to make the necessary arrangements at the first opportunity.

Inquiries for bulk sales may be solicited at: jaypee@jaypeebrothers.com

Algorithms in Infertility and Reproductive Medicine

First Edition: **2024**

ISBN: 978-93-5696-048-0

Dedicated to
Our patients who teach us practice everyday

Contributors

Aashna Arora MBBS MS (Obs & Gyne)
Consultant
Sukhmani Hospital
Gurugram, Haryana, India

Abha Majumdar MS MBBS FICS
Emeritus Consultant
Department of Obstetrics and
Gynecology
Sir Ganga Ram Hospital
New Delhi, India

Ajitabh Shukla MD DNB FNB
IVF Consultant
Department of Obstetrics and
Gynecology
Genome—The Fertility Center
Kolkata, West Bengal, India

Anshu Dhar MBBS MD (Obs & Gyne)
Fellow Reproductive Medicine
Milann Hospital
Bengaluru, Karnataka, India

Bhawani Shekhar MD DNB MRCOG
Clinical Associate
Center of IVF and Human Reproduction
Sir Ganga Ram Hospital
New Delhi, India

Chaitra Nayak
MBBS MS (Obs & Gyne) FNB (Rep Med)
Consultant
Department of Reproductive Medicine
Cloud Nine Hospitals
Bengaluru, Karnataka, India

Deepika Krishna
MBBS MS Fellowship in Reproductive Medicine
Senior Consultant IVF
Milann Fertility Center
Bengaluru, Karnataka, India

Devi R
MBBS MS (Obs & Gyne) Fellowship in
Reproductive Medicine
Clinical Head and Fertility Specialist
Oasis Fertility
Bengaluru, Karnataka, India

Divya Sardana
MD DNB (Obs & Gyne) FNB (Rep Med)
Senior Consultant (IVF)
Cloudnine Hospital
Gurugram, Haryana, India

Divyashree PS MBBS MS DNB FNB
(Rep Med) PGDMLE
Medical Director
Genia Fertility Center
Bengaluru, Karnataka, India

G Rani Aishwarya MBBS MS
Consultant Reproductive Medicine
Milann Fertility and Birthing Centre
Bangaluru, Karnataka, India

Harpreet Kaur
MBBS MD DNB FNB (Rep Med) MRCOG (UK)
Associate Professor
Department of Obstetrics and
Gynecology
All India Institute of Medical Sciences
Bilaspur, Himachal Pradesh, India

Harsh Nihlani
MCh (Reproductive Medicine and Surgery) MD
(Obs & Gyne)
Senior Resident
Department of Obstetrics and
Gynecology
Sri Ramachandra Institute of Higher
Education and Research (SRIHER)
Chennai, Tamil Nadu, India

Jasneet Kaur MBBS MS FRM
Consultant and Clinical Director
(Reproductive Medicine)
Milann—The Fertility Center
Chandigarh, India

JB Sharma MD FRCOG FAMS PhD
Professor
Department of Obstetrics and
Gynecology
All India Institute of Medical Sciences
New Delhi, India

Kamini A Rao
MBBS DGO MCh FRCOG FNAMS FICOG PGDMLE
Medical Director
Milann Fertility Center
Bengaluru, Karnataka, India

Madhuri
MBBS MD FNB (Reproductive Medicine)
Consultant
Milann Fertility Center
Bengaluru, Karnataka, India

Mamta Dighe
MBBS MD DNB FNB (Reproductive Medicine)
FCPS DGO
Director
Xenith Advanced Fertility Centre
Pune, Maharashtra, India

Mandeep Kaur
MBBS MD FNB (Reproductive Medicine)
Medical Director
Star Fertility
Jalandhar, Punjab, India

Manishi Mittal
MD (Obs & Gyne) Fellowship in Reproductive
Medicine
Consultant
Department of Obstetrics and
Gynecology
Mittal Maternity and Superspecialty
Hospital
Yamunanagar, Haryana, India

Mansi Deoghare
MBBS MD (Obs & Gyne)
Senior Resident
Department of Obstetrics and
Gynecology
All India Institute of Medical Sciences
New Delhi, India

Mohammed Ashraf C
Masters (Medical Anatomy) PhD (Clinical
Embryology)
Associate Director and Senior
Embryologist
Milann Fertility Center
Bengaluru, Karnataka, India

Monika Rajput MD DNB DM
Resident
Reproductive Medicine
Department of Obstetrics and
Gynecology
All India Institute of Medical Sciences
New Delhi, India

Ms Lakshmishree BR
MSc in Clinical Embryology
Embryologist
Milann Fertility Hospitals
Bangaluru, Karnataka, India

Contributors

Neena Malhotra MD DNB FRCOG
Professor and Head of Unit
ART Centre
All India Institute of Medical Sciences
New Delhi, India

Nivedita Shetty
MBBS MD (OBG) FRCOG (UK)
Fellowship in Reproductive Medicine (National Board)
Director of the ART Unit
Manipal Hospital
Mysuru, Karnataka, India

Pallavi Kalghatgi MBBS DGO DNB
ICOG Certificate Course Reproductive Medicine
Consultant
Xenith Advanced Fertility Centre
Pune, Maharashtra, India

Plabani Sarkar MBBS MS
Obstetrician, Infertility Specialist
Department of Obstetrics and Gynecology
Postgraduate Institute of Medical Education and Research
Chandigarh, India

Prakash B Savannur
MBBS FRCOG DGO CCT(UK)
Consultant
Department of Obstetrics and Gynecology
Manipal Hospital
Mysuru, Karnataka, India

Pratibha S Malik
MD (Obs & Gyne) DNB (Obs & Gyne) FNB (Reproductive Medicine) MRCOG (UK)
Consultant Reproductive Medicine
Cloudnine Hospital
Gurugram, Haryana, India

Priyanka Kar MBBS MD
Department of Reproductive Medicine
Fellow at Matritava Advanced IVF and Training Centre
New Delhi, India

Rahul Kumar Gupta MSc Biotechnology
Head Embryologist
Motherhood Hospital
Gurugram, Haryana, India

Reeta Mahey MD DNB
Additional Professor
Department of Obstetrics and Gynecology
All India Institute of Medical Sciences
New Delhi, India

Rohitha Cheluvaraju MD DNB DM
Resident
Reproductive Medicine
Department of Obstetrics and Gynecology
All India Institute of Medical Sciences
New Delhi, India

Ruma Satwik DGO DNB FNB
Consultant
Centre of IVF and Human Reproduction
Associate Professor
Ganga Ram Institute of Postgraduate Medical Education and Research (GRIPMER)
Sir Gangaram Hospital
New Delhi, India

Runa Acharya MBBS MD
Clinical Director and Senior Consultant
Medicover Fertility Solutions
Hyderabad, Telangana, India

Rutvij Dalal
MBBS DGO DNB FNB Reproductive Medicine
IVF Specialist, Janini IVF
New Delhi, India

Saloni Kamboj MS DNB
Senior Research Associate
ART Centre
All India Institute of Medical Sciences
New Delhi, India

Sandhya Krishnan
DNB FNB (Reproductive Medicine) PGDMLE
Senior Consultant
N-CARE IVF
Kozhikode, Kerala, India

Sangita Sharma
MD DNB FNB (Reproductive Medicine) MNAMS
Unit Head and Consultant
Manipal Fertility
Jaipur, Rajasthan, India

Sapna Yadav MD
Embryologist
Cloudnine Hospitals
Noida, Uttar Pradesh, India

Saumya Prasad MBBS MD
Senior Consultant
Fellow at Matritava Advanced IVF and Training Centre
New Delhi, India

Shalini Gainder MBBS MD
Professor
Department of Obstetrics and Gynecology
Postgraduate Institute of Medical Education and Research
Chandigarh, India

Shallu Gupta
MBBS MD DNB FNB (Rep Med) MNAMS
Senior Consultant and IVF Specialist
Cloudnine Hospital
Gurugram, Haryana, India

Shikha Sardana MBBS MS DNB FRM
Consultant Reproductive Medicine
Milann Fertility Center
Chandigarh, India

Shivani Singh Kapoor
MBBS MD DNB FNB (Rep Med) MNAMS
Clinical Director
Srijan Fertility (A Unit of JK Hospital)
New Delhi, India

Shrinkhla Khandelwal MBBS MD
Department of Reproductive Medicine
Fellow at Matritava Advanced IVF and Training Centre
New Delhi, India

Snehal Dhobale Kohale
MS DNB (Obs & Gyne) MRCOG (UK)
Fellowship in Reproductive Medicine
Consultant
Fertility Specialist and Clinical Director
Ova Fertility and Women Care
Thane, Maharashtra, India

Sona Dharmendra MD
Consultant
Department of Obstetrics and Gynecology
All India Institute of Medical Sciences
New Delhi, India

Sonal Agarwal
MBBS MS DNB FNB (Rep Med) FMAS PGDLM
Senior Infertility Specialist
Creations World IVF Center
Noida, Uttar Pradesh, India

Sowmya Dinesh HR
MS FRCOG (UK) Fellowship in Reproductive Medicine
Chief Fertility Specialist and Gynec Endoscopic Surgeon
Medical Director SSM Multispeciality Hospital Pvt Ltd
Hassan Santasa IVF and EndoSurgery Institutes
Mysore, Karnataka, India

Sudha Prasad MBBS MD
Director
Deptartment of Reproductive Medicine
Fellow at Matritava Advanced IVF and Training Centre
New Delhi, India

Sujata Siwatch MBBS MD
Associate Professor
Department of Obstetrics and
Gynecology
Postgraduate Institute of Medical
Education and Research
Chandigarh, India

Sweta Gupta
MBBS MD (Obs & Gyne) MRCOG (London)
DFSRH (UK) FRCOG (London) MSc (Reproduction
and Development, Bristol, UK) Fellowship in
Reproductive Medicine and ART (London)
Medical Director
Crysta IVF
New Delhi, India

T Shilpa Reddy
MBBS MD (OBG) MRCOG (UK) FRM
Consultant
Reproductive Medicine Milann Fertiltiy
Bengaluru, Karnataka, India

Umesh Nandani Jindal MBBS MD
Director
Jindal IVF and Sant Memorial Nursing
Home
Chandigarh, India

Vanita Suri MBBS MD
Professor and Head
Department of Obstetrics and
Gynecology
Postgraduate Institute of Medical
Education and Research
Chandigarh, India

Vasani Nidhi N MD DNB (Obs & Gyne)
Post-Doctoral Fellowship (Reproductive
Medicine) FICOG
IVF Consultant and Director
Sahaj Gastro Care and Sarjan Fertility
Centre
Bhavnagar, Gujarat, India

Veronica Irene Yuel
MD DNB FRM FICOG
ART Consultant/Gynec Laparoscopic
Surgeon/Obstetrician and Gynecologis
NNH-MMI Superspecialty Hospital
Raipur, Chhattisgarh, India

Vivek Kakkad
MCh (Reproductive Medicine and Surgery)
MD (Obs & Gyne) Clinical Andrology Training
(Miami, USA)
Scientific Director
ART Fertility Clinics – India
Consultant Reproductive Medicine and
Surgery
Ahmedabad, Gujarat, India

Yogita Dogra MBBS MD DM (Rep Med)
Senior Consultant and Director
Arriva IVF Superspecialty Centre
Shimla, Himachal Pradesh, India

Preface

Infertility is a worldwide problem, affecting couples in their reproductive age which causes considerable social, emotional, and psychological stress not only for the couples but also their families. It affects up to one in six couples and remains a major cause of distress in both men and women. Concerns about fertility continue to grow across the world, since lifestyle choices and social pressures have caused couples to delay childbirth. The increase in the mean age at which couples decide to plan a pregnancy has also led to a substantial increase in the requirements for infertility solutions. In recent decades, steady progress has been made in the treatment of infertility and the number of centers offering infertility treatment has burgeoned throughout the world.

It was in this context that we felt the need to bring out a book on Algorithms in Infertility and Reproductive Medicine. Understanding gyne-endocrinology and reproductive medicine can be difficult and therefore to make it more reader-friendly, we conceptualized the idea of adding maximum algorithms to the diagnostic work-up and management plan of the problems which clinicians come across in their day-to-day practice. The simple format makes this book an excellent choice and a ready-reckoner for practicing fertility specialists of all spectrums. The book is aimed at practicing clinicians as well as at students of Gynecology and Reproductive Medicine.

The readers of this text will encounter a comprehensive and perspicacious view of the discipline of reproductive medicine as revealed by practicing fertility specialists of the day. The book has been designed to keep a balance of text and algorithms/flowcharts/diagrams, so as to provide comprehensive information in a concise and easy-to-understand format. Also, the memory for such diagrammatic presentation is long-lasting and it acts as a ready-reckoner for clinicians in practice and students for their examinations. The contents are mainly practical problems faced by clinicians in day-to-day practice and the chapters have been contributed by experienced doctors working in the field of infertility and reproductive medicine incorporating their vast practical experience. The information provided in the textbook is based on evidence-based guidelines and clinical experience.

We are extremely thankful to all the authors for contributing their chapters as well as for their constant support during the execution of this project. Our huge thanks to M/s Jaypee Brothers Medical Publishers (P) Ltd and their team for their dedicated efforts. We hope that this book will provide a concise guide to fertility practice for trainees as well as for specialists. Hope readers will enjoy reading this book and gain maximum from the experienced authors who have contributed to this book.

Kamini A Rao
Harpreet Kaur

Contents

1. **Work-up of a Case of Infertility** 1
   Snehal Dhobale Kohale

2. **Tubal Evaluation Methods and Assessment of Tubal Factor Infertility** 8
   Vasani Nidhi N

3. **Hysterolaparoscopy: Indications and Usage** 12
   Madhuri, Anshu Dhar

4. **Disorders of Puberty** 21
   Yogita Dogra

5. **Disorders of Sexual Development** 33
   Reeta Mahey, Monika Rajput, Rohitha Cheluvaraju

6. **Thyroid Disorders and Fertility** 50
   Shikha Sardana

7. **Hyperprolactinemia and Infertility: An Algorithm-based Approach** 54
   Sonal Agarwal, Rutvij Dalal

8. **Amenorrhea—Work-up and Management** 61
   Harpreet Kaur

9. **Management of the Hypogonadotropic Hypogonadism Male and Female** 67
   Ruma Satwik

10. **Management of Müllerian Anomalies** 77
    Vanita Suri, Sujata Siwatch

11. **Pelvic TB—Work-up and Management** 86
    JB Sharma, Mansi Deoghare, Sona Dharmendra

12. **Asherman's Syndrome** 89
    Saloni Kamboj, Neena Malhotra

13. **Management of Endometriosis** 99
    Mamta Dighe, Pallavi Kalghatgi

14. **Management of Fibroids and Adenomyosis in Infertility** 108
    Sangita Sharma

15. **Management of PCOS: Infertility and Long-term Management** 118
    Devi R, G Rani Aishwarya

16. **Management of Hirsutism** 131
    Chaitra Nayak

17. **Ovulation Induction Protocols for Intrauterine Insemination** 135
    Shivani Singh Kapoor, Shalu Gupta

18. **Sperm Selection in IUI and IVF** 144
    Mohammed Ashraf C, Ms Lakshmishree BR

19. **Controlled Ovarian Stimulation Protocols for In Vitro Fertilization** 161
    Pratibha S Malik

20. **Management of Ovarian Hyperstimulation Syndrome** 170
    Deepika Krishna

21. **Pregnancy of Unknown Location** 180
    Veronica Irene Yuel

22. **Diagnosis and Management of Ovarian Torsion** 185
    Divya Sardana, Aashna Arora

23. **Work-up and Management of Thin Endometrium** 190
    Runa Acharya

24. **Endometrial Preparation for Frozen Embryo Transfer** 196
    Manishi Mittal, Umesh Nandani Jindal

25. **Work-up of Azoospermia** 207
    Divyashree PS

26. **Ejaculatory/Erectile Dysfunction—Work-up and Management** 215
    Vivek Kakkad, Harsh Nihlani

27. **Dyspareunia—Work-up and Management** 220
    Sudha Prasad, Saumya Prasad, Shrinkhla Khandelwal, Priyanka Kar

28. **Work-up and Management of Premature Ovarian Insufficiency** 226
    Nivedita Shetty, Prakash B Savanur

29. **Recurrent Pregnancy Loss: Work-up and Management** 231
    Shalini Gainder, Plabani Sarkar

30. **Recurrent Implantation Failure—Work-up and Management** 239
    Mandeep Kaur, Ajitabh Shukla

31. **Lifestyle Factors in Infertility** 250
    T Shilpa Reddy

32. **Luteal Phase Support—What and Till When** 256
    Sandhya Krishnan

33. **Fertility Preservation Techniques** 260
    Jasneet Kaur

34. **Third Party Reproduction** 269
    Sowmya Dinesh HR

35. **PGT: When and Where to Offer** 279
    Abha Majumdar, Bhawani Shekhar

36. **Viral Infections and IVF—Hepatitis B, Hepatitis C, and HIV** 285
    Sweta Gupta, Sapna Yadav, Rahul Kumar Gupta

Index *293*

CHAPTER 1

Work-up of a Case of Infertility

Snehal Dhobale Kohale

INTRODUCTION

According to the American Society of Reproductive Medicine, if there is a failure to achieve pregnancy within 12 months of unprotected sexual intercourse or therapeutic donor insemination in women <35 years or within 6 months if women >35 years is considered as "infertility".[1,2] Incidence of infertility is approximately up to 15% of couples (one in six couples).[3]

WHEN TO SEEK HELP OF FERTILITY EXPERT?

- Couples as per above definition
- Couples having a high risk of infertility.

INDICATIONS OF IMMEDIATE EVALUATION FOR INFERTILITY[4]

- Age of women >40 years
- Age of women >35 years and failed attempts of 6 months
- If any of the following conditions:
  - Oligomenorrhea or amenorrhea
  - Known or suspected uterine/tubal/peritoneal disease
  - Stage III or stage IV endometriosis
  - Known or suspected male infertility
  - Previous history of surgery of reproductive organs.

CAUSES OF INFERTILITY

Infertility can be due to male factors, female factors, or a combination of both **(Table 1)**.[5-8]

TABLE 1: Factors causing infertility and its incidence.

Factors of infertility	Incidence
Male factor	25–30%
Ovulatory dysfunction	21–25%
Tubal factor	15–20%
Other (cervical, peritoneal, and uterine abnormalities)	10–13%
Combined	40%
Unexplained	25–28%

It is very important to offer detailed information and counseling to couples facing problems to conceive, as a part of the evaluation. Because the anxiety related to infertility tends to cause more stress, decreased libido and thus complicating the issue, thorough counseling plays a vital part in managing cases of infertility.[8]

Work-up of infertility should be carried out for both the partners at the same time and it should involve ruling out all the etiologies one by one **(Table 2)**.

TABLE 2: Work-up of infertility.

Female evaluation	Male evaluation
History	History
Physical examination	Semen analysis
Prepregnancy evaluation—to optimize a woman's health and control any comorbidities, if any	Others (only if required): • Hormonal evaluation • Imaging • Sperm DNA fragmentation index • Genetic tests

Evaluation of cause of infertility
 • Ovulatory factor:
   – Hormonal tests (AMH; baseline FSH, LH, and estradiol levels)
   – Transvaginal ultrasonography (for antral follicle count and to rule out any abnormality of reproductive organs)
   – TSH and prolactin
 • Tubal factor:
   – Hysterosalpingography
   – Hysterosalpingo-contrast-sonography
   – Saline sonography
   – Laparoscopy and hysteroscopy
 • Uterine factor:
   – Transvaginal sonography
   – Sonohysterography
   – Hysterosalpingography
   – Hysteroscopy
	Testicular biopsy

(AMH: anti-Müllerian hormone; DNA: deoxyribonucleic acid; FSH: follicle-stimulating hormone; LH: luteinizing hormone; TSH: thyroid-stimulating hormone)

FEMALE EVALUATION

History

Clinical history involves following points which generally direct further investigations:[3]
- Age of the female partner
- Coinhabiting the partner or not/trying since when?
- Duration of infertility
- Prior evaluation and its results
- History of prior treatment of infertility
- *Menstrual history:* Cycle length, regularity, duration and amount of the flow, pain associated with cycle, and premenstrual symptoms
- *Obstetric history:* Prior pregnancies and outcomes, time taken to conceive, fertility treatment for conception, complications, and mode of delivery
- History of contraception
- *Sexual history:* Timing and frequency of intercourse, any sexual dysfunction
- *Gynecological history:* History of polycystic ovarian syndrome, pelvic inflammatory disease, sexually transmitted disease, endometriosis, and fibroids
- *Medical history:* History of any illness, hospitalization, long-term medications, and allergies
- *Surgical history:* Previous history of surgeries, especially abdominal and pelvic procedures, indication, surgical details, and outcomes
- History of thyroid disease, galactorrhea, hirsutism, dyspareunia, and pelvic or abdominal pain
- *Family history:* History of medical problems, birth defects, developmental delay, early menopause, any fertility-related issues
- Occupational history, any known environmental hazard
- *Substance abuse:* Tobacco or nicotine-related products, alcohol, and recreational drugs.

Physical Examination

It includes general examination, pelvic examination, and thyroid and breast examination.
- *General examination:* Vitals (pulse and blood pressure) and body mass index (BMI) (height and weight)
- *Thyroid examination:* Nodule, enlargement, or tenderness
- *Breast examination:* Any secretions, its character, and nodularity
- Signs of androgen excess
- Tanner staging of breast, axillary, and pubic hairs (in cases of amenorrhea)
- *Pelvic examinations:* Vaginal and cervical secretions or abnormality; uterine size, shape, position, mobility, pelvic, or adnexal mass, tenderness, pouch of Douglas—tenderness and nodularity.

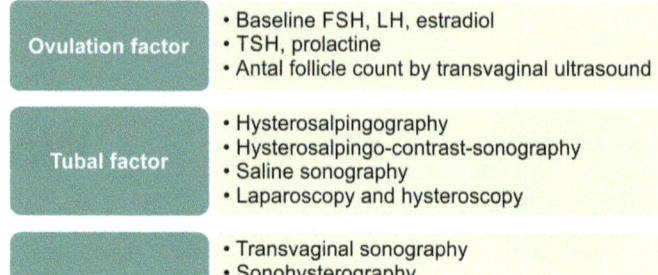

Fig. 1: Evaluation related to etiology of infertility. (FSH: follicle-stimulating hormone; LH: luteinizing hormone; TSH: thyroid-stimulating hormone)

Evaluation Related to Etiology of Infertility (Fig. 1)

These tests focus on structured problems, ovulatory dysfunction, and ovarian reserve. These include laboratory and imaging tests. Even though cervical factor plays minor role, test for evaluation of cervical mucus is not reliable and is not helpful for management of infertility in clinical practice.[6]

Tests of Ovarian Reserve

Ovarian reserve represents number of oocytes available for potential fertilization at a point of time. It predicts response to ovarian stimulation.[9] The tests of ovarian reserve are interpreted in the background of patient's age.

Hormonal Tests for Ovarian Reserve

- *Day 2 to day 5 serum estradiol and serum follicle-stimulating hormone (FSH):*
  - FSH value >10 IU/L is associated with low response to ovarian stimulation.[10]
  - Basal estradiol level should be <60–80 pg/mL.
  - High estradiol level suppresses FSH level. So high estradiol and normal FSH is associated with diminished ovarian reserve.[3]
- *Serum anti-Müllerian hormone (AMH):* AMH is produced by granulosa cells of preantral and antral follicles thus it specifically correlates with egg reserve. It does not fluctuate in the menstrual cycle so can be assessed on any day of the cycle.[11,12] AMH and antral follicle count (AFC) has the similar abilities to predict ovarian stimulation response and live birth.[9]
- *Ultrasound assessment AFC:*
  - AFC is the number of follicles measuring between 2 and 10 mm diameter in the ovaries on a transvaginal sonography done during baseline scan.
  - AFC below 5–7 is considered as low and is associated with poor response to stimulation.[13]

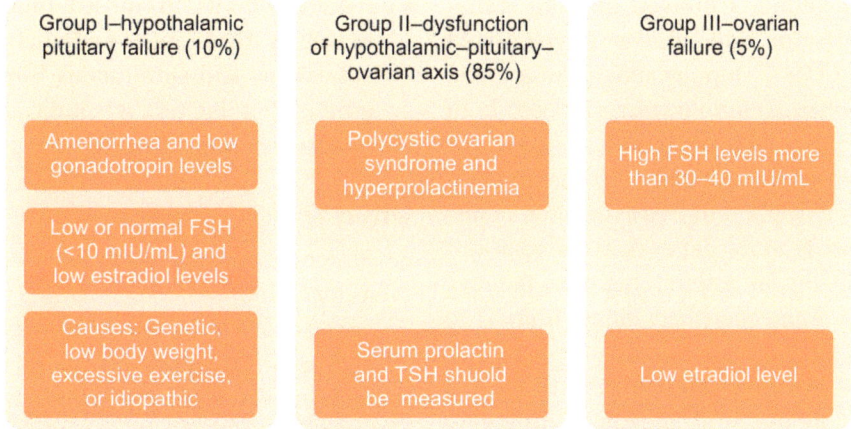

Fig. 2: Categories of ovulatory dysfunction as per the World Health organization (WHO). (FSH: follicle-stimulating hormone; TSH: thyroid-stimulating hormone)

- But AFC is relatively poor indication for prediction of future fertility.[10]
- AFC is elevated in polycystic ovary syndrome (PCOS) and decreased in women with hypothalamic amenorrhea and those taking hormonal contraceptive pills[14]

Ovarian reserve tests are good predictors of response to ovarian stimulation but poor results do not necessarily predict inability to achieve a live birth.[3,15,16]

Tests for Ovulatory Dysfunction

Generally menstrual history is enough to predict ovulatory function. Majority of ovulatory cycles will have regular menstrual periods between 25 and 35 days along with premenstrual symptoms. Even with the regular cycle, up to one-third of women may be anovulatory. So, ovulation needs to be confirmed with various tests.[17]

Ovulation can be objectively detected by:
- Cervical mucus changes
- Biphasic basal body temperature
- Positive luteinizing hormone kit
- Midluteal progesterone measurement.

In women of regular menstrual cycles, serum progesterone is tested at day 21 for confirmation of ovulation.[8] In women with irregular cycles, testing is done 7 days prior to presumed date of onset of periods and repeated weekly till periods resume. Ovulation is confirmed with progesterone level of 5 ng/mL or more.[6,18]

In cases of anovulation; obesity, hypothalamic-pituitary dysfunction, PCOS, and other causes have to be ruled out.

The World Health Organization (WHO) categorizes ovulatory dysfunction into three groups **(Fig. 2).**[8]
- PCOS is most common cause of ovulatory infertility.[19,20]
- Thyroid disease and hyperprolactinemia can cause ovulatory dysfunction ranging from luteal phase insufficiency, oligomenorrhea to anovulation, and amenorrhea.

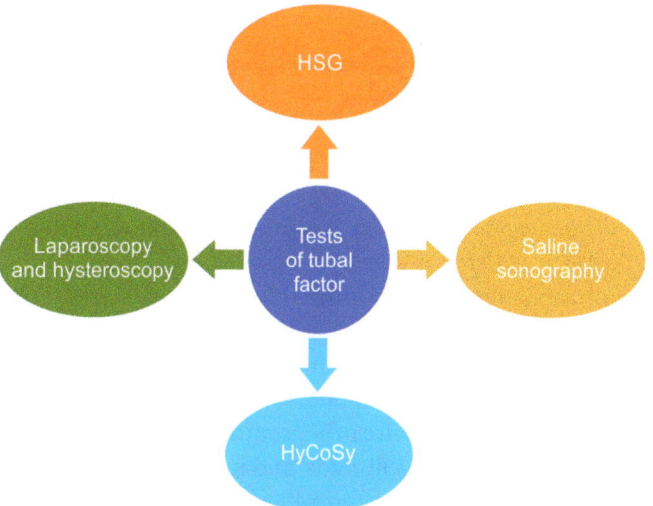

Fig. 3: Tests of tubal factor. (HSG: hysterosalpingography; HyCoSy: hysterosalpingo-contrast-sonography)

- In women with ovarian insufficiency or failure on elevated FSH level before 40 years, fragile X carrier screening is recommended to rule out *FMR 1* gene premutation.[21]

Tests of Tubal Factor (Fig. 3)

- *Hysterosalpingography (HSG):* It is most commonly used procedure for determining tubal patency. Radio-opaque contrast medium is injected through the cervix. Uterus and tubes are evaluated through fluoroscopy. It can detect proximal and distal tubal occlusions, peritubal adhesions, and salpingitis isthmica nodosa.

Following are predictive values of HSG for demonstrating tubal patency:[22]
- Positive predictive value 38%
- Negative predictive value 94%

As it has low positive predictive value, HSG showing nonpatency of tube may require further tests like laparoscopy to confirm tubal occlusion.[23]

- *Saline sonography:* Saline is infused through transcervical catheter. Uterus and adnexa is visualized ultrasonographically. Use of Doppler adds accuracy to it.
- *Hysterosalpingo-Contrast-Sonography (HyCoSy):* In this test, contrast agent with air bubbles is used for visualization of tubes sonographically. The agents used are perflutren lipid microsphere as well as agitated saline. Accuracy of this test is more dependent on operator experience. Its sensitivity for determining tubal patency ranges from 76 to 96% and specificity ranges from 67 to 100%.[24,25]
- *Laparoscopy and hysteroscopy:* Women with risk factors for tubal obstruction like endometriosis, previous pelvic infection, or ectopic pregnancy might require laparoscopy to rule out other pelvic pathology. It allows diagnosis and treatment at the same time for structural abnormalities of uterus like fibroids.

Tests for Uterine Factor (Fig. 4)

Uterine factors contributing to infertility are endometrial polyp, intrauterine adhesions, submucous fibroids, and Müllerian anomalies.

- *Transvaginal ultrasonography:* It helps in detection of fibroids distorting endometrial cavity. Use of three-dimensional ultrasonography improves detection of Müllerian anomalies and is comparable to pelvic magnetic resonance imaging (MRI) for accurate diagnosis of this condition.[26]
- *Sonohysterography:* It can be used to diagnose endometrial polyps, submucous fibroids, and intrauterine adhesions. It has 91% sensitivity and 84% specificity for diagnosing polyp or fibroid.
- *HSG:* It has limited ability to diagnose uterine cavity masses or adhesions as these structures are not radio-opaque. It has only 50% sensitivity for diagnosing polypoid lesions.[27]

- *Hysteroscopy:* It is the most definitive method of diagnosis as well as treatment of endometrial polyps, intrauterine adhesions, and submucous fibroids. Though it is not used as first-line test, it is indicated to confirm and treat intracavity lesions detected by other imaging techniques.

Other Tests

- Postcoital cervical mucus test is no longer recommended as it cannot predict the inability to conceive as well as it does not affect clinical treatment of patient.[28]
- Endometrial biopsy is nowadays not used as histological endometrial dating as neither it is reliable nor it is predictive of infertility. It should be performed only in women with suspected pathology like chronic endometritis or neoplasia and to rule out genital tuberculosis.[6,22]

EVALUATION OF MALE

About 40–50% of infertile couples may have male factor infertility.[29] Minimum evaluation of male includes reproductive history and semen analysis.[30] Any abnormalities in basic evaluation requires examination by specialist—reproductive urologist or andrologist.[30]

History

Following key points are noted in history:[30]
- Duration of infertility
- Prior fertility
- Coital frequency and timing
- Any evidence of sexual dysfunction including erectile or ejaculatory problems
- Developmental history
- Childhood illness
- History of previous surgery (e.g., cryptorchidism with or without surgery)
- Medication use e.g., anabolic steroids and supplements like testosterone
- History of sexually transmitted diseases
- History of allergies
- History of exposure to gonadal trauma or toxins
- Smoking, alcohol, or substance abuse.

Physical Examination

- *General examination:*
  - Built, height, weight, and BMI
  - Hair distribution
  - Rule out any gynecomastia
- *Local examination:*
  - Bilateral testis—size and consistency
  - Epididymis (any fullness/nodularity/tenderness)
  - Presence of bilateral vas deferens
  - Any evidence of genital infections.

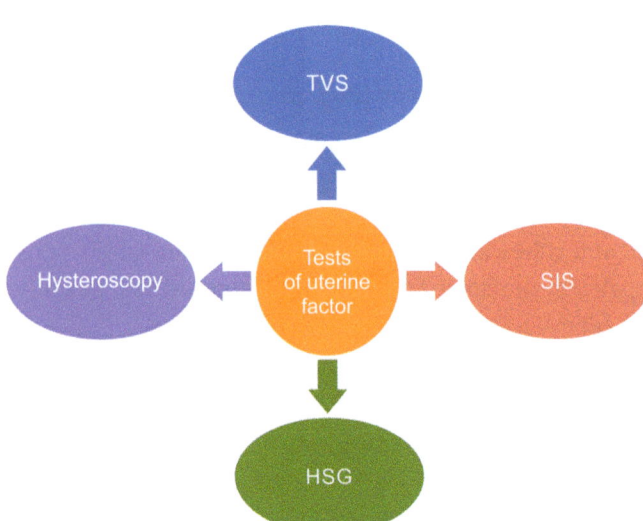

Fig. 4: Tests for uterine factor. (HSG: hysterosalpingography; SIS: saline infusion sonography TVS: transvaginal scan)

TABLE 3: The WHO 2010 semen analysis reference guidelines.[31]

Semen characteristic	Lower reference limit
Volume, mL	1.5
Sperm concentration, 10^6/mL	39
Total sperm number, 10^6	15
Total motility (PR + NP), %	40
Progressive motility (PR), %	32
Vitality (live spermatozoa), %	58
Sperm morphology (normal forms), %	4
pH	≥7.2
Seminal fructose, μmol/ejaculate	≥13

(PR: progressive motility; NP: non-progressive motility)
(*Source:* WHO laboratory manual)

Semen Analysis

It is the quantitative microscopic evaluation of sperm parameters. Semen sample is obtained by masturbation in laboratory collection room with 2-5 days of abstinence. As sperm generation time is just over 2 months, it is recommended to wait for 3 months before repeat sampling.[8]

The WHO 2010 guidelines are currently followed for determining normality of semen parameters **(Table 3)**.[31]

Abnormalities in Semen Analysis

- *Oligospermia:* Sperm count <15 million per mL
- *Asthenozoospermia:* Total sperm motility <40% or rapid progressive motility <32%
- *Teratozoospermia:* Normal morphology <4% (as per strict Krugerberg criteria)
- If an individual has all three low sperm conditions, it is known as *oligoasthenoteratozoospermia (OAT) syndrome*, which is typically associated with an increased likelihood of genetic etiology of the infertility.
- *Azoospermia:* Absence of sperms in semen

In cases of abnormal semen parameters further evaluation is needed. Hypogonadism is suspected when there is oligospermia or azoospermia.

- *Primary hypogonadism:* Decreased level of total testosterone (morning level) and increased level of FSH
- *Secondary hypogonadism:* Decreased level of total testosterone and decreased level of FSH (normal ranges: total testosterone—240-950 ng/dL; FSH—1.5-12.4 mIU/mL).

Sperm Deoxyribonucleic Acid Fragmentation Index

The integrity of deoxyribonucleic acid (DNA) present in the sperm is very crucial for the process of fertilization and normal embryo development. It has been observed that the sperm DNA fragmentation (SDF) is higher in infertile men compared to fertile men. When the DNA which carries the genetic material with all the instructions to the baby is fragmented, it can lead to poor fertilization, poor embryo development, and miscarriage. Also, if the fertilization happens with the DNA fragmented sperm, there is a high risk of genetic disease in the baby.

Fragmented DNA is usually can be caused by various reasons such as:
- Infection
- Smoking and alcohol
- Use of recreational drugs and medications
- Stress
- Increased BMI and poor diet
- Exposure to toxins and radiation
- Advanced age
- Varicocele (enlarged veins inside the scrotum)
- Increased testicular temperature.

Semen analysis is the standard test to assess the sperm quality. But it is not a fool proof test as it neither provides information regarding all the sperm functions nor the fertility potential of sperm. In addition to semen analysis, SDF test can be done to measure the sperm integrity and the damage to the DNA.

Sperm DNA Fragmentation Index (%)

- 15% or less fragmentation—excellent sperm DNA integrity
- 15-25% DNA fragmentation index (DFI)—good to fair
- 25-50% DFI—fair to poor
- 50% or greater DFI—extremely poor sperm DNA integrity.

Other Tests

- *Semen culture:* Assessment of semen sample for bacterial infections:
  - It is indicated in patients with clinical signs of genitourinary infections or leukocytes >1 million/mL in semen analysis.
- *Hormonal evaluation:* Assessment of FSH, LH, and testosterone levels
  - It is indicated in patients showing abnormal semen parameters like severe OAT or azoospermia.
- *Genetic testing—karyotyping, Y chromosome microdeletion, single gene defect testing, and cystic fibrosis transmembrane regulator (CFTR) mutation:*
  - Genetic testing is done when examination is showing Klinefelter phenotype (small testes, tall stature, gynecomastia, and learning disabilities)
  - Y chromosome microdeletion is done in cases of azoospermia or severe oligoasthenospermia.
  - CFTR gene mutation is tested when clinical examination shows the absence of vas deferens.

- *Testicular biopsy:*
  - It is done in cases of azoospermia (to know the cause of nonobstructive azoospermia by histology of testicular tissue).

Postcoital testing and antisperm antibody testing are not considered useful in male evaluation.[28,32]

Unexplained infertility may be diagnosed in as many as 30% of infertile couples. At a minimum, these patients should have evidence of ovulation, tubal patency, and a normal semen analysis.

Principles of Evaluation

- It should be systematic, expeditious, and cost-effective manner.
- It should identify all relevant factors.
- The initial emphasis should be on least invasive methods for detection of most common causes.
- The investigations which are chosen should be tailored to the needs of the individual patient.

Key Learning Points

- Infertility work-up is offered to the couple fulfilling "infertility" definition criteria or having a high risk of infertility and it should be offered to both the partners at the same time.
- Immediate evaluation is needed in women older than 40 years or those having conditions known to cause infertility.
- A comprehensive medical history and targeted physical examination for the partner is the key to offer appropriate investigations to the couple and thus ruling out causes of infertility one by one.
- Female partner's tests focus on ovarian reserve, ovulation test, checking for ovulatory dysfunction, structural abnormalities of reproductive organ, and tubal patency.
- Male is referred to reproductive urologist or andrologist if indicated from history or having abnormal semen parameters.
- A careful history and physical examination can identify symptoms or signs suggesting a specific cause for infertility and thereby help to focus subsequent diagnostic evaluation on the factor(s) most likely responsible.

REFERENCES

1. Practice Committee of American Society for Reproductive Medicine. Definitions of infertility and recurrent pregnancy loss: a committee opinion. Fertil Steril. 2013;99:63.
2. American College of Obstetricians and Gynecologists. reVitalize. Gynecology data definitions (version 1.0). Washington, DC: American College of Obstetricians and Gynecologists; 2017.
3. Practice Committee of the American Society for Reproductive Medicine. Diagnostic evaluation of the infertile female: a committee opinion. Fertil Steril. 2015;103:e44-50.
4. American College of Obstetricians and Gynecologists. Female age-related fertility decline. Committee Opinion No. 589. Obstet Gynecol. 2014;123:719-21.
5. Gutmacher AF. Factors effecting normal expectancy of conception. J Am Med Assoc. 1956;161(9):855-60.
6. Practice Committee of American Society for Reproductive Medicine. Diagnostic evaluation of the infertile female: a committee opinion. Fertil Steril. 2012;98(2):302-7.
7. Thonneau P, Marchand S, Tallec A, Ferial ML, Ducot B, Lansac J, et al. Incidence and main causes of infertility in a resident population (1,850,000) of three French regions (1988-1989). Hum Reprod. 1991;6(6):811-6.
8. National Collaborating Centre for Women's and Children's Health. Fertility: assessment and treatment for people with fertility problems. London, United Kingdom: National Institute for Health and Clinical Excellence (NICE); 2013. pp. 1-63.
9. Practice Committee of the American Society for Reproductive Medicine. Testing and interpreting measures of ovarian reserve: a committee opinion. Fertil Steril. 2015;103: e9-17.
10. Broekmans FJ, Kwee J, Hendriks DJ, Mol BW, Lambalk CB. A systematic review of tests predicting ovarian reserve and IVF outcome. Hum Reprod Update. 2006;12:685-718.
11. La Marca A, Stabile G, Artenisio AC, Volpe A. Serum anti-Mullerian hormone throughout the human menstrual cycle. Hum Reprod. 2006;21:3103-7.
12. Gracia CR, Shin SS, Prewitt M, Chamberlin JS, Lofaro LR, Jones KL, et al. Multi-center clinical evaluation of the Access AMH assay to determine AMH levels in reproductive age women during normal menstrual cycles. J Assist Reprod Genet. 2018;35:777-83.
13. Ferraretti AP, La Marca A, Fauser BC, Tarlatzis B, Nargund G, Gianaroli L. ESHRE consensus on the definition of "poor response" to ovarian stimulation for in vitro fertilization: the Bologna criteria. ESHRE working group on Poor Ovarian Response Definition. Hum Reprod. 2011;26:1616-24.
14. D'Arpe S, Di Feliciantonio M, Candelieri M, Franceschetti S, Piccioni MG, Bastianelli C. Ovarian function during hormonal contraception assessed by endocrine and sonographic markers: a systematic review. Reprod Biomed Online. 2016;33:436-48.
15. Scott RT Jr, Elkind-Hirsch KE, Styne-Gross A, Miller KA, Frattarelli JL. The predictive value for in vitro fertility delivery rates is greatly impacted by the method used to select the threshold between normal and elevated basal follicle-stimulating hormone. Fertil Steril. 2008;89:868-78.
16. ACOG Committee Opinion No. 773: The use of antimüllerian hormone in women not seeking fertility care. Obstet Gynecol. 2019;133:275-9.
17. Prior JC, Naess M, Langhammer A, Forsmo S. Ovulation prevalence in women with spontaneous normal-length menstrual cycles—a population-based cohort from HUNT3, Norway. PLoS One. 2015;10:e0134473.
18. Rowe PJ, Comhaire FH, Hargreave TB, Mellows HJ. WHO Manual for the Standardized Investigation and Diagnosis of the Infertile Couple. New York, NY: Cambridge University Press; 1993.
19. American College of Obstetricians and Gynecologists' Committee on Practice Bulletins—Gynecology. ACOG Practice Bulletin No. 194. Polycystic Ovary Syndrome. Obstet Gynecol. 2018;131:e157-71.
20. Fauser BC, Tarlatzis BC, Rebar RW, Legro RS, Balen AH, Lobo R, et al. Consensus on women's health aspects of polycystic ovary syndrome (PCOS): the Amsterdam ESHRE/

ASRM-Sponsored 3rd PCOS Consensus Workshop Group. Fertil Steril. 2012;97:28-38.e25.
21. Committee Opinion No. 691: Carrier screening for genetic conditions. Obstet Gynecol. 2017;129:e41-55.
22. Coutifaris C, Myers ER, Guzick DS, Diamond MP, Carson SA, Legro RS, et al. Histological dating of timed endometrial biopsy tissue is not related to fertility status. Fertil Steril. 2004;82(5):1264-72.
23. Technology Assessment No. 12: Sonohysterography. Obstet Gynecol. 2016;128:38-42.
24. Luciano DE, Exacoustos C, Luciano AA. Contrast ultrasonography for tubal patency. J Minim Invasive Gynecol. 2014;21:994-8.
25. Maheux-Lacroix S, Boutin A, Moore L, Bergeron ME, Bujold E, Laberge P, et al. Hysterosalpingosonography for diagnosing tubal occlusion in subfertile women: a systematic review with meta-analysis. Hum Reprod. 2014;29:953-63.
26. Graupera B, Pascual MA, Hereter L, Browne JL, Ubeda B, Rodriguez I, et al. Accuracy of three-dimensional ultra-sound compared with magnetic resonance imaging in diagnosis of Müllerian duct anomalies using ESHRE-ESGE consensus on the classification of congenital anomalies of the female genital tract. Ultrasound Obstet Gynecol. 2015;46:616-22.
27. Soares SR, Barbosa dos Reis MM, Camargos AF. Diagnostic accuracy of sonohysterography, transvaginal sonography, and hysterosalpingography in patients with uterine cavity diseases. Fertil Steril. 2000;73:406-11.
28. Oei SG, Helmerhorst FM, Bloemenkamp KW, Hollants FA, Meerpoel DE, Keirse MJ. Effectiveness of the postcoital test: randomised controlled trial. BMJ. 1998;317(7157):502-5.
29. Kumar RM, Shahul S. Role of breast-feeding in transmission of hepatitis C virus to infants of HCV-infected mothers. J Hepatol. 1998;29:191-7.
30. Practice Committee of the American Society for Reproductive Medicine. Diagnostic evaluation of the infertile male: a committee opinion. Fertil Steril. 2015;103:e18-25.
31. Cooper TG, Noonan E, von Eckardstein S, Auger J, Gordon Baker HW, Behre HM, et al. World Health Organization reference values for human semen characteristics. Hum Reprod Update. 2010;16(3):231-45.
32. Kamel RM. Management of the infertile couple: an evidence-based protocol. Reprod Biol Endocrinol. 2010;8:21.

CHAPTER 2

Tubal Evaluation Methods and Assessment of Tubal Factor Infertility

Vasani Nidhi N

INTRODUCTIONV

Infertility is defined as the failure to achieve a successful pregnancy after ≥12 months of regular, unprotected intercourse.[1] Among the various causes of infertility, tubal and peritoneal pathology remains the most commonly encountered. Tubal factor accounts for 25–35% of female infertility.[2] The fallopian tubes not only make a vital portal for transport of gametes and embryos, but also provide an important holding action. Hence, only the patency of fallopian tubes is not important. The tubal function and tubo-ovarian relationship play an important role in reproduction.

TUBAL EVALUATION METHODS (FLOWCHART 1)

What are the characteristics of an ideal method?
- Easily available
- Cost-effective
- Acceptable
- No complications
- High sensitivity and specificity.

Flowchart 1: Algorithmic approach to tubal evaluation for infertility.

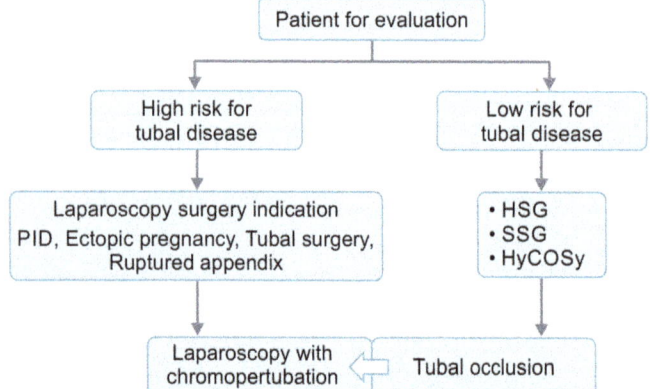

(HSG: Hysterosalpingography; HyCoSy: hysterosalpingo-contrast sonography; PID: pelvic inflammatory disease; SSG: sono-hysterosalpingography)

But such an ideal method is still illusive. The following are currently available methods:
- Hysterosalpingography (HSG)
- Sonohysterosalpingography (SSG)
- Hysterosalpingo-contrast sonography (HyCoSy)
- Laparoscopy with chromopertubation
- Chlamydia antibody test (CAT).

Hysterosalpingography and laparoscopy are the most widely used methods for tubal patency evaluation. These two tests are complementary rather than being mutually exclusive.[3]

Hysterosalpingography

Hysterosalpingography is a widely used technique which uses image intensification fluoroscopy **(Figs. 1 to 3)**.

Timing

Mid-proliferative phase (day 6–10 of a regular menstrual cycle).

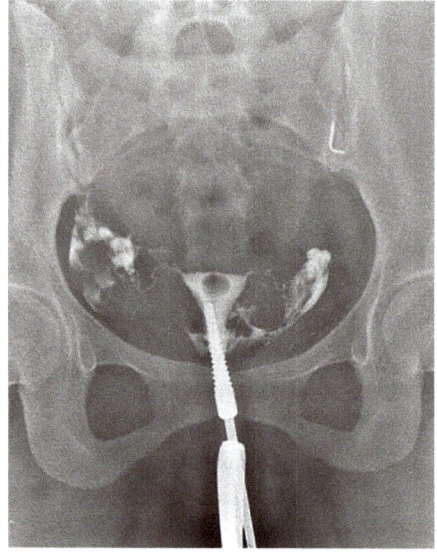

Fig. 1: Normal hysterosalpingogram with bilateral spill (indicating patent fallopian tubes)

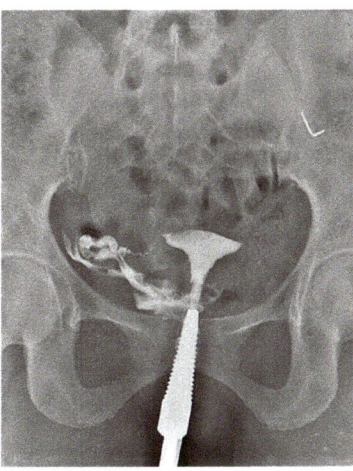

Fig. 2: Hysterosalpingogram suggesting left tubal block.

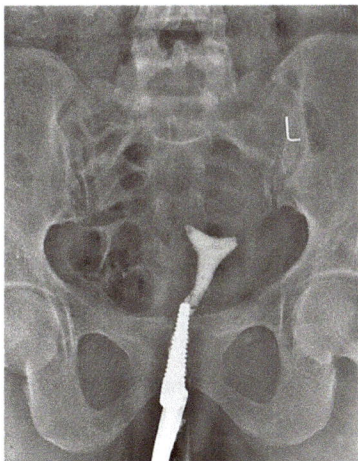

Fig. 3: Hysterosalpingogram suggesting bilateral tubal block.

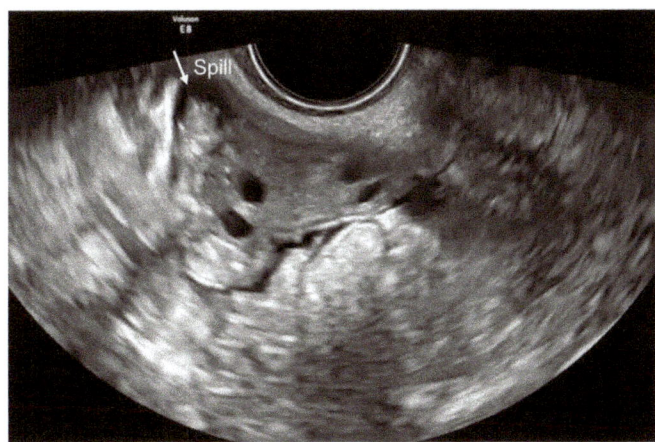

Fig. 4: Two-dimensional image of uterus and left ovary. Fluid collection marked by arrow indicates spill on saline sonosalpingogram.

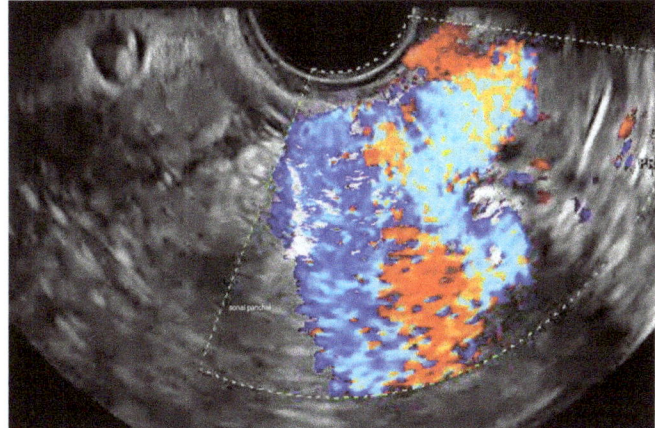

Fig. 5: Two-dimensional color Doppler image of uterus and left ovary. Periovarian color blush indicates patent tube on power Doppler during saline sonosalpingogram.

Advantages
- Cost-effective
- Outpatient procedure
- No anesthesia required
- Relatively safe
- Good delineation of fallopian tubes, tubal patency, uterine cavity, and peritubal adhesions.

Disadvantages
- Painful
- Radiation exposure
- Requirement of a radiologist
- High false-negative rate.[4]

In conclusion, when HSG demonstrated tubal patency, there is little chance that the tube is actually occluded (approximately 5%). But when HSG reveals tubal blockage, there is a high probability that the tube is open (approximately 60%).

Sonohysterosalpingography

Transvaginal ultrasound (TVS) is an inseparable component of female infertility evaluation. The only disadvantage of TVS is the nonvisualization of fallopian tubes. In SSG, fluid is introduced transcervically, using a catheter to visualize the fallopian tubes by ultrasound (**Figs. 4 and 5**).

Timing
Mid-proliferative phase (day 6–10 of a regular menstrual cycle).

Advantages
- Safe
- Noninvasive
- Cost-effective
- Easily available
- Outpatient procedure
- No radiation exposure
- Does not require radiologist
- Results correlate positively with laparoscopy in 97% of cases and with HSG in 93% of cases.[5]

Disadvantages

- Not always possible to delineate spill from individual tube
- Fluid in pouch of Douglas is suggestive of at least unilateral tubal patency
- Minor chance of pelvic infection
- Failure of procedure completion in 7% of patients.[6]

Several modifications have been made in SSG to improve diagnostic accuracy:[7]
- Using pulse Doppler
- Using color Doppler
- Combining air and saline
- Three-dimensional SSG.

Hysterosalpingo-contrast Sonography

Hysterosalpingo-contrast sonography is used for determining tubal patency and evaluating the uterine cavity by TVS after introduction of saline mixed with air into the uterine cavity and fallopian tubes. Currently, various other contrast agents have been used such as SonoVue (Bracco), Ecovist and Levovist (Schering AG, Berlin) **(Figs. 6 to 8)**.

Timing

Mid-proliferative phase (day 6–10 of a regular menstrual cycle).

Advantages

- Safe
- Cost-effective
- Noninvasive
- Outpatient procedure
- Avoids ionizing radiation
- No requirement for radiologist
- Better concomitant detection of intrauterine pathologies, visualization of ovaries, and myometrium providing a complete assessment.

Disadvantages

- Requires greater operator expertise
- Requires high-end ultrasound machine
- Not widely available.

Currently various modifications such as using pulse Doppler and three-dimensional pulse Doppler have been used for better reconstruction of images.

In a study comparing HyCoSy and laparoscopy with chromopertubation, there was a high degree of correlation in the assessment of tubal patency.[8]

Laparoscopy with Chromopertubation

It is the definitive test of tubal patency. It is still considered the gold standard for tubal factor evaluation **(Fig. 9)**.[9]

Timing

Mid-proliferative phase (day 6–10 of a regular menstrual cycle).

Advantages

- Provides a panoramic view of the reproductive anatomy
- Can identify milder decrease of distal tubal occlusion, pelvic or adnexal adhesions, and endometriosis

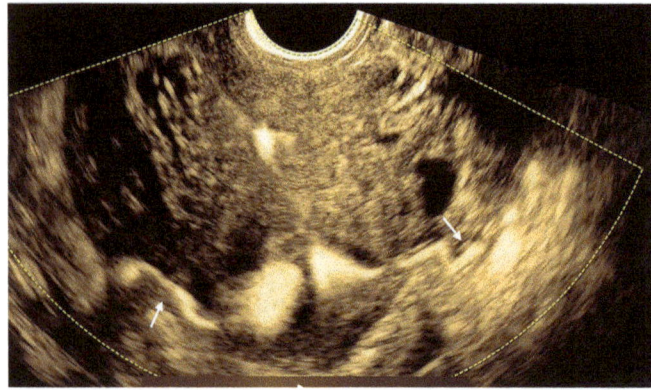

Fig. 6: Two-dimensional hysterosalpingo-contrast sonography (HyCoSy) showing endometrium and bilateral tubes.

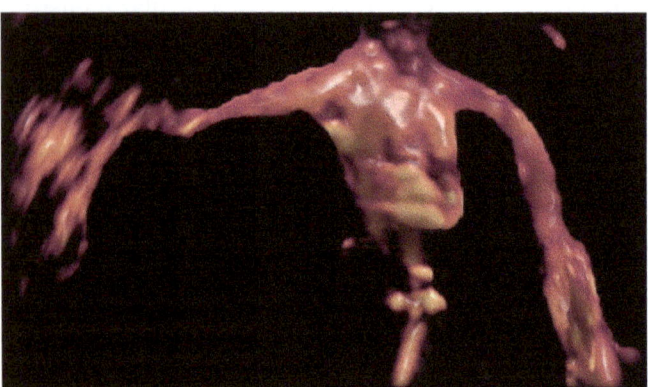

Fig. 7: Three-dimensional power Doppler rendered image of hysterosalpingo-contrast sonography (HyCoSy) showing normal endometrial cavity, both tubes, fimbrial end with spill.

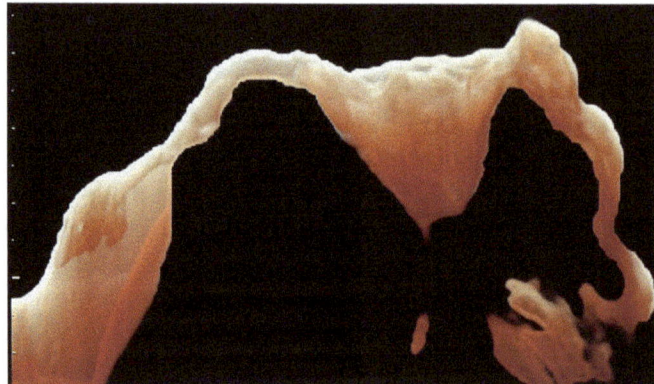

Fig. 8: High-definition (HD) live rendered image of three-dimensional hysterosalpingo-contrast sonography (HyCoSy) showing normal endometrial cavity, both tubes, fimbrial end with spill.

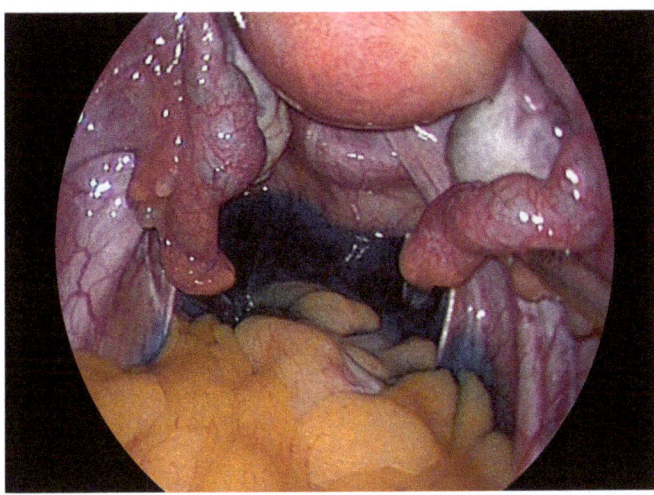

Fig. 9: Laparoscopic chromopertubation showing bilateral tubal spill.

- Opportunity to see and treat the disease at the same time
- A better predictor of future fertility.

Disadvantages

- Invasive
- Expensive
- Inpatient procedure
- Requires anesthesia
- Requires expert operator.

This investigation has stood the test of time and is very useful in determining the best option for future treatment.

Chlamydia Antibody Test

Role of CAT has not been adequately defined. It can be used as a pretest to select women who may require earlier or more detailed evaluation. Negative CAT usually suggests absence of disease, but a positive CAT requires further evaluation.

Timing

Can be done at patient's convenience, irrespective of day of menstrual cycle.

Advantages

- Easy to perform
- Noninvasive
- Cost-effective.

Disadvantages

- Diagnostic performance is limited
- Performance of different tests varies widely with the assay method
- Lacks clinical utility to predict tubal patency.

ACKNOWLEDGMENT

Dr Ravi Patel, MD, Ravi Sono-X-Ray Clinic, Bhavnagar, Gujarat for **Figures 1 to 3** and Dr Sonal Panchal, MD, Ahmedabad, Gujarat for **Figures 4 to 8**.

REFERENCES

1. Practice committee of the American Society of Reproductive Medicine. Fertility evaluation of infertile women: a committee opinion. Fertil Steril. 2021;116:1255-64.
2. Honoré GM, Holden AE, Schenken RS. Pathophysiology and management of proximal tubal blockage. Fertil Steril. 1999;71(5):785-95.
3. Taylor Hugh S, Fritz Marc A, Seli Emre. Speroff's Clinical Gynecologic Endocrinology and Infertility, 9th edition. Philadelphia (PA): Wolters Kluwer; 2020.
4. Maheux-Lacroix S, Boutin A, Moore L, Bergeron M-È, Bujold E, Laberge P, et al. Hysterosalpingosonography for Diagnosing Tubal Occlusion in Subfertile Women: A Systematic Review with Meta-Analysis. Human Reprod. 2014;29:953-63.
5. Seal SL, Ghosh D, Saha D. Comparative evaluation of sonosalpingography, hysterosalpingography and laparoscopy for determination of tubal patency. J Obstet Gynecol India. 2007;57(2):158-61.
6. de Kroon C, de Bock GH, Dieben S, Jansen FW. Saline contrast hysterosonography in abnormal uterine bleeding: a systematic review and meta-analysis. BJOG. 2003;110:938-47.
7. Panchal S, Nagori C. Imaging techniques for assessment of tubal status. J Hum Reprod Sci. 2014;7(1):2-12.
8. Lucaino DE, Exacoustos C, Johns DA. Transabdominal saline contrast sonohysterography: Can it replace hysterosalpingography in low resource countries? Am J Obstet Gynecol. 2011;204:79.
9. Patil M. Assessing tubal damage. J Hum Reprod Sci. 2009;2:2-11.

CHAPTER 3

Hysterolaparoscopy: Indications and Usage

Madhuri, Anshu Dhar

INTRODUCTION

In the present era, mastering the art of minimally invasive surgery is indispensable, not only to provide optimal care to the patient but also to survive in an age where increasingly complex procedures are being dealt with laparoscopically. With its advantage of lesser morbidity, early recovery, lesser risk of adhesions, lesser blood loss, the decreased requirement of postoperative analgesia and early resumption of routine activity as compared to the laparotomy, laparoscopic surgery is becoming the standard of care for patients. The role of minimally invasive surgery in the field of infertility cannot be overemphasised. In the next few pages, we have tried to briefly describe the indications and usage of hysteroscopy and laparoscopy against a background of infertility.

INSTRUMENTS

Instruments for Laparoscopy

- Laparoscope-parts **(Fig. 1) (Table 1)**
- *Primary trocars*—with trumpet valves to prevent dissipation of pneumoperitoneum created, at the time of withdrawal of instrument.
- *Secondary trocars*—(various sizes ranging from 3 to 20 mm, with 5 mm being the most commonly used)
- *Veress needle*—for initial creation of pneumoperitoneum before the insertion of primary trocar. It is made up of blunt-tipped, spring-loaded inner stylet covered by a sharp outer needle **(Fig. 2)**.

Parts of Hysteroscope (Fig. 3)

Hysteroscope is an endoscope used to visualize the uterine cavity directly. It is available as 0°, 15°, 30°, and 70°. The 0° provides a panoramic view whereas the angled ones are useful in visualizing uterine anomalies as well as the *uterine ostia*.

It is further of two types **(Table 2)**.

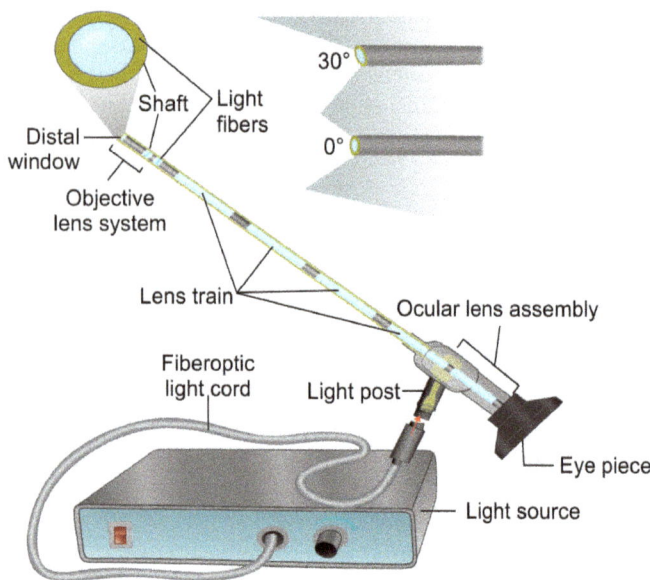

Fig. 1: Parts of laparoscope.

TABLE 1: Parts of laparoscope.	
Light port	**Attachment of fiber optic cord**
Light fiber	Glass fibers carrying light from the light port to distal end of the scope (light source—Xenon)
Objective lens system	Collection of lenses, windows, and/or prisms at the distal end of the scope. The distal objective can have angles from 0 to 120°, enabling the visualization of areas which might otherwise be out of view
Lens train	Series of glass rod lenses and spacers used to transfer the image through the shaft
Shaft	Stainless steel tube—accommodates the lens train
Ocular lens assembly	Focusing lens of the scope at proximal end of the scope
Eyepiece	Located at the proximal end of the scope. The image either seen through the scope, or the eyepiece attached to a camera coupler to visualize the image on an external monitor

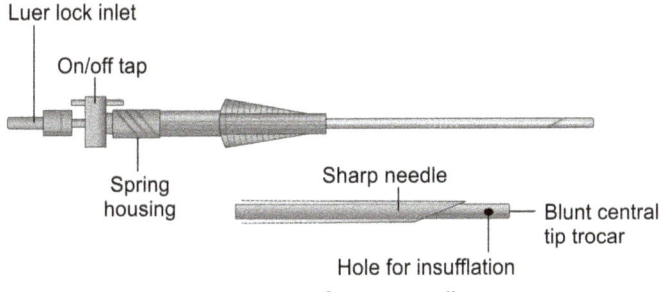

Fig. 2: Parts of Veress needle.

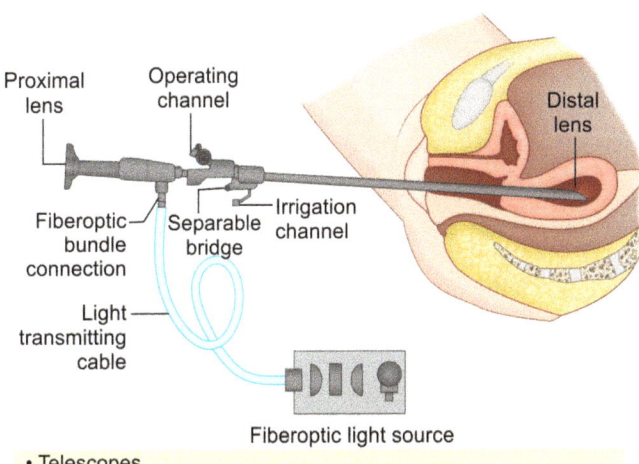

- Telescopes
- *Light source:* Tungsten, metal halide, halogen, or Xenon (best)
- *Camera:* Three-chip cameras HD cameras
- Diagnostic and operative sheaths
- Accessory instruments

Fig. 3: Parts of hysteroscope.

■ INDICATIONS

See **Tables 3 and 4**.

■ PROCEDURE

Laparoscopy

Procedure of laparoscopy involves following steps:
- Position of patient
- Technique of entry **(Flowchart 1)**
- Confirmation of proper positioning of Veress needle if used **(Box 1) (Flowchart 2)**
- Creation of pneumoperitoneum
- Insertion of primary trocar
- Insertion of secondary trocars-to be done perpendicular to the skin under vision after transillumination of inferior epigastric vessels to avoid injury.

Hysteroscopy

It comprises of insertion of a rigid or flexible hysteroscope through the cervical canal into the uterus followed by the utilization of distending media **(Table 5)** to enable distension and comprehensive assessment of the endometrial cavity **(Box 2)**.

TABLE 2: Types of hysteroscope.

Rigid hysteroscope	Flexible hysteroscope
• In patient/OT hysteroscope • Mini telescopes can be used for office hysteroscopy	Office hysteroscope
• Telescope diameter 4 mm with outer diameter >5 mm for standard rigid hysteroscopes • Telescope diameter between 1.2 and 3 mm for mini telescopes having diagnostic and operative sheaths with outer diameter <5 mm.	• A semirigid 3.2 mm fiber optic mini hysteroscope • It consists of a 1.8 mm telescope with a 0° angle of vision and a single disposable outer sheath. • Tip deflection of 120–160°
Better image quality and visualization	A reduced image size on the monitor screen compared with full-size standard hysteroscopy
Better durability	flexible

TABLE 3: Indications of hysteroscopy in infertile patient.

Diagnostic	Operative
Endometrial polyps	Polypectomy
Chronic endometritis	Endometrial biopsy
Leiomyoma	Myomectomy
Intrauterine synechia	Adhesiolysis
Müllerian anomalies	Septoplasty
Unexplained infertility	Tubal cannulation

TABLE 4: Indications of laparoscopy in infertility.

Diagnostic uses	Therapeutic uses
• Tubal block on HSG • Suspected peritubular adhesions • Suspected endometriosis • Mullerian anomaly • Unexplained infertility • Ovarian cyst	• Adhesiolysis • Myomectomy • Ovarian cystectomy • Management of hydrosalpinx—salpingectomy or tubal clipping • Endometriosis • Laparoscopic ovarian drilling in PCOS • Tubal reanastomosis

(HSG: hysterosalpingogram; PCOS: polycystic ovary syndrome)

Fluid overload:
- Isotonic solution—2,500 mL
- Hypotonic solution—1,000 mL.

Fertiloscopy is the visualization of the posterior pelvis via introduction of an optical device in the pouch of Douglas, through the posterior fornix of vagina, under general or local anesthesia.

Usage of Hysteroscopy

Hysteroscopic characteristics of normal uterus are enumerated in **Table 6**.

Flowchart 1: Laparoscopic entry techniques.

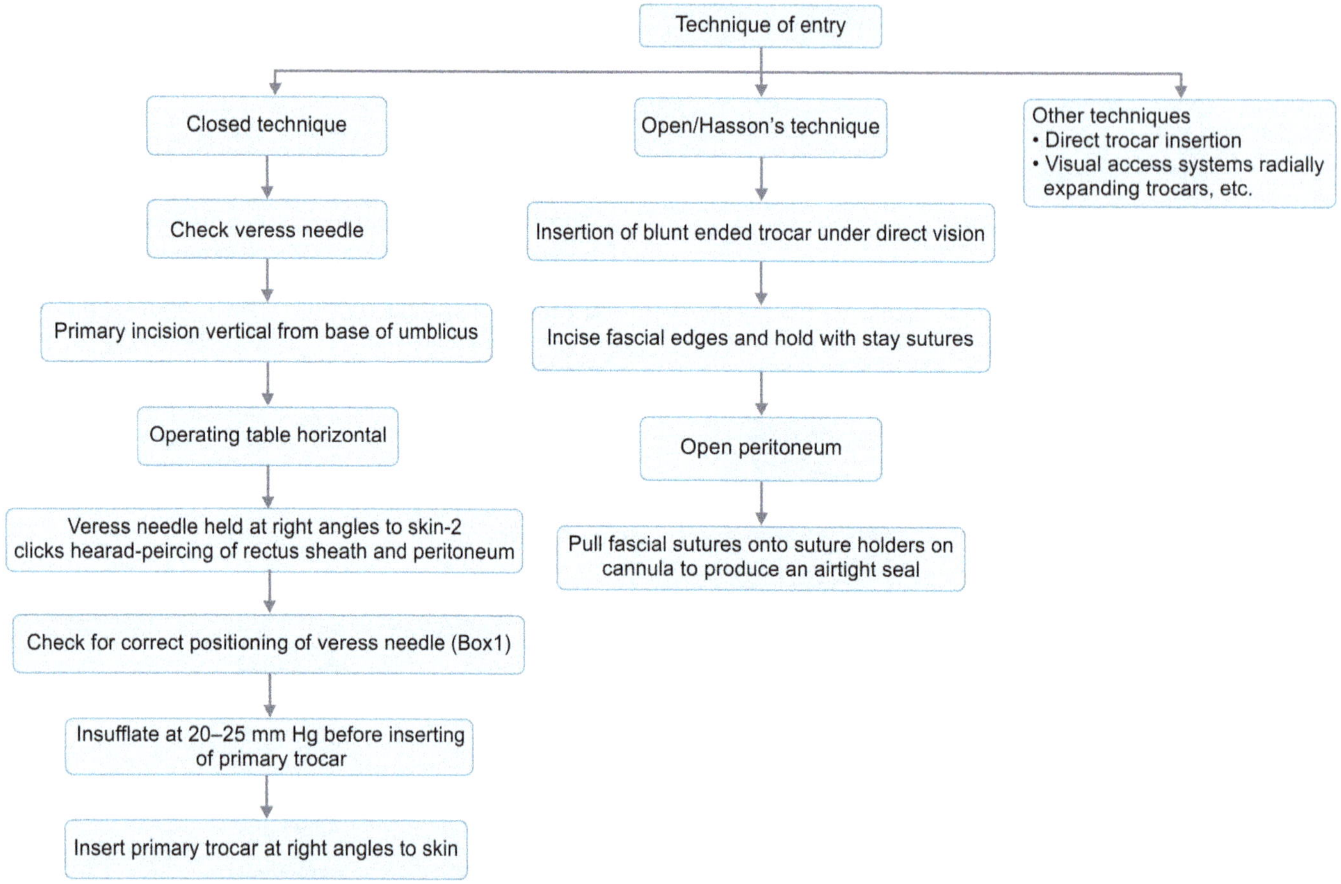

Technique of entry
Closed technique
Check veress needle
Primary incision vertical from base of umblicus
Operating table horizontal
Veress needle held at right angles to skin-2 clicks hearad-peircing of rectus sheath and peritoneum
Check for correct positioning of veress needle (Box1)
Insufflate at 20–25 mm Hg before inserting of primary trocar
Insert primary trocar at right angles to skin
Open/Hasson's technique
Insertion of blunt ended trocar under direct vision
Incise fascial edges and hold with stay sutures
Open peritoneum
Pull fascial sutures onto suture holders on cannula to produce an airtight seal
Other techniques
• Direct trocar insertion
• Visual access systems radially expanding trocars, etc.

BOX 1: Confirmation of proper positioning of Veress needle.

Proper positioning of Veress needle can be confirmed by the following:[1]

- Fluid injection and aspiration through the needle
- During the insufflation, the liver dullness would be lost
- An unconstrained needle rotation could help in diagnosing anterior abdominal wall adhesions
- Air entering and free flow of air through the Veress needle
- with inspiratory and expiratory diaphragmatic motions
- Reflection of the variation in pressure gauge needle
- Hanging drop test

Flowchart 2: Sites for insertion of primary trocar/Veress needle.

Sites of primary trocar/veress
Umblical
Palmar's point* in case of abdominal adhesions like prior abdominal surgeries
• Other sites not usually preferred
• Posterior fornix
• Suprapubic
• Uterine fundus

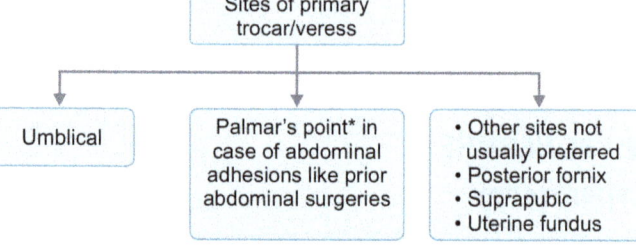

*3 cm below the left costal margin in the midclavicular line

TABLE 5: Types of distension media.[2]

Distension media	***Electrolytes***	***Osmolarity***	***Procedure***	***Energy device type***
Normal saline	Present	285 mOsm/L (iso-osmolar)	Diagnostic and operative hysteroscopy	Mechanical, bipolar, laser (electrolyte containing media cannot be used with monopolar because of dissipation of energy without surgical effect on tissues)
Ringer's lactate	Present	279 mOsm/L (iso-osmolar)	Diagnostic and operative hysteroscopy	Mechanical, bipolar, and laser
Mannitol	Absent	274 mOsm/L (iso-osmolar	Operative hysteroscopy	Monopolar
Glycine 1.5%	Absent	200 mOsm/L (hypo-osmolar)	Operative hysteroscopy	Monopolar
Dextrose 5%	Absent	Hypo-osmolar	Operative Hysteroscopy	Monopolar
Sorbitol 3%	Absent	165 mOsm/L (hypo-osmolar)	Operative Hysteroscopy	Monopolar

BOX 2: Hysteroscopic assessment of uterus.

Assessment of uterus
Parameters of endometrium:
- Thickness
- Surface
- Color
- Vasculature
- Glandular openings

Uterocervical characteristics:
- Cervical canal
- Uterine axis, size, and shape
- Any focal lesions

TABLE 6: Hysteroscopic characteristics of normal uterus.

	Menstruation (1–4 days)	Proliferative (5–14 days)	Early luteal (14–21 days)	Late luteal (21–28 days)
Color	Red	Pink	White	White
Surface	Irregular	Smooth	Wavy	Spongy
Glands	Not seen	White spots	Prominent	Not seen
Notch	Not seen	Hemorrhagic	Avascular	Serous
Vessels	Not seen	Thin vessels	Not seen	Not seen

BOX 3: Hysteroscopic appearance of polyps.

Hysteroscopic appearance:
- *Gross appearance:* Discrete outgrowth of endometrium moving with flow of distension media. Note the number and site
- *Covering endometrium:* Thin (appearing translucent with a delicate vascular network) or thick (obliterating surface vascularity)
- Can be vascular (reddish pink) or fibrous (whitish)
- Surface can be regular or irregular and necrotic (yellowish)
- Distinguished from fibroids by the movement with distension media and indention of surface with the tip of optical instrument

BOX 4: Management of polyps.

Management:
- Expectant especially if polyp is <1 cm (spontaneous regression in 25% cases)
- Hysteroscopic polypectomy for larger polyps or those obstructing the cornu
- In context of infertility, hysteroscopic scissors preferred for removal. Cautery may be used in case of bleeding

Hystero-Laparoscopic Findings in Various Pathologies

- *Endometrial polyps* **(Boxes 3 and 4):** Up to 10–32% of women with unexplained infertility may have endometrial polyps.[3,4]

BOX 5: Hysteroscopic features of submucosal fibroids.

Hysteroscopic features of uterine fibroids:
- Protrusions of solid, dense, regular, and whitish tissue into uterine cavity
- Stretched endometrium over fibroid surface revealing thin fragile surface blood vessels-whitish vascular appearance
- Multiple intramural fibroids may give an undulating appearance to cavity

TABLE 7: European Society for Gynecological Endoscopy (ESGE) classification of fibroids.

Type	Degree of intramural extension
0	None
1	<50%
2	≥50%

- *Submucosal fibroids* **(Box 5):** The submucosal fibroids **(Table 7)** are well known to affect implantation and hence fertility. Management of fibroids with submucosal component can be guided by the STEP W classification[5] **(Table 8)**. The various devices for the same have been enumerated in **Table 9**.
- *Intrauterine synechiae:* The classification of intrauterine adhesions[6] have been presented in **Table 10** while causes, presentation and management have been described in **Boxes 6 to 8**.
- *Chronic endometritis:* It is defined as persistent inflammation of endometrial lining diagnosed with hysteroscopy and histopathology. Presenting features are enumerated in **Box 9**. Hysteroscopic features are enumerated in the **Box 10**. The most common pathogens associated include mycoplasma and chlamydia.
- *Müllerian anomalies*[7]*:* Hysteroscopy can serve as a useful tool for evaluation of congenital uterine anomalies due to abnormal development or fusion of the Müllerian (paramesonephric) ducts during embryonic development.

The hysteroscopic characteristics of these abnormalities are described in **Table 11**.

- *Adenomyosis:* Diagnostic hysteroscopy cannot establish a definitive diagnosis of adenomyosis, considering that its field of vision is restricted to the endometrial surface layer. However, some findings are indicative of adenomyosis **(Box 11)**.

Adenomyosis has been variously associated with a lower implantation rates. The challenge in surgical management of adenomyosis is that there is no demarcation between the adenomyoma and the uterus. The various techniques available for adenomyomectomy are described in **Table 12**.

If the adenomyoma is distorting cavity or if the uterus is too bulky, then the debulking surgery is to be done.

TABLE 8: Step W or Lasmar classification.[5]

	Size (cm)	Topography	Extension of the base	Penetration	Lateral wall	Total
0	<2	Low	<1/3	0		
1	>2 a5	Middle	>1/3 – 2/3	<50%	+1	
2	>5	Upper	>2/3	>50%		
Score	+	+	+	+	+	+

Score	Group	Complexity and therapeutic options
0–4	I	Low complexity hysteroscopic myomectomy
5–6	II	High complexity hysteroscopic myomectomy. Consider gonadotropin-releasing hormone (GnRH) use? Consider two-step hysteroscopic myomectomy
7–9	III	Consider alternative to the hysteroscopic technique

TABLE 9: Devices used for hysteroscopic myomectomy.

Methods of hysteroscopic myomectomy	
Mechanical	Cut stalk (this is mainly used for prolapsed fibroid through the cervix)
Resection (using resectoscope)	Used for electrocautery and monopolar energy
Versapoint®	Bipolar energy, vaporization, and dissection. Used mainly for small lesions
MyoSure® TruClear™	Hysteroscopic tissue removal systems with fast cutting blade and tissue retrieval technology
Laser (rarely used)	Vaporize, morcellate, dissect, and myolysis

BOX 7: Presentation of intra uterine adhesions.

Presentation:
- Menstrual disturbances such as oligomenorrhea, hypomenorrhea
- Infertility or subfertility
- Failure to bleed even after estrogen and progesterone challenge

BOX 8: Management of intrauterine adhesions.

Management:
- Hysteroscopic adhesiolysis with scissors
- Avoid cautery
- Prevention of recurrence—hormone replacement therapy (hrt), intrauterine devices, antiadhesion agents like autocross-linked collagen, pediatric foley's for 7 days

TABLE 10: Classification of intra uterine adhesions.

Characteristics			
Extent of cavity involved	<1/3 1	<1/3–2/3 2	<2/3 4
Type of adhesions	Flimsy 1	Filmy and Dense 2	Dense 4
Menstrual pattern	Normal 0	Decreased 2	Amenorrhea 4
Prognostic classification		HSG score	Hysteroscopy score
Stage I (Mild)	1–4		
Stage II (Moderate)	5–8		
Stage III (Severe)	9–12		

BOX 9: Presentation of chronic endometritis.

Presentation:
- Asymptomatic
- Chronic pelvic pain
- Menstrual irregularities
- Persistent white discharge per vaginum
- Infertility, subfertility, and implantation failure

BOX 10: Hysteroscopic features of chronic endometritis.

Hysteroscopic features:
- Mucosal edema
- Hyperemia
- Micropolyps <1 mm
- Hypervascularity
- Sunshine sign—suspicion of chronic salpingitis

BOX 6: Causes of intrauterine adhesions.

Causes:
- Curettage of uterine walls following surgical evacuation, termination of pregnancy or following post partum hemorrhage
- Infections like tuberculosis
- Surgeries involving damage to basal endometrium like myomectomy

- *Endometriosis:* Endometriosis is a common clinical entity encountered by reproductive medicine practitioners.
    - *Peritoneal endometriosis* **(Table 13)**
    The peritoneal endometriosis may have varied appearances.
    However, one should also remember the possibility of "invisible" lesions. The treatment options include

TABLE 11: Hysteroscopic features of müllerian anomalies.			
Anomaly	Cavity	Cornu tubal ostia	Remarks
Arcuate uterus	Gently bulges into uterine cavity	Cornual recesses become pronounced	Believed to be a normal variant
Bicornuate uterus	Two chambered uterus with central division extending INTO UTERINE CAVITY	Diagnosis suspected when only one ostium or cornual recess visibe in cylindrical uterus	• Has to be distinguished from septate uterus which can be done laparoscopically by observing the uterine fundus which has slight or no indentation in septate uterus while an external indentation in present in bicornuate uterus • Hysteroscopic appearance has to be distinguished from unicornuate and hypoplastic uterus
Unicornuate uterus	Single uterine cavity	Single ostium	• Draw hysteroscope out carefully and move it towards the contralateral side to look for any communication with the other 'half' of the uterus • Careful vaginoscopic inspection of the upper vagina along with a pelvic examination so as not to overlook a complete uterine septum or uterine didelphys
Septate uterus	Septum covered with endometrial mucosa,	In complete septum, the other ostia may not be visualized	The more the septum projects into the uterine cavity, the easier it may be for the other half of cavity to be overlooked

BOX 11: Hysteroscopic features of adenomyosis.
- Irregular endometrium with tiny openings seen on the endometrial surface
- Pronounced hypervascularization and endometrial "strawberry" pattern
- Hemorrhagic cystic lesions assuming a dark blue or chocolate brown appearance

TABLE 12: Techniques of adenomyomectomy.	
Osada's triple-flap technique[8]	Double-flap technique[9]
A sagittal incision is given	Useful in diffuse adenomyoma
Debulking is done with 1 cm margin of serosa and 1 cm myometrium above endometrium	Modification of Osada's triple flap technique, the two-flaps are overlapped such that the serosa of the underlying wall is excised, hence only myometrial walls are overlapped
Suture endometrium and 2 flaps	Intermittent 3–0 sutures for endometrium
Third-flap should cover the 2 flaps	

laparoscopic excision, vaporization, and coagulation **(Box 12)**.
- *Ovarian endometriosis*
  The ovarian endometrioma can be superficial or deep. The management of ovarian endometrioma can be done by vaporization or excision. Principles of management are presented in the **Box 13**.
- *Tubal factors*[10]
  - Proximal tubal block **(Flowchart 3)**
  - Distal tubal block—*hydrosalpinx*: Hydrosalpinx may decrease the pregnancy rates associated with assisted reproductive technology (ART).

Management in cases of infertility is described in the **Flowchart 4**.

TABLE 13: Types of peritoneal endometriosis.		
Red	black	White
Most active lesions	Relatively older lesions	Look-like peritoneal scarring or confined patches
They are commonly seen at broad ligaments and the uterosacral ligaments	Brownish to black due to the blood pigment collected within	Usually, subovarian adhesions
On histopathological examination (HPE)—numerous glandular excrescences are seen	On HPE—glands, stroma, and intraluminal debris are noted	On HPE—occasional retroperitoneal structure and scanty stroma

BOX 12: Treatment options for peritoneal endometriosis.
- Endometriotic excision—with of scissors. Excision technique involves less risk of recurrence
- Vaporization—with CO_2 laser, the effervesce/bubble formation during vaporization is a sign that the peritoneal fat is reached and vaporization is complete
- Coagulation—using bipolar cautery is not as safe as vaporization because of difficulty in assessing the depth of penetration and nonavailability of tissue for histopathological diagnosis

BOX 13: Principles of surgery for ovarian endometrioma.
- Incision preferably with scissors over antimesenteric border, away from hilus of ovary
- The hydrodissection technique to remove the cyst wall from the ovarian stroma
- A continuous counter traction during dissection of the ovarian endometrioma
- Remove through the 10 mm of trocar
- Use of Endo bag to avoid spillage
- The ovarian wall need not be sutured
- Minimal use of cautery is to be done to preserve ovarian reserve

Flowchart 3: Causes and management of proximal tubal block.

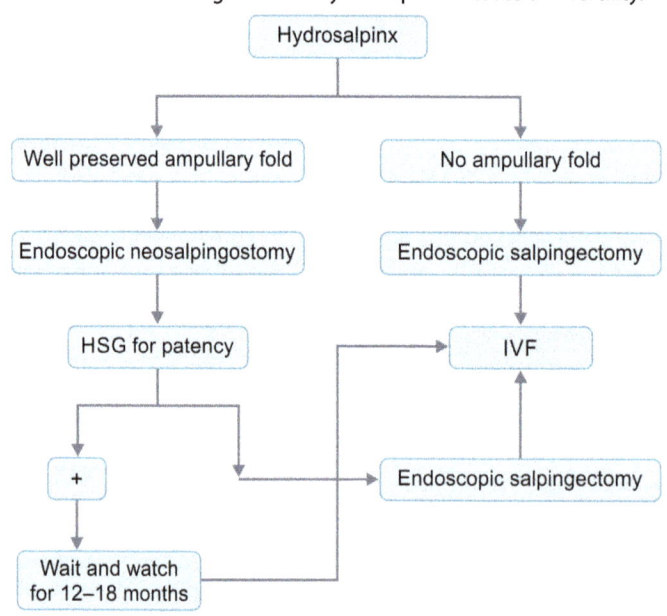

Flowchart 4: Management of hydrosalpinx in cases of infertility.

TABLE 14: Genital tuberculosis—sites.					
Site	**Fallopian tubes**	**uterus**	**Ovaries**	**Cervix**	**Vagina, vulva**
Affected in % of cases	More than 90%	70%	20-30%	5%	Rare
Pathology	Endosalpingitis, exosalpingitis, interstitial TB salpingitis, salpingitis isthmica nodosa, and hydrosalpinx	Multiple ulcers and Asherman's syndrome	Cysts, tubo-ovarian mass, and adhesions	Ulcers and polypoidal growth	Hypertrophic ulcer, mass or as fistulas

- *Tuberculosis*[11]: The most common etiological agent involved in female genital tuberculosis is *Mycobacterium tuberculosis*, although rarely it may be caused by *Mycobacterium bovis*, atypical mycobacteria. The infection spread can occur by hematogenous, lymphatic or direct spread **(Table 14)**.

Tuberculosis is a cause of both primary and secondary infertility in almost 40–80% of cases. The etiology of infertility is presented in **Flowchart 5**.

In patients with tuberculosis, low pregnancy rates are reported, up to 19%. The treatment to be offered depends on the organ affected **(Flowchart 6)**.

Flowchart 5: Etiology of infertility in genital tuberculosis.

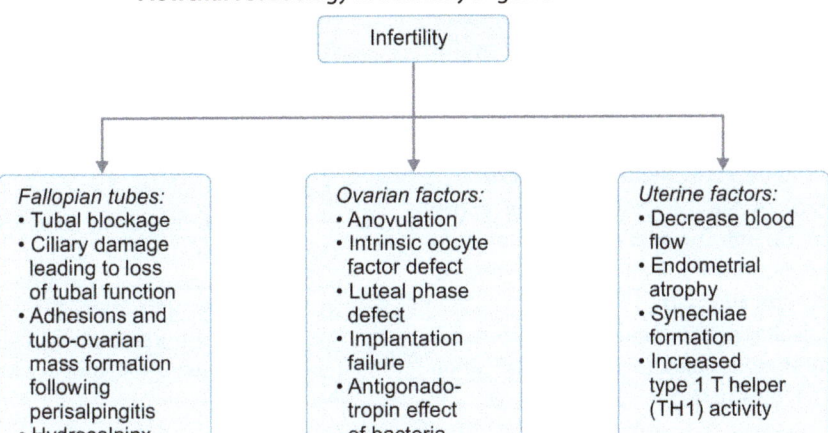

Flowchart 6: Management of genital TB.

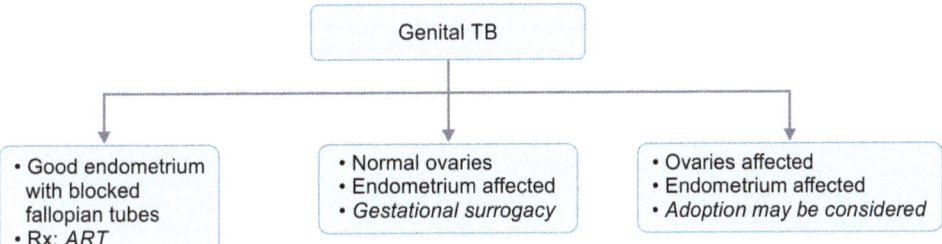

BOX 14: Hysteroscopic findings in TB.
Hysteroscopy: • Pale looking cavity • Tubercles (small white caseous nodules) • Variable grades of synechiae • Cavity may be shrunken

BOX 15: Laparoscopic findings in TB.
• Subacute stage—congestion, edema, and miliary tubercles over the peritoneum or adnexa or uterus • Chronic stage—fimbrial, midtubal or cornual block, tubal beading, hydrosalpinx, and pyosalpinx • On injecting methylene blue alternate constrictions and dilatations of fallopian tubes in female genital tuberculosis (FGTB) (Sharma's blue python sign) • Fusion of fimbrial ends due to caseous material (Sharma's kissing fallopian tube sign) • Calcified tubes like a dried tree branch (Sharma's dried tree branch sign) • Perihepatic synechiae (Fitz–Hugh–Curtis syndrome) may be seen in about 48% of cases

Hence a vigilant and prudent use of hysteroscopy and laparoscopy can be helpful in increasing the success rates in infertile patients **(Boxes 14 and 15)**.

Key Learning Points

- Endoscopic surgery is a powerful tool in the hands of an infertility specialist which can facilitate unravelling an enigmatic diagnosis as well as treat pathologies.
- With the advent of high resolution and 3-D ultrasonography, the role of laparoscopy solely for the purpose of diagnosis has become questionable.
- It is important to be well-versed with laparoscopic instruments and media to make optimum use of laparoscopy and avoid complications.
- To be aware of the various hystero-laparoscopic findings in different pathologies and their implications can serve as a guide to plan further management and achieve best results in terms of pregnancy rates in infertile patients.

REFERENCES

1. Nezhat C, Nezhat F, Nezhat C. Nezhat's operative gynecologic laparoscopy and hysteroscopy. Cambridge: Cambridge University Press; 2008.
2. Umranikar S, Clark TJ, Saridogan E, Miligkos D, Arambage K, Torbe E, et al. BSGE/ESGE guideline on management of fluid distension media in operative hysteroscopy. Gynecol Surg. 2016;13(4):289-303.
3. Hinckley MD, Milki AA. 1000 office-based hysteroscopies prior to in vitro fertilization: feasibility and findings. JSLS. 2004;8(2):103-107.

4. Shalev J, Meizner I, Bar-Hava I, Dicker D, Mashiach R, Ben-Rafael Z. Predictive value of transvaginal sonography performed before routine diagnostic hysteroscopy for evaluation of infertility. Fertil Steril. 2000;73(2):412-7.
5. Lasmar RB, Xinmei Z, Indman PD, Celeste RK, Sardo AD. Feasibility of a new system of classification of submucous myomas: a multicenter study. Fertil Steril. 2011;95(6):2073-7.
6. AAGL Elevating Gynecologic Surgery. AAGL practice report: practice guidelines on intrauterine adhesions developed in collaboration with the European Society of Gynaecological Endoscopy (ESGE). Gynecol Surg. 2017;14(1):6.
7. Pfeifer SM, Attaran M, Goldstein J, Lindheim SR, Petrozza JC, Rackow BW, et al. ASRM müllerian anomalies classification 2021. Fertil Steril. 2021;116(5):1238-52.
8. Osada H, Silber S, Kakinuma T, Nagaishi M, Kato K, Kato O. Surgical procedure to conserve the uterus for future pregnancy in patients suffering from massive adenomyosis. Reprod Biom Online. 2011;22(1):94-9.
9. Huang X, Huang Q, Chen S, Zhang J, Lin K, Zhang X. Efficacy of laparoscopic adenomyomectomy using double-flap method for diffuse uterine adenomyosis. BMC Womens Health. 2015;15:24.
10. Practice Committee of the American Society for Reproductive Medicine. Role of tubal surgery in the era of assisted reproductive technology: a committee opinion. Fertil Sterility. 2015;103(6):e37-43.
11. Sharma JB, Sharma E, Sharma S, Dharmendra S. Female genital tuberculosis: Revisited. Indian J Med Res. 2018;148(Suppl 1):S71-83.

CHAPTER 4

Disorders of Puberty

Yogita Dogra

INTRODUCTION

Puberty is a stage of cognitive, psychological, and biological development. Although growth and the appearance of secondary sexual characteristics are the most obvious markers of the onset of puberty, changes in body composition and cognitive development are also significant.[1] Although puberty occurs naturally, it may be a difficult changeover for many teenagers, and it offers even more obstacles when it occurs prematurely or late.

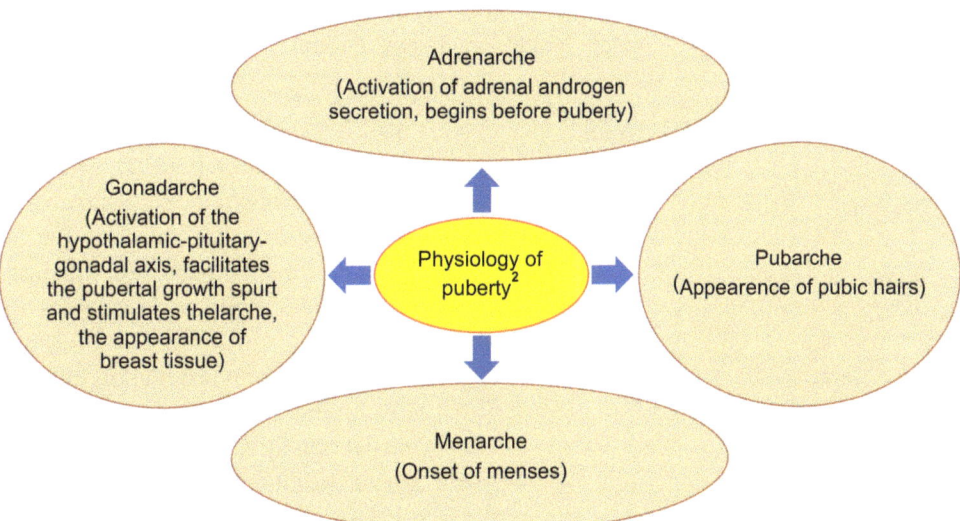

Puberty is characterized by a set of predictable occurrences that differ in time, chronology, and pace. In most teenage females, the first symptom of puberty is an increase in development, followed by breast development (thelarche), the formation of pubic hair (pubarche), and, lastly, commencement of menstruation (menarche).[2]

Marshall and Tanner described the most commonly used staging methods for describing puberty's physical changes in 1969 (for girls)[3] (**Fig. 1**) and 1970 (for boys).[4]

Breast development (thelarche) follows a well-defined timeline.[2]
- *Tanner stage I:* No glandular breast tissue palpable.
- *Tanner stage II:* Breast budding seen as expansion and spreading of the areolae.
- *Tanner stage III:* The breast expands and rises above the areolae.
- *Tanner stage IV:* Areolae and nipple produce secondary mounds.
- *Tanner stage V:* The breast attains an adult shape.

Pubarche follows thelarche in the majority of teenagers. In a considerable proportion of individuals, however, pubarche precedes thelarche. In every situation, the two are interdependent and advance simultaneously.[2]
- *Tanner stage I:* No hairs
- *Tanner stage II:* Tiny quantity of long, generally straight hair
- *Tanner stage III:* The hair subsequently becomes curlier and coarser as it grows outward
- *Tanner stage IV:* Hair expands farther to cover the entire triangle over the pubic region
- *Tanner stage V:* Adult pattern with expansion across the medial thigh.

22 Disorders of Puberty

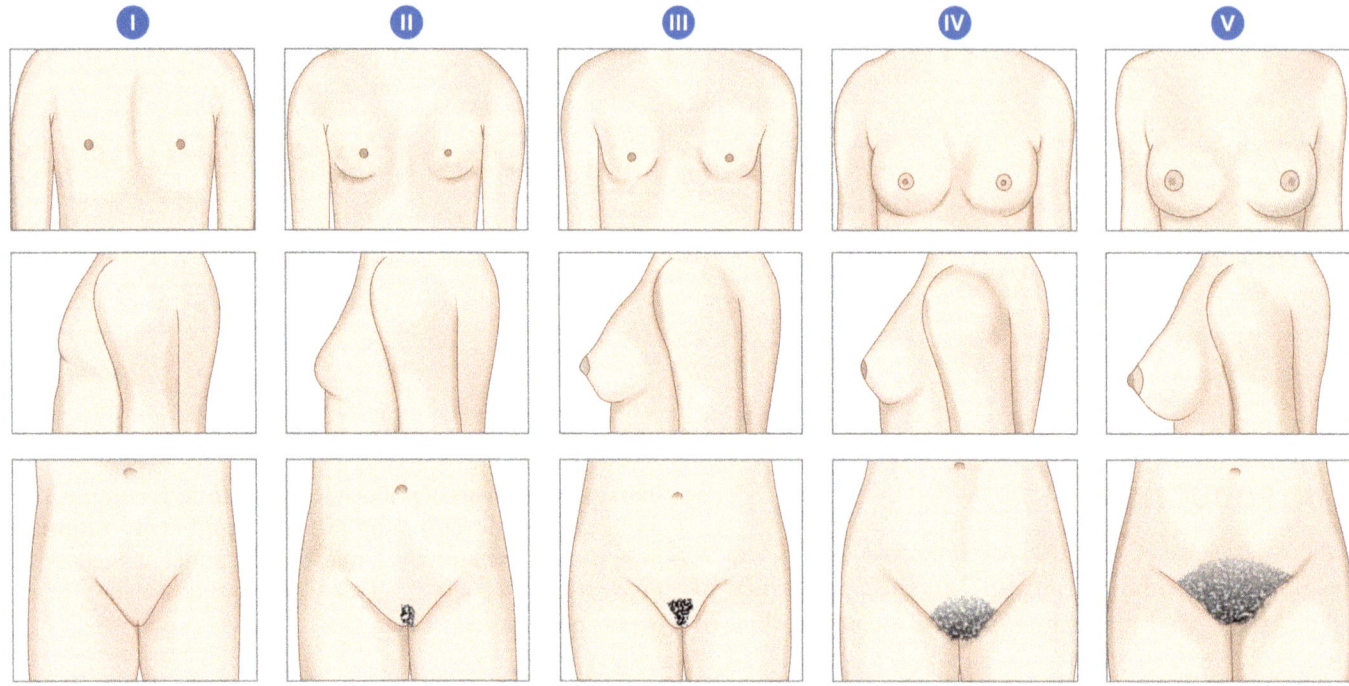

Fig. 1: Illustration of the Tanner scale for females.
(*Courtesy:* Michał Komorniczak, Poland)

■ SEQUENCE OF PUBERTAL MILESTONES[2]

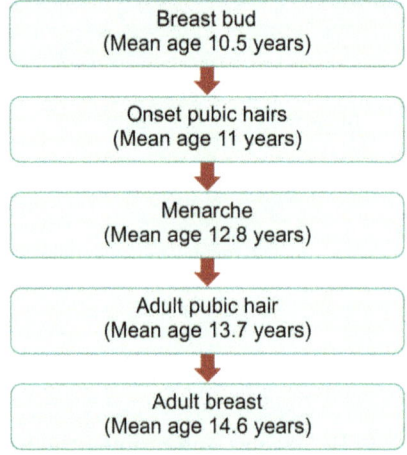

■ SUMMARY OF PUBERTAL EVENTS[2]

- During fetal life, the hypothalamic-pituitary-gonadal axis differentiates and develops, becoming completely functioning prior to birth.
- Pulsatile secretion of hypothalamic gonadotropin-releasing hormone (GnRH) is greatly reduced to extremely low levels of activity starting in late infancy and continuing through childhood as a result of central inhibitory mechanisms and, to a lesser extent, a considerable sensitivity to low levels of gonadal steroid feedback.
- Adrenal androgen production increases (adrenarche) in late childhood, continues to rise consistently thereafter, and eventually encourages pubarche.
- After a decade of inactivity, pulsatile GnRH production escalates and the hypothalamic-pituitary-gonadal axis (gonadarche) is revived.
- Before 10 years of age, gonadotropin [follicle-stimulating hormone (FSH) and luteinizing hormone (LH)] levels escalate gradually, followed by a steady rise in estradiol levels, which promote thelarche.
- Gonadal estrogen production increases significantly at midpuberty to drive endometrial development, resulting in the commencement of menstruation (menarche).

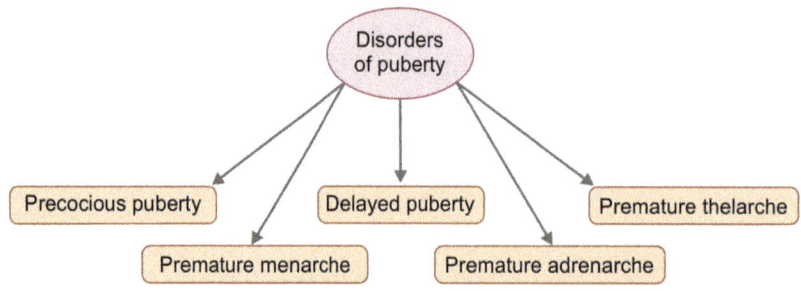

PRECOCIOUS PUBERTY

Precocious puberty refers to pubertal development that occurs at a younger age than would be predicted based on recognized standard norms, i.e., before 8 years in girls and before 9 years in boys. Its causes are numerous, ranging from typical developmental deviations such as early adrenarche to major disease such as malignant brain neoplasms. Precocious puberty in children requires rigorous investigation to determine the reason and, if necessary, prompt intervention to dodge the psychological and developmental repercussions of unusually early sexual maturity.[2]

Indications for Evaluation[2]

- Pubertal changes >2.5 SD earlier than the mean age
- Girls <6 years of age with breast or pubic hair development
- Girls <8 years of age with both breast and pubic hair development

Classification of Precocious Puberty[2]

- Gonadotropin-dependent precocious puberty
- Gonadotropin-independent precocious puberty
- Incomplete precocious puberty

Gonadotropin-dependent or True Precocious or Central Precocious Puberty

- Results from early developement of the hypothalamic-pituitary-gonadal axis
- In girls, it is characterised by the developement of breast and pubic hair, whereas in boys, it is characterised by pubic hair development as well as testicular volume >4 mL or 2.5 cm in diameter[2]
- More prevalent in girls than in boys[5]
- In majority it is idiopathic and diagnosis is made by exclusion[6,7]
- Can be linked to a wide range of central nervous system disorders, including trauma, tumors, cysts, irradiation, inflammatory illnesses, hydrocephalus, and midline developmental anomalies like septo-optic dysplasia[7-9]
- Ependymomas, hamartomas, pineal tumors, astrocytomas, and optic and hypothalamic gliomas are among the cancers linked with gonadotropin-dependent premature puberty[2]
- Girls with severe primary hypothyroidism may experience early puberty, breast growth, galactorrhea, and episodic menstrual bleeding[2]

Gonadotropin-independent or Pseudoprecocious or Peripheral Precocious Puberty

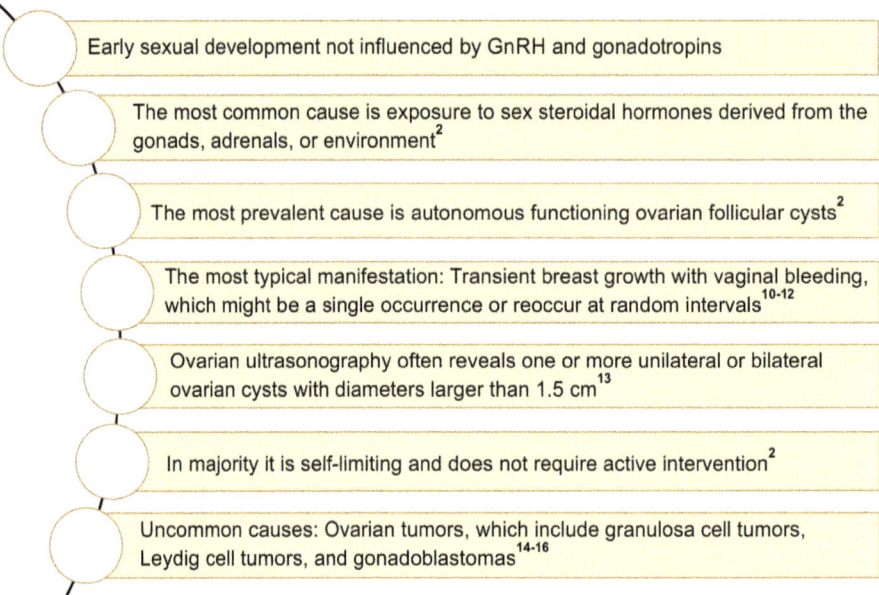

- Early sexual development not influenced by GnRH and gonadotropins
- The most common cause is exposure to sex steroidal hormones derived from the gonads, adrenals, or environment[2]
- The most prevalent cause is autonomous functioning ovarian follicular cysts[2]
- The most typical manifestation: Transient breast growth with vaginal bleeding, which might be a single occurrence or reoccur at random intervals[10-12]
- Ovarian ultrasonography often reveals one or more unilateral or bilateral ovarian cysts with diameters larger than 1.5 cm[13]
- In majority it is self-limiting and does not require active intervention[2]
- Uncommon causes: Ovarian tumors, which include granulosa cell tumors, Leydig cell tumors, and gonadoblastomas[14-16]

Incomplete Precocious Puberty[2]

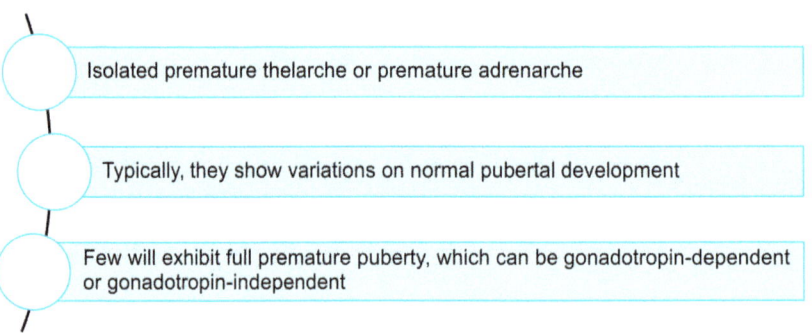

- Isolated premature thelarche or premature adrenarche
- Typically, they show variations on normal pubertal development
- Few will exhibit full premature puberty, which can be gonadotropin-dependent or gonadotropin-independent

Evaluation of Precocious Puberty in Girls[17]

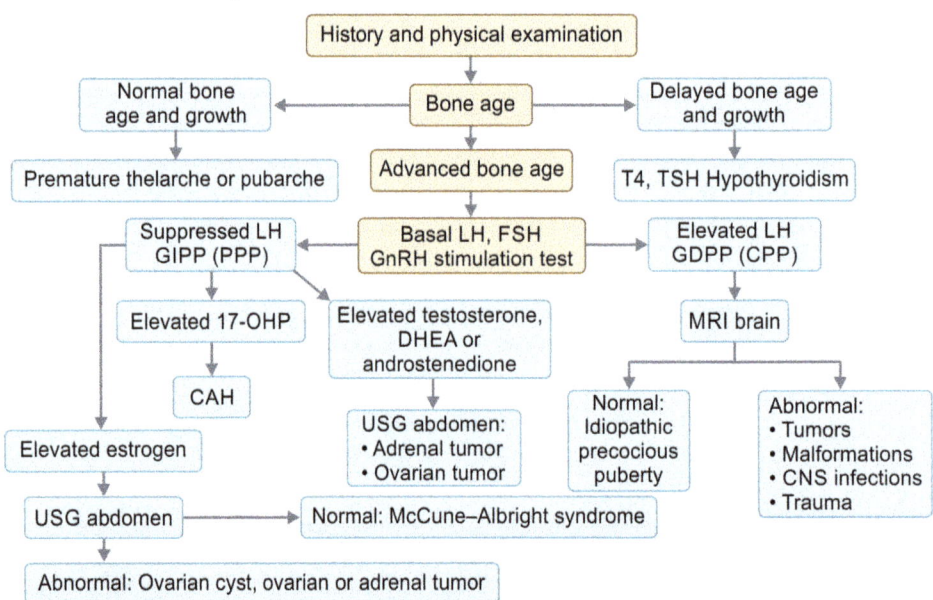

(CAH: congenital adrenal hyperplasia; CNS: central nervous system; CPP: central precocious puberty; DHEA: dehydroepiandrosterone; FSH: follicle-stimulating hormone; GDPP: gonadotropin-dependent precocious puberty; GIPP: gonadotropin-independent precocious puberty; GnRH: gonadotropin-releasing hormone; LH: luteinizing hormone; PPP: peripheral precocious puberty; T4: thyroxine; TSH: thyroid-stimulating hormone; USG: ultrasonography; 17-OHP: 17-hydroxyprogesterone)

Evaluation of Precocious Puberty in Boys[17]

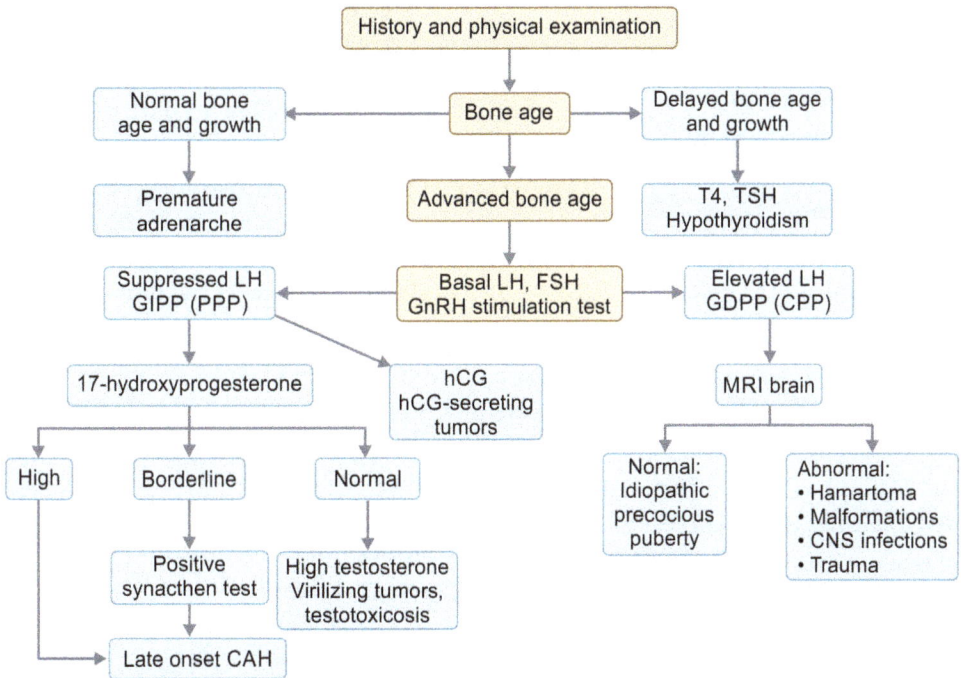

(CAH: congenital adrenal hyperplasia; CPP: central precocious puberty; DHEA: dehydroepiandrosterone; FSH: follicle-stimulating hormone; GDPP: gonadotropin-dependent precocious puberty; GIPP: gonadotropin-independent precocious puberty; GnRH: gonadotropin-releasing hormone; hCG: human chorionic gonadotropin; LH: luteinizing hormone; MRI: magnetic resonance imaging; PPP: peripheral precocious puberty; T4: thyroxine; TSH: thyroid-stimulating hormone; 17-OHP: 17-hydroxyprogesterone)

- A complete history and physical examination, as well as bone age evaluation, to see whether there is a corresponding increase in linear growth.
- The medical history to determine when the physical change(s) were first observed in the patient's siblings and parents. Look for evidence of growth acceleration, rule out any previous history of neurologic disease or trauma, or exposure to sex steroids, and identify any associated symptoms of headache, seizures, or abdominal pain.[2]
- Height, weight, and growth velocity (cm/year) should also be measured during the physical examination, as this is typically an early indicator of developing premature puberty.[18]
- To identify papilledema, a symptom of elevated intracranial pressure, a fundoscopic examination should be conducted.[2]
- Look out for any café au lait spots, which raise the suspicion of McCune–Albright syndrome.[2]
- Tanner staging of pubic hair and/or breast development should be undertaken.
- The glandular breast tissue's diameter should be assessed and to exclude the adipose tissue from glandular tissue.

Imaging and Endocrine Evaluation

- Basal and GnRH-stimulated serum gonadotropin levels to distinguish gonadotropin-dependent from gonadotropin-independent precocious puberty.
- The GnRH stimulation test is carried out by taking blood samples before and 30–40 minutes after a single intravenous dose of GnRH (100 g).[2]
- The most effective diagnostic measure is the stimulated serum LH levels.
- A head MRI is recommended in children with gonadotropin-dependent precocious puberty (as shown by high baseline or stimulated serum LH levels) to rule out a cerebral mass lesion.[19,20]
- Thyroid function tests (TSH and free T4) should be conducted in case of suspicion of hypothyroidism.
- Serum concentrations of estradiol, testosterone, and hCG (functional ovarian cysts and tumors, functional adrenal tumors), late afternoon cortisol (Cushing syndrome), DHEA-S (premature adrenarche), and 17-OHP (CAH) should be evaluated in children with gonadotropin-independent precocious puberty (as identified by normal basal and stimulated serum LH levels), and 17-OHP (CAH).[2]
- Abdominal and pelvic ultrasonography is recommended in all precocious puberty females to diagnose functioning ovarian cysts or tumors.[2]

Treatment of Precocious Puberty[2]

The primary aims of therapy are to halt or restrict growth until normal pubertal age, optimize adult height, and lower the risk of psychological difficulties associated with early sexual maturation.

Indications for Medical Management

- When sexual maturity advances to next stage in a span of 3–6 months.
- Accelerated growth, >6 cm in a year.
- Bone age is advanced by a year or more.
- When estimated adult height falls below the specified range or decreases with repeated measurements.[20]

Treatment of Gonadotropin-dependent Precocious Puberty[2]

- The management of gonadotropin-dependent precocious puberty is planned by the underlying disease as well as the rate of sexual development.
- If an intracranial lesion has been diagnosed, therapy should be tailored to the lesion, if feasible.
- The decision to treat patients with no intracranial lesion should primarily be based on the pace of progression and the estimated adult height.

> Growth spurt should be observed for minimum of 3–6 months before opting for treatment[21]

> Long-acting GnRH agonists (depot preprations) are effacacious for the treatment[19]

> - Buserelin 6.3 mg every 2 months
> - Goserelin 3.6 mg every month or 9.8 mg every 3 months
> - Histrelin 50 mg implant every year
> - Leuprolide 3.75–7.5 mg monthly or 11.25 mg every 3 months
> - Triptorelin 3.0–3.75 mg monthly or 11.25 mg every 3 months[22-24]

- The efficacy of GnRH agonist therapy may be easily determined by measuring serum LH concentrations every 30–60 minutes following repeated injections of the agonist. Following acute GnRH agonist stimulation, the LH level should be <3,0 IU/L, which is comparable with prepubertal norms.[25]
- GnRH agonist treatment should be monitored at 3–6 month intervals with serial physical examinations to identify any progressing pubertal development; bone age should also be checked routinely.[19]
- Breast development should cease, and growth pace and bone age progression should decelerate.[26]
- Treatment with GnRH agonists appears to have no deleterious long-term effects on hypothalamic-pituitary-gonadal axis function.[27]

Treatment of Gonadotropin-independent Precocious Puberty[2]

> Based on underlying disease

> Girls having functioning tumors of the ovaries or adrenals are surgically managed

> Depending on the nature and location of the tumor, hCG-secreting tumors may additionally require adjuvant radiation or chemotherapy

> Solitary unilateral functioning ovarian cysts can also be surgically removed

Treatment of McCune–Albright Syndrome in Girls

> Intended to prevent aromatization and estrogen production

> As an alternative, antiestrogens like tamoxifen have been used successfully to treat the vaginal bleeding that often accompanies excess estrogen[26]

> Bone pain and fractures can be alleviated with bisphosphonate medication for patients with fibrous dysplasia[28]

> Supplemental treatment with a GnRH agonist may be useful for those who, like individuals with idiopathic gonadotropin-dependent precocious puberty, develop a gonadotropin-dependent component to their precocious development as a result of persistent early exposure to sex steroids[29]

■ PREMATURE ADRENARCHE[2]

Increased adrenal androgens have been linked to the unexpected appearance of vaginal hair at a young age.

- A serum DHEA-S concentration >40 ug/dL is the strongest predictor of adrenarche.

Bone age and growth rate are often above normal, although they are not excessive.

- When describing the clinical extremity of premature adrenarche, the term "exaggerated adrenarche" is sometimes used.

Benign condition and requires no specific treatment.

■ PREMATURE PUBARCHE[2]

Generally the outcome of an early adrenarche.

- Without an accompanying rise in adrenal androgen production, idiopathic premature pubarche is likely caused by an increased sensitivity of hair follicles to baseline androgen levels.

Premature puberty is unlikely if the sexual hair is sparse and slow-growing and the bone age is normal, thus expectant care with regular re-evaluation at 6 months is advised.

- Serum testing for testosterone and DHEA-S can be performed as part of a limited endocrine evaluation and compared to age-adjusted norms.

Benign condition and requires no specific treatment.

PREMATURE THELARCHE[2,30,31]

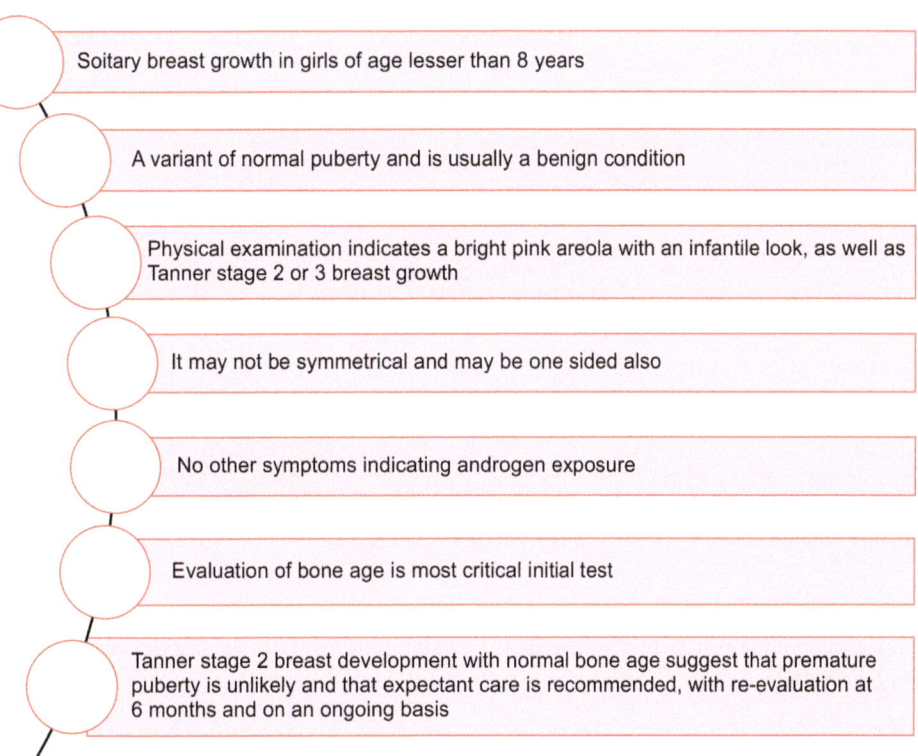

- Premature thelarche is followed by gonadotropin-dependent precocious puberty in around 15–20% of females, with a mean bone age of 9.0 ± 1.1 years and a mean age of 7.1 ± 0.7 years.

DELAYED PUBERTY

- When sexual development has not begun by the age at which 95% of children of the same sex begin pubertal development, we say that puberty has been delayed.[2]
- Delay in breast development by 13 years, a delay of over 4 years between thelarche and the completion of puberty,

or the lack of menarche by 16 years are all indicative of delayed puberty in females. For males, this condition manifests itself when testicular development is delayed past the age of 14 years or when there is an interval of >5 years between the beginning of testicular development and the end of puberty.[32,33]

- Hypogonadism, the medical term for delayed puberty, can result from either an inactive hypothalamic-pituitary axis (hypogonadotropic hypogonadism) or an intrinsic failure of the testes (hypergonadotropic hypogonadism).[2]

Causes of Hypogonadotropic Hypogonadism[2]

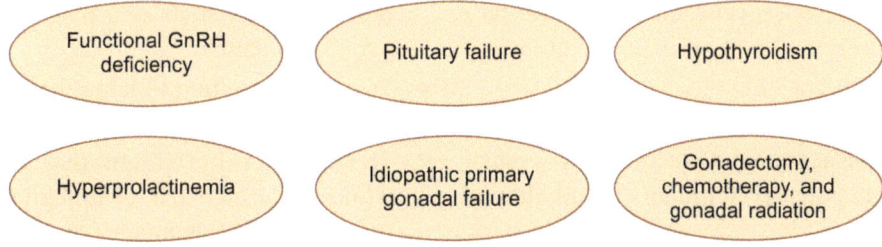

Evaluation of Delayed Pubertal Development[2,3]

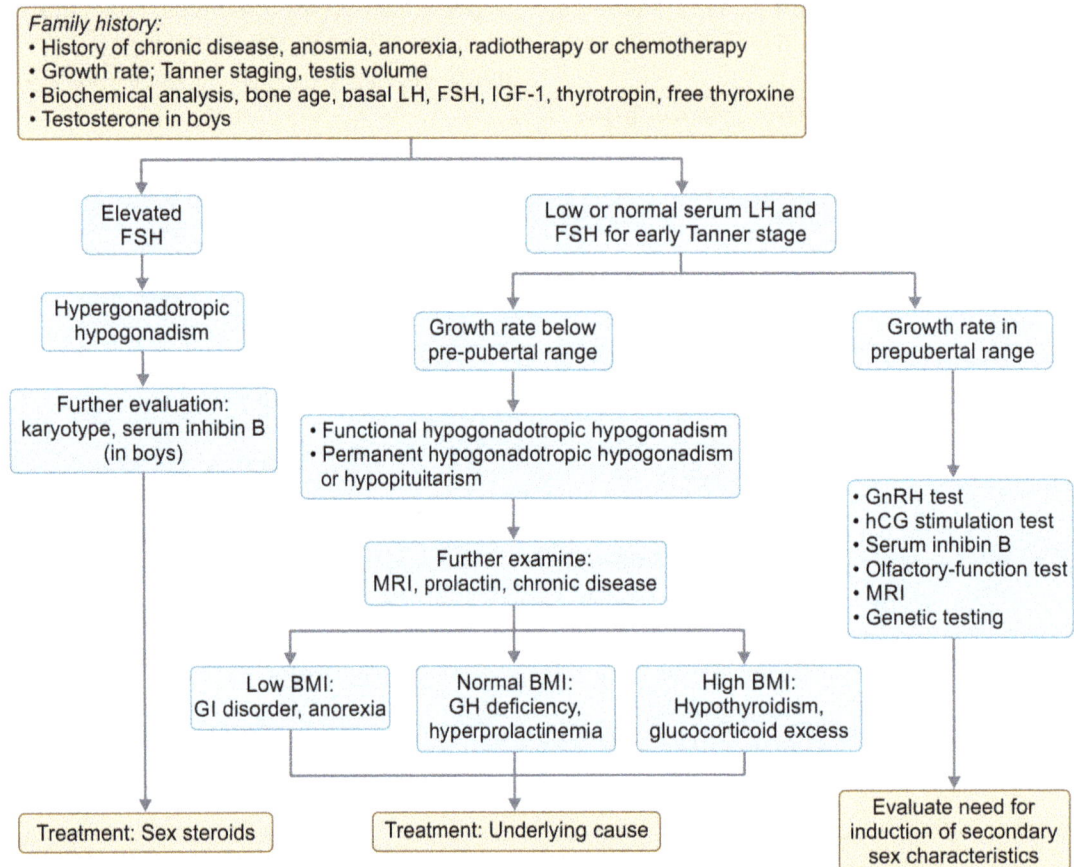

(BMI: body mass index; CDGP: constitutional delay of growth and puberty; FSH: follicle-stimulating hormone; GH: growth hormone; GnRH: gonadotropin-releasing hormone; hCG: human chorionic gonadotropin; IGF-1: insulin-like growth factor-1; LH: luteinizing hormone; MRI: magnetic resonance imaging)

- The medical history should reveal if pubertal development has not yet begun or has begun and then stopped.
- This may be determined by a combination of a physical examination, a history of any relevant illnesses, and a measurement of the patient's bone age.
- In addition to dietary and activity patterns, significant diseases and medications that might delay or slow the onset of puberty are also important contextual variables.
- Delayed puberty may be an early indicator of a metabolic disorder such inflammatory bowel disease or hypothyroidism.
- Most people with constitutional delay have a similar history in other family members, so it is important to have a full family history, paying special attention to the ages at which older siblings and parents reached important developmental milestones.
- It is important to measure more than just height and weight during a physical examination; the Tanner staging of breast and pubic hair development should also be taken into account.

Imaging and Laboratory Evaluation[2]

- Measurements of blood FSH, LH, and estradiol concentrations are commonly used to make this distinction between primary (hypergonadotropic) and secondary (hypogonadotropic) hypogonadism.
- Once this difference has been identified, additional laboratory assessment can focus on identifying the underlying etiology of hypogonadotropic or hypergonadotropic hypogonadism.

Hypergonadotropic Hypogonadism[2]

- To rule out chromosomal abnormalities, a karyotype should be performed on all women with hypergonadotropic hypogonadism unless there is a good reason not to, such as a history of chemotherapy or gonadal radiation.
- Turner syndrome (45,X) is the template for the most prevalent condition of this sort, gonadal dysgenesis.
- Those with a Y chromosome (e.g., 46,XY, Swyer syndrome) who have a high risk of malignant transformation in occult testicular elements (20–30%) will be identified by

karyotype in addition to those with other structural X chromosomal abnormalities (e.g., deletions, rings, and isochromosomes).
- Individuals with hypergonadotropic hypogonadism with a normal (46,XX) karyotype may be tested for 17-hydroxylase deficiency, an uncommon steroidogenic enzyme defect associated with sexual infantilism and hypertension, and other odd causes of primary ovarian failure.

Hypogonadotropic Hypogonadism[2]
- In females with hypogonadotropic hypogonadism, serum prolactin levels should be measured to identify those with hyperprolactinemia.
- Hyperprolactinemia is a reason for MRI imaging, unless it is clearly ascribed to medicines.
- Other laboratory tests, such as complete blood count (CBC), erythrocyte sedimentation rate (ESR), and liver function test (LFT) to identify patients who may have an undetected chronic disease.
- Although pelvic ultrasonography can be used to determine whether or not a uterus is present in a female who is a virgin, this procedure should be performed with caution.
- An MRI of the head to detect mass lesions.
- The presence or absence of olfactory bulbs and tracts can also be determined by imaging, as they are absent in Kallmann syndrome.

Treatment of Delayed Puberty[2]
- When possible, treating the underlying cause is the best course of action, such as in the cases of hypothyroidism (with thyroid hormone treatment), hyperprolactinemia (with dopamine agonist therapy), and the removal of a craniopharyngioma or other operable central lesion.
- Those with unexplained delays in puberty should be evaluated for congenital GnRH insufficiency apart from those with constitutional puberty delay.
- Both hormone replacement therapy and expectant care, including reassurance and psychological support, are options for patients with congenital GnRH deficiency or constitutional puberty delay.
- Management with sex hormones to be reserved for females above the age of 12 years who show no or few indicators of sexual maturity that cause substantial anguish or worry.
- Long-term goals for individuals with isolated GnRH insufficiency include maintaining sex hormone levels within the normal physiologic range and, if and when fertility is a concern, stimulating ovulation with exogenous gonadotropin therapy.
- Complete sexual maturation is targeted to occur within 2–3 years after starting oral or transdermal estrogen medication (0.25–0.5 mg oral micronized estradiol or its equivalent) and increasing gradually dependent on response (Tanner stage and bone age).
- Addition of a progestin to the treatment plan is not recommended since it may have an unfavorable impact on breast growth and/or appearance.
- After menstruation has begun or after 12–24 months of estrogen therapy, progestin medication can be started safely.
- Hormone medication can be discontinued for periods of 1–3 months once breast development is complete and menstruation has begun to assess the likelihood of spontaneous menstruation, which is typical in females with constitutional puberty delay.
- Persistent hypogonadism after the age of 18 strongly indicates congenital GnRH insufficiency.
- Only patients with a confirmed GH deficiency should get GH medication. It is common for patients with constitutional delayed puberty to have low serum GH and IGF-I levels; however, these levels often increase with estrogen treatment and are typically normal in those with congenital GnRH impairment.

GROWTH DISORDERS IN ADOLESCENT AGE

One of the worst aspects of teenage development issues is the way it may make a young person feel "strange". The adolescent probably hates being different more than anybody else. Height gain occurs constantly, although in an atypically nonlinear fashion.[2] There are three distinct phases of maturation.

1. The first is the newborn stage, when a child's height increases by 30–35 cm in just 2 years.
2. The second stage, childhood, sees growth remain relatively constant around 5–7 cm/year; however, it usually slows in late childhood.
3. The third and final phase, puberty, is characterized by a growth spurt of 8–14 cm each year due to elevated levels of both GH and sex steroid hormones.[23,34]

Short Stature

A kid is considered to be of short stature if they are two or more standard deviations below the mean height for children of the same gender and chronological age on a standard growth chart. The direction of progress is more important than any specific value. The most important finding is the mitigation of irregular increases in size (percentile). Children should average at least 5 cm of growth every year from the age of 4 years until the onset of puberty.[2]

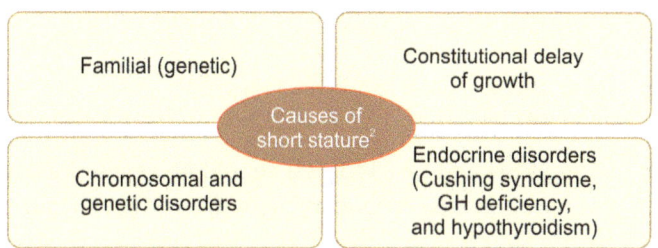

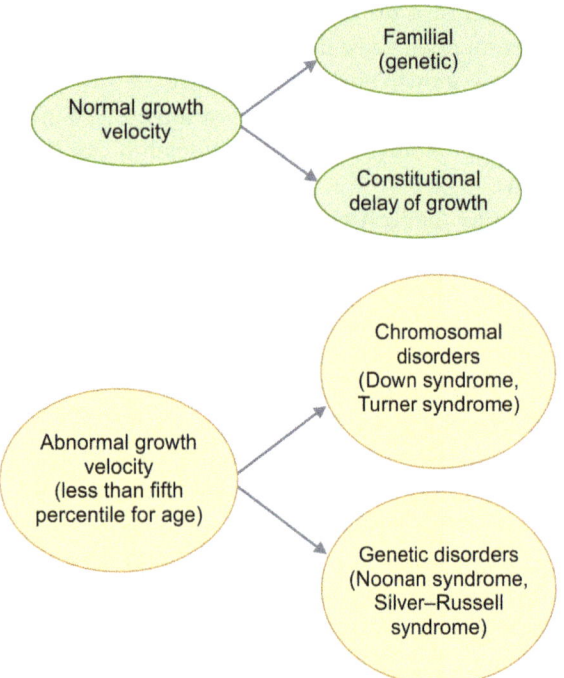

Children with short stature due to endocrine problems are typically overweight for their height.

Idiopathic short stature is defined as when a kid is underweight for his or her age and has a height that is more than two standard deviations below the mean for that age. The growth rates of these kids are often below average, yet their blood levels of IGF-I are normal. People with constitutional growth delay have a delayed bone age than those with hereditary or familial short stature but nonetheless have a predicted adult height within the normal range.[2]

Evaluation[2]

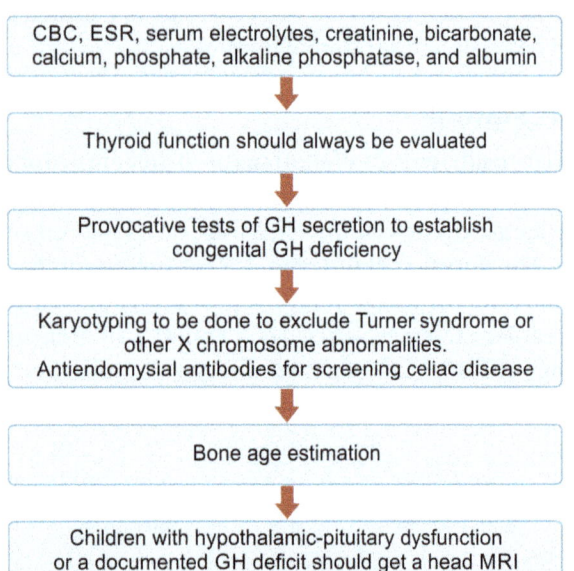

- Serum TSH and free T4 levels should be checked since both primary and secondary hypothyroidism can cause growth failure.

- Hypercortisolism (Cushing syndrome) in children is unusual unless brought on by an overdose of glucocorticoids.
- Severe growth failure, a delayed bone age, and extremely low blood concentrations of IGF-I and its primary binding protein, IGFBP-3, are classic symptoms of congenital GH insufficiency in young children.

Treatment

- If a female patient's height is >2.25 standard deviations below the mean for her age, her epiphyses are not closed, and her projected adult height is <59 inches, then GH medication is indicated for the treatment of idiopathic short stature.[2]
- Most kids with idiopathic short stature, especially those who have a constitutional growth delay, make up for lost time throughout the teen years even without treatment.[35]
- The best time to begin therapy is between the ages of 5 and early adolescence.[36]
- Although GH treatment appears promising, it should be reserved for children whose short stature is a significant disability and whose confidence and social skills are expected to considerably benefit from a significant increase in height.[37]
- A long-acting GnRH agonist may be used as an alternate therapy to postpone pubertal growth and epiphyseal fusion.[2]

Tall Stature[2]

Tall stature is defined as two or more standard deviations above the mean height for children of the same gender and chronological age.

Height over average that is tall stature is more socially acceptable and less often recognized as a problem than height below average (short stature).

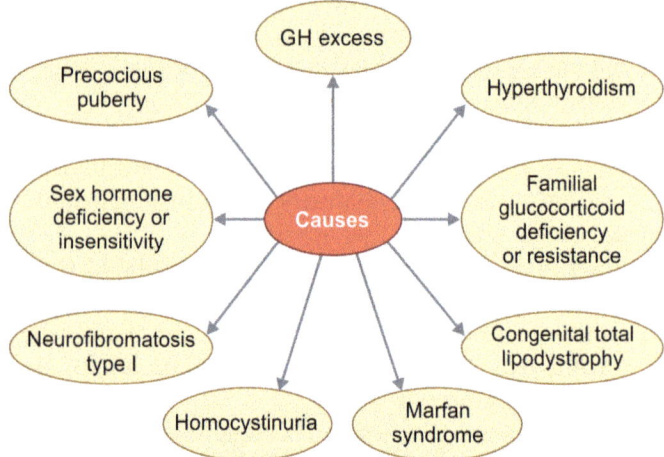

- Family history and the lack of dysmorphic characteristics separate familial or constitutional long height from problems of excessive development.

- A comprehensive physical examination along with family history and bone age are usually enough to establish the diagnosis and give reassurance in most tall but otherwise normal youngsters.

Treatment

- Treatment should be restricted to people whose tall height is causing serious psychological concerns.
- For decades, sex steroids are being prescribed to kids who are particularly tall in the hopes that their bones will fuse sooner.[38,39]
- The puberty growth surge happens before menarche, thus therapy needs to start before menarche to be effective, making the stage of secondary sexual development crucial.[40]
- The average age for starting therapy is between 10 and 12 years.
- Even if treatment is initiated after menarche, it is possible to achieve a reduction of 1 inch in height.[41,42]
- A low-dosage oral contraceptive tablet with 15–30 g of ethinylestradiol is a common starting dose.[43]
- Taking serial measurements of bone age every 6–12 months throughout therapy can demonstrate that treatment has been successful in closing the epiphyses.[43]
- A recent study including adult women with inherited tall height indicated that those treated with estrogen as teenagers had a considerably greater risk of future infertility and cycle fecundity was lowered by around 40% compared to those who were not treated.[44]

Key Learning Points

- Central precocious puberty typically starts before 8 years of age.
- It is important to differentiate between the central precocious puberty and peripheral precocious puberty.
- The gold standard for management of central precocious puberty is GnRH analogs.
- Management of peripheral precocious puberty is directed at its etiology.
- Delayed puberty is characterized by the absence of breast development by 13 years in females and by a lack of testicular enlargement by 14 years.
- When feasible, treating the underlying cause of delayed puberty should be the primary focus of treatment.

REFERENCES

1. Dahl RE. Adolescent brain development: a period of vulnerabilities and opportunities. Keynote address, Ann N Y Acad Sci. 2004;1021(1):1-22.
2. Taylor HS, Pal L, Seli E. Speroff's Clinical Gynecologic Endocrinology and Infertility, 9th edition. Philadelphia: Wolters Kluwer; 2020. pp. 734-820.
3. Marshall WA, Tanner JM. Variations in pattern of pubertal changes in girls. Arch Dis Child. 1969;44(235):291-303.
4. Marshall WA, Tanner JM. Variations in the pattern of pubertal changes in boys. Arch Dis Child. 1970;45(239):13-23.
5. Pescovitz OH, Comite F, Hench K, Barnes K, McNemar A, Foster C, et al. The NIH experience with precocious puberty: diagnostic subgroups and response to short-term luteinizing hormone releasing hormone analogue therapy. J Pediatr. 1986;108(1):47-54.
6. Bridges NA, Christopher JA, Hindmarsh PC, Brook CG. Sexual precocity: sex incidence and aetiology. Arch Dis Child. 1994;70(2):116-8.
7. Chemaitilly W, Trivin C, Adan L, Gall V, Sainte-Rose C, Brauner R. Central precocious puberty: clinical and laboratory features. Clin Endocrinol. 2001;54(3):289-94.
8. Chalumeau M, Chemaitilly W, Trivin C, Adan L, Breart G, Brauner R. Central precocious puberty in 5-7 girls: an evidence-based diagnosis tree to predict central nervous system abnormalities. Pediatrics. 2002;109:61-7.
9. Ng SM, Kumar Y, Cody D, Smith CS, Didi M. Cranial MRI scans are indicated in all girls with central precocious puberty. Arch Dis Child. 2003;88(5):414-8.
10. Rodriguez-Macias KA, Thibaud E, Houang M, Duflos C, Beldjord C, Rappaport R. Follow up of precocious pseudo-puberty associated with isolated ovarian follicular cysts. Arch Dis Child. 1999;81(1):53-6.
11. de Sousa G, Wunsch R, Andler W. Precocious pseudopuberty due to autonomous ovarian cysts: a report of ten cases and long-term follow-up. Hormones. 2008;7(2):170-4.
12. Pienkowski C, Baunin C, Gayrard M, Lemasson F, Vaysse P, Tauber M. Ovarian cysts in prepubertal girls. Endocr Dev. 2004;7:66-76.
13. Fakhry J, Khoury A, Kotval PS, Noto RA. Sonography of autonomous follicular ovarian cysts in precocious pseudo-puberty, J Ultrasound Med. 1988;7(11):597-603.
14. Lack EE, Perez-Atayde AR, Murthy AS, Goldstein DP, Crigler JF Jr, Vawter GF. Granulosa theca cell tumors in premenarchal girls: a clinical and pathologic study of ten cases. Cancer. 1981;48(8):1846-54.
15. Young RH, Dickersin GR, Scully RE. Juvenile granulosa cell tumor of the ovary. A clinicopathological analysis of 125 cases. Am J Surg Pathol. 1984;8(8):575-96.
16. Arhan E, Cetinkaya E, Aycan Z, Aslan AT, Yucel H, Vidinlisan S. A very rare cause of virilization in childhood: ovarian Leydig cell tumor. J Pediatr Endocrinol Metab. 2008;21(2):181-4.
17. Menon PSN, Vijayakumar M. Precocious puberty. In: Vasudev AS, Shah NK (Eds). Algorithms in Puberty. New Delhi: Jaypee Brothers Medical Publishers (P) Ltd.; 2017. pp. 535-42.
18. Papadimitriou A, Beri D, Tsialla A, Fretzayas A, Psychou F, Nicolaidou P. Early growth acceleration in girls with idiopathic precocious puberty. J Pediatr. 2006;149(1):43-6.
19. Carel JC, Eugster EA, Rogol A, Ghizzoni L, Palmert MR; ESPE-LWPES GnRH Analogs Consensus Conference Group. Consensus statement on the use of gonadotropin-releasing hormone analogs in children. Pediatrics. 2009;123(4):e752-62.
20. Carel JC, Leger J. Precocious puberty. N Engl J Med. 2008;358(22):2366-77.
21. Comite F, Cutler GB Jr, Rivier J, Vale WW, Loriaux DL, Crowley WF Jr. Short-term treatment of idiopathic precocious puberty with a long-acting analogue of luteinizing hormone-releasing hormone. A preliminary report. N Engl J Med. 1981;305(26):1546-50.
22. Antoniazzi F, Zamboni G. Central precocious puberty: current treatment options. Paediatr Drugs. 2004;6(4):211-31.

23. Lahlou N, Carel JC, Chaussain JL, Roger M. Pharmacokinetics and pharmacodynamics of GnRH agonists: clinical implications in pediatrics. J Pediatr Endocrinol Metab. 2000;13(Suppl 1):723-38.
24. Partsch CJ, Sippell WG. Treatment of central precocious puberty. Best Pract Res Clin Endocrinol Metab. 2002;16(1):165-89.
25. Bhatia S, Neely EK, Wilson DM. Serum luteinizing hormone rises within minutes after depot leuprolide injection: implications for monitoring therapy. Pediatrics. 2002;109(2):E30.
26. Wierman ME, Beardsworth DE, Crawford JD, Crigler JF Jr, Mansfield MJ, Bode HH, et al. Adrenarche and skeletal maturation during luteinizing hormone releasing hormone analogue suppression of gonadarche. J Clin Invest. 1986;77(1):121-6.
27. Cassio A, Bal MO, Orsini LF, Balsamo A, Sansavini S, Gennari M, et al. Reproductive outcome in patients treated and not treated for idiopathic early puberty: long-term results of a randomized trial in adults. J Pediatr. 2006;149(4):532-6.
28. Lala R, Matarazzo P, Bertelloni S, Buzi F, Rigon F, de Sanctis C. Pamidronate treatment of bone fibrous dysplasia in nine children with McCune-Albright syndrome. Acta Paediatr. 2000;89(2):188-93.
29. Haddad N, Eugster E. An update on the treatment of precocious puberty in McCune-Albright syndrome and testotoxicosis. J Pediatr Endocrinol Metab. 2007;20(6):653-62.
30. Pasquino AM, Pucarelli I, Passeri F, Segni M, Mancini MA, Municchi G. Progression of premature thelarche to central precocious puberty. J Pediatr. 1995;126(1):11-4.
31. Zhu SY, Du ML, Huang TT. An analysis of predictive factors for the conversion from premature thelarche into complete central precocious puberty. J Pediatr Endocrinol Metab. 2008;21(6):533-8.
32. Bozzola M, Bozzola E, Montalbano C, Stamati FA, Ferrara P, Villani A. Delayed puberty versus hypogonadism: a challenge for the pediatrician. Ann Pediatr Endocrinol Metab. 2018;23(2):57-61.
33. Palmert MR, Dunkel L. Delayed puberty. N Engl J Med. 2012;366:443-53.
34. Kerrigan JR, Rogol AD. The impact of gonadal steroid hormone action on growth hormone secretion during childhood and adolescence. Endocr Rev. 1992;13(2):281-98.
35. Leschek EW, Rose SR, Yanovski JA, Troendle JF, Quigley CA, Chipman JJ, et al. Effect of growth hormone treatment on adult height in peripubertal children with idiopathic short stature: a randomized, double-blind, placebo-controlled trial. J Clin Endocrinol Metab. 2004;89(7):3140-8.
36. Cohen P, Rogol AD, Deal CL, Saenger P, Reiter EO, Ross JL, et al. Consensus statement on the diagnosis and treatment of children with idiopathic short stature: a summary of the Growth Hormone Research Society, the Lawson Wilkins Pediatric Endocrine Society, and the European Society for Paediatric Endocrinology Workshop. J Clin Endocrinol Metab. 2008;93(11):4210-7.
37. Sandberg DE, Bukowski WM, Fung CM, Noll RB. Height and social adjustment: are extremes a cause for concern and action? Pediatrics. 2004;114(3):744-50.
38. Bierich JR. Estrogen treatment of girls with constitutional tall stature. Pediatrics 1978;62(6):1196-201.
39. Sorgo W, Scholler K, Heinze F, Heinze E, Teller WM. Critical analysis of height reduction in oestrogen-treated tall girls. Eur J Pediatr. 1984;142(4):260-5.
40. Drop SL, De Waal WJ, De Muinck Keizer-Schrama SM. Sex steroid treatment of constitutionally tall stature. Endocr Rev. 1998;19:540-58.
41. Schoen EJ, Solomon IL, Warner O, Wingerd J. Estrogen treatment of tall girls. Am J Dis Child. 1973;125(1):71-4.
42. Daniel Jr WA, Wettenhall HN, Cahill C, Roche AF. Tall girls: a survey of 15 years of management and treatment. J Pediatr. 1975;86(4):602-10.
43. de Waal WJ, Greyn-Fokker MH, Stijnen T, van Gurp EA, Toolens AM, de Munick Keizer-Schrama SM, et al. Accuracy of final height prediction and effect of growth-reductive therapy in 362 constitutionally tall children. J Clin Endocrinol Metab. 1996;81(3):1206-16.
44. Venn A, Bruinsma F, Werther G, Pyett P, Baird D, Jones P, et al. Oestrogen treatment to reduce the adult height of tall girls: long-term effects on fertility. Lancet. 2004;364(9444):1513-8.

CHAPTER 5

Disorders of Sexual Development

Reeta Mahey, Monika Rajput, Rohitha Cheluvaraju

INTRODUCTION

Sex of the individual has a fundamental role in determining our physical structure, brain orientation, behaviour (sexual and social) and self-concept. This chapter begins with the elaboration of normal sexual differentiation to provide basic understanding to readers about the physiological processes involved and recognize the cause and type of abnormal sexual development. Affected individuals may be recognized at birth by ambiguous genitalia or may present later with postnatal virilization, delayed/absent puberty, amenorrhea or infertility. These conditions are associated with variations in genes, developmental programming, and hormones.

Unlike physical development; discussion on psychosexual health in patients with disorders of sex development (DSD) remains neglected by family and clinicians. This chapter enlightens comprehensive approach and individualised management in these patients. The individual DSD has been described in an algorithmic manner for easy learning. Clinical presentation and systematic approach to an individual with DSD along with detailed endocrine profile, indications of karyotype, hormonal therapy, fertility issues and role of assisted reproduction is discussed here.

DEFINITION

The term "disorders/differences of sex development" (DSD) is used for the congenital anomalies in which development of chromosomal, gonadal, or phenotypic sex (including external genitalia/internal genitalia) is atypical.[1,2] It includes all the disorders where chromosomal, gonadal, phenotypic, or psychological sex are incongruent.

INCIDENCE

Global incidence is approximately 1 in 4,500–5,500 newborns.[1] The incidence of DSD in 46,XY individuals is around 1 in 20,000 births while in 46,XX individuals is estimated to be 1 in 14,000–15,000 live births.[3]

CLINICAL PRESENTATION OF DIFFERENCES OF SEX DEVELOPMENT

Differences of sex developments may be identified at different times of the life cycle:
- Ambiguous genitalia at birth
- *In phenotypic females:*
  - Delayed puberty
  - Primary amenorrhea
  - Unexpected virilization
  - Precocious puberty
  - Infertility
  - Inguinal masses
  - Gonadal tumors
- *In phenotypic males:*
  - Gynecomastia
  - Under virilized male
  - Infertility
  - Undescended testis/coital problems
  - Moderate to severely affected sperm parameters
  - Gonadal tumors.

REVISED NOMENCLATURE (TABLE 1)

- It is vital to use "precise and appropriate terms" when applying definitions and diagnostic labels.

TABLE 1: Revised nomenclature as per Chicago Consensus.[1]

Previous	Proposed
Intersex	Disorders of sexual development (DSD)
• Male pseudohermaphrodite • Under virilisation of XY male • Under masculinisation of XY male	46,XY DSD
• Female pseudohermaphrodite • Over virilisation of XX female • Masculinisation of XX female	46,XX DSD
True hermaphrodite	Ovo testicular DSD
• XX male or XX sex reversal • XY sex reversal	• 46,XX testicular DSD • 46,XY complete gonadal dysgenesis

- The ideal nomenclature should be sufficiently flexible and robust to incorporate new information and to maintain consistency.
- Terms used by clinicians should be sensible and descriptive enough to reflect genetic etiology and the spectrum of phenotypical variation.
- *Terms such as intersex, pseudohermaphrodites, hermaphrodites, and sex reversal are abandoned.*

NORMAL SEXUAL DIFFERENTIATION (FLOWCHART 1)

Normal sexual differentiation is a dynamic and sequential process that starts with establishment of chromosomal sex at the time of fertilization; and is described in **Flowchart 1** as per classical Jost's paradigm.[4] The fate of bipotential gonads into testes or ovaries is governed by the presence of pro testicular factors (SRY, SOX9, and FGF9), and pro ovarian factors (WNT4, Dax1, Foxl2 and RSPO1) respectively.

Important Points

- The development of one side Wolffian system along with regression of Müllerian duct system will happen only in presence of ipsilateral fully functional testis.
- Müllerian duct system will develop on one side even in the presence of a streak gonads (as this does not require any hormonal influence so functional female gonads are not required for the development of ipsilateral Müllerian structures).

Psychosexual Development

This is a vital part of final sexual orientation of an individual. Sexual differentiation of genitalia occurs in the first 2 months of pregnancy but sexual differentiation of brain occurs in second half of pregnancy, so both processes may be dissociated. Sexual orientation of brain may be affected by prenatal and postnatal hormones exposure, extent of virilization, genetic factors, environmental, psychological, and family factors. The three components of psychosexual development may be discordant in individuals with DSD **(Flowchart 2)**.

Flowchart 1: Normal sexual differentiation.

```
Chromosomal sex ──── At the time of fertilization ──── XY or XX (variations: XO, XXY, and mosaicism)

Gonadal sex ──── Bipotential gonadal ridge ──── Testis/ovary (variations ovotestis; streak gonads)
                    │                    │
                SRY gene +           SRY gene –
                    │                    │
          Sertoli and leydig cells    Ovarian development
                    │
        Hormones secreted from the gonads
                    │                                    (in absence of any hormonal influence)
   Sex phenotype (internal and external genitalia)

Leydig cells: Testosterone—                      No testosterone:
Wolffian duct differentiation into Vas           Regression of Wolffian duct
deference, epidiymis, and seminal vesicles       development of female external genitalia

Sertoli cells: Anti-Müllerian hormone (AMH)—     No AMH:
suppression of Müllerian duct                    Müllerian duct develops into uterus;
                                                 fallopian tube upper two-thirds of vagina
Dihydrotestosterone (from testosterone)
• Male external genitalia and closure of urethral folds
  development of scrotum and prostate
• Suppresses the development of sinovaginal bulb

Insulin-like peptide-3-testicular descent

Psychological sex

Androgen—masculinization of brain in second half    • Genital tubercle—clitoris
of pregnancy (gender identity)                      • Urethral folds—labia minora
                                                    • Labioscrotal swellings—labia majora

          Male                                              Female
```

Flowchart 2: Psychosexual development and components.

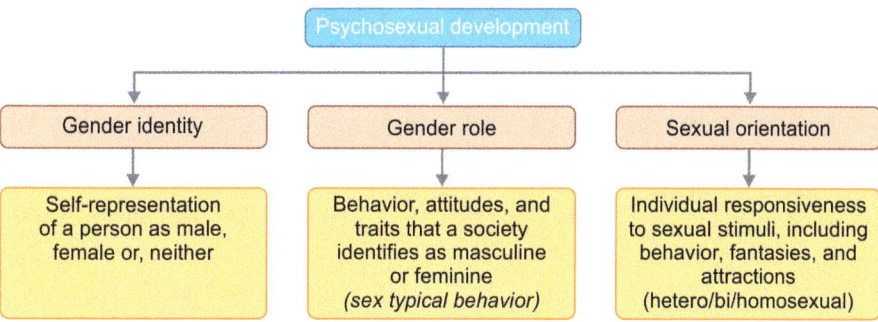

TABLE 2: Classification of abnormal sexual differentiation.[1]

Sex chromosome DSD	46,XY DSD	46,XX DSD
45,XO Turner syndrome	• Disorders of testicular development 　– Complete gonadal dysgenesis (Swyer syndrome) 　– Partial gonadal dysgenesis 　– Gonadal regression 　– Ovotesticular DSD	• Disorders of ovarian development 　– Ovotesticular DSD 　– Testicular DSD (SRY+ male) 　– Gonadal dysgenesis
47,XXY Klinefelter syndrome and variants	• Disorders in androgen synthesis or action 　– Androgen biosynthesis defect (17-HSD deficiency, 5-α-reductase and STAR mutations) 　– Defect in androgen action (complete and partial AIS) 　– LH receptor defects 　– Disorders of AMH and AMH receptor (persistent Müllerian duct syndrome)	• Androgen excess 　– Fetal cause (21-hydroxylase deficiency and 11-hydroxylase deficiency) 　– Fetoplacental (aromatase deficiency) 　– Maternal (luteoma and drug exposure)
45,XO/46,XY (mixed gonadal dysgenesis and ovotesticular DSD)	Others (like severe hypospadias and cloacal exstrophy)	Others (such as cloacal exstrophy, vaginal atresia, and MURCS)
46,XX/46,XY (ovotesticular DSD)		
Rare: SRY gene positive 46,XX testicular DSD (de la Chapelle syndrome)		

(AIS: androgen insensitivity syndrome; AMH: anti-Müllerian hormone; DSD: disorders of sexual development; LH: luteinizing hormone; MURCS: Müllerian duct aplasia–renal agenesis–cervicothoracic somite dysplasia; STAR: steroid hormone acute regulatory protein)

Gender Dissatisfaction

This is still a poorly understood entity. This along with homosexual orientation is not considered as DSD and is not considered an indication of incorrect gender assignment).

Gender Dysphoria

This is characterized by marked incongruence between the assigned gender and experienced/expressed gender, which is associated with clinically significant functional impairment (it can occur in the presence or absence of DSD). **Table 2** describes the classification of DSD mainly sex chromosome DSD, 46,XX and 46,XY DSDs.

Disorders of Sexual Differentiation

Table 2 describes the classification of DSD disorders mainly sex chromosome DSD, 46,XX and 46,XY DSDs.

Sex Chromosome DSD

Turner syndrome (45,XO)

- This DSD presents as female phenotype with absence/aneuploidy or structural rearrangement of X chromosome.
- Majority have 45,XO karyotype with others having various mosaics involving 46,XX/45,XO or 45,XO/46,XY cells

- Incidence of 45,XO karyotypes is approximately 1 in 2,500 live borne phenotypic female births and is mostly sporadic type of mutation **(Fig. 1)**.[5]
- **Figure 2** describes the clinical stigmata of Turner syndrome. The patient given in the figure is a case of Turner mosaic (45,XX; 45,XO) who presented with primary amenorrhea and had severe hypertension.
- Women over the age of 50 years with <5% 45,X cells and phenotypic males with 45,X/46,XY are not included in Turner syndrome.[9]
- *Clinical presentation:* Importance of karyotyping at various age groups is depicted in **Figure 1**.

Indications: Indications for chromosome analysis to diagnose Turner syndrome:[8]
- *As the only clinical feature:*
    - Fetal cystic hygroma or hydrops, especially
    - Severe idiopathic short stature
    - Obstructive left-sided congenital heart defect
    - Unexplained delayed puberty/menarche

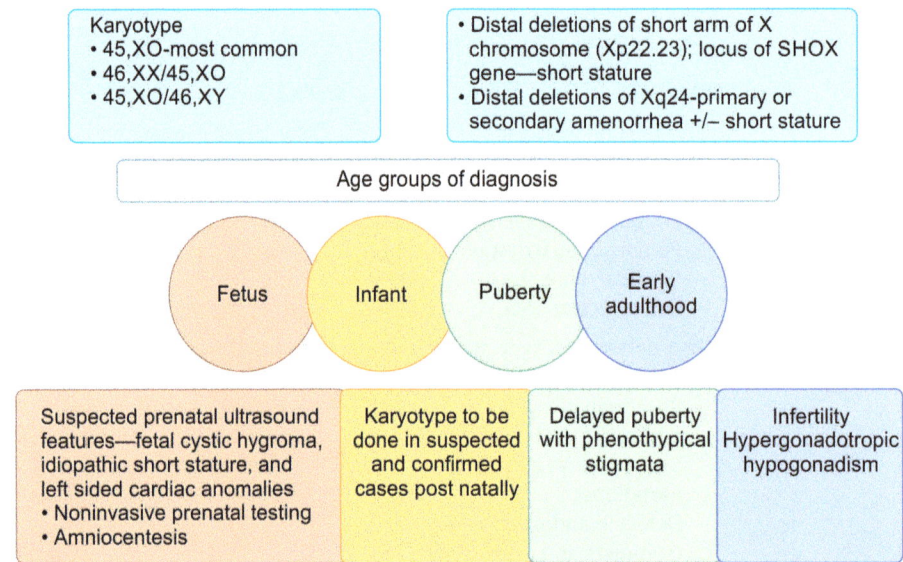

Fig. 1: Description of chromosomal abnormalities, various age groups at diagnosis and importance of karyotyping in turner syndrome[6-8,10,11]

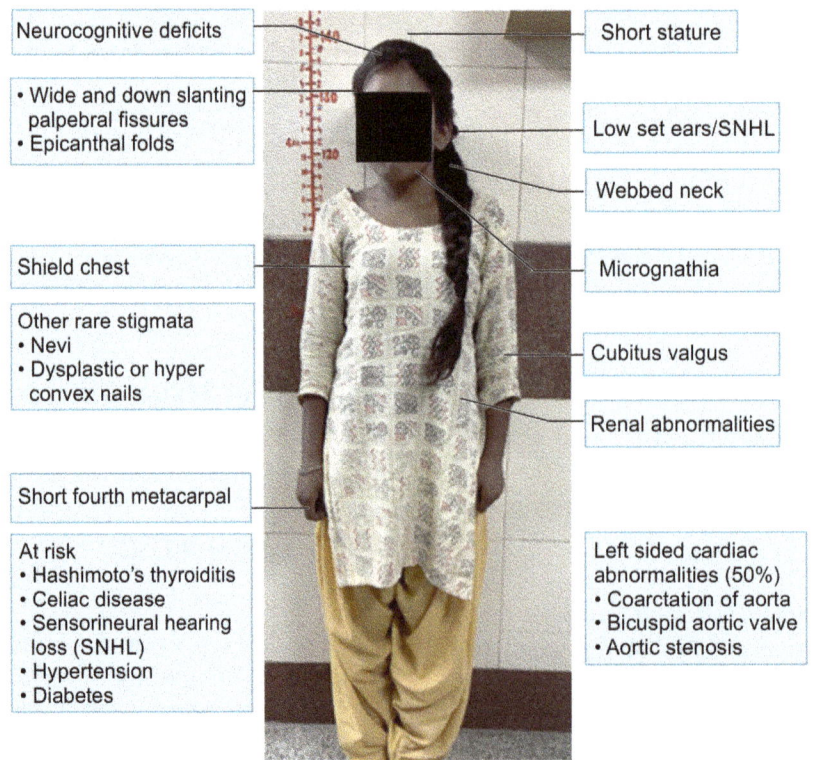

Fig. 2: Clinical characteristics of turner syndrome.

- *Couple with infertility*
- Characteristic features in a female
- Hypergonadotropic hypogonadism.
- *At least two of the following:*
  - Renal anomaly (horseshoe, absence, or hypoplasia) Madelung deformity
  - Neuropsychological problems and/or psychiatric issues
  - Multiple typical or melanocytic nevi
  - Dysplastic or hyperconvex nails
  - Other congenital heart defects
  - Hearing impairment <40 years of age together with short stature.

Management of Turner syndrome:
- Establishment of growth potential
- Induction of puberty
- Fertility management
- Addressing associated systemic comorbidities.

Hormonal therapy in Turner syndrome **(Flowchart 3)**.

Natural fertility and assisted reproductive technologies (ART) in TS **(Table 3)**.[8,13]

Pregnancy and Turner syndrome:[8]

- Transthoracic echocardiogram (TTE) should be performed in women with TS without aortic dilatation or other risk factors (hypertension, bicuspid aortic valve, coarctation, previous aortic surgery) at least once during pregnancy and approximately 20 weeks of gestation.
- Women with TS with an ascending ASI >2.0 cm/m² or any risk factor (hypertension, bicuspid aortic valve, coarctation, and previous AoD or surgery) should be monitored frequently, including TTE at 4-8 weeks interval during pregnancy and during the first 6 months postpartum.
- Cardiac magnetic resonance scan (CMR) imaging (without gadolinium) should be performed during pregnancy when there is a suspicion of disease of the distal ascending aorta, aortic arch, or descending aorta.

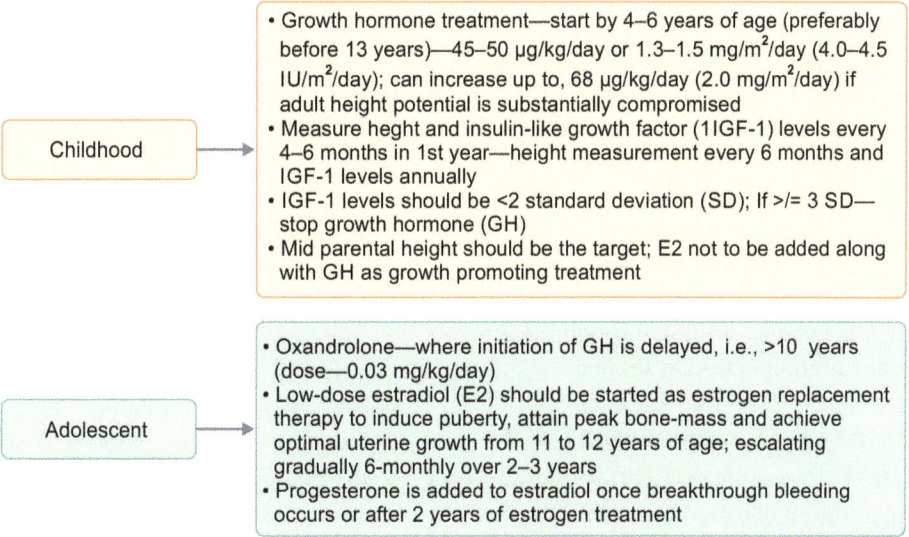

Flowchart 3: Hormonal therapy in Turner syndrome.[8,12,13]

Childhood
- Growth hormone treatment—start by 4–6 years of age (preferably before 13 years)—45–50 µg/kg/day or 1.3–1.5 mg/m²/day (4.0–4.5 IU/m²/day); can increase up to, 68 µg/kg/day (2.0 mg/m²/day) if adult height potential is substantially compromised
- Measure heght and insulin-like growth factor (1IGF-1) levels every 4–6 months in 1st year—height measurement every 6 months and IGF-1 levels annually
- IGF-1 levels should be <2 standard deviation (SD); If >/= 3 SD—stop growth hormone (GH)
- Mid parental height should be the target; E2 not to be added along with GH as growth promoting treatment

Adolescent
- Oxandrolone—where initiation of GH is delayed, i.e., >10 years (dose—0.03 mg/kg/day)
- Low-dose estradiol (E2) should be started as estrogen replacement therapy to induce puberty, attain peak bone-mass and achieve optimal uterine growth from 11 to 12 years of age; escalating gradually 6-monthly over 2–3 years
- Progesterone is added to estradiol once breakthrough bleeding occurs or after 2 years of estrogen treatment

TABLE 3: Fertility and pre pregnancy management in TS	
Infertility	*Pre pregnancy*
• Probability of spontaneous pregnancy—4.8–7.6% • Fertility decreases with age • Fertility preservation in adolescent girls – ovarian tissue cryopreservation can be offered, but still in research settings • Post pubertal girls with mosaicism - oocyte cryopreservation can be offered • ART option for TS female with no ovarian reserve is Donor-oocyte IVF • Other ART options like adoption and surrogacy should be discussed during preconception counselling	• Imaging of the thoracic aorta and heart with a transthoracic echocardiography (TTE) and CT/cardiac magnetic resonance scan (CMR) within 2 years to be done before conception/IVF • ART or spontaneous conception is contraindicated if ascending aortic size index (ASI) of >2.5 cm/m² or an ascending ASI 2.0–2.5 cm/m² with associated risk factors for aortic dissection (AoD), which include bicuspid aortic valve, elongation of the transverse aorta, coarctation of the aorta and hypertension • Exercise testing before pregnancy reveals exercise induced hypertension, especially in women with coarctation

TABLE 4: Mode of delivery in TS as per ASI.		
ASI (cm/m²)	Preferred	Considered
<2	Vaginal delivery	
2–2.5	Vaginal with cut short second stage with epidural analgesia	Caesarean section
>2.5	Caesarean	Vaginal with cut short second stage with epidural analgesia

- Blood pressure control to be strict (<135/85 mm Hg) in all pregnant women with TS.
- During pregnancy prophylactic surgery is reasonable in case of a dilated aorta with rapid increase in diameter.

Mode of delivery in Turner syndrome with aortic dissection **(Table 4)**:
- In women with TS with a history of AoD, a cesarean section should be performed.

As the mutation of Turner syndrome are sporadic, so chances of second baby having TS or risk to offspring are negligible.

Risk to fetus:[14] Mothers with mosaic Turner syndrome (MTS) have inherent higher risk of transmission of total/partial X chromosome absence to the fetus and miscarriage rates because of which preimplantation genetic testing for aneuploidy (PGT-A) has an important role in improving reproductive potential by transferring euploid embryos. Although oocyte donation seems to be the best option in terms of cumulative live-birth rates.

Health surveillance for comorbidities throughout lifespan of Turner syndrome is enumerated in **Table 5**.

Klinefelter Syndrome (Sex Chromosome DSD)

Klinefelter syndrome (KS) affects only males. This syndrome is not inherited, as an addition of extra X chromosome and occurs during the formation of gametes in one of the affected parents. KS usually goes undiagnosed till adolescence or adulthood in most of the cases.

Prevalence and chromosomal abnormalities in Klinefelter's syndrome is depicted in **Flowchart 4**.

46,XY DSD (UNDERVIRILISED MALE)

Diagnosis and clinical presentation of Klinefelter syndrome at different age groups are depicted in **Flowchart 5**.

Karyotyping in Klinefelter syndrome is depicted in **Flowchart 6**.

Investigations and therapeutic approaches from infancy, childhood, and adolescence in KS.
- High attention to management of undescended testes as early as possible since preservation of testicular function is closely linked to descended testes.

TABLE 5: Health surveillance for comorbidities throughout life span of turner syndrome.[8]	
Audiometry	At diagnosis and 5 yearly
TSH, T4	At diagnosis and annually
HbA1c with or without fasting plasma glucose	10 years and then annually
Lipid profile	18 years and then annually
Dental/orthodontic evaluation	At diagnosis
Comprehensive ophthalmological examination	12 and 18 months of age or at the time of diagnosis
Scoliosis	Every 6 months during GH therapy/ otherwise annually until growth is completed
Serum 25-hydroxyvitamin D	9 and 11 years of age and every 2–3 years thereafter
DEXA scan	If HRT is discontinued
Transglutaminase antibodies	2–3 years of age at a frequency of every 2 years
LFT	10 years and then annually
Renal USG	At diagnosis

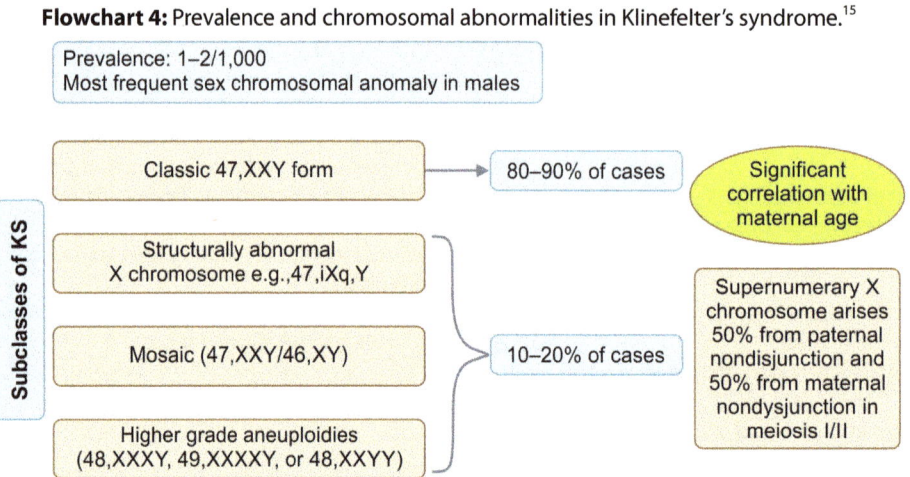

Flowchart 4: Prevalence and chromosomal abnormalities in Klinefelter's syndrome.[15]

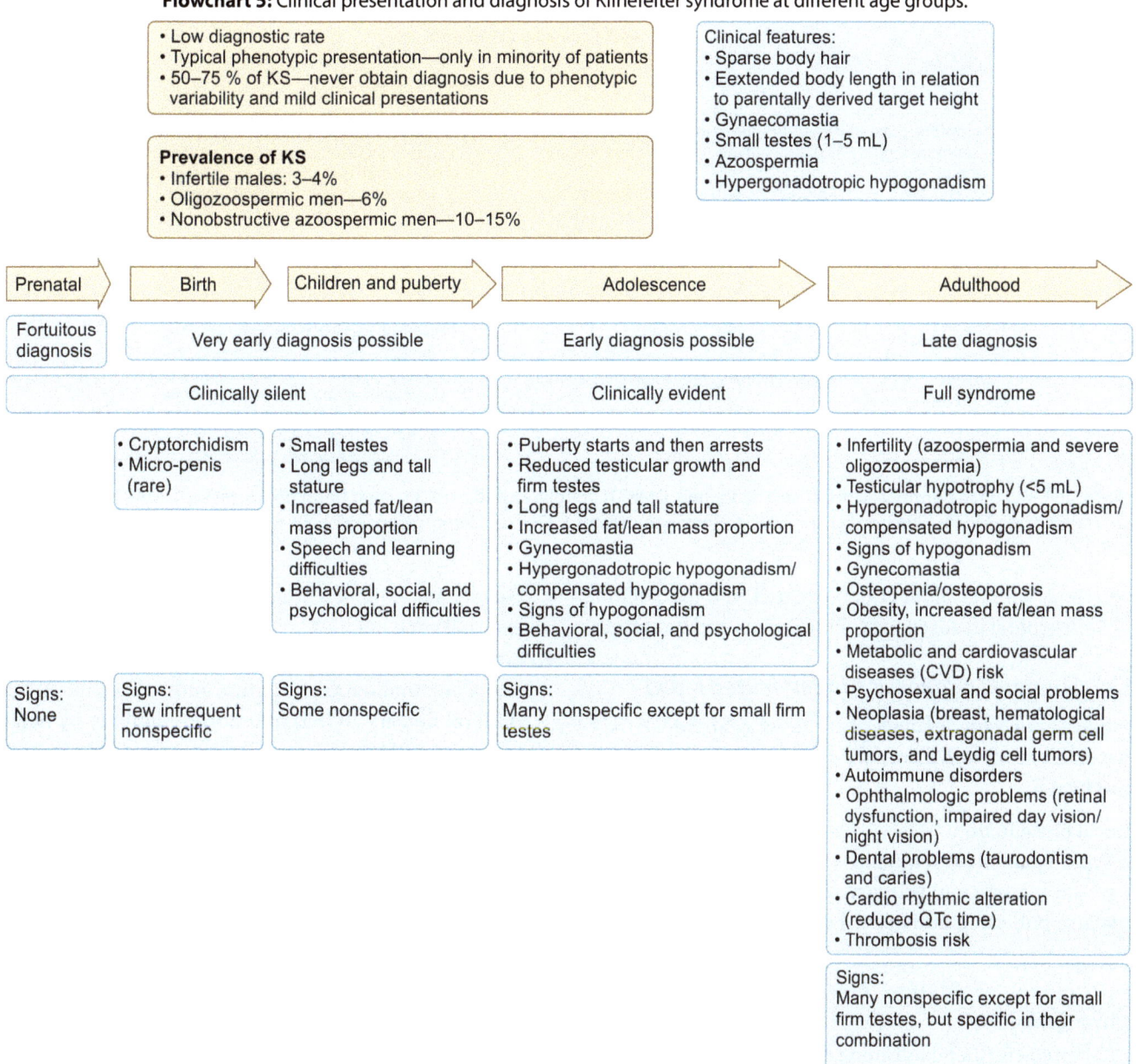

Flowchart 5: Clinical presentation and diagnosis of Klinefelter syndrome at different age groups.[15]

- Treated cryptorchidism does not reduce the chances for positive sperm retrieval in patients with KS.
- The postnatal surge of sex hormones during the so-called mini-puberty represents a diagnostic window in first 3 months of birth for evaluating the hypothalamic-pituitary-testicular axis in infancy and recognize poor testicular function and hypogonadism.
- Recommend speech therapist control and therapy, monitoring learning disabilities, social training and psychological support in pre-pubertal children with KS

Long-term surveillance in KS.[15]

Metabolic disorders, body composition, cardiovascular risk, and thrombosis.

Psychological and psychiatric conditions/gender incongruence.

Testosterone replacement therapy:[15]
- Assessment of fertility status is required before starting testosterone therapy.
- Theoretically, testosterone treatment may suppress any remaining spermatogenesis if the endogenous LH levels are low or may even maintain or improve spermatogenesis by increasing serum and intratesticular testosterone. In absence of robust evidence; the given recommendations from European Society of Endocrinology are to be followed.
  - Testosterone supplementation is prescribed in males with delayed puberty and/or hypogonadism with low-normal testosterone and high-normal serum LH concentrations to improve secondary sexual-features, libido, and bone-health.

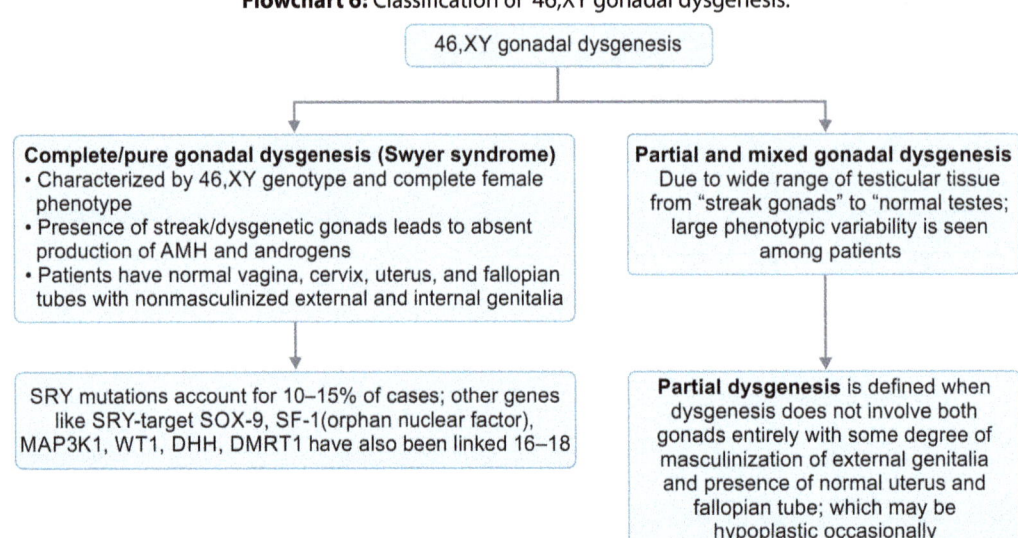

Flowchart 6: Classification of 46,XY gonadal dysgenesis.

(AMH: anti-Müllerian hormone; DHH: desert hedgehog; DMRT1: doublesex and mab-3 related transcription factor 1; MAP3K1: mitogen-activated protein kinase kinase kinase 1; SF-1: steroidogenic factor 1; SRY: sex determining region on Y; SOX-9: SRY-related HMG box 9)

- Boys with KS should not be treated with testosterone in general in absence of clinical signs and symptoms.

46,XY Gonadal Dysgenesis (Undervirilized Male)

Complete/pure gonadal dysgenesis (Swyer syndrome)[20-22]
Classification of 46,XY gonadal dysgenesis is depicted in **Flowchart 6**.

Clinical presentation:
- Typical patient presentation is after puberty with delayed sexual maturation, primary amenorrhea with normal/sparse pubic hair and normal breast development.

Investigations:
- Hormonal evaluation reveals hypergonadotropic hypogonadism
- Karyotype further confirming diagnosis.
- Chromosomal sex—46,XY; sex of rear/phenotypic sex—female

Management:
- Gonadectomy is indicated as soon as diagnosis is established due to high risk (20–30%) of germ cell tumors in occult testicular tissue.[23]
- Estrogen therapy to induce breast development followed by the progesterone (cyclic or combined) also for growth of uterus before planning in vitro fertilization (IVF).
- Fertility option—assisted reproduction by IVF using donor-oocytes.

Partial and mixed gonadal dysgenesis:
- Patients with mixed dysgenesis have both Müllerian and Wolffian structures with asymmetric virilization of external and internal genitalia depending on ipsilateral testicular tissue.[24]
- Gender assignment is done as per degree of virilization of external genitalia.
- Sex steroid replacement is given at puberty to complete sexual maturation, growth spurt, and attain optimal bone mineral density (BMD) monitored regularly by height, weight and BMD measurement by yearly DEXA scan.
- Gonadectomy is indicated in the cases who identify themselves as females.

Disorders of Androgen Synthesis

Steroidogenesis and its enzymes, as well as the deficiencies of the enzymes involved in the formation of androgens from universal precursor cholesterol, can manifest anywhere in the adrenal gland and in the testis. Genital ambiguity hence depends on the level of the stop in steroidogenesis pathway as depicted in **Flowchart 10**.[25]

Steroid 5-α-reductase deficiency (SRD5α-2):[25] Diagnosis and management of steroid 5-α-reductase deficiency (SRD5α2) are depicted in **Flowchart 7**.

17-α-hydroxylase deficiency/17,20-lyase:[26] CYP17A1 gene encodes for both above mentioned enzymes which are further required for cortisol, androgens and estrogens in both adrenals and gonads as depicted in **Flowchart 10**.
- Mutation in CYP17A1 gene results in cortisol and sex-steroid deficiency shunting the steroidogenic pathway towards mineralocorticoid synthesis (11-deoxy steroids) due to compensatory increase in adrenocorticotropic hormone (ACTH) levels.
- In this autosomal recessive disorder
  - *Affected males (46,XY):* Reared as females; may present at birth with ambiguous genitalia with absent

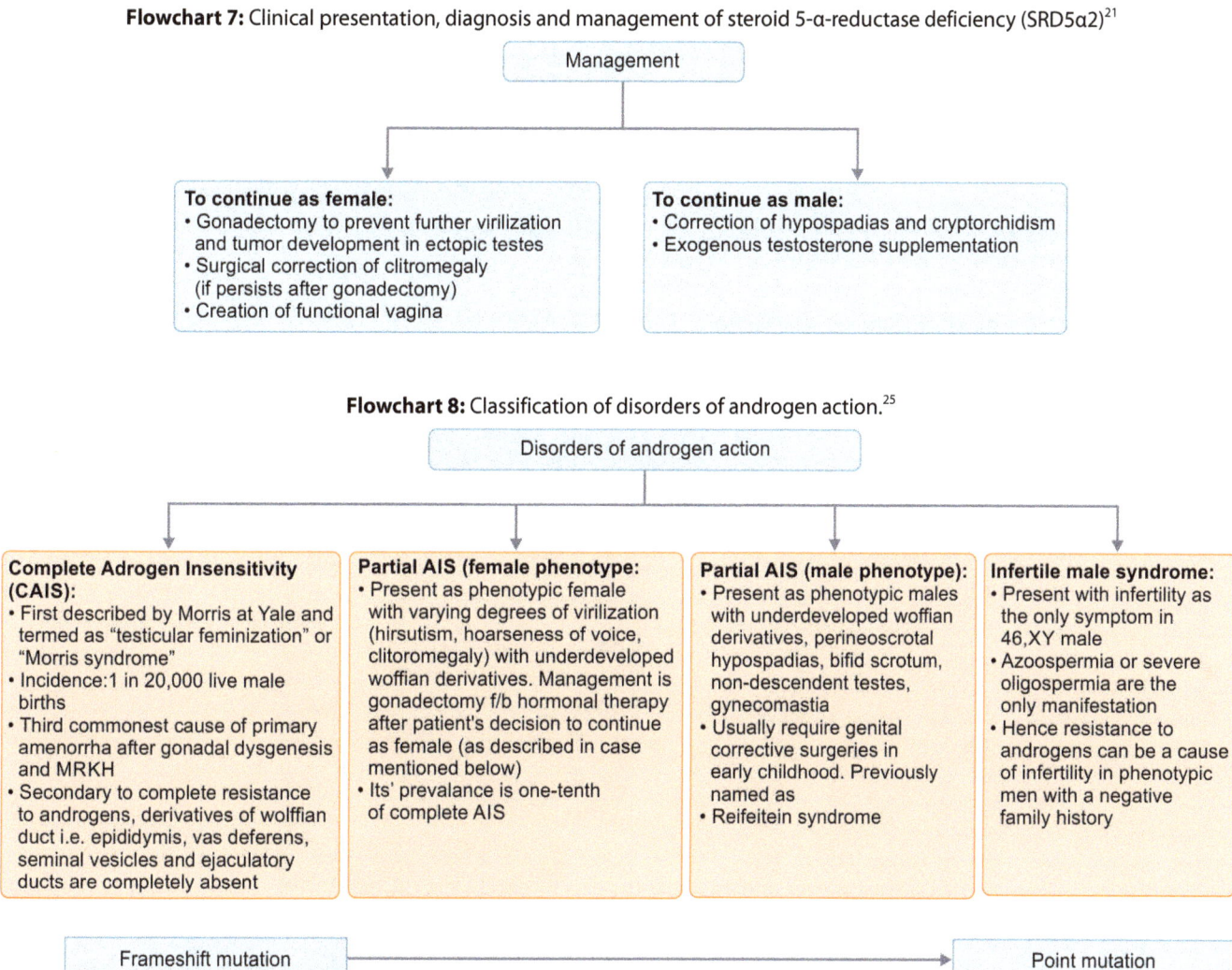

Flowchart 7: Clinical presentation, diagnosis and management of steroid 5-α-reductase deficiency (SRD5α2)[21]

Flowchart 8: Classification of disorders of androgen action.[25]

(AIS: androgen insensitivity syndrome; MRKH: Mayer–Rokitansky–Küster–Hauser; partial androgen insensitivity syndrome)

Müllerian structures and intra-abdominal testes or at puberty, they present with delayed puberty, primary amenorrhea, hypergonadotropic hypogonadism along with low-renin hypertension and hypokalemia (mineralocorticoid effect)

- *Affected genotypic females (46,XX):* Present in late adolescent with delayed puberty or primary amenorrhea.

- Diagnosis: It is made by decreased serum concentrations of 17-hydroxyprogesterone (17-OHP), cortisol, dehydroepiandrosterone (DHEA), dehydroepiandrosterone sulfate (DHEAS), androstenedione, testosterone, and estradiol and increased serum progesterone levels.

- *Management* requires physiologic levels of glucocorticoids along with estrogen therapy at the time of diagnosis.
  - Progesterone needs to be added with estrogen in 46,XX female having well-formed uterus.
  - 46,XY individuals who are reared as females—gonadectomy to be done at puberty followed by estrogen therapy.

Disorders of Androgen Action

Mutation in gene encoding for androgen receptor (AR) results in end-organ resistance to the action of both testosterone and DHT hormone; in the presence of normal gonads and biosynthesis.

AR gene is located on X chromosome (Xq12), thus exhibiting X-linked recessive pattern of inheritance, though 40% cases represent de-novo mutations with no family history.[27]

Creates diverse phenotypic spectrum as shown underneath ranging from unambiguous XY female to phenotypic XY male correlating with degree of gene mutation.

Classification of disorders of androgen action **(Flowchart 8)**.

Spectrum of presentation of androgen insensitivity syndrome (AIS) is depicted in **Flowchart 9**.

Flowchart 9: Presentation and management of CAIS.[25]

CAIS characterized by:
- Functional testicular tissue (in abdomen, inguinal canal, or labia majora)
- Absent Mullerian structures
- Short and blind vagina
- Normal female external genitalia
- Normal clitoris

Classic phenotype:
- Female with absent axillary and pubic hair with well-formed breast
- Female pattern distribution of body fat
- Usually presents at puberty with primary amenorrhea with inguinal hernia or labial masses at puberty

Diagnosis: guided by normal or moderately raised testosterone concentrations (normal for male range); raised LH levels, normal serum FSH levels
- 46,XY karyotype confirms the diagnosis

Management: estrogen therapy after gonadectomy is performed
- Creation of functional vagina through vaginal dilation and vaginoplasty
- Psychological support

Gonadectomy best delayed till puberty is completed (around 16–18 years): as endogenous hormones assist more smoothly in attaining puberty plus the risk of germ-cell tumour is low (5–10%)[25]

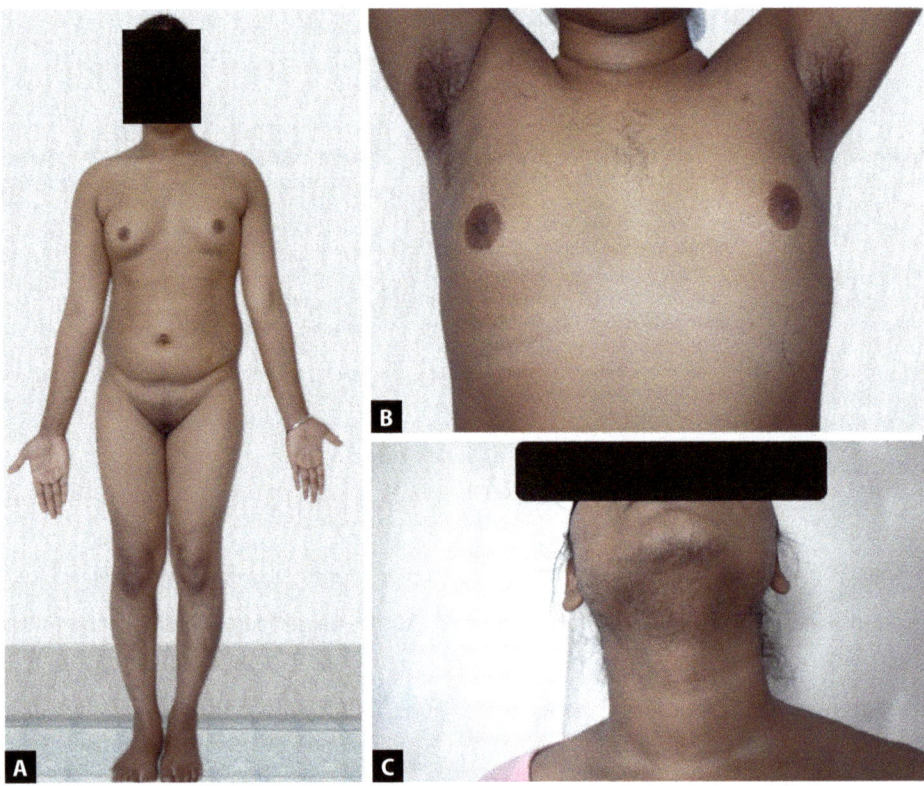

Figs. 3A to C: Partial AIS (female phenotype). (A) 16-year-old athlete reared as female with c/o primary amenorrhea. She had Tanner II breasts (B), excessive facial hair (C), Karyotype showed 46,XY confirming the diagnosis of Partial AIS (female phenotype).

Figures 3A to C and describes the clinical picture of a case of partial AIS who was reared as female and presented to us with primary amenorrhea, excessive hair growth, and clitromegaly.

Figure 4A to D describes the intraoperative findings of laparoscopic gonadectomy.

Figure 4 depicts clinical presentation in a case of complete AIS (CAIS) who presented only with primary amenorrhea, primary infertility, and blind vagina on examination. This patient also underwent gonadectomy.

Figure 11 depicts clinical presentation of a case of partial AIS who was reared as male and had undergone genital corrective surgery.

46,XX Disorder (Overvirilized Female)

46,XX ovotesticular DSD:
- Previously named as "true hermaphroditism"
- A rare combination of mixed ovarian and testicular tissue with bilateral ovotestes (20% cases) or an ovotestes and contralateral ovary or testes (50% cases).
- Majority of patients have 46,XX genotype; while one-third are mosaics and 7% of patients have 46,XY genotype.[30]
- Degree of internal genitalia corresponds with the ipsilateral gonad and external genitalia development depends on level of androgen production and exposure.
- Phenotypic females have hypoplastic uterus (though half patients menstruate at puberty), normal adnexa and vagina.

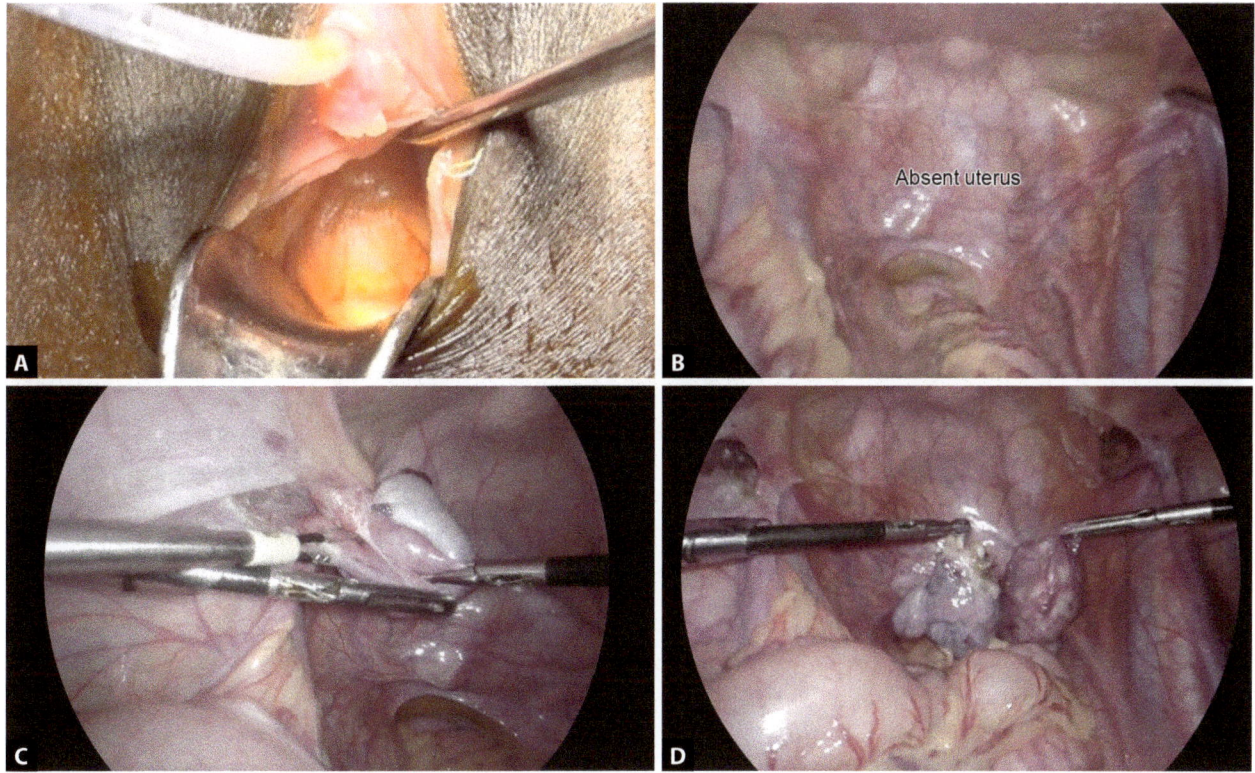

Figs. 4A to D: Complete AIS- (A) Normal female external genitalia and blind vagina; (B) Laparoscopic view showing absent uterus and bilateral gonads in the inguinal canal; (C) and (D)- steps of gonadectomy.

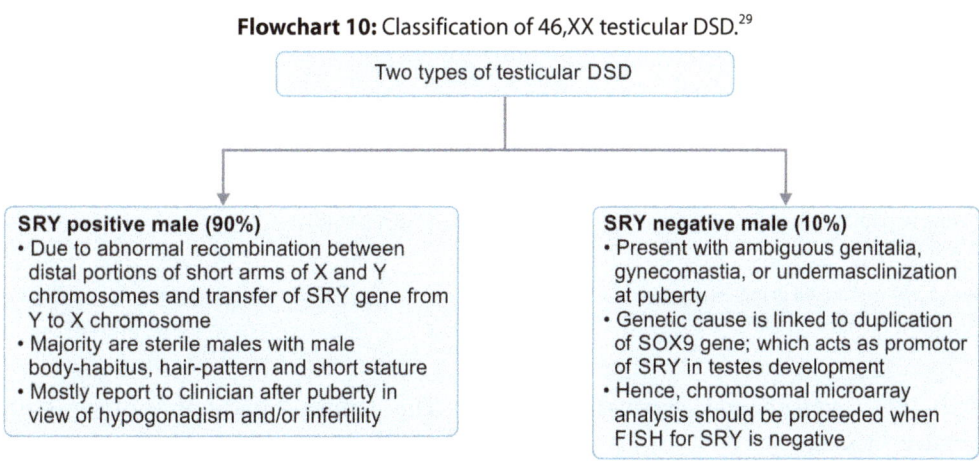

- Phenotypic males are more common secondary to sufficient virilization and three-fourths experience change in gender-assignment due to gynecomastia and menses at puberty.
- Ovotesticular DSD males have normal levels of serum FSH, LH, estradiol, T and DHT.
- Diagnosis is further enhanced by pelvic ultrasound, serum AMH, and FISH analysis for *SRY* gene.
- Management is guided by the sex of rearing.
- Ovotesticular DSD females have reported normal pregnancy till term.
- Ovotesticular DSD males are usually azoospemic; achieving fertility with the help of ART.

46,XX testicular DSD/46,XX male:
- A rare "sex reversal" syndrome where chromosomal sex (XX) does not correspond to gonadal sex (testes).
- Was first described by de la Chapelle in 1964.[31]
- Different from ovotesticular DSD in terms of phenotype being predominantly male with no genital ambiguity; with hypergonadotropic hypogonadism depicted by raised serum levels of FSH and LH, decreased T and DHT concentrations.
- No risk of developing gonadoblastoma as there is complete absence of Y chromosome.

Classification of 46,XX testicular DSD is depicted in **Flowchart 10**.

Disorders of Sexual Development

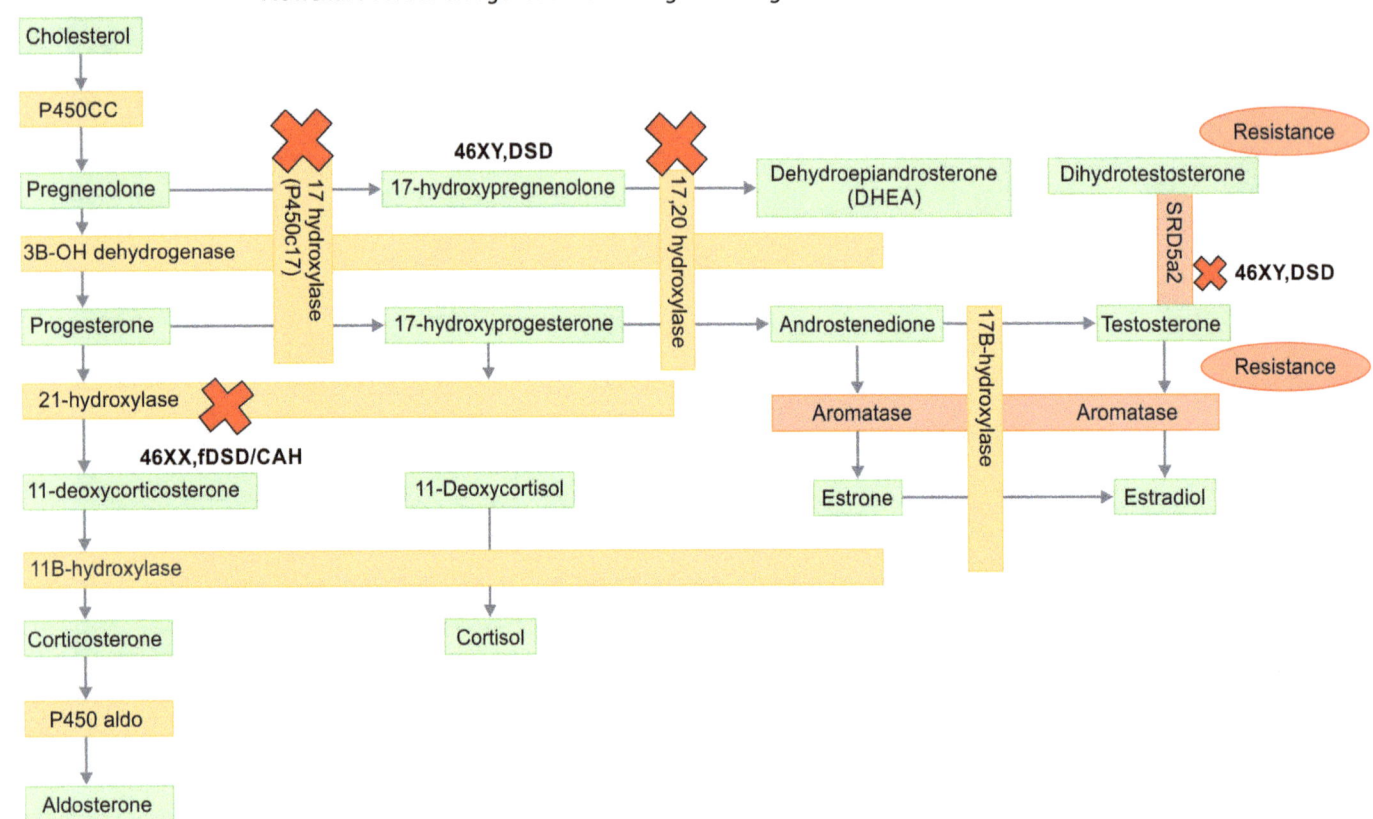

Flowchart 11: Steroidogenesis in adrenal gland and gonads and different levels of blocks.

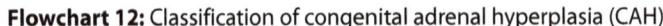

Flowchart 12: Classification of congenital adrenal hyperplasia (CAH).

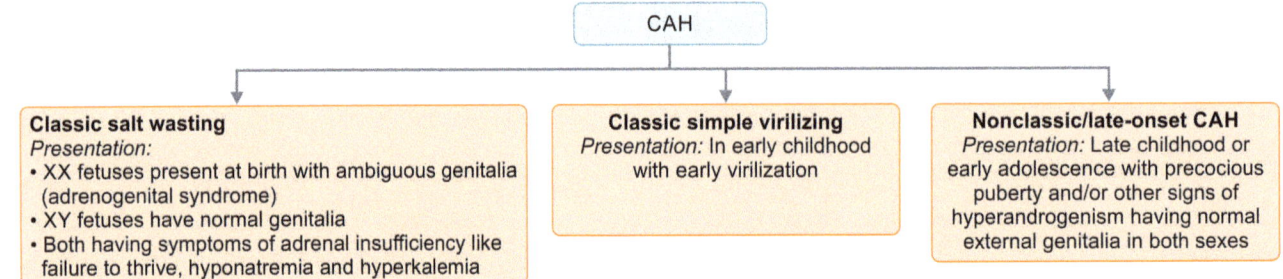

Androgen excess DSD—congenital adrenal hyperplasia:
- Autosomal recessive disorder
- Virilizing congenital adrenal hyperplasia (CAH) can manifest in both 46,XX and 46,XY genotypes.
- Prevalence varies with ethnicity being more common among Mediterranean, Eastern European Jewish, and Hispanics.
- High abnormal levels of intrauterine androgens due to enzyme defects in adrenal steroidogenesis result in varying degrees of clitoral enlargement, "scrotalization" of labia, urogenital sinus, and phallic urethra along with well-formed Müllerian structures.
- The most common cause of CAH and neonatal ambiguity is deficiency of 21-hydroxylase (CYP21 A2) and rest due to 11B-hydroxylase and 3B-HSD.
  Steroidogenesis in adrenal gland and gonads and different levels of blocks (**Flowchart 11**).
- The common pathophysiology is decreased cortisol production with compensatory increase in ACTH hormone leading to adrenal hyperplasia and raised levels of steroid hormones proximal to enzyme block seeking alternative metabolic pathway raising androgen production.

Classification of congenital adrenal hyperplasia (CAH) is depicted in **Flowchart 12**.

Clinical presentation, diagnosis, and management of classic and nonclassic CAH are depicted in **Flowchart 13**.

Approach to a Patient with DSD (Flowchart 14)

History of the individual:
- Age of the patient
- Chief complaint (ambiguous genitalia may or may not be the presenting or only complaint in DSD)
- Has menarche set or not

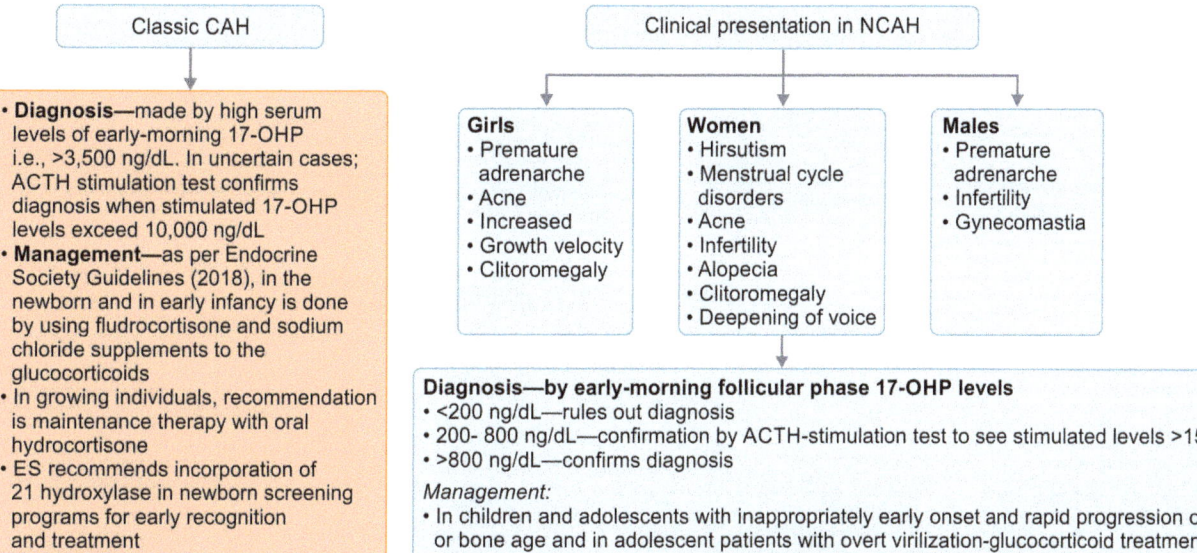

Flowchart 13: Clinical presentation, diagnosis and management of classic and nonclassic CAH.

- If yes—age of menarche, spontaneous or hormone induced, pattern of bleeding, and need to take regular hormonal (combined or progesterone pills)
- Marital status
- Psychosexual orientation of the individual; sexual arousal history
- What are the choices of individual pertaining to psychosexual performances?

Family and past history:
- Was the mother exposed to any known teratogens, environmental disrupting agents or medications?
- Are there other family members with similar/atypical presentation?
- Enquiring about consanguinity is helpful when autosomal-recessive disorder is suspected.
- What was the sex assigned at birth?
- Is there any corrective surgery or medical/hormonal treatment taken in past?

General physical examination:
- Vital signs—blood pressure and pulse rate
- Anthropometric parameters [height, weight, weight/height ratio, and body mass index (BMI)]
- Examination of secondary sexual characteristics
  - Breast examination and Tanner staging
  - Presence/absence of axillary hair
  - Pubic hair examination and Tanner staging
  - Detailed examination of external genitalia (Prader's classification for various degree of virilization in females).[3]
- Per abdomen examination—for any abnormal mass palpation, inguinal masses (testis/gonads in the inguinal canal), and cough impulse.

INDICATION OF KARYOTYPE TESTING (FLOWCHART 15)

- Newborn with atypical/ambiguous genitalia
- Adult presenting with primary amenorrhea and hormonal analysis revealing hypergonadotropic hypogonadism
- Signs of virilization (hirsutism, deepening of voice, and clitoromegaly) and masculinization
- Abnormal anthropometric examination parameters
- Inadequate development of secondary sexual characteristics (sparse pubic hair; poor breast development)
- Clinical findings not fitting into a single pathology (>1 pathology may be present rarely)
- Family history of primary amenorrhea or DSD.

WHICH GENETIC TESTING?

- First-line genetic tests performed is either karyotyping with G-banding technique and/or FISH analysis for X and Y probe; but since many genes involved in gonadal development have a dosage-effect (with loss-of-function or gain-of-function) DSD may be caused by copy-number variations (CNV) that goes undetected by conventional karyotype and FISH analysis.
- Two innovative molecular tests; chromosomal microarray analysis with array comparative genomic hybridization (aCGH) and Next-generation sequencing including whole genome sequencing (WGS) and whole exome sequencing (WES) have emerged as novel future diagnostic tools.

GENITAL SURGERIES

- *Early in 1950s' genital surgery was done to create an anatomy matching with the sex of rearing and traditional decision makers were the family and clinician.*

Disorders of Sexual Development

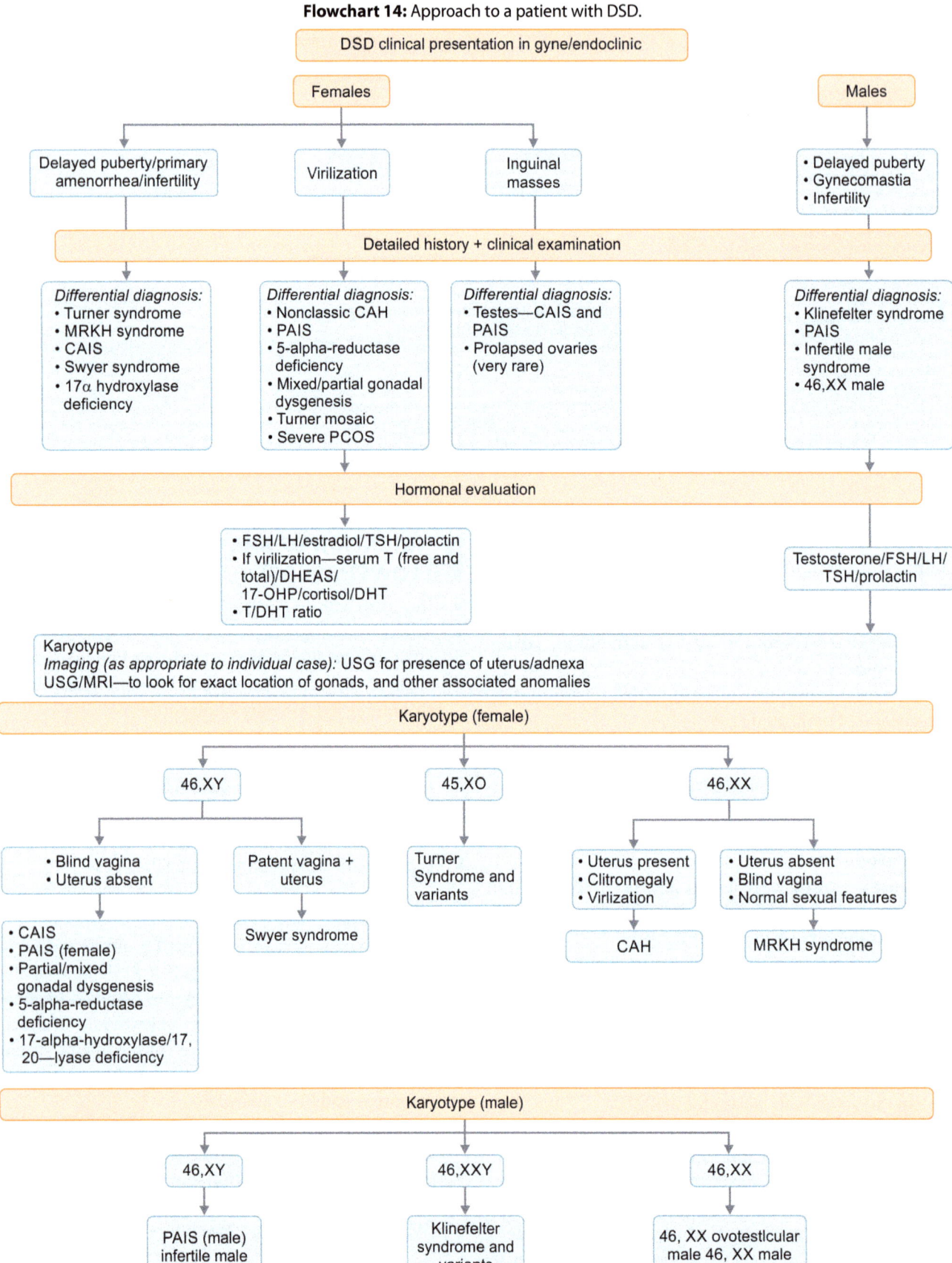

Flowchart 14: Approach to a patient with DSD.

(AMH: anti-Müllerian hormone; CAH: congenital adrenal hyperplasia; CAIS: complete androgen insensitivity syndrome; DHEAS: dehydroepiandrosterone sulfate; DHT: dihydrotestosterone; DSD: differences of sex development; FSH: follicle-stimulating hormone; LH: luteinizing hormone; MRKH: Mayer-Rokitansky-Küster-Hauser syndrome; PAIS: partial androgen insensitivity syndrome; PCOS: polycystic ovary syndrome; OHP: hydroxyprogesterone)

Flowchart 15: Indications of Karyotyping in Klinefelter syndrome.

Prenatal → Birth → Children and puberty → Adolescence → Adulthood

- Indicated if elder sibling/father/family history of KS
- Noninvasive prenatal testing (NIPT)—not a diagnostic test, requires confirmation; high false positive results
- Amniocentesis (Chorionic villus sampling (CVS)
- Genetic counseling of parents

- Conventional karyotyping indicated in suspicious cases especially in bilateral cryptorchidism after 1 year of life
- Karyotype recommended in men with nonobstructive azoospermia or (severe) oligozoospermia (total sperm count $<10 \times 10^6$/ejaculate or sperm concentration $<5 \times 10^6$/mL
- Karyotype recommended in men with primary hypogonadism (low serum levels of testosterone) and elevated serum levels of gonadotropins [LH and follicle-stimulating hormone (FSH)] combined with small testicular volumes (<5 mL per testis)

TABLE 6: Hormonal parameters in XY DSD.

Hormonal parameters	Swyer's syndrome	CAIS	5 alpha reductase deficiency	PAIS
FSH	↑	Normal	Normal	Normal
LH	↑	Normal to high	Normal	Normal to high
Testosterone (T)	↓	Normal to high	Normal	Normal to high
Dihydrotestosterone (DHT)	↓	NA	Low to undetectable	Normal
T/DHT ratio	NA	NA	↑	Normal

- *2005 consensus statement changed the insight and suggested to avoid early surgeries in infancy.*[1]
- Only surgeons with expertise in the surgery of DSD should undertake these procedures.
- Surgery should be considered in cases of severe virilization (Prader III, IV, and V) with emphasis to retain orgasmic function and erectile sensation rather than a cosmetic appearance.
- In females with gonadal dysgenesis and Y chromosome material; bilateral gonadectomy is to be performed soon after the diagnosis to prevent malignancy.
- Clitoroplasty is indicated in major degrees of clitoral hypertrophy. Usually deferred in minor degrees since it is associated with high rate of complications and injuries.
- Vaginal dilatation and vaginoplasty should not be undertaken until patient is psychologically mature, motivated and wants to initiate sexual activity.
- The testes in patients with CAIS and PAIS; raised as female, should be removed to prevent malignancy in adulthood.
- Patients with bilateral ovotestes are potentially fertile from functional ovarian tissue.[1] Separation of ovarian and testicular tissue can be technically difficult and should be undertaken in early life.

Hormonal parameters in XY DSD are enumerated in **Table 6**.

Management of DSD is summarized in **Table 7**.

Summary of neoplastic disorders in DSD is enumerated in **Table 11**.

CONCLUSION

DSD present as a wide spectrum of chromosomal and clinical presentations. Detailed conceptual understanding of different aspects (genetic sex, gonadal sex, phenotypic sex, sex of rearing and individual preference) are important before planning any medical or surgical intervention. Psychosexual orientation must not be ignored while counselling these individuals. Addressal of preferences of individual is prioritized than preferences of family members.

SUMMARY

Differences of sex development present as a wide spectrum of chromosomal and clinical presentations. Detailed conceptual understanding of different aspects (genetic sex, gonadal sex, phenotypic sex, sex of rearing, and individual preference) are important before planning any medical or surgical intervention. Psychosexual orientation must not be ignored while counseling these individuals. Addressal of preferences of individual is prioritized than preferences of family members.

TABLE 7: Summarized management of DSD.

Summary	Turner syndrome	Klinefelter syndrome	CAIS	PAIS with female phenotype	PAIS with male phenotype	NCCAH	Swyer's syndrome	5-α reductase deficiency – if identifies herself as female	5-α reductase deficiency – if identifies herself as male
Gender assignment at puberty	• Female at birth • Female at puberty	• Male at birth • Male at puberty	• Female at birth • Female at puberty	• Female at birth • Gender reassignment option given at puberty	• Male at birth • Male at puberty	• Female at birth • Female at puberty	• Female at birth • Female at puberty	• Female at birth • Female at puberty	• Female at birth • Male at puberty
Hormonal therapy	GH E + P therapy	Testosterone replacement therapy	Estrogen therapy after gonadectomy	Estrogen therapy after gonadectomy	Testosterone therapy – for SSC and spermatogenesis	Glucocorticoids-symptomatic and pregnancy	E + P therapy	Estrogen therapy after gonadectomy	Topical DHT cream on face and external genitalia
Gonadectomy	Only when Y material detected	NA	Gonadectomy at 16–18 years	Gonadectomy at diagnosis	Orchidopexy with genital reconstructive surgery	NA	At diagnosis	At diagnosis	Orchidopexy and hypospadias correction; gonads retained
Fertility options	OTC Oocyte cryopreservation IVF with self/donor oocyte	Sperm cryopreservation TESE	Surrogacy with donor oocyte/adoption	Surrogacy with donor oocyte/adoption	TESE Donor sperm IVF	Spontaneous fertility resumes	Donor oocyte IVF	Surrogacy with donor oocyte	TESE Donor sperm IVF

(GH: growth hormone; OTC: ovarian tissue cryopreservation; TESE: testicular sperm extraction; SSC: secondary sexual characteristics; NCCAH: non-classical congenital adrenal hyperplasia; IVF: in-vitro fertilization; DHT: Dihydrotestosterone)

REFERENCES

1. Hughes IA, Houk C, Ahmed SF, Lee PA, LWPES Consensus Group, ESPE Consensus Group. Consensus statement on management of intersex disorders. Arch Dis Child. 2006;91 (7):554-63.
2. ECPS_Syllabus_-_Index.pdf [Internet]. [cited 2022 Jul 22]. Available from: https://www.essm.org/wp-content/uploads/publications/textbooks/ECPS_Syllabus_-_Index.pdf
3. Pang SY, Wallace MA, Hofman L, Thuline HC, Dorche C, Lyon IC, et al. Worldwide experience in newborn screening for classical congenital adrenal hyperplasia due to 21-hydroxylase deficiency. Pediatrics. 1988;81 (6):866-74.
4. Problems of Fetal Endocrinology - the Gonadal and Hypophyseal Hormones – ScienceOpen [Internet]. [cited 2022 Jul 22]. Available from: https://www.scienceopen.com/document?vid=042cc5d3-472a-48e9-8ee5-a9b72cb6ac4d
5. Stochholm K, Juul S, Juel K, Naeraa RW, Gravholt CH. Prevalence, incidence, diagnostic delay, and mortality in Turner syndrome. J Clin Endocrinol Metab. 2006;91 (10):3897-902.
6. Rao E, Weiss B, Fukami M, Rump A, Niesler B, Mertz A, et al. Pseudoautosomal deletions encompassing a novel homeobox gene cause growth failure in idiopathic short stature and Turner syndrome. Nat Genet. 1997;16 (1):54-63.
7. Rappold G, Blum WF, Shavrikova EP, Crowe BJ, Roeth R, Quigley CA, et al. Genotypes and phenotypes in children with short stature: clinical indicators of SHOX haploinsufficiency. J Med Genet. 2007;44 (5):306-13.
8. Gravholt CH, Andersen NH, Conway GS, Dekkers OM, Geffner ME, Klein KO, et al. Clinical practice guidelines for the care of girls and women with Turner syndrome: proceedings from the 2016 Cincinnati International Turner Syndrome Meeting. Eur J Endocrinol. 2017;177 (3):G1-70.
9. Russell LM, Strike P, Browne CE, Jacobs PA. X chromosome loss and ageing. Cytogenet Genome Res. 2007;116 (3):181-5.
10. Hook EB. Exclusion of chromosomal mosaicism: tables of 90%, 95% and 99% confidence limits and comments on use. Am J Hum Genet. 1977;29(1):94-7.
11. Wiktor AE, Van Dyke DL. Detection of low level sex chromosome mosaicism in Ullrich-Turner syndrome patients. Am J Med Genet A. 2005;138A(3):259-61.
12. Gault EJ, Perry RJ, Cole TJ, Casey S, Paterson WF, Hindmarsh PC, et al. Effect of oxandrolone and timing of pubertal induction on final height in Turner's syndrome: randomised, double blind, placebo controlled trial. BMJ. 2011;342:d1980.
13. Bryman I, Sylvén L, Berntorp K, Innala E, Bergström I, Hanson C, et al. Pregnancy rate and outcome in Swedish women with Turner syndrome. Fertil Steril. 2011;95(8):2507-10.
14. Giles J, Meseguer M, Mercader A, Rubio C, Alegre L, Vidal C, et al. Preimplantation genetic testing for aneuploidy in patients with partial X monosomy using their own oocytes: is this a suitable indication? Fertil Steril. 2020;114(2):346-53.
15. Zitzmann M, Aksglaede L, Corona G, Isidori AM, Juul A, T'Sjoen G, et al. European academy of andrology guidelines on Klinefelter Syndrome Endorsing Organization: European Society of Endocrinology. Andrology. 2021;9(1):145-67.
16. Bogani D, Siggers P, Brixey R, Warr N, Beddow S, Edwards J, et al. Loss of mitogen-activated protein kinase kinase kinase 4 (MAP3K4) reveals a requirement for MAPK signalling in mouse sex determination. PLoS Biol. 2009;7(9):e1000196.
17. McElreavy K, Vilain E, Abbas N, Costa JM, Souleyreau N, Kucheria K, et al. XY sex reversal associated with a deletion 5' to the SRY 'HMG box' in the testis-determining region. Proc Natl Acad Sci U S A. 1992;89(22):11016-20
18. Assumpção JG, Benedetti CE, Maciel-Guerra AT, Guerra G, Baptista MTM, Scolfaro MR, et al. Novel mutations affecting SRY DNA-binding activity: the HMG box N65H associated with 46,XY pure gonadal dysgenesis and the familial non-HMG box R30I associated with variable phenotypes. J Mol Med Berl Ger. 2002;80(12):782-90.
19. Cools M, Stoop H, Kersemaekers AMF, Drop SLS, Wolffenbuttel KP, Bourguignon JP, et al. Gonadoblastoma arising in undifferentiated gonadal tissue within dysgenetic gonads. J Clin Endocrinol Metab. 2006;91(6):2404-13.
20. Migeon CJ, Wisniewski AB. Human sex differentiation and its abnormalities. Best Pract Res Clin Obstet Gynaecol. 2003;17(1):1-18.
21. Peterson RE, Imperato-McGinley J, Gautier T, Sturla E. Male pseudohermaphroditism due to steroid 5-alpha-reductase deficiency. Am J Med. 1977;62(2):170-91.
22. New MI. Male pseudohermaphroditism due to 17α-hydroxylase deficiency. J Clin Invest. 1970;49(10):1930-41.
23. Hiort O, Sinnecker GH, Holterhus PM, Nitsche EM, Kruse K. Inherited and de novo androgen receptor gene mutations: investigation of single-case families. J Pediatr. 1998;132(6):939-43.
24. Hughes IA, Davies JD, Bunch TI, Pasterski V, Mastroyannopoulou K, MacDougall J. Androgen insensitivity syndrome. The Lancet. 2012;380(9851):1419-28.
25. Lumbroso S, Paris F, Sultan C, Jeandel C, Terouanne B, Belon C, et al. Disorders of Androgen Action. Semin Reprod Med. 2002;20(3):217-28.
26. Nordenström A, Falhammar H. MANAGEMENT OF ENDOCRINE DISEASE: Diagnosis and management of the patient with non-classic CAH due to 21-hydroxylase deficiency. Eur J Endocrinol. 2019 Mar;180(3):R127-R145. doi: 10.1530/EJE-18-0712. PMID: 30566904
27. Krob G, Braun A, Kuhnle U. True hermaphroditism: geographical distribution, clinical findings, chromosomes and gonadal histology. Eur J Pediatr. 1994;153(1):2-10.
28. Queipo G, Zenteno JC, Peña R, Nieto K, Radillo A, Dorantes LM, et al. Molecular analysis in true hermaphroditism: demonstration of low-level hidden mosaicism for Y-derived sequences in 46,XX cases. Hum Genet. 2002;111(3):278-83.
29. Dupuy O, Palou M, Mayaudon H, Sarret D, Bordier L, Garcin JM, et al. [De La Chapelle syndrome]. Presse Medicale Paris Fr 1983. 2001;30(8):369-72.

CHAPTER 6

Thyroid Disorders and Fertility

Shikha Sardana

INTRODUCTION

Thyroid disorders are one of the most common endocrine disorders. *In the reproductive age group women, the prevalence of thyroid disorders is between 5 and 7% for subclinical hypothyroidism (SCH), 2 and 4.5% for overt hypothyroidism (OH), and 0.5 and 1% for hyperthyroidism.*[1]

HYPOTHYROIDISM AND FEMALE INFERTILITY

Hypothyroidism can be easily identified by evaluating hormonal levels. A slightly elevated thyroid-stimulating hormone (TSH) level with normal free thyroxine (FT4) and free triiodothyronine (FT3) levels indicates SCH whereas high TSH level along with low FT4 and FT3 levels indicates OH.

Thyroid dysfunction affects ovulation and fertility through direct and indirect interactions with the hypothalamic-pituitary-ovarian axis and the reproductive organs **(Table 1)**.

TABLE 1: Direct and indirect effects of hypothyroidism on reproductive system.

Direct effects	Indirect effects

Via thyroid hormone receptors: Thyroid hormone receptors are present along the reproductive system and *contribute an important role in the ovarian function regulation*	*Via hormonal changes*[2]:
	• Prolactin and gonadotropin-releasing hormone levels
	  In hypothyroidism:
	  – Prolactin levels ↑
	  – Pulsatile secretion of gonadotropin-releasing hormone ↓
	  This can cause ovulatory dysfunction and corpus luteum insufficiency resulting in low progesterone production.
	• Serum testosterone and estradiol levels
	  In hypothyroidism:
	  – Peripheral aromatization ↑
	  – Metabolic clearance ↓
	  – Sex hormone-binding globulin (SHBG) ↓
	  All these result in:
	• Serum testosterone (total) and estradiol levels ↓
	• The unbound fractions of serum testosterone and estradiol ↑

THYROID AUTOIMMUNITY AND FERTILITY

Thyroid autoimmunity (TAI) is the most common autoimmune disorder in women of reproductive age. *The prevalence varies in different ethnic backgrounds but typically it is around 10%.*[3] Thyroid peroxidase antibodies (TPOAb) are elevated in TAI and this can lead to higher TSH concentrations. *TAI is one of the main causes of SCH.*

Thyroid autoimmunity is more common in subgroups of women with idiopathic infertility, polycystic ovarian syndrome (PCOS), diminished ovarian reserve (DOI), and premature ovarian insufficiency (POI). The connecting mechanisms between TAI and idiopathic infertility remain speculative till date. Various proposed theories are:

- Thyroid hormone-dependent effects might disturb fertility as TAI predisposes to hypothyroidism, especially during pregnancy.[4] However, commencing levothyroxine treatment before pregnancy has not shown any benefits in euthyroid women with TAI facing infertility.[5,6]
- TAI might reflect a general immune dysfunction that can affect embryo implantation.
- A recent study delineated that endometrium and placenta express thyroid peroxidase (TPO) at gene and protein levels. This might explain why infertility and miscarriages are more frequent in patients with TAI.[7]

IMPACT OF OVARIAN STIMULATION ON THYROID FUNCTION

During the assisted reproductive technology (ART) procedure, ovaries are stimulated in order to collect an optimal number of oocytes. Ovarian stimulation induces a rapid and supraphysiologic increase of serum estradiol. Estradiol rise results in an increase in thyroxine-binding globulin (TBG) levels and ultimately a decrease in free thyroid hormone levels.

Subsequent to ovarian stimulation, patients with TAI are more prone to develop elevated TSH and diminished FT4 levels with respect to patients without TAI **(Fig. 1)**.[8] This is attributable to impaired thyroid function reserve in TAI.

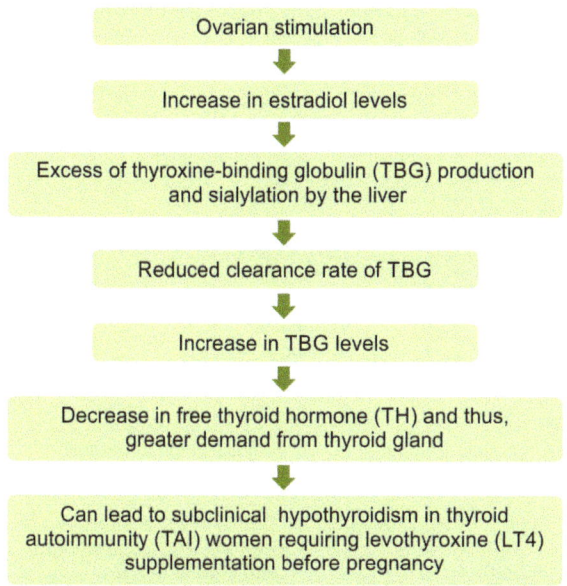

Fig. 1: Effect of ovarian stimulation on women with thyroid autoimmunity.

A similar negative effect of ovarian stimulation on thyroid function is observed in hypothyroid women. This effect seems to last till 3 months after ovarian stimulation. However, in a euthyroid state and in absence of TAI, the net impact of ovarian stimulation on thyroid function is considered insignificant.

Considering the negative effect of ovarian stimulation on thyroid function, *thyroid hormones should be serially evaluated after ovarian stimulation in women with hypothyroidism or TAI*. This will help prevent adverse pregnancy outcomes related to poorly controlled or unrecognized maternal hypothyroidism. The subsequent assessment of thyroid function should start from 6 weeks after commencing ovarian stimulation or 3 weeks after ovulation induction.[2]

WORK-UP AND MANAGEMENT OF THYROID DISORDERS IN INFERTILE COUPLES (FLOWCHART 1)

All women presenting with infertility should be systematically screened for serum TSH and TPOAb.[2] **Flowchart 1** depicts the workflow for diagnosing and managing thyroid disorders in infertile couples starting ART.

Impaired fertilization rates and embryo quality are reported in women with TSH >4.0 mIU/L and this may be improved with levothyroxine treatment.[9,10] In a meta-analysis, levothyroxine treatment improved clinical pregnancy outcomes of ART cycles in women with TSH levels >4.0 mIU/L.[11] Thus in overt thyroid dysfunction (when TSH values are >4.0 mIU/L or upper limit reference range), levothyroxine treatment should be started promptly. The treatment should be started independent of the presence of TAI and the target is to maintain serum TSH levels <2.5 mIU/L.

Likewise, hypothyroid women on levothyroxine treatment before ART should have a serum TSH level of <2.5 mIU/L. They should adapt the required dosage of levothyroxine at least 4 weeks prior to ovarian stimulation.

In women with TSH levels between 2.5 and 4 mIU/L and TAI, treatment decisions should be individualized. Other causes of female infertility, history of previous unsuccessful ART treatments, or previous pregnancy loss should be taken into consideration.[2]

In a recent meta-analysis investigating the impact of TAI on in vitro fertilization/intracytoplasmic sperm injection (IVF/ICSI) outcomes, live birth rates were not influenced in TAI women who were euthyroid.[12]

HYPERTHYROIDISM AND FEMALE INFERTILITY

The extent to which hyperthyroidism affects fertility is not well known as there is limited data in the literature. However, increased levels of sex hormone-binding globulin (SHBG) and estradiol (E2) have been identified in women with thyrotoxicosis compared to euthyroid women. Hyperthyroidism can also lead to menstrual irregularities.[7] Further, increased risks of maternal and fetal complications have been identified in women with hyperthyroidism.[2] *Thus for infertile women with hyperthyroidism, euthyroidism should be restored before ART treatment (Flowchart 1).*

THYROID DISORDERS AND MALE INFERTILITY

In males of infertile couples, the prevalence of thyroid disorders has been reported to be 7.4% for SCH and 3.7% for subclinical hyperthyroidism.[13]

Sperm morphology and motility gets disturbed in cases of prolonged OH and hyperthyroidism in adults. This adverse effect of thyroid disorders on male fertility comes through the influence of thyroid hormones on Sertoli cell maturation, Leydig cell differentiation, and steroidogenesis in fetal, early neonatal, and adult life.[14]

Additionally, erectile function seems to be dependent on thyroid hormone as hypothyroidism is associated with delayed ejaculation and hyperthyroidism is associated with premature ejaculation.

Thus, men with ejaculatory and erectile dysfunction, and/or altered semen parameters should be screened for thyroid dysfunction (TSH). However, it is not advisable to screen all the males of infertile couples for thyroid dysfunction.[2] In case of thyroid disorder, ART treatment (IVF/ICSI) should not be deferred if sperm parameters are not severely affected.[2]

Flowchart 1: Work-up and management algorithm for thyroid disorders in women of infertile couples starting an ART procedure.

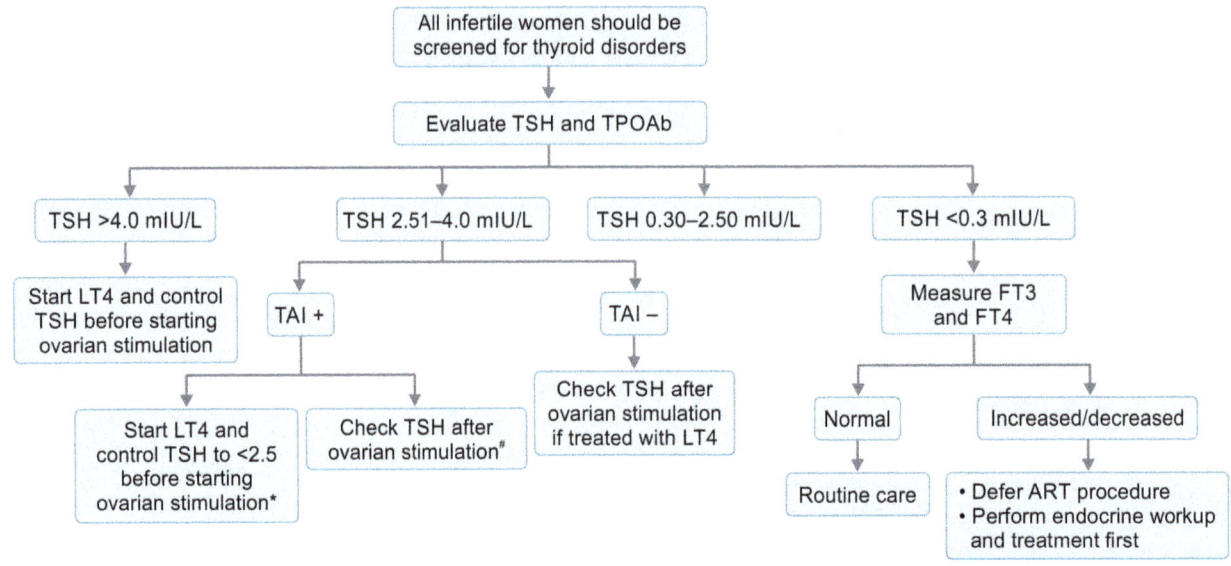

*Treatment decisions should be individualized. Other causes of female infertility, history of previous unsuccessful ART treatments, or previous pregnancy loss should be taken into account.[2]
#In case of pregnancy, 6 weeks after commencing ovarian stimulation or 3 weeks following ovulation induction.
(ART: assisted reproductive technology; FT3: free triiodothyronine; FT4: free thyroxine; LT4: levothyroxine; mIU/L: milli-international units per liter; TAI: thyroid autoimmunity; TPOAb: thyroid peroxidase antibodies)

Key Learning Points

- Thyroid dysfunction and TAI have often been associated with infertility and poor reproductive outcomes.
- In overt thyroid dysfunction (when TSH values are >4.0 mIU/L or upper limit reference range), levothyroxine treatment should be started promptly. The treatment should be started independent of the presence of TAI and the target is to maintain serum TSH levels <2.5 mIU/L.
- Women with hypothyroidism treated with levothyroxine prior to ART should have a serum TSH level <2.5 mIU/L.
- In women with TSH levels between 2.5 and 4 mIU/L and TAI, treatment decision should be individualized. Other causes of female infertility, history of previous unsuccessful ART treatments, or previous pregnancy loss should be taken into consideration.[2]
- Ovarian stimulation in ART treatment leads to high estradiol levels, which may lead to a decrease in free thyroid hormones and thus, increased demand on thyroid gland in women with TAI or hypothyroidism. Thus, serial evaluation of thyroid hormones should be performed in such women undergoing ovarian stimulation.
- Screening for thyroid dysfunction (TSH) in males of infertile couples should be limited to male subsets with ejaculatory and erectile dysfunction and/or altered semen parameters.[2]

REFERENCES

1. Valdes S, Maldonado-Araque C, Lago Sampedro A, Lillo JA, Garcia-Fuentes E, Perez-Valero V, et al. Population-based national prevalence of thyroid dysfunction in Spain and associated factors: Diabetes study. Thyroid. 2017;27(2):156-66.
2. Poppe K, Bisschop P, Fugazzola L, Minziori G, Unuane D, Weghofer A. 2021 European Thyroid Association Guideline on Thyroid Disorders prior to and during Assisted Reproduction. Eur Thyroid J. 2021;9(6):281-95.
3. Hollowell JG, Staehling NW, Flanders WD, Hannon WH, Gunter EW, Spencer CA, et al. Serum TSH, T(4), and thyroid antibodies in the United States population (1988 to 1994): National Health and Nutrition Examination Survey (NHANES III). J Clin Endocrinol Metab. 2002;87(2):489-99.
4. Krassas GE, Poppe K, Glinoer D. Thyroid function and human reproductive health. Endocr Rev. 2010;31(5):702-55.
5. Wang H, Gao H, Chi H, Zeng L, Xiao W, Wang Y, et al. Effect of levothyroxine on miscarriage among women with normal thyroid function and thyroid autoimmunity undergoing in vitro fertilization and embryo transfer: a randomized clinical trial. JAMA. 2017;318(22):2190-8.
6. Dhillon-Smith RK, Middleton LJ, Sunner KK, Cheed V, Baker K, Farrell-Carver S, et al. Levothyroxine in women with thyroid peroxidase antibodies before conception. N Engl J Med. 2019;380(14):1316-25.
7. Rahnama R, Mahmoudi AR, Kazemnejad S, Salehi M, Ghahiri A, Soltanghoraee H, et al. Thyroid peroxidase in human endometrium and placenta: a potential target for anti-TPO antibodies. Clin Exp Med. 2021;21(1):79-88.
8. Poppe K, Glinoer D, Tournaye H, Schiettecatte J, Devroey P, van Steirteghem A, et al. Impact of ovarian hyperstimulation on thyroid function in women with and without thyroid autoimmunity. J Clin Endocrinol Metab. 2004;89(8):3808-12.
9. Velkeniers B, Van Meerhaeghe A, Poppe K, Unuane D, Tournaye H, Haentjens P. Levothyroxine treatment and pregnancy outcome in women with SCH undergoing assisted reproduction technologies: systematic review and meta-analysis of RCTs. Hum Reprod Update. 2013;19(3):251-8.
10. Kim CH, Ahn JW, Kang SP, Kim SH, Chae HD, Kang BM. Effect of levothyroxine treatment on in vitro fertilization and pregnancy outcome in infertile women with subclinical hypothyroidism

undergoing in vitro fertilization/intracytoplasmic sperm injection. Fertil Steril. 2011;95(5):1650-4.
11. Velkeniers B, Van Meerhaeghe A, Poppe K, Unuane D, Tournaye H, Haentjens P. Levothyroxine treatment and pregnancy outcome in women with SCH undergoing assisted reproduction technologies: systematic review and meta-analysis of RCTs. Hum Reprod Update. 2013;19(3):251-8.
12. Busnelli A, Paffoni A, Fedele L, Somigliana E. The impact of thyroid autoimmunity on IVF/ ICSI outcome: a systematic review and meta-analysis. Hum Reprod Update. 2016; 22(6):775-90.
13. Lotti F, Maseroli E, Fralassi N, Degl'Innocenti S, Boni L, Baldi E, et al. Is thyroid hormones evaluation of clinical value in the work-up of males of infertile couples? Hum Reprod. 2016;31(3):518-29.
14. Mendis-Handagama SM, Ariyaratne HB. Effects of thyroid hormones on Leydig cells in the postnatal testis. Histol Histopathol. 2004;19(3):985-97.

CHAPTER 7

Hyperprolactinemia and Infertility: An Algorithm-based Approach

Sonal Agarwal, Rutvij Dalal

INTRODUCTION

- Hyperprolactinemia (HPRL) is a condition of elevated prolactin (PRL) levels in blood above 10–28 ng/mL in women and 5–10 ng/mL in men.
- It can be physiological, pathological, or idiopathic in origin.[1]
- Prevalence is <1% of the general population to 17% in women with reproductive disorders.
- 30% of infertile women suffer from HPRL.
- It is a cause of secondary amenorrhea in 30% of women.
- 20% of women suffer from galactorrhea with a normal basal PRL level during their lifetime.[2]

REGULATION OF PROLACTIN SECRETION

Unlike other tropic hormones secreted by the anterior pituitary gland, PRL secretion is controlled primarily by inhibition from the hypothalamus and there is no negative feedback from the periphery **(Fig. 1)**.

Dual Hypothalamic Regulation

- *PRL releasing factors:* Thyrotropin-releasing hormone and vasoactive intestinal peptide
- *Prolactin inhibitory factors (PIFs):* Dopamine (DA) is primary.
- PIF activity is dominant—PRL is under tonic inhibition by the hypothalamus. If the stalk is cut, PRL levels rise whereas other hormone levels fall.[3]
  - PIF is synthesized in the hypothalamic neurons, particularly in the dorsal portion of arcuate nucleus (ARC) and inferior portion of ventromedial nucleus, transported via axonal neurons to median eminence (TI pathway). It binds to D2 receptors on lactotrophs and inhibits PRL secretion.
  - Prolactin via a short loop has a negative feedback on its own secretion.[4]
  - Gonadotropin-releasing hormone (GnRH)-associated peptide also has inhibitory influence on PRL secretion.

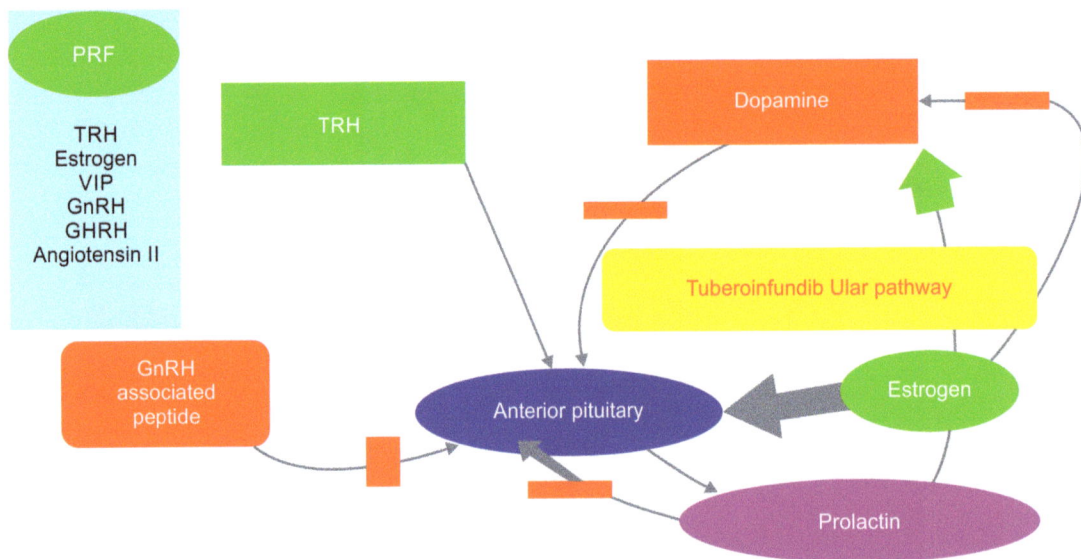

Fig. 1: Prolactin neuroregulation.
(GHRH: growth hormone–releasing hormone; GnRH: gonadotropin-releasing hormone; PRF: prolactin releasing factor; TRH: thyrotropin-releasing hormone; VIP: vasoactive intestinal peptide)

Prolactin Secretion

- Released in pulsatile fashion
- Diurnal variation (highest levels during sleep)
- *Pulse generator:* Suprachiasmatic nucleus of hypothalamus
- Pulse frequency ranges between 14 pulses/day in the late follicular phase and 9 pulses/day in the luteal phase.[5]
- Pulse amplitude increases from early to late follicular phase due to increase in estrogen.
- Lowest levels are in midmorning after the subject awakes and highest levels in sleep.
- Levels increase 1 hour after the onset of sleep and continue to rise after the peak values are reached between 5 and 7 AM.
- Maximum rise is seen during rapid eye movement (REM) sleep.[6]

CAUSES OF HYPERPROLACTINEMIA (FIG. 2)

- *Prolactinomas:*
  - Most frequent cause of persistent HPRL
  - It is the presence of a microprolactinoma (<10 mm diameter) or macroprolactinoma >10 mm diameter.
  - Either these secrete excessive amount of PRL or disrupt dopamine secretion control.
- *Idiopathic hyperprolactinemia:*
  - Accounts for 30–40% of cases where there is no obvious cause for the disorder and hypothalamic pituitary anatomy is normal.
- *Macroprolactinemia:*
  - A condition where >60% of circulating PRL is made up of macroprolactin, which has low biologic activity instead of the normal 5–10%.
  - HPRL due to macroprolactin is because of its lower renal clearance and longer half-life.
  - Control over hypothalamic dopaminergic tone may also occur.
  - Asymptomatic generally
  - No medication or tests are needed further in this scenario.

EFFECT OF HYPERPROLACTINEMIA ON FEMALE FERTILITY

- Inhibits GnRH activity by interacting with hypothalamic DA and opioid system via the short-loop feedback mechanism—leading to anovulation (Fig. 3).
- Kisspeptin is expressed in ARC and anteroventral periventricular nucleus (AVPV).[7]
- Kisspeptins in ARC mediate sex steroid feedback regulation of GnRH secretion while those in AVPV mediate estrogen-induced ovulatory surge of GnRH in females.
- Sonigo et al. noticed reduced kisspeptin in ARC and AVPV in the hyperprolactinemic mouse model, thus proving the role of kisspeptins in anovulation and hypogonadotropic hypogonadism (HH) induced by HPRL.
- Kisspeptin neurons also express PRL receptors.
- Exogenously administered kisspeptins or kisspeptin agonists may have potential therapeutic implications in HPRL.[8]
- There is role in induction of luteinizing hormone (LH) receptors to maintain progesterone synthesis.
- Prolactin is necessary for complete luteinization. However, a very high PRL level in the early phase of follicular growth inhibits progesterone secretion (by inhibiting corpus luteal steroidogenesis).

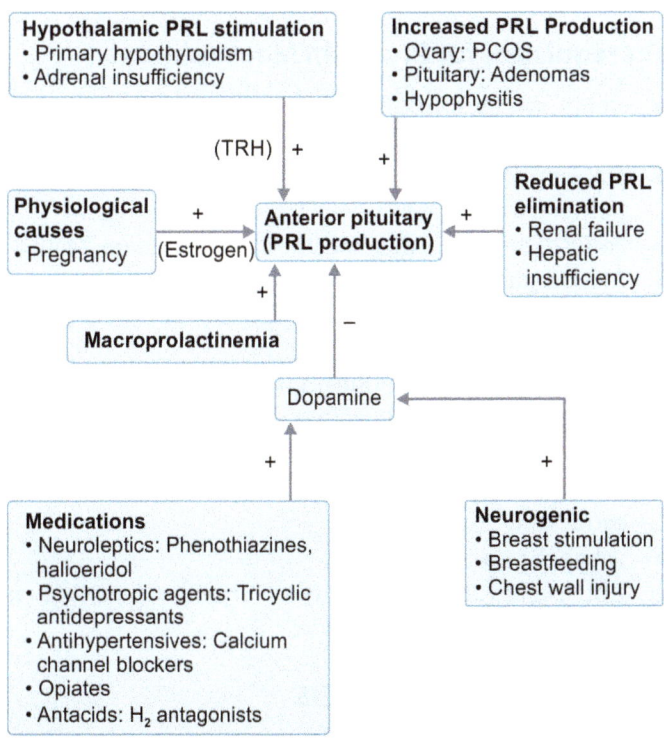

Fig. 2: Causes of hyperprolactinemia.
(PCOS: polycystic ovary syndrome; PRL: prolactin; TRH: thyrotropin-releasing hormone)

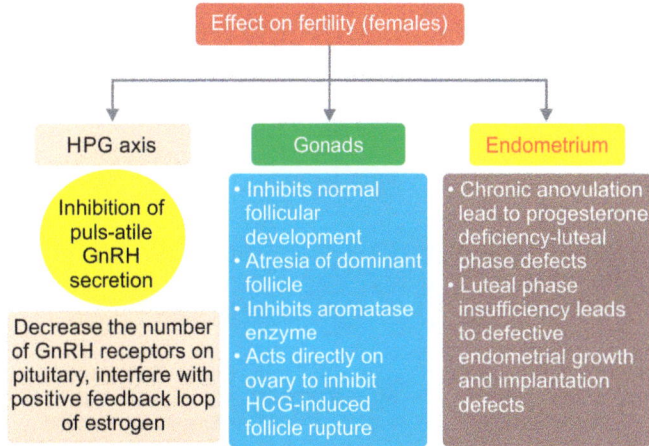

Fig. 3: Effect of hyperprolactinemia on female fertility.
(GnRH: gonadotropin-releasing hormone; HPG: hypothalamic-pituitary-gonadal)

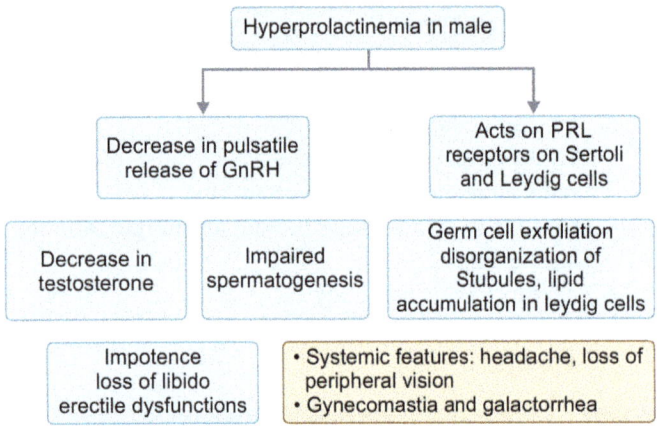

Fig. 4: Effect of hyperprolactinemia on male fertility. (GnRH: gonadotropin-releasing hormone; PRL: prolactin; S: seminiferous)

EFFECT OF HYPERPROLACTINEMIA ON MALE FERTILITY

- HPRL can cause primary or secondary hypogonadism and is responsible for infertility in about 11% of males with oligospermia **(Fig. 4)**.
- There is 88% prevalence of sexual dysfunction in men with HPRL.
- Most common sexual dysfunction is erectile dysfunction (ED) followed by reduced sexual desire and impaired orgasm.[9,10]
- Nearly half of the patients with ED with HPRL show a normal serum testosterone level.
- In males with HPRL, serum sex hormone-binding globulin is low. This in turn increases unbound proportion of testosterone and attenuates the biological impact of low total testosterone.
- Galactorrhea is less common in men than in women because the glandular breast tissue in men has not been made sensitive to PRL by precedent stimulation of estrogen and progesterone.

CLINICAL FEATURES[11,12]

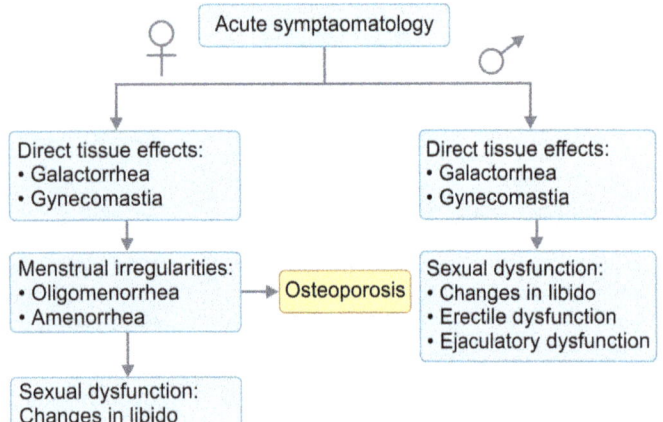

TABLE 1: Prolactin levels and their effect on females.

Prolactin levels[13]	Reproductive changes
Normal: 10–25 ng/mL	
20–50 ng/mL	Short luteal phase
50–100 ng/mL	Amenorrhea/oligomenorrhea
>100 ng/mL	Overt hypogonadism

Evaluation of Hyperprolactinemia

- *History:*
  - Rule out possibility of pregnancy.
  - Ask for history of (H/o) intake of medications.
  - Ask for visual symptoms, headache, galactorrhea, and signs of hypothyroidism.
- *Physical examination:*
  - Visual field examination
  - Signs of hypothyroidism or hypogonadism
  - Breast examination—galactorrhea and gynecomastia
  - Chest wall injury
- *Laboratory evaluation* **(Table 1)**:
  - Since PRL is a dynamic hormone, caution must be exercised before taking a blood sample for analysis.
  - Check thyroid stimulating hormone (TSH) levels.

National Institute for Health and Care Excellence (NICE) guidelines on infertility (2004) state that fertility assessment should not routinely include assessment of PRL levels and this should be offered to women with ovulatory disorders, galactorrhea, or pituitary tumors.

Prerequisites for Prolactin Measurement

- Being awake 2 hours before extraction and without making any physical effort
- On empty stomach, after rest, in comfort, preferably between 6 and 8 AM
- Avoid high-protein diet from the day before the extraction.
- Avoid high-fat diet from the day before the extraction.
- Avoid breast stimulation from the day before the extraction.
- Be in 8–10 hours of fasting prior to extraction
- Do not take medications that may increase or decrease prolactin.
- Be relaxed and rested for at least 30 minutes before extraction.
- Do not be under stress.

PRL levels >200 ng/mL may occur with drugs such as risperidone and metoclopramide.[14]

PITFALLS IN DIAGNOSIS

- *Macroprolactinemia* **(Flowchart 2)**:
  - Found in 10% of cases
  - High levels of big PRL molecules[15]

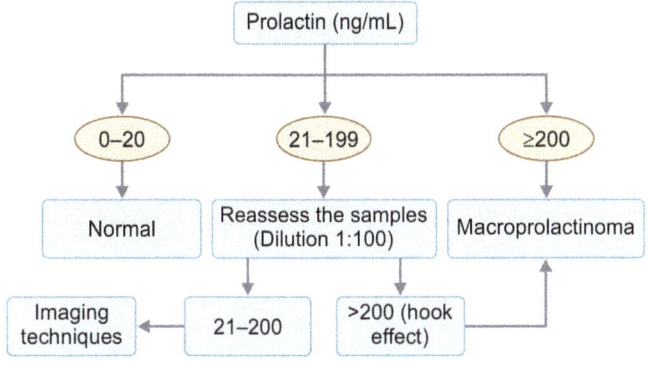

Flowchart 2: Prolactin levels and pitfalls in diagnosis.

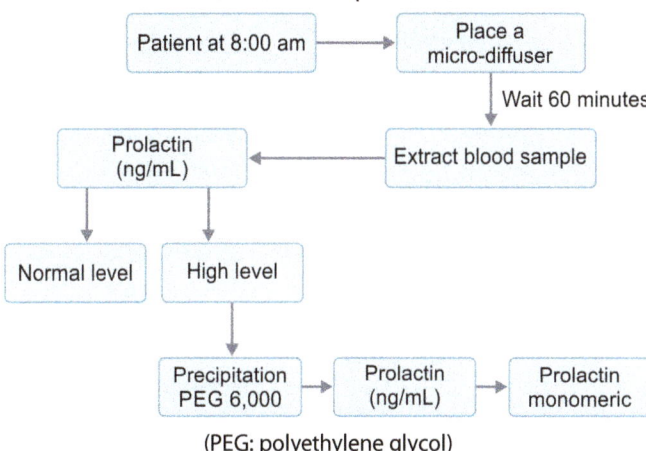

Flowchart 3: Macroprolactinemia.

(PEG: polyethylene glycol)

- Immunoreactive but biologically inactive
- Although a smaller proportion of patients with macroprolactinemia may have symptoms of HPRL, it should be suspected when typical symptoms of HPRL are absent. As macroprolactinemia is a common cause of HPRL, routine screening for macroprolactinemia could eliminate unnecessary diagnostic testing as well as treatment.[16]
- Investigation for macroprolactin should always be done in cases of asymptomatic hyperprolactinemic subjects. Many commercial assays do not detect macroprolactin. Polyethylene glycol precipitation is an inexpensive way to detect the presence of macroprolactin in the serum **(Flowchart 3)**.[17]
- *Hook effect:*
  - Macroadenoma with modest elevation
  - In this even though the test diagnoses hyperprolactinemia, the biological protein is normal and thus lacks clinical symptoms.
  - The intensity of an antigen–antibody interaction depends primarily on the relative proportion of the antigen and the antibody. A relative excess of either will impair adequate immune complex formation. This is called the "high-dose hook effect" or the "prozone phenomenon".
  - It can be corrected with serial dilutions.

Imaging Technique

- The magnetic resonance imaging (MRI) with gadolinium gives the most precise anatomical details.[18]
- If MRI is normal, after excluding other HPRL causes, think of idiopathic HPRL.
- Serum concentrations of >100 ng/mL are diagnostic of a pituitary microadenoma and lower concentrations (<100 ng/mL) have only 20% risk of having tumor.
- However, there is no consensus as to when radiological investigations should be done.
  Some recommend that computed tomography (CT) or MRI should be done in all patients with HPRL, while others suggest that these need to be done only when serum PRL exceeds 100 ng/mL or there are signs suggestive of an intracranial space occupying lesion (SOL).

■ MANAGEMENT

- *Group 1:* Idiopathic or microadenoma-associated hyperprolactinemia. These cases can be managed medically alone.
- *Group 2:* HPRL with macroadenoma. This group needs fertility management in combination of drugs and surgery/radiotherapy.
- *Group 3:* Miscellaneous group which involves HPRL due to systemic disorders, drugs, pituitary hypersecretion (other than adenomas), and hypothalamic-pituitary stalk damage. Treating the underlying etiology brings PRL levels back to normal.

Medical Management

Drugs

- Bromocriptine
- Cabergoline.
  Their mechanism, dose, and side effects are explained in **Table 2**.

Monitoring (Flowcharts 4 and 5)

Microadenoma:
- No treatment required for asymptomatic microadenomas
- Dose of DA can be reduced after 1 year of treatment if serum PRL is normal.
- MRI monitoring at 1st, 2nd, and 5th year[26]
- Therapy may be tapered and discontinued in patients who have been treated with dopamine agonists for at least 2 years if normal serum PRL and no visible tumor remnant on MRI.

Macroadenoma:
- Visual field examination to be reassessed at 1 month of start of therapy.

TABLE 2: Drugs given in hyperprolactinemia.		
Drug	Bromocriptine	Cabergoline
Class	Antiparkinsonian and dopamine (DA) agonist	Long-acting selective receptor agonist [high affinity for dopamine 2 (D2) receptors][23]
Mechanism of action	Activates polysynaptic DA receptor to inhibit prolactin secretion	Directly stimulates D2 receptors and inhibits synthesis of prolactin (PRL) secretion
Dose	2.5 mg twice bd Maximum 10 mg/day	• 0.25 mg twice weekly every 4 weeks • Maximum 2 mg/week
Side effect	Hypotension, constipation, nausea, vomiting, dizziness, headache, and fatigue[24,25]	Nausea is less common than bromocriptine and pergolide

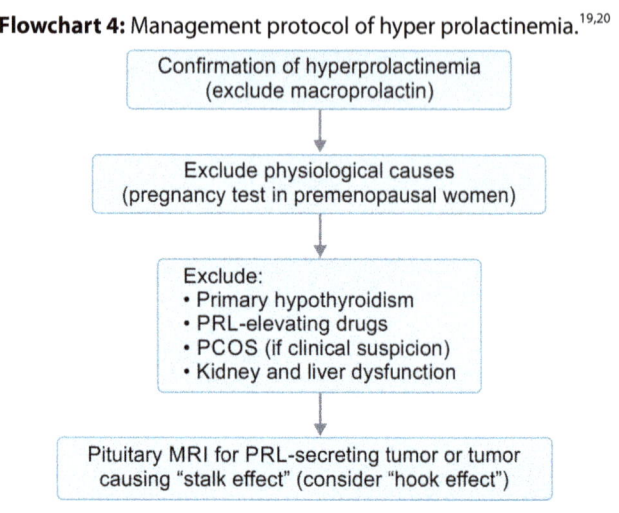

Flowchart 4: Management protocol of hyper prolactinemia.[19,20]

(PEG: polyethylene glycol; MRI: magnetic resonance imaging; PCOS: polycystic ovary syndrome; PRL: prolactin)

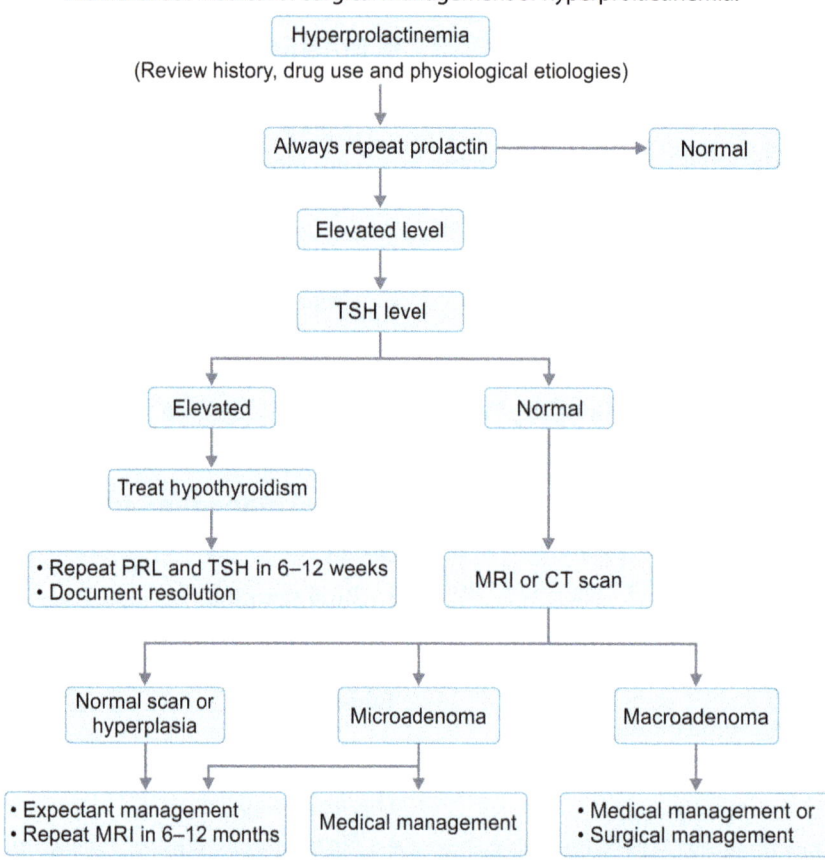

Flowchart 5: Medical or surgical management of hyperprolactinemia.[21,22]

(CT: computed tomography; MRI: magnetic resonance imaging; PRL: prolactin; TSH: thyroid stimulating hormone)

- Repeat MRI at 6 months, 12 months, 2 years, and 5 years.[27]
- If serum PRL levels have been normal for 1 year and adenoma has decreased in size, the dose of DA can be decreased, if PRL levels are normal in serum **(Table 2)**.
- Treatment can be only discontinued in those whose macroadenoma <1.5 cm, with normal serum PRL levels, and no adenoma visualized on MRI.[28,29]
- Discontinuation should not be considered if adenoma was initially >2 cm, or can be visualized on MRI, and if PRL levels have not been normalized on treatment.

Surgical Treatment

To be done in patients:
- Who do not tolerate DA therapy

- Who do not respond to medical management or show progression after an initial response to medical treatment
- With large macroadenomas desirous of pregnancy, even when their tumor responds to medical treatment
- To prevent excessive growth of adenomas in pregnancy in woman with giant lactotroph adenoma.

Drawbacks of Surgical Resection

- Incomplete resection
- Persistent HPRL
- Surgical risk
- Risk of hypopituitarism
- Recurrence of the adenoma (50% at 4 years) and HPRL (39% at 5 years).

MANAGEMENT FOR PATIENTS HAVING HYPERPROLACTINEMIA DUE TO SYSTEMIC DISORDERS (GROUP 3)

- Around 40% patients with primary hypothyroidism have mild elevation of PRL levels that can be normalized by thyroid hormone replacement.
- Medications that can cause HPRL should be discontinued for 48–72 hours if it is safe to do so and serum PRL level repeated.
- Sometimes, the causative agent is essential for the patient's health (e.g., a psychotropic agent) but it may cause symptomatic hypogonadism. In these patients, treatment with a dopamine agonist should be avoided since it might compromise the effectiveness of the psychotropic drug and the patient should simply be treated with replacement of sex steroids.
- About 30% patients with chronic renal failure and up to 80% patients on hemodialysis have raised PRL levels. This is probably due to either decreased clearance or increased production of PRL as a result of disordered hypothalamic regulation of PRL secretion. Correction of the renal failure by transplantation results in normal PRL levels.

MANAGEMENT FOR PREGNANT WOMEN

- Over 80–85% of females with HPRL with/without adenoma achieve pregnancy on DA treatment.
- Risk of tumor growth in pregnancy is 1–2% in microadenoma and 15–20% in macroadenoma.
- Serial PRL measurement is not necessary during pregnancy.
- Regardless of the size of adenoma, there is no indication for treatment with DA or for imaging during pregnancy in the absence of symptoms.[30]
- Women with prolactinomas should discontinue DA treatment as soon as pregnancy is recognized, except for patients with invasive macroadenomas or adenomas abutting optic chiasma.[30]
- Breastfeeding poses no risk for tumor growth in females with microadenomas/macroadenomas that remains asymptomatic during pregnancy, but is contraindicated in those with neurological symptoms during pregnancy.[31]

REFERENCES

1. Biller BM. Hyperprolactinemia. Int J Fertil Womens Med. 1999;44(2):74-7.
2. Melmed S, Jameson JL. Disorders of the anterior pituitary and hypothalamus. In: Kasper DL, Braunwald E, Fauci AS, Hauser SL, Longo DL, Jameson JL, (Eds). Harrison's Principles of Internal Medicine, 16th edition. New York: McGraw Hill; 2008. pp. 2076-97.
3. Freeman ME, Kanyicska B, Lerant A, Nagy G. Prolactin: structure, function, and regulation of secretion. Physiol Rev. 2000;80(4):1523-631.
4. Benker G, Jaspers C, Häusler G, Reinwein D. Control of prolactin secretion. Klin Wochenschr. 1990;68(23):1157-67.
5. Verhelst J, Abs R. Hyperprolactinemia: pathophysiology and management. Treat Endocrinol. 2003;2(1):23-32.
6. Escobar-Morreale HF. Macroprolactinemia in women presenting with hyperandrogenic symptoms: Implications for the management of polycystic ovary syndrome. Fertil Steril. 2004;82(6):1697-9.
7. George JT, Veldhuis JD, Roseweir AK, Newton CL, Faccenda E, Millar RP, et al. Kisspeptin-10 is a potent stimulator of LH and increases pulse frequency in men. J Clin Endocrinol Metab. 2011;96(8):E1228-36.
8. Luciano AA. Clinical presentation of hyperprolactinemia. J Reprod Med. 1999;44 (12 Suppl):1085-90.
9. Boyd AE 3rd, Reichlin S, Turksoy RN. Galactorrhea-amenorrhea syndrome: diagnosis and therapy. Ann Intern Med. 1977;87(2):165-75.
10. Urman B, Yakin K. Ovulatory disorders and infertility. J Reprod Med. 2006;51(4):267-82.
11. Bachelot A, Binart N. Reproductive role of prolactin. Reproduction. 2007;133(2):361-9.
12. Díaz S, Seron-Ferre M, Croxatto HB, Veldhuis J. Neuroendocrine mechanisms of lactational infertility in women. Biol Res. 1995;28(2):155-63.
13. Ugwa EA, Ashimi AO, Abubakar MY, Takai IU, Lukman OT, Lawal HA, et al. An assessment of serum prolactin levels among infertile women with galactorrhea attending a gynecological clinic North-West Nigeria. Niger Med J. 2016;57(3):178-81.
14. Glezer A, Soares CR, Vieira JG, Giannella-Neto D, Ribela MT, Goffin V, et al. Human macroprolactin displays low biological activity via its homologous receptor in a new sensitive bioassay. J Clin Endocrinol Metab. 2006;91(3):1048-55.
15. Donadio F, Barbieri A, Angioni R, Mantovani G, Beck-Peccoz P, Spada A, et al. Patients with macroprolactinaemia: clinical and radiological features. Eur J Clin Invest. 2007;37(7):552-7.
16. Fahie-Wilson MN, John R, Ellis AR. Macroprolactin; high molecular mass forms of circulating prolactin. Ann Clin Biochem. 2005;42(Pt 3):175-92.
17. McKenna TJ. Should macroprolactin be measured in all hyperprolactinaemic sera? Clin Endocrinol (Oxf). 2009; 71(4):466-9.

18. Isik S, Berker D, Tutuncu YA, Ozuguz U, Gokay F, Erden G, et al. Clinical and radiological findings in macroprolactinemia. Endocrine. 2012;41(2):327-33.
19. Ono M, Miki N, Amano K, Kawamata T, Seki T, Makino R, et al. Individualized high-dose cabergoline therapy for hyperprolactinemic infertility in women with micro- and macroprolactinomas. J Clin Endocrinol Metab. 2010; 95(6):2672-9.
20. Crosignani PG. Management of hyperprolactinemia in infertility. J Reprod Med. 1999;44(12 Suppl):1116-20.
21. Wang AT, Mullan RJ, Lane MA, Hazem A, Prasad C, Gathaiya NW, et al. Treatment of hyperprolactinemia: a systematic review and meta-analysis. Syst Rev. 2012;1:33.
22. Essaïs O, Bouguerra R, Hamzaoui J, Marrakchi Z, Hadjri S, Chamakhi S, et al. Efficacy and safety of bromocriptine in the treatment of macroprolactinomas. Ann Endocrinol (Paris). 2002;63(6 Pt 1):524-31.
23. Melmed S, Casanueva FF, Hoffman AR, Kleinberg DL, Montori VM, Schlechte JA, et al. Endocrine Society. Diagnosis and treatment of hyperprolactinemia: an Endocrine Society clinical practice guideline. J Clin Endocrinol Metab. 2011;96(2):273-88.
24. Gillam MP, Molitch ME, Lombardi G, Colao A. Advances in the treatment of prolactinomas. Endocr Rev. 2006;27(5): 485-534.
25. Casanueva FF, Molitch ME, Schlechte JA, Abs R, Bonert V, Bronstein MD, et al. Guidelines of the Pituitary Society for the diagnosis and management of prolactinomas. Clin Endocrinol (Oxf). 2006;65(2):265-73.
26. Brue T, Lancranjan I, Louvet JP, Dewailly D, Roger P, Jaquet P. A long-acting repeatable form of bromocriptine as long-term treatment of prolactin-secreting macroadenomas: a multicenter study. Fertil Steril. 1992;57(1):74-80.
27. Passos VQ, Souza JJ, Musolino NR, Bronstein MD. Long-term follow-up of prolactinomas: normoprolactinemia after bromocriptine withdrawal. J Clin Endocrinol Metab. 2002; 87(8):3578-82.
28. Di Sarno A, Landi ML, Cappabianca P, Di Salle F, Rossi FW, Pivonello R, et al. Resistance to cabergoline as compared with bromocriptine in hyperprolactinemia: prevalence, clinical definition, and therapeutic strategy. J Clin Endocrinol Metab. 2001;86(11):5256-61.
29. Schlechte JA. Long-term management of prolactinomas. J Clin Endocrinol Metab. 2007;92(8):2861-5.
30. Almalki MH, Alzahrani S, Alshahrani F, Alsherbeni S, Almoharib O, Aljohani N, et al. Managing Prolactinomas during Pregnancy. Front Endocrinol (Lausanne). 2015;26;6:85.
31. Molitch ME. Endocrinology in pregnancy: Management of the pregnant patient with a prolactinoma. Eur J Endocrinol. 172(5):R205-13.

CHAPTER 8

Amenorrhea—Work-up and Management

Harpreet Kaur

DEFINITION

Amenorrhea is defined as absence of menstruation by 16 years of age in the presence of secondary sexual organs or no menstruation by 14 years of age in the absence of secondary sexual characters.[1] In a woman who has been menstruating previously, absence of menses for over 6 months or for an interval equivalent to previous three cycles defines amenorrhea.

The possibility of a pregnancy as a reason for amenorrhea should always be considered.

PRIMARY AMENORRHEA

Primary amenorrhea describes a woman who has never menstruated whereas secondary amenorrhea describes those who have menstruated previously.[1]

The work-up of amenorrhea, like any other medical problems, follows the standard principles of thorough history and detailed examination and is aided by investigations.[2,3] The diagnostic work-up of a case of primary amenorrhea is shown in **Flowchart 1**.

Amenorrhea can be congenital, acquired, or multifactorial. The systematic evaluation of amenorrhea should ideally start from the lower compartment and progress to the higher level until the cause is determined.[2,3] The normal menstrual pathways and various cases of amenorrhea are shown in **Figure 1**.

Detailed medical history:
- *Menstrual history:* It is self-explanatory in primary amenorrhea.
  - Cyclical pain (cryptomenorrhea) occurs.
  - In secondary amenorrhea, preceding events such as dilation and curettage (D&C), removal of submucous myoma, and uterine sepsis are observed.
- Symptoms of hyperandrogenism such as acne and hirsutism in polycystic ovary syndrome (PCOS)/androgen-secreting tumors
- Symptoms of hormonal deficiency such as hot flushes and mood swings in primary ovarian insufficiency (POI)[4,5]
- Symptoms of thyroid disturbances/prolactin disorders such as headache or galactorrhea[6-8]
- Chronic medical illness, lifestyle, general illness, and drug intake

Physical examination:
- General body habitus, body mass index (BMI)—to look for gonadal dysgenesis, rule out hypothalamic causes such as eating disorders, obesity, and high waist-to-hip ratio in PCOS.[9,10]
- Axillary hair and Tanner staging
- Thyroid examination
- Breast development, Tanner staging, any galactorrhea
- Any suprapubic abdominal mass
- Pubic hair development and Tanner staging
- External genitalia: Look for imperforate hymen/bluish discoloration of hymen and patency of vagina.[2]
- The American Society for Reproductive Medicine (ASRM) practice committee has published a flow diagram for evaluation of amenorrhea **(Flowchart 2)**.[3]

The genital outflow tract can be checked by normal hormone [estrogen/progesterone (E/P)] challenge test or ultrasonography. In cases of suspected genital outflow tract

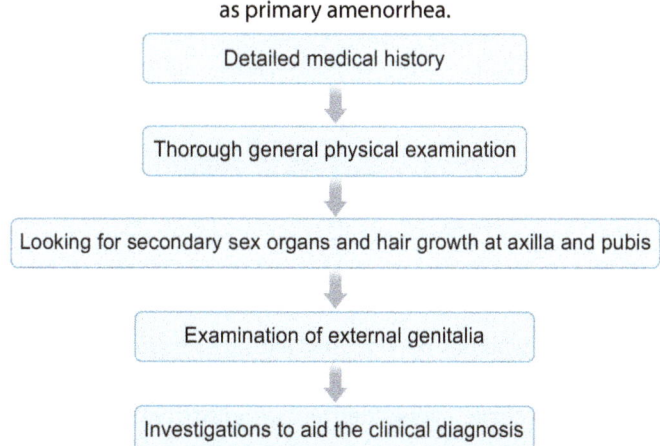

Flowchart 1: Diagnostic work-up of a case defined as primary amenorrhea.

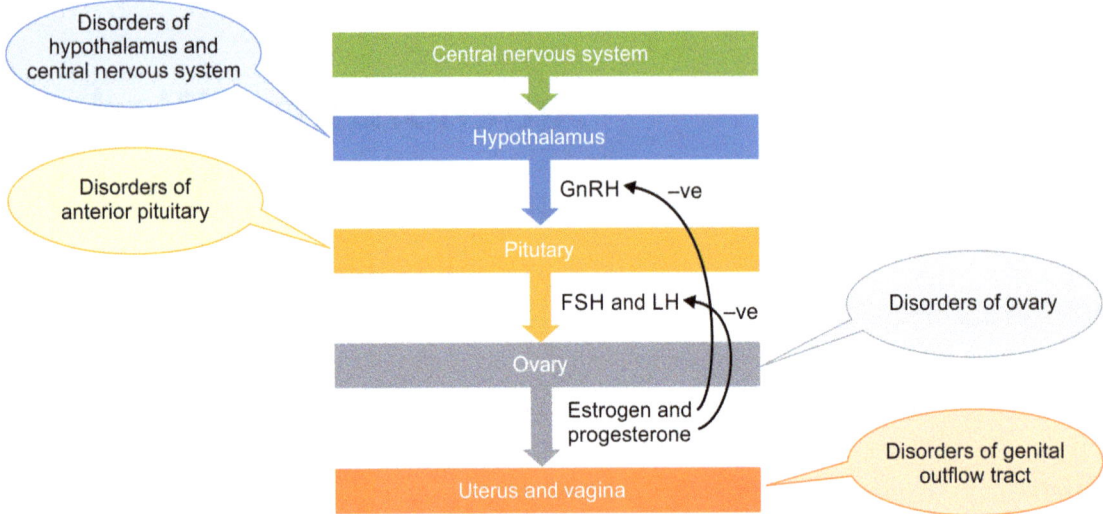

Fig. 1: Normal menstrual pathway and various causes of amenorrhea.
(FSH: follicle stimulating hormone; GnRH: gonadotropin releasing hormone; LH: luteinizing hormone)

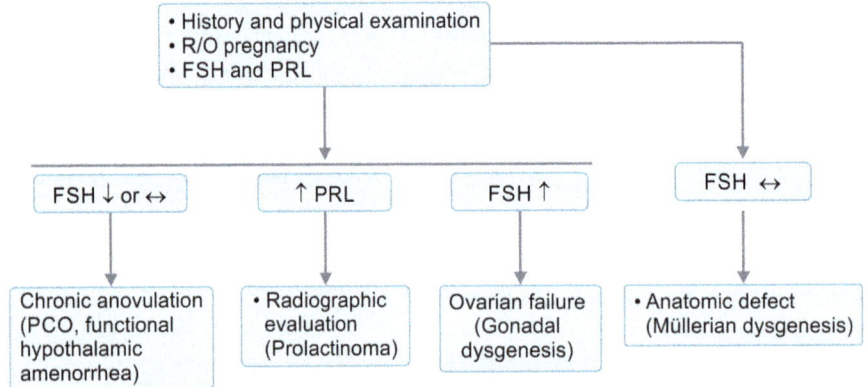

(FSH: follicle stimulating hormone; PCO: polycystic ovary; PRL: prolactin)
Source: Adapted from Practice Committee of American Society for Reproductive Medicine.

Flowchart 3: Suspected genital outflow tract obstruction.

```
                    Blind or absent vagina
                    /                    \
        Symptoms of                    Asymptomatic
     obstructed menses                 /           \
       /         \            Normal pubic hair   Scant/absent
  Imperforate  Transverse           |              pubic hair
    hymen     vaginal septum    Müllerian              |
                                agenesis      Androgen insensitivity
                                                   syndrome
```

abnormality, MRI is further suggested to delineate the type of abnormality **(Flowchart 3)**.

After thorough history and physical examination, a set of investigations are recommended depending upon the suspected pathology **(Flowchart 4)**.

SECONDARY AMENORRHEA

In a woman who has been menstruating previously, absence of menses for over 6 months or for an interval equivalent to previous three cycles defines amenorrhea. Secondary amenorrhea means a woman has menstruated previously.

Flowchart 4: Investigations in primary amenorrhea.[9,11,12]

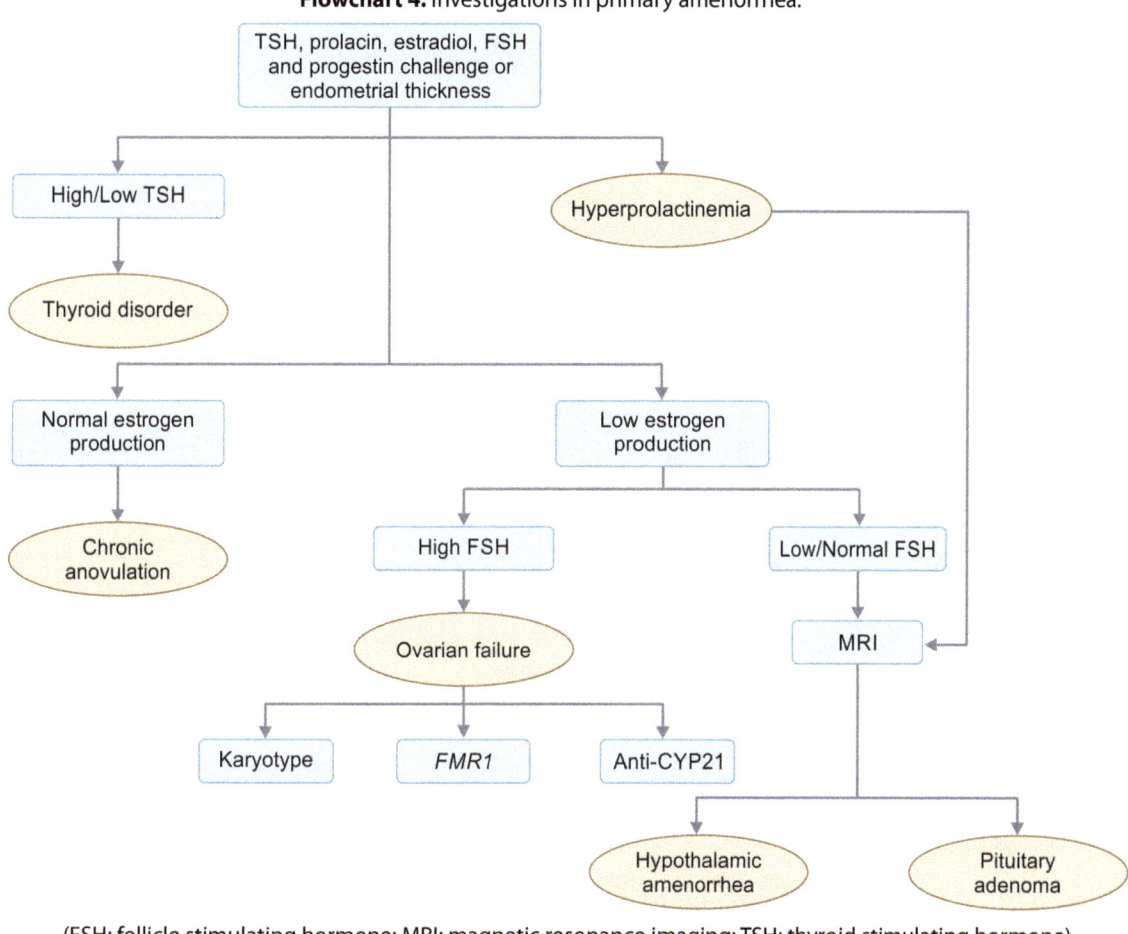

(FSH: follicle stimulating hormone; MRI: magnetic resonance imaging; TSH: thyroid stimulating hormone)

Flowchart 5 describes the possible causes and work-up of a case of secondary amenorrhea.

GENITAL OUTFLOW TRACT OBSTRUCTION

Outflow obstruction can occur at various levels with resultant variation in presentation. Majority of obstructions are congenital but most of them go unrecognized until puberty. Asherman syndrome is an important cause for acquired outflow obstruction **(Fig. 2)**.[13,14]

- *Müllerian agenesis* (Mayer-Rokitansky-Küster-Hauser syndrome): It is characterized by normal, symmetrical breast and pubic hair development and normal female karyotype (46,XX).
- *Androgen insensitivity syndrome (AIS)* (testicular feminization/male pseudohermaphrodite): They have normal male karyotype (46,XY). They have normal breast development but scant/absent pubic hair.[15]
- *Asherman syndrome* (intrauterine adhesions): It is most commonly seen following instrumentation of uterine cavity. Diagnosis is based on a high index of suspicion, history, and no withdrawal on E+P. This is further aided by thin, irregular endometrium on ultrasonography (USG), hysterosalpingography (HSG), saline infusion sonography, and hysteroscopy.[16,17]

OVARIAN CAUSES OF AMENORRHEA (FIG. 3)[11,12]

- *Turner syndrome:* This syndrome has typical stigmata with 45,X) or mosaic 46,XX/45,X0 karyotype. Once diagnosed, these patients need additional investigations such as echocardiography, audiometry, renal function tests, and USG. Thyroid evaluation and complete blood count are done at regular intervals.[18,19]
- *Swyer syndrome:* The patient needs gonadectomy soon after diagnosis is made due to a significant risk of malignant transformation in occult testicular tissue (20-30%).
- Ovarian failure following chemotherapy/radiation therapy.[20]
- Autoimmune causes
- Familial cases as in *FMR1* mutations.

CENTRAL NERVOUS SYSTEM CAUSES OF AMENORRHEA (FLOWCHART 6)

Pituitary adenoma and eating disorders are the important causes of amenorrhea in this category.[21,22] Management includes medical, psychosocial, or surgical treatment depending upon the cause. Rarely hypothalamic amenorrhea can be due to congenital gonadotropin releasing hormone

64 Amenorrhea—Work-up and Management

Flowchart 5: Work-up of secondary amenorrhea.

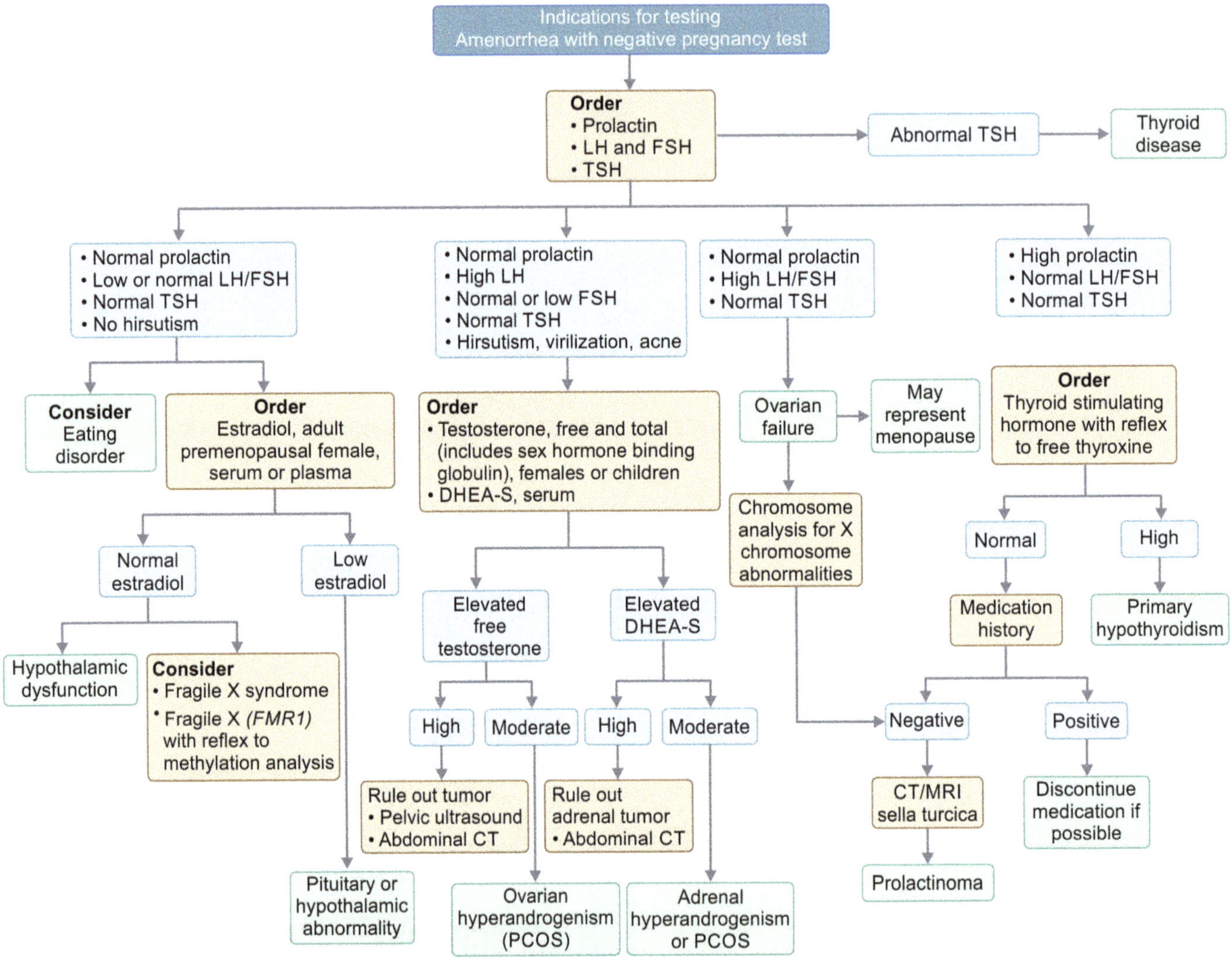

```
Indications for testing
Amenorrhea with negative pregnancy test
                │
              Order
            • Prolactin
            • LH and FSH ─────────→ Abnormal TSH ─→ Thyroid disease
            • TSH
```

- **Normal prolactin, Low or normal LH/FSH, Normal TSH, No hirsutism**
  - Consider Eating disorder
  - **Order** Estradiol, adult premenopausal female, serum or plasma
    - Normal estradiol → Hypothalamic dysfunction
    - Low estradiol → **Consider** Fragile X syndrome; Fragile X (*FMR1*) with reflex to methylation analysis

- **Normal prolactin, High LH, Normal or low FSH, Normal TSH, Hirsutism, virilization, acne**
  - **Order** Testosterone, free and total (includes sex hormone binding globulin), females or children; DHEA-S, serum
    - Elevated free testosterone
      - High / Moderate → Rule out tumor • Pelvic ultrasound • Abdominal CT
        - High → Pituitary or hypothalamic abnormality
        - Moderate → Ovarian hyperandrogenism (PCOS)
    - Elevated DHEA-S
      - High / Moderate → Rule out adrenal tumor • Abdominal CT
        - Moderate → Adrenal hyperandrogenism or PCOS

- **Normal prolactin, High LH/FSH, Normal TSH**
  - Ovarian failure → May represent menopause
  - Chromosome analysis for X chromosome abnormalities

- **High prolactin, Normal LH/FSH, Normal TSH**
  - **Order** Thyroid stimulating hormone with reflex to free thyroxine
    - Normal → Medication history
      - Negative → CT/MRI sella turcica → Prolactinoma
      - Positive → Discontinue medication if possible
    - High → Primary hypothyroidism

(CT: computed tomography; DHEA-S: dehydroepiandrosterone sulfate; FSH: follicle stimulating hormone; LH: luteinizing hormone; MRI: magnetic resonance imaging; PCOS: polycystic ovary syndrome; TSH: thyroid stimulating hormone)

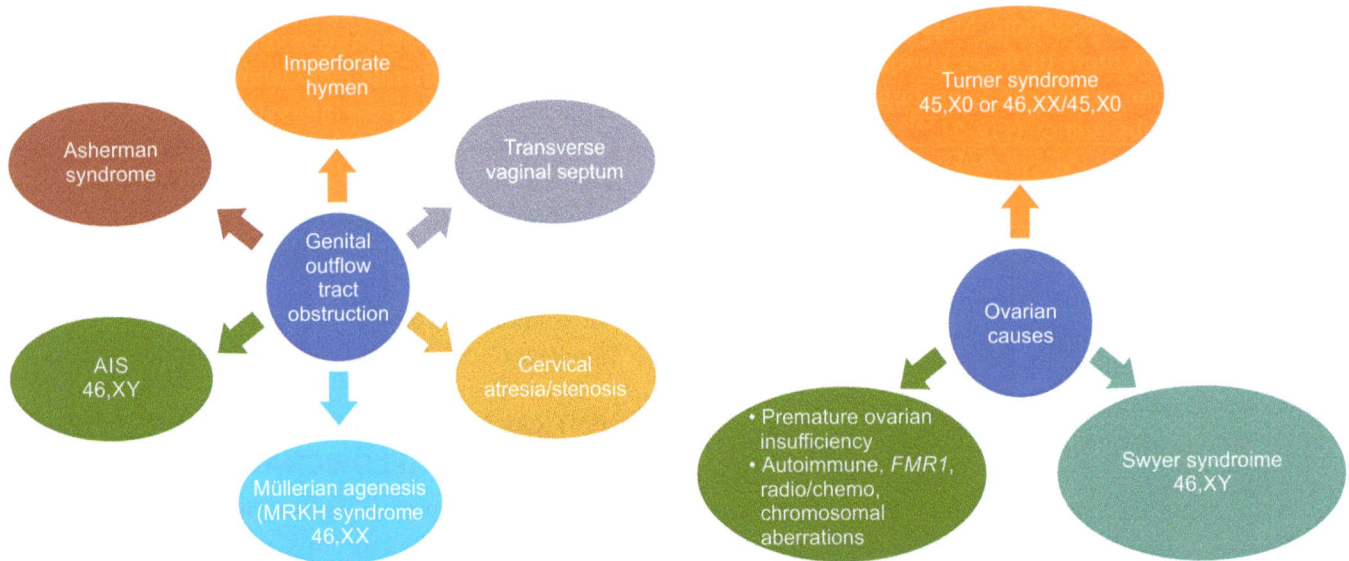

Fig. 2: Important causes for genital tract outflow obstruction.
(AIS: androgen insensitivity syndrome; MRKH syndrome: Mayer–Rokitansky–Küster–Hauser–syndrome)

Fig. 3: Ovarian causes of amenorrhea.

Flowchart 6: Central nervous system causes of amenorrhea.

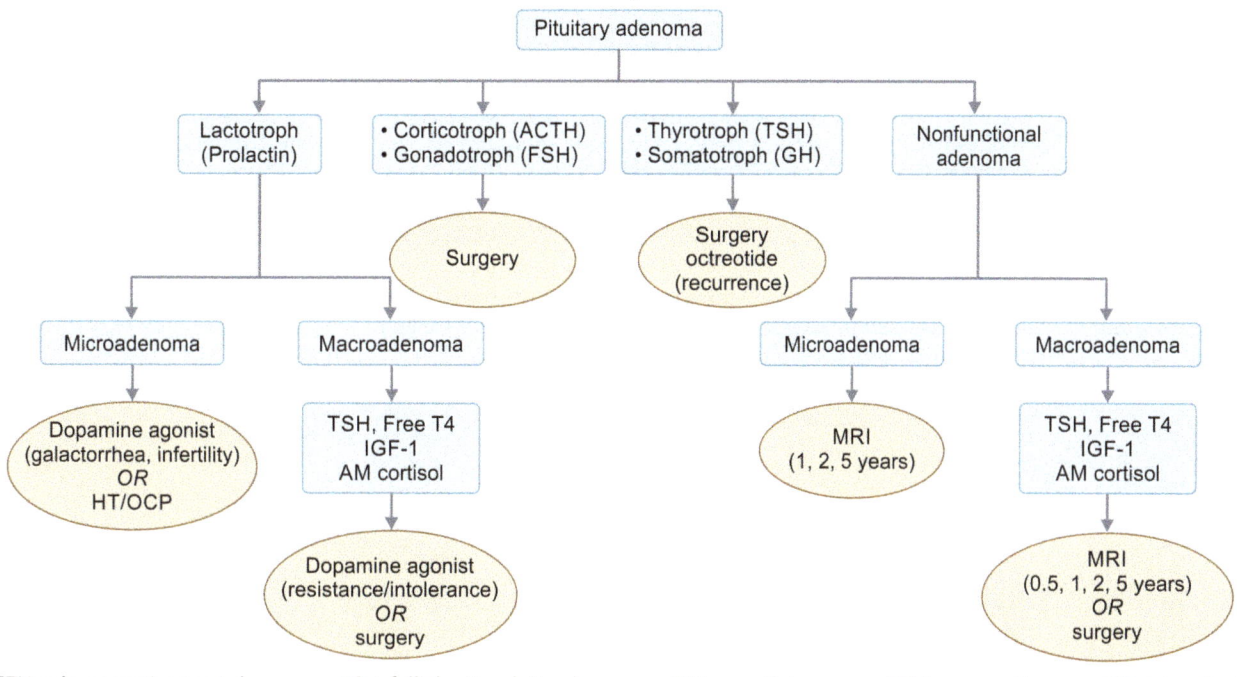

(ACTH: adrenocorticotropic hormone; FSH: follicle stimulating hormone; GH: growth hormone; HT: hormone therapy; IGF-1: insulin-like growth factor 1; MRI: magnetic resonance imaging; OCP: oral contraceptive pill; TSH: thyroid stimulating hormone; T4: thyroxine)

(GnRH) deficiency, e.g., Kallmann syndrome which can be attributed to various genetic causes[23,24] or mutations in GnRH receptor.[25]

Key Learning Points

- In all reproductive-age women, the possibility of pregnancy as a cause for amenorrhea should be considered.
- The work-up of amenorrhea, like any other medical problem, follows the standard principles of a thorough history and detailed examination and is aided by investigations.
- Amenorrhea can be congenital, acquired, or multifactorial. The systematic evaluation of amenorrhea should ideally start from the lower compartment and progress to the higher level until the cause is determined.
- A positive progesterone challenge test can be a simple test to rule out genital outflow tract obstruction and CNS cause of amenorrhea.

REFERENCES

1. Taylor HS, Pal L, Seli E. Amenorrhea. In: Speroff's Clinical Gynecologic Endocrinology and Infertility Textbook, 9th edition. Argentina: Wolters Kluwer; 2020. pp. 821-940.
2. Klein DA, Poth MA. Amenorrhea: an approach to diagnosis and management. Am Fam Physician. 2013;87(11):781-8.
3. Practice Committee of American Society for Reproductive Medicine. Current evaluation of amenorrhea. Fertile Steril. 2008;90(Suppl 5);S219-25.
4. Welt CK. Primary ovarian insufficiency: a more accurate term for premature ovarian failure. Clin Endocrinol (Oxf). 2008;68(4):499-509.
5. Rebar RW, Connolly HV. Clinical features of young women with hypergonadotropic amenorrhea. Fertil Steril. 1990;53(5):804-10.
6. Contreras P, Generini G, Michelson H, Pumarino H, Campino C. Hyperprolactinemia and galactorrhea: spontaneous versus iatrogenic hypothyroidism. J Clin Endocrinol Metab. 1981;53(5):1036-9.
7. Poretsky L, Garber J, Kleefield J. Primary amenorrhea and pseudoprolactinoma in a patient with primary hypothyroidism. Am J Med. 1986;81(1):180-2.
8. Yazigi RA, Quintero CH, Salameh WA. Prolactin disorders. Fertil Steril. 1997;67:215.
9. Manuel M, Katayama KP, Jones HW Jr. The age of occurrence of gonadal tumors in intersex patients with a Y chromosome. Am J Obstet Gynecol. 1976;124(3):293-300.
10. Troche V, Hernandez E. Neoplasia arising in dysgenetic gonads. Obstet Gynecol Surv. 1986;41(2):74-9.
11. Wittenberger MD, Hagerman RJ, Sherman SL, McConkie-Rosell A, Welt CK, Rebar RW, et al. The FMR1 premutation and reproduction. Fertil Steril. 2007;87(3):456-65.
12. Hoek A, Schoemaker J, Drexhage HA. Premature ovarian failure and ovarian autoimmunity. Endocr Rev. 1997;18(1):107-34.
13. Dane C, Dane B, Erginbas M, Cetin A. Imperforate hymen—a rare cause of abdominal pain: two cases and review of the literature. J Pediatr Adolesc Gynecol. 2007;20:245-7.
14. Letterie GS, Wilson J, Miyazawa K. Magnetic resonance imaging of müllerian tract abnormalities. Fertil Steril. 1988;50(2):365-6.
15. Rutgers JL, Scully RE. The androgen insensitivity syndrome (testicular feminization): a clinicopathologic study of 43 cases. Int J Gynecol Pathol. 1991;10(2):126-44.
16. Berman JM. Intrauterine adhesions. Semin Reprod Med. 2008;26(4):349-55.
17. Yu D, Wong YM, Cheong Y, Xia E, Li TC. Asherman syndrome—one century later. Fertil Steril. 2008;89(4):759-79.
18. Saenger P, Wikland KA, Conway GS, Davenport M, Gravholt CH, Hintz R, et al. Recommendations for the diagnosis and

management of Turner syndrome. J Clin Endocrinol Metab. 2001;86(7):3061-9.
19. Oktay K, Bedoschi G, Berkowitz K, Bronson R, Kashani B, McGovern P, et al. Fertility preservation in women with Turner syndrome: a comprehensive review and practical guidelines. J Pediatr Adolesc Gynecol. 2016;29(5):409-16.
20. Lo Presti A, Ruvolo G, Gancitano RA, Cittadini E. Ovarian function following radiation and chemotherapy for cancer. Eur J Obstet Gynecol Reprod Biol. 2004;113(Suppl 1):S33.
21. Keski-Rahkonen A, Hoek HW, Susser ES, Linna MS, Sihvola E, Raevuori A, et al. Epidemiology and course of anorexia nervosa in the community. Am J Psychiatry. 2007;164(8):1259-65.
22. Norre J, Vandereycken W, Gordts S. The management of eating disorders in a fertility clinic: clinical guidelines. J Psychosom Obstet Gynaecol. 2001;22(2):77-81.
23. Bhagavath B, Layman LC. The genetics of hypogonadotropic hypogonadism. Semin Reprod Med. 2007;25(4):272-86.
24. Hardelin JP, Dode C. The complex genetics of Kallmann syndrome: KAL1, FGFR1, FGF8, PROKR2, PROK2, et al. Sex Dev 2008;2(4-5):181-93.
25. Bedecarrats GY, Kaiser UB. Mutations in the human gonadotropin-releasing hormone receptor: insights into receptor biology and function. Semin Reprod Med. 2007;25(5):368-78.

CHAPTER 9

Management of the Hypogonadotropic Hypogonadism Male and Female

Ruma Satwik

■ INTRODUCTION

The initiation and maintenance of reproductive capacity in humans involve action at various levels. Pulsatile secretion of the hypothalamic gonadotropin-releasing hormone (GnRH) initiates synthesis and release of gonadotropins: follicle-stimulating hormone (FSH) and luteinizing hormone (LH) from the pituitary gland which in turn stimulate the gonads to complete gametogenesis and steroidogenesis. This hormonal axis from the brain to the gonads is referred to as the hypothalamic–pituitary–gonadal axis (HPG axis). The gonadal steroids: testosterone in men and estrogen in women are responsible for the maturation and maintenance of internal and external genitalia in form and function, whereas gametogenesis renders an individual fertile. The deficient production, secretion, or action of GnRH or less commonly, FSH and LH, leads to the clinical condition of hypogonadotropic hypogonadism (HH) characterized by delayed puberty, infertility, and loss of estrogenization and virilization in women and men, respectively.

This chapter deals with the different types, etiology, clinical features, diagnosis, and management of HH.

■ PREVALENCE, TYPES, AND ETIOLOGY

Hypogonadotropic hypogonadism is a rare condition, prevalent in 0.3–1% of men referred for infertility work-up.[1,2] In women with amenorrhea, 3–4% would have HH.

It can be divided into the congenital type and the acquired type based on its etiological origins (**Flowchart 1**).

Congenital hypogonadotropic hypogonadism (CHH) is a clinically heterogeneous condition detectable in 1–10 newborns per 100,000 live births.[3] CHH has a male predominance of 3–5 male:1 female. About two-thirds of CHH is associated with hyposmia or anosmia in which case it is called Kallmann's syndrome. This is a well-characterized syndrome that may additionally be associated with midline facial defects such as cleft lip and palate, dental agenesis, and less commonly with synkinesis, unilateral renal agenesis, ear agenesis, or neurosensory deafness.[4] The remaining third have normo-osmic CHH and have variously been called isolated GnRH deficiency (IGD) or idiopathic CHH in the past.

Although rare in occurrence the reproductive endocrinologist should also be aware of the coexistence of HH state with some well-characterized syndromes such as congenital pituitary hormone deficiency; CHARGE syndrome (coloboma, heart defects, choanal atresia, growth retardation, genital abnormalities, and ear abnormalities);[5] adrenal hypoplasia congenita (salt wasting, hyperpigmentation, muscular dystrophy, and hypogonadism);[6] Waardenburg syndrome (congenital sensorineural deafness and abnormal pigmentation of the iris, hair, and skin);[7] Bardet-Biedl-Moon syndrome (a rare autosomal recessive disorder associated with five fundamental characteristics: retinitis

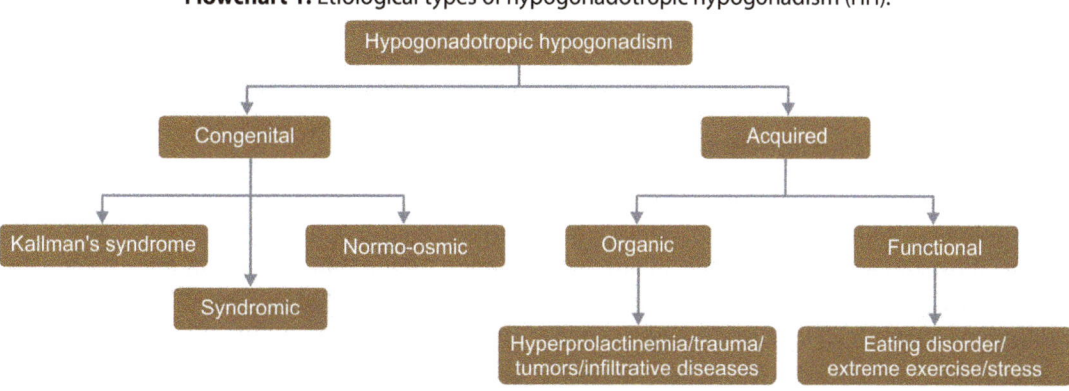

Flowchart 1: Etiological types of hypogonadotropic hypogonadism (HH).

pigmentosa, polydactyly, obesity, hypogonadism, and mental retardation);[8] Gordon Holmes syndrome (an autosomal recessive adult-onset neurodegenerative disorder characterized by progressive cognitive decline, dementia, ataxia, and chorea),[9] and others.

A genetic cause may be detectable in approximately 50% of individuals with CHH (both in syndromic and non-syndromic cases) when using the next-generation sequencing (NGS) platform.[10] CHH is genetically heterogeneous with approximately 40 genes identified at different loci to date.[11] These genes encode for either (1) GnRH neuronal migration from the olfactory placode to the preoptic hypothalamic nucleus during embryonal development, such as *KAL1*, *FGF8*, *FGFR1*, *PROK2*, or *PROK2R* gene; (2) GnRH peptide synthesis such as the *KISS1* or *GNRH1* gene; (3) GnRH receptor synthesis or its action, such as *GNRHR* gene; or (4) synthesis of anterior pituitary hormones. CHH is mostly a monogenic disorder, but digenic or oligogenic forms are known to exist too.[12] Both sporadic (de novo mutations) and familial cases are known. Familial cases have a monogenetic alteration and transmission can be X-linked (most common) through the *KAL1* gene, autosomal dominant through the *FGF8*, *FGFR1*, *CHD7*, or the *SOX10* gene, or autosomal recessive through the *GNRH1R*, *KISS1R*, *PROK2*, or *PROKR2* gene.[13] Variability in inheritance pattern is additionally introduced by variable gene penetrance and expressivity.

Acquired type of HH could arise due to exogenous steroid use,[14] pituitary tumors such as prolactinomas (the most common cause), pituitary trauma, infiltrative diseases such as sarcoidosis, hemochromatosis, or amyloidosis, iatrogenic causes such as surgeries or radiation, or developmental abnormalities like cysts, aneurysms, etc., leading to panhypopituitarism.[15] The cause could also be functional such as severe malnutrition due to an eating disorder, extreme stress or physical activity, or a severe chronic illness.

■ CLINICAL FEATURES

Although CHH is present from birth onward, its diagnosis may be missed at birth. Most patients with CHH are diagnosed late in adolescence (15–19 years) or early in adulthood as CHH is challenging to differentiate from other causes of delayed puberty. The acquired causes may present before or during puberty but much more commonly present as an adult onset disorder.

Neonatal Congenital Hypogonadotropic Hypogonadism

A history of cryptorchidism or the presence of a micropenis at birth may point to the diagnosis of CHH in male infants. No specific clinical signs of CHH are present in female neonates. Lack of minipuberty, a physiological state that persists in young infants due to an active GnRH pulse generator from the fetal period, could also point to the diagnosis of CHH. Reproductive hormones in normal infants at 2–4 months are in the normogonadotropic range for adults before settling into the hypogonadotropic range by age one. At months 2–4, gonadotropic hormones in the undetectable range point to a diagnosis of CHH. Genetic tests are initiated when clinical features and hormonal tests suggest the presence of CHH or when infants are born to HH parents with identifiable genetic mutations.[16]

Adolescent Congenital Hypogonadotropic Hypogonadism

In adolescence, HH manifests as delayed, absent, or incomplete puberty. A delay in puberty in boys is classically defined as lack of testicular enlargement by age 14 (testicular volumes <4 mL). In girls, a lack of breast development (Tanner's stage 2 or less) by age 13 or amenorrhea by age 15 would constitute delayed puberty. In addition, virilization, marked by voice change, facial hair and libido, is lacking in HH boys. In the absence of gonadal steroid induced growth spurts boys and girls continue to grow at steady rates. Similarly, in the absence of gonadal steroid induced epiphyseal closure their long bones gain eunuchoidal proportions with arm spans being longer than their vertical heights. These adolescents in later life manifest infertility in the absence of therapy due to their anovulatory and azoospermic states. Adolescents and young adults with CHH often have low self-esteem, distorted body image, and, in some cases, problems with sexual identity.[17]

Adult-onset Hypogonadotropic Hypogonadism

It is less common and attributable to acquired causes. It manifests as secondary amenorrhea, infertility, and loss of libido in women and with increasing severity of oligozoospermia, infertility, and libido loss in men. In long-standing cases there may be regression of signs of virilization and estrogenization and bone mineral density loss in both sexes.

■ DIFFERENTIAL DIAGNOSES AND WORK-UP

A complete diagnostic work-up is presented in **Table 1**.

A careful *history* of symptoms, its onset, symptoms of headache, visual and olfactory defects, personal history of exercise, eating disorder, presence of chronic illness, drug intake, prior brain surgeries, radiation or chemotherapy, and family history of similar syndromes or delayed puberty should be elicited from the affected individual. A sexual history, questions on libido, fertility, and menstrual history should additionally be elicited from adults. An *examination* to rule out morphological defects involving the lip, palate, teeth, and ears along with an assessment of height, weight, arm span, testicular volume using orchidometer, secondary

TABLE 1: Diagnostic work-up in a suspected hypogonadotropic hypogonadal individual.

Diagnostic modality	What to look for	Additional features
History	• Symptom details (with a focus on menstruation in women) and onset • Symptoms of headache, visual and olfactory defect • Past history: Brain surgeries, radiation or chemotherapy, trauma, chronic illnesses • Family history of similar syndromes • Current or past medicines • Exercise schedule and present eating habits	• Sexual history (wherever appropriate), questions on libido • Shaving frequency in men • Reproductive history • Questions to identify low self-esteem, depression
Examination	Height, weight, arm span, facies, palate, secondary sexual characteristics, systemic and local examination, testicular volume in men	Visual, olfactory, and hearing tests where indicated
Ultrasound	Small size uterus with normal morphology, small volume ovaries, low antral follicle count	If cryptorchidism, ultrasound to locate testes
Seminogram (in men)	Low volume ejaculate, azoospermia, pH >7.2, and positive fructose	
Hormones	• Low estrogen and low testosterone • Low to normal gonadotropins • Normal prolactin and TSH • High prolactin and low TSH in acquired causes of HH	• GAST to distinguish between pituitary and hypothalamic causes of HH • AMH and inhibin B are low but not used for diagnosis in isolation
Brain MRI	Macro- or microadenoma of the pituitary fossa, granuloma, abscesses, tumors, other SOLs	Olfactory placode hypoplasia
Genetic tests	HH gene panel	Whole exome sequencing

(AMH: anti-müllerian hormone; GAST: GnRH agonist stimulation test; HH: hypogonadotropic hypogonadism; SOLs: space occupying lesions; TSH: thyroid-stimulating hormone)

sexual characteristics and a perineal, and pelvic and systemic examination is essential to the cause of making a diagnosis. The sense of smell, hearing, and peripheral field vision should be checked using olfactometry, hearing tests, and visual field tests, respectively when indicated by history.

Ultrasonography of the abdomen with specific focus on the pelvic organs and kidneys will help identify an infantile uterus, small volume ovaries in women with reduced antral follicle count and any coexisting renal defects in both sexes. Ultrasound pelvis may also be able to locate testes in cryptorchidism.

The *reproductive hormones* in HH are at levels less than the fifth centile for normal. Typically, in complete forms of CHH, the gonadotropic hormones would be at *FSH* <1.2 mIU/mL[18] and *LH* <0.65 mIU/mL.[19] Another study finds higher cutoff for females with serum basal LH <0.85 IU/L and basal FSH <2.43 IU/L showing moderate sensitivity (80.0% or 100.0%) and specificity (75.0% or 50.0%) in the diagnosis of HH in females.[20] Basal inhibin B is low, typically <30 ng/dL in both sexes.[21] Basal *anti-müllerian hormone (AMH)* is low as well though it cannot be used for diagnosis in isolation. Low basal AMH does not reflect a poor ovarian reserve as preantral and small antral follicular pool that generates AMH is nonexistent and AMH value is likely to improve with FSH therapy as more and more FSH regulated preantral and small antral follicles are recruited into the pool.[22] The gonadal hormones would be at estradiol <20 pg/mL, progesterone <1 ng/mL in women and total testosterone <100 ng/dL in men. It is essential to run a *prolactin test* to rule out a prolactinoma or other pituitary macro- or microadenomas, and a *thyroid profile* to test anterior pituitary function.

A *GnRH agonist stimulation test (GAST)* helps in distinguishing between a hypothalamic (more common) and a pituitary origin (less common) for this condition. An intravenous injection of 100 µg/m^2 or 2.5 µg/kg of GnRH agonist buserelin or leuprolide or 1 µg/kg of nafarelin is administered and blood is tested for FSH and LH at baseline and half hourly for four to eight samples till peak FSH and LH levels are reached. The levels of FSH and LH should typically rise in healthy individuals with an intact hypothalamic-pituitary axis, in the first couple of hours before falling.[23] Individuals with a pituitary cause for HH will not respond to GnRH agonists whereas those with a hypothalamic cause will respond.

Additionally, GAST can also help distinguish between CHH and constitutional delay in growth and development (CDGP), a more common cause of delayed puberty. Making this distinction in adolescence is a challenging task since both conditions present with delayed puberty and similar basal hormonal characteristics. On follow-up, CDGP adolescent will go through normal puberty albeit at a later age than a normal adolescent. An HH adolescent will not go through puberty at all. Hence it is necessary to distinguish between these similar profiles individuals to be able to take the right management decision (reassure the former and start steroidal therapy in the latter).

The gonadotropin rise seen after GAST is typically to a mean of 22 mIU/mL for LH and to a mean of 12 mIU/mL for FSH in adolescents with CDGP. In CHH, LH peaks remain under 9 mIU/mL.[24] FSH peaks as a rule are lower in CHH than in CDGP, but there is a considerable overlap in values between the two groups and hence FSH peaks post-GAST cannot be used to discriminate between CDGP and CHH.[25] Toward the same cause, using *radiographs for bone age* as a key part of the work-up helps in differentiating between CDGP adolescents (bone age <13) and HH adolescents (bone age >13).[26]

Once a diagnosis of HH has been made based on clinical profile and hormonal testing, the next step is to establish a cause for this state. If the cause is correctable, attention is focused on its alleviation following which the HH state autocorrects itself.

A *brain MRI* reliably rules out a pituitary micro- or macroadenoma, craniopharyngioma, aneurysms, Rathke pouch cysts, central nervous system (CNS) tumors, granulomas, abscesses, and infiltrative lesions of the pituitary. It may also identify olfactory placode aplasia or hypoplasia where these exist.

Genetic tests have a high yield in cases with normal MRI scans. The purpose of genetic tests is to be able to counsel individuals about heritability of the condition and its transmission risks.[27] This is best done by ordering an HH gene panel or in recent years, by whole genome sequencing using the NGS platform.

MANAGEMENT OF THE HYPOGONADOTROPIC HYPOGONADAL MALE

There are two states of concern to the individual: delayed puberty and infertility. Both have separate management algorithms and are discussed separately.

Induction of Puberty and Maintenance of Secondary Sexual Characteristics

The aim of treatment is to induce virilization and normal sexual function, stimulate stature growth, promote bone health, and address psychological and emotional wellbeing.

Typically, testosterone replacement therapy (TRT) is utilized to achieve these aims. The dosage and preparation chosen are appropriate to the sexual developmental stage the individual is in and the target stage aimed at. For young boys between 12 and 16 years with the right diagnosis and after ruling out other causes, treatment begins with low dose testosterone **(Table 2)**. This is gradually increased in dose and frequency every 6–9 months over 24 months. Once the boy enters Tanner's stage IV development, full adult dose may be commenced. Such regimen helps mimic natural puberty and maximize stature growth while affording time for psychosexual development and minimizing the risk of precocious sexual activity.

For young adults presenting for the first time for TRT, a more aggressive approach may be adopted with starting dose being higher than in boys and stepped up more frequently at 3–6 monthly interval to reach the final adult dose over 1 year. Dosing frequency is guided by trough serum testosterone measurement (preinjection testosterone levels) targeting the lower end of the normal range typically 350–400 ng/dL. Long-acting injections cause a huge difference between peak testosterone values seen usually in the first-week post-injection and trough values, seen at the end of the injection interval. These huge fluctuations in serum testosterone levels cause alternate states of hypergonadism and hypogonadism. Smaller more frequent dosing can avoid this issue but introduces the issue of frequent needle pricks. Transdermal patches and gels may be the best for maintaining steady levels of testosterone but are limited by their costs and skin allergies in some men. The choice of preparation and dosing should be individualized in every case.[28]

Side effects associated with TRT include gynecomastia, weight gain, acne, erythrocytosis, hepatotoxicity, and development/worsening of obstructive sleep apnea, worsening of lower urinary tract symptoms and increased risk of prostate cancer with long-term usage.

Monitoring patients on TRT as per the Endocrine Society Guideline 2018,[29] should be with assessment of change in voice, testicular size, facial and body hair growth, shaving

TABLE 2: Hormone therapy for induction of puberty and maintenance of reproductive maturation in males.

Preparation	Dose	Frequency	Route
For boys between 12 and 16 years (puberty induction)			
Testosterone enanthate	50 mg	4 weeks	Intramuscular
Transdermal testosterone	10 mg	Every other day	Transdermal
Testosterone undecanoate	40 mg	Daily	Oral
For adults (induction or maintenance)			
Testosterone enanthate	150–200 mg	2–4 weeks	Intramuscular
Testosterone undecanoate	750 mg	10–14 weeks	Intramuscular
Testosterone gel	50–100 mg (1%) 25–50 mg (2%)	Daily	Transdermal
Testosterone patch	4 mg	Daily	Transdermal

frequency, change in libido, erection and ejaculation frequency, and sleep patterns. Preinjection total testosterone levels, complete blood count (CBC) and liver function test (LFT) should be ordered at each visit to monitor response to therapy and development of adverse effects. Bone densitometry is ordered for changes in osteoporotic status every 1-2 years after initiation of TRT. Prostate-specific antigen (PSA) is ordered for older hypogonadal individuals above 40 years of age. Additional tests may be ordered as per the clinical situation.

Testosterone replacement therapy ideally is administered lifelong to attain optimal benefit and does not lead to gonadal size increment or improvement in fertility. The patient and their relatives need to be informed of these facts. If while on testosterone therapy, men report an increase in testicular size, the physician should consider two possibilities: testicular tumor or a spontaneous reversal of CHH with return of HPG axis activity. A reversal has been seen in 10-20% of individuals.[30] In either case, the physician should stop the TRT and investigate through appropriate tests.

Contraindications to TRT as per the Endocrine Society are untreated prostate or breast cancer, uninvestigated prostate nodule, or a PSA >4, congestive heart failure grade 3-4, hematocrit >54%, severe obstructive sleep apnea, myocardial infarction or stroke within the past 6 months, and a current desire for fertility. Pulsatile GnRH or a combination of human chorionic gonadotropin (hCG) and FSH may be used to induce or maintain virilization in such patients.

Treatment of Infertility in Males

Irrespective of HH etiology, it is one of the most medically treatable causes of nonobstructive azoospermia. Identifiable acquired causes need to be addressed separately. Hyperprolactinemia responds to dopamine agonist therapy or in intractable cases to surgery. Anabolic steroid-induced hypogonadal state responds to cessation within 3-6 months. Functional causes such as eating disorders, extremely low weight, and excess stress respond to appropriate behavioral interventions. Pituitary tumors, abscesses, sarcoidosis, and hemochromatosis can respond to appropriate medical or surgical intervention. In those with idiopathic HH or those with an acquired cause not responsive to specific therapy, the treatment protocol to induce fertility in men as specified by the European Consensus on management of CHH is shown in **Flowchart 2**.

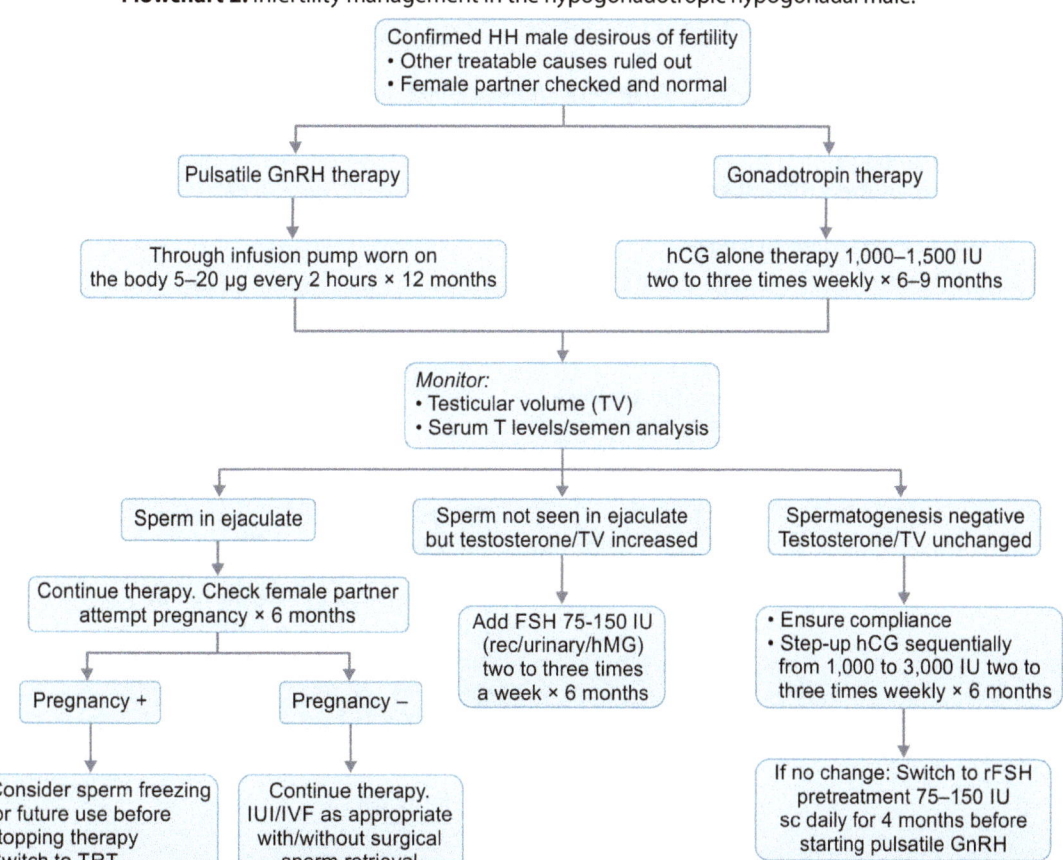

Flowchart 2: Infertility management in the hypogonadotropic hypogonadal male.

(FSH: follicle-stimulating hormone; GnRH: gonadotropin-releasing hormone; hCG: human chorionic gonadotropin; HH: hypogonadotropic hypogonadism; hMG: human menopausal gonadotropin; IUI: intrauterine insemination; IVF: in vitro fertilization; rFSH: recombinant follicle-stimulating hormone TRT: testosterone replacement therapy)

A GnRH therapy is as effective as gonadotropin therapy in achieving spermatogenesis and pregnancy in patients with hypothalamic disorders who have intact pituitary function. However, due to its cumbersome nature and its ineffectiveness in men with panhypopituitarism, pulsatile GnRH is less likely to be used than gonadotropin therapy. Dose titration should be guided by mean testosterone levels. Response to therapy is quicker in men who have signs of puberty at the time of treatment initiation. Those with a history of cryptorchidism and prepubertal onset of HH usually have less response rates and may take up to 2 years to respond. In severe cases, a reversal of treatment order involving FSH pretreatment for 4 months followed by pulsatile GnRH for 18–24 months has been tried successfully.[31]

Clomiphene citrate 25 mg daily has been tried in select men with idiopathic HH and with intact pituitary function with two pregnancies resulting in partners of 10 men treated this way.[32] However, there are inconsistencies in literature with respect to the effect of clomiphene and cannot be recommended for routine use in men with idiopathic HH men.

About 75% of patients initiated on gonadotropin therapy will have a response in the form of sperm in ejaculate at 12 months. Clinicians should remember that even with long-term therapy, sperm counts rarely return to normal with a mean sperm count of 5.9×10^6/mL (range: $4.7–7.1 \times 10^6$/mL) for gonadotropin therapy and 4.3×10^6/mL (range: $1.8–6.7 \times 10^6$/mL) for GnRH therapy reported in a 2014 meta-analysis.[33] And yet, this low mean sperm count begets natural fertility.[34] The pregnancy rates for gonadotropin and GnRH therapy are between 30 and 50%. Only a minority of pregnancies require assisted reproductive technology (ART). Sperm may be obtained through the ejaculate or in the face of persisting azoospermia but with testicular volume and hormone improvements, through surgical retrieval.

MANAGEMENT OF THE HYPOGONADOTROPIC HYPOGONADAL FEMALE

Induction of Puberty and Maintenance of Secondary Sexual Characteristics

The aim of treatment is to induce estrogenization: normal breast and uterine growth, establishment of menses, promote bone and cardiovascular health, and to address psychological and emotional wellbeing. The treatment guidelines as per the Expert European Consensus on treatment of CHH female are as given in **Table 3**.

TABLE 3: Hormone therapy for induction puberty and maintenance of reproductive maturation.

Estradiol preparation	Dosage	Frequency	Progesterone	Purpose	Period
Young girls (10–13 years with no prior breast development)					
Transdermal estradiol	• 0.05–0.07 µg/kg • Stepped up every 6 months to a maximum of 0.8–1.2 µg/kg • Maximum daily dose 50 µg/day	Daily at bed time	–	• Induction of puberty • Breast development	• 12–24 months • Till full breast development or • Till first menstrual bleed
Oral estradiol	• 0.1–0.2 mg • Stepped up every 6 months by 0.1 mg/day • To a maximum of 1–2 mg/day	Daily	–		
After growth spurt and breast development to at least Tanner's stage 3 (Choose a combination of any one estrogen and any one progesterone)					
Transdermal estrogen	50–100 µg	Daily	• Medroxyprogesterone acetate • 2.5–5 mg daily continuously or • 10 mg for 12 days a month	• Maintenance of reproductive maturation • Maintaining cyclic menstrual bleeding • Bone health • Reducing cardiovascular risk • Psychosexual well-being	• Till age of natural menopause or • As per symptoms of woman after risk-benefit assessment
Oral estrogen	1–2 mg	Daily	• Micronized progesterone • 100 µg daily continuously or • 200 µg for 12 days a month		
Conjugated equine estrogen	0.625–1.2 mg	Daily	Levonorgestrel (LNG) intrauterine device		
Estradiol gel	One to two pumps of 0.06%	Daily	–		

Puberty can be induced by oral or preferably transdermal estradiol using low dose preparations with the goal of mimicking estradiol levels during gonadarche. The estradiol dose is slowly increased over 12–24 months, after which time cyclic progesterone is added or after the first menstrual bleed whichever is earlier, in order to maximize breast development. In adulthood, higher estradiol doses are used and progesterone is added either continuously or sequentially to avoid endometrial hyperplasia. Estrogen treatment increases uterine size and combined estrogen and progestin therapy induces monthly withdrawal bleeding, but does not induce ovulation.

Another common approach is the use of combined hormonal contraceptives, which may allow for ease of administration compared with a hormone replacement therapy (HRT) regimen. However, the dose of estrogen and progestin in combined hormonal contraceptives is not replacement dosage; these hormonal preparations are significantly more potent than the aforementioned hormone therapy (HT) options.

Data on HT use in hypogonadal women and its link with breast cancer is scarce and indirect. Based on the premise that HT uses low doses meant to attain physiological levels of steroids in the body, the adverse cardiovascular event risk and cancer risk should not be affected. Hence the confidence in prolonged usage of HT is high. However, combined oral contraceptives (COCs) which use supraphysiological doses of hormones and not in a physiological order and prolonged use of COCs especially when given to postmenopausal women may be thought to be detrimental. A 2017 prospective nationwide cohort involving >10 lakh women between 15 and 49 years of age revealed that, the overall relative risk of invasive breast cancer among women who were current or recent users of any hormonal contraception was 1.20 [95% confidence interval (CI), 1.14–1.26] compared with women who never used hormonal contraception. Relative risk increased with duration of use, ranging from 1.09 (95% CI, 0.96–1.23) for <1 year of use to 1.38 (95% CI, 1.26–1.51) for use longer than 10 years. In general, risk was similar among different formulations or preparations of COCs.[35]

Treatment of Infertility in Females

A GnRH deficiency leads to incomplete development of follicles especially from stages that are FSH dependent such as preantral, small, and midantral follicular stage. A histopathological examination of HH ovaries would reveal the ovarian cortex studded with primordial, primary, and secondary follicles but lacking in of antral follicles.[36] This leads to the combination of small ovaries, decreased antral follicular count, and low circulating AMH concentrations observed in women with CHH.[22] It could wrongly suggest an alteration in ovarian reserve and a poor fertility prognosis and the woman should be made aware that this is not the case. With adequate duration of GnRH or gonadotropin therapy, follicular growth and maturation commences and ovarian sizes, antral follicular counts, and AMH start to rise. Fertility is usually not an issue.

The algorithm for management of the infertile hypogonadotropic hypogonadal female is given in **Flowchart 3**.

Prior checking of uterine morphology, adnexal pathology, tubal patency, and partner seminogram is advisable before commencing ovulation induction. Acquired causes need attention and treatment as per etiology detailed in the section on male HH should be initiated.

Women respond equally well to pulsatile GnRH therapy just as to gonadotropin therapy.

Pulsatile GnRH therapy in women mimics physiological pulses of GnRH with frequency and amplitude set as per the menstrual phase. Typically a dose of 75 ng/kg per pulse is given through an intravenous infusion pump. The dose for subcutaneously administered pulsatile GnRH therapy is twice as high as the intravenous route. A pulse frequency of 90 minutes is set in the early follicular phase and this is reduced to 60 minutes in the periovulatory (late follicular, ovulatory, and early luteal) period. These pulses increase to 120 minutes in the mid and late luteal phase.[37] The major advantage of pulsatile GnRH therapy compared with gonadotropin treatment is the physiological way of causing folliculogenesis and ovulation, absence of a need for exogenous ovulatory trigger or luteal phase support, decreased risk of multiple pregnancy and ovarian hyperstimulation and reduced need for monitoring. The disadvantages are the inconvenience of having to wear these pumps over the body during the course of treatment sometimes for periods as long as 1–2 years, complications of phlebitis or cellulitis and lack of easy availability of these pumps.

Gonadotropin therapy is the preferred therapy for its easier availability and convenience of usage. GnRH deficiency leads to absence of both FSH and LH and hence a preparation having LH activity is preferable over pure FSH alone. Both human menopausal gonadotropins (hMGs) and recombinant FSH + recombinant LH preparations in ratios of 2:1 have been used. In a two-arm randomized controlled trial involving 70 HH women, 70% of r-FSH/r-LH treated patients achieved ovulation versus 88% in hMG-HP group ($p = 0.11$). However, pregnancy rate in r-hFSH/r-hLH group was 55.6% compared to 23.3% in hMG-HP group ($p = 0.01$).[38] Other retrospective studies have not shown this benefit at all but shown hMG outperforming recombinant gonadotropins in terms of pregnancy rates.[39]

When using hMG, it is normal practice to start with 75 IU IM of hMG and response is monitored with ultrasound folliculometry at 7–10 days. Dose is titrated up after 14 days if ovaries remain nonresponsive or titrated down if a hyperresponse is seen.[40] It is not unusual to see long follicular phase lengths with typical durations being between 15 and

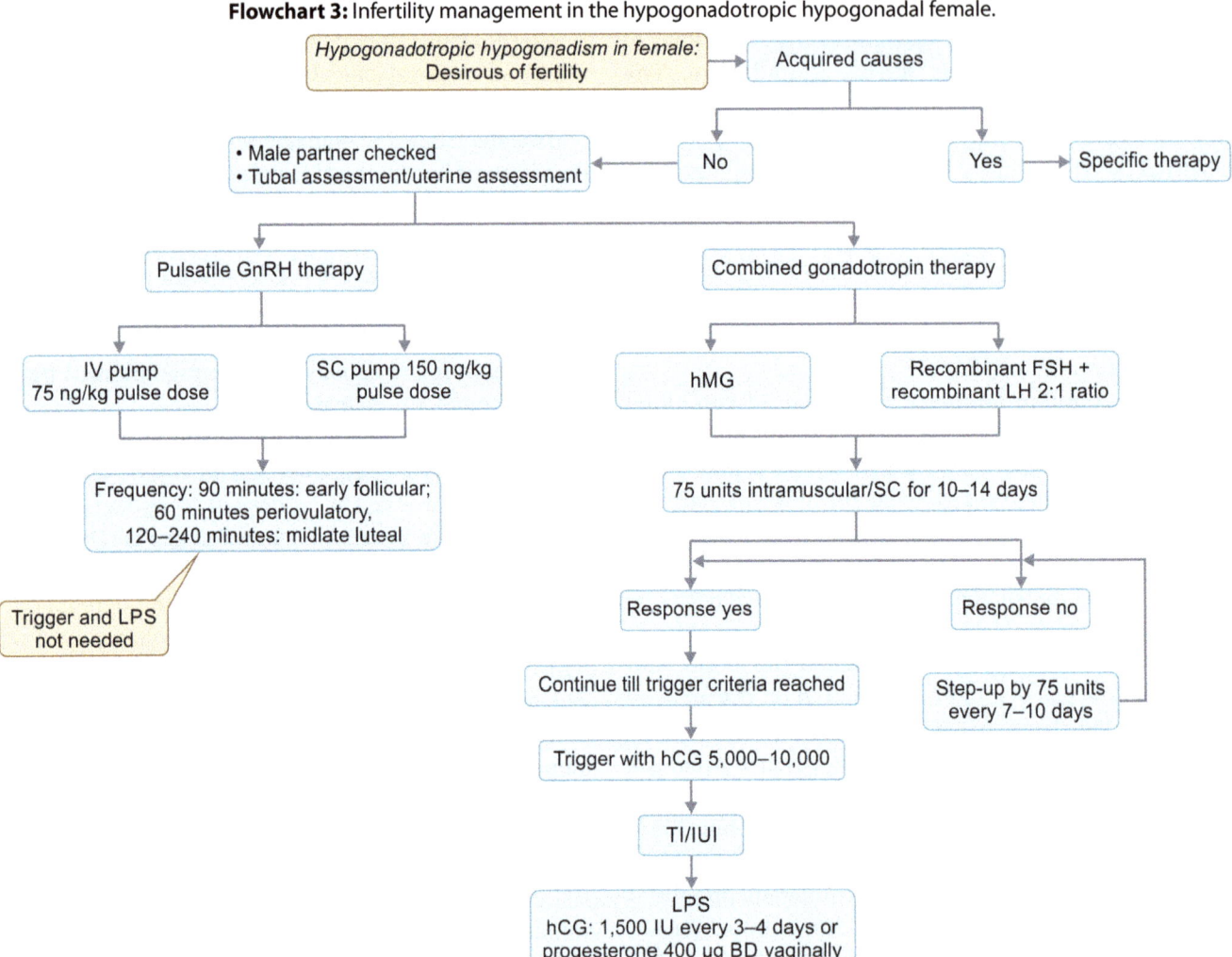

Flowchart 3: Infertility management in the hypogonadotropic hypogonadal female.

(FSH: follicle-stimulating hormone; GnRH: gonadotropin-releasing hormone; hCG: human chorionic gonadotropin; hMG: human menopausal gonadotropin; IUI: intrauterine insemination; IV: intravenous; LH: luteinizing hormone; LPS: luteal phase support; SC: subcutaneous; TI: timed intercourse)

20 days. A duration of 60 days to achieve follicular dominance has also been described during the first stimulation and physicians and women should have this knowledge to persist with treatments patiently. Subsequent cycles seem to require fewer injections.[39]

After follicular sizes of 18 mm or more are achieved, final ovulation trigger is given with an hCG injection (5,000–10,000 IU urinary or 250 μg of recombinant). GnRH agonist trigger may be used as well but would not work with pituitary causes of HH. Luteal phase needs to be supported with hCG injection 1,500–2,000 IU twice weekly if there is no risk of ovarian hyperstimulation syndrome (OHSS) or with exogenous progesterone either given vaginally (400 μg twice daily) or intramuscularly (100 mg once daily) when there is an OHSS risk. The ovulatory response rates are to the tune of 90% and pregnancy rates per cycle of about 12–27% have been achieved.[28,39] Cumulative pregnancy rates of 89% after six treatment cycles have been reported in two small series of hypogonadotropic women.[41]

If pregnancy occurs, luteal phase needs to be supported with exogenous progesterone till luteoplacental transition, which typically occurs at 8 weeks of pregnancy. Rates of multiple pregnancies are high, at about 30% and this fact alone can make HH pregnancies at high risk for preterm labor.[41] There is no evidence to suggest, however, that the course of a singleton pregnancy in the HH female is any different from a normally ovulating female.

Key Learning Points

- HH is a rare cause of infertility in men and women.
- It can be congenital or due to acquired causes.
- The congenital form manifests as absent puberty in both sexes. The acquired form manifests most commonly as secondary amenorrhea in women and azoospermia and regression of signs of virilization in men.
- When fertility is not the issue, age-appropriate doses of sex steroidal hormones are the treatment of choice in men and women.

- When fertility is the primary concern, gonadotropins or pulsatile GnRH therapy is used.
- Gonadotropins are more easily acceptable and available though could lead to multiple pregnancies and OHSS in women.
- Pulsatile GnRH therapy is a physiological way of inducing ovulation and spermatogenesis and is devoid of the side effects of multiple pregnancies and OHSS, but its use is limited by its availability and the inconvenience of having to have a pump worn over the body.

REFERENCES

1. Sigman M, Jarow JP. Endocrine evaluation of infertile men. 1997;50(5):659-64.
2. Hwang K, Walters RC, Lipshultz LI. Contemporary concepts in the evaluation and management of male infertility. Nat Rev Urol. 2011;8:86-94.
3. Bianco SD, Kaiser UB. The genetic and molecular basis of idiopathic hypogonadotropic hypogonadism. Nat Rev Endocrinol. 2009;5(10):569-76.
4. Fraietta R, Zylberstejn DS, Esteves SC. Hypogonadotropic hypogonadism revisited. Clinics (Sao Paulo). 2013; 68(Suppl 1):81-8.
5. Xu C, Cassatella D, van der Sloot AM, Quinton R, Hauschild M, De Geyter C, et al. Evaluating CHARGE syndrome in congenital hypogonadotropic hypogonadism patients harboring CHD7 variants. Genet Med. 2018;20(8):872-81.
6. Peter M, Viemann M, Partsch CJ, Sippell WG. Congenital Adrenal Hypoplasia: Clinical Spectrum, Experience with Hormonal Diagnosis, and Report on New Point Mutations of the DAX-1 Gene. J Clin Endocrinol Metab. 1998;83(8):2666-74.
7. Rojas RA, Kutateladze AA, Plummer L, Stamou M, Keefe DL Jr, Salnikov KB, et al. Phenotypic continuum between Waardenburg syndrome and idiopathic hypogonadotropic hypogonadism in humans with SOX10 variants. Genet Med. 2021;23(4):629-36.
8. Forsythe E, Beales PL. Bardet-Biedl syndrome. Eur J Hum Genet. 2013;21(1):8-13.
9. Salgado P, Carvalho R, Brandão AF, Jorge P, Ramos C, Dias D, et al. Gordon Holmes syndrome due to compound heterozygosity of two new PNPLA6 variants—a diagnostic challenge. eNeurologicalSci. 2019;14:9-12.
10. Cioppi F, Rosta V, Krausz C. Genetics of Azoospermia. Int J Mol Sci. 2021;22(6):3264.
11. Cangiano B, Swee DS, Quinton R, Bonomi M. Genetics of congenital hypogonadotropic hypogonadism: Peculiarities and phenotype of an oligogenic disease. Hum Genet. 2021;140:77-111.
12. Sykiotis GP, Plummer L, Hughes VA, Au M, Durrani S, Nayak-Young S, et al. Oligogenic basis of isolated gonadotropin-releasing hormone deficiency. Proc Natl Acad Sci USA. 2010;107:15140-4.
13. Thakker S, Persily J, Najari BB. Kallman syndrome and central non-obstructive azoospermia. Best Pract Res Clin Endocrinol Metab. 2020;34:101475.
14. Park HJ, Anabolic steroid-induced hypogonadism: a challenge for clinicians. J Exerc Rehabil. 2018;14(1):2-3.
15. Salenave S, Trabado S, Maione L, Brailly-Tabard S, Young J. Male acquired hypogonadotropic hypogonadism: diagnosis and treatment. Ann Endocrinol (Paris). 2012;73(2):141-6.
16. Boehm U, Bouloux PM, Dattani MT, de Roux N, Dodé C, Dunkel L, et al. Expert consensus document: European Consensus Statement on congenital hypogonadotropic hypogonadism—pathogenesis, diagnosis and treatment. Nat Rev Endocrinol. 2015;11:547-64.
17. Huffer V, Scott WH, Connor TB, Lovice H. Psychological studies of adult male patients with sexual infantilism before and after androgen therapy. Ann Intern Med. 1964;61:255-68.
18. Grinspon RP, Ropelato MG, Gottlieb S, Keselman A, Martínez A, Ballerini MG, et al. Basal follicle-stimulating hormone and peak gonadotropin levels after gonadotropin-releasing hormone infusion show high diagnostic accuracy in boys with suspicion of hypogonadotropic hypogonadism. J Clin Endocrinol Metab. 2010;95:2811-8.
19. Sequera AM, Fideleff HL, Boquete HR, Pujol AB, Suárez MG, Ruibal GF. Basal ultrasensitive LH assay: a useful tool in the early diagnosis of male pubertal delay? J Pediatr Endocrinol Metab. 2002;15(5):589-96.
20. Sun QH, Zheng Y, Zhang XL, Mu YM. Role of Gonadotropin-releasing Hormone Stimulation Test in Diagnosing Gonadotropin Deficiency in Both Males and Females with Delayed Puberty. Chin Med J (Engl). 2015;128(18):2439-43.
21. Pitteloud N, Hayes FJ, Dwyer A, Boepple PA, Lee H, Crowley WF Jr. Predictors of outcome of long-term GnRH therapy in men with idiopathic hypogonadotropic hypogonadism. J Clin Endocrinol Metab. 2002;87(9):4128-36.
22. Bry-Gauillard H, Larrat-Ledoux F, Levaillant JM, Massin N, Maione L, Beau I, et al. Anti-Müllerian Hormone and Ovarian Morphology in Women with Isolated Hypogonadotropic Hypogonadism/Kallmann Syndrome: Effects of Recombinant Human FSH. J Clin Endocrinol Metab. 2017;102(4):1102-11.
23. Besser GM, McNeilly AS, Anderson DC, Marshall JC, Harsoulis P, Hall R, et al. Hormonal responses to synthetic luteinizing hormone and follicle stimulating hormone-releasing hormone in man. Br Med J. 1972;3(5821):267-71.
24. Zamboni G, Antoniazzi F, Tatò L. Use of the gonadotropin-releasing hormone agonist triptorelin in the diagnosis of delayed puberty in boys. J Pediatr. 1995;126(5 Pt 1):756-8.
25. Harrington J, Palmert MR. Distinguishing Constitutional Delay of Growth and Puberty from Isolated Hypogonadotropic Hypogonadism: Critical Appraisal of Available Diagnostic Tests. J Clin Endocrinol Metab. 2012;97(9):3056-67.
26. Bozzola M, Bozzola E, Montalbano C, Stamati FA, Ferrara P, Villani A. Delayed puberty versus hypogonadism: a challenge for the pediatrician. Ann Pediatr Endocrinol Metab. 2018;23(2):57-61.
27. Practice Committee of the American Society for Reproductive Medicine. Management of nonobstructive azoospermia: a committee opinion. Fertil Steril. 2018;110(7):1239-45.
28. Young J, Xu C, Papadakis GE, Acierno JS, Maione L, Hietamäki J, et al. Clinical Management of Congenital Hypogonadotropic Hypogonadism. Endocr Rev. 2019;40(2):669-710.
29. Bhasin S, Brito JP, Cunningham GR, Hayes FJ, Hodis HN, Matsumoto AM, et al. Testosterone Therapy in Men With Hypogonadism: An Endocrine Society Clinical Practice Guideline. J Clin Endocrinol Metab. 2018;103(5):1715-44.
30. Raivio T, Falardeau J, Dwyer A, Quinton R, Hayes FJ, Hughes VA, et al. Reversal of idiopathic hypogonadotropic hypogonadism. N Engl J Med. 2007;357(9):863-73.

31. Dwyer AA, Sykiotis GP, Hayes FJ, Boepple PA, Lee H, Loughlin KR, et al. Trial of recombinant follicle-stimulating hormone pretreatment for GnRH-induced fertility in patients with congenital hypogonadotropic hypogonadism. J Clin Endocrinol Metab. 2013;98(11):E1790-5.
32. Whitten SJ, Nangia AK, Kolettis PN. Select patients with hypogonadotropic hypogonadism may respond to treatment with clomiphene citrate. Fertil Steril. 2006;86(6):1664-8.
33. Rastrelli G, Corona G, Mannucci E, Maggi M. Factors affecting spermatogenesis upon gonadotropin-replacement therapy: a meta-analytic study. Andrology. 2014;2(6):794-808.
34. Burris AS, Clark RV, Vantman DJ, Sherins RJ. A low sperm concentration does not preclude fertility in men with isolated hypogonadotropic hypogonadism after gonadotropin therapy. Fertil Steril. 1988;50:343-7.
35. Mørch LS, Skovlund CW, Hannaford PC, Iversen L, Fielding S, Lidegaard Ø. Contemporary hormonal contraception and the risk of breast cancer. N Engl J Med. 2017;377:2228-39.
36. Pask AJ, Kanasaki H, Kaiser UB, Conn PM, Janovick JA, Stockton DW, et al. A Novel Mouse Model of Hypogonadotrophic Hypogonadism: N-Ethyl-N-Nitrosourea-Induced Gonadotropin-Releasing Hormone Receptor Gene Mutation. Mol Endocrinol. 2005;19(4):972-81.
37. Filicori M, Santoro N, Merriam GR, Crowley WF Jr. Characterization of the physiological pattern of episodic gonadotropin secretion throughout the human menstrual cycle. J Clin Endocrinol Metab. 1986;62(6):1136-44.
38. Carone D, Caropreso C, Vitti A, Chiappetta R. Efficacy of different gonadotropin combinations to support ovulation induction in WHO type I anovulation infertility: clinical evidences of human recombinant FSH/human recombinant LH in a 2:1 ratio and highly purified human menopausal gonadotropin stimulation protocols. J Endocrinol Invest. 2012;35(11):996-1002.
39. Huseyin K, Berk B, Tolga K, Eser O, Ali G, Murat A. Management of ovulation induction and intrauterine insemination in infertile patients with hypogonadotropic hypogonadism. J Gynecol Obstet Hum Reprod. 2019;48(10):833-8.
40. Yasmin E, Davies M, Conway G, Balen AH. British Fertility Society: 'Ovulation induction in WHO Type 1 anovulation: Guidelines for practice' Produced on behalf of the BFS Policy and Practice Committee. Hum Fertil (Camb). 2013;16(4):228-34.
41. Tadokoro N, Vollenhoven B, Clark S, Baker G, Kovacs G, Burger H, et al. (1997). Cumulative pregnancy rates in couples with anovulatory infertility compared with unexplained infertility in an ovulation induction programme. Hum Reprod. 1997;12:1939-44.

CHAPTER 10: Management of Müllerian Anomalies

Vanita Suri, Sujata Siwatch

INTRODUCTION

Müllerian duct anomalies are abnormalities that emerge during the process of embryogenesis resulting in the abnormal development of genital tract from the paramesonephric ducts and urogenital sinus.

The prevalence of müllerian anomalies is rare and exact prevalence is unknown. Prevalence of congenital uterine anomalies has been reported as 6.7%, 7.3%, and 16.7% in general population, sterile women, and women with recurrent miscarriages respectively.[1] Septate uterus is the most common anomaly found in sterile women, while arcuate uterus is the most common among women with recurrent abortions.[1]

EMBRYOLOGY

The female reproductive tract consists of the ovaries, fallopian tubes, uterus, cervix, and vagina.[2] The müllerian or paramesonephric ducts give rise to the uterus, fallopian tubes, cervix, and upper two-thirds of the vagina while the lower vagina develops from the sinovaginal bulbs **(Fig. 1)**.[2] The embryological development of müllerian duct derivatives is completed in three phases: organogenesis or formation of two müllerian ducts, fusion of the ducts to form the uterus and resorption of the central septum. The failure of the first results in agenesis/hypoplasia of the uterus or a unicornuate uterus, defects of the second result in bicornuate or didelphys uterus and problems in the resorption result in septate or arcuate uterus.

CLASSIFICATION

There are many classification systems proposed for the classification of the müllerian duct anomalies such as the most commonly used The American Fertility Society (AFS) classification 1988, Vagina Cervix Uterus Adnexa-associated Malformation (VCUAM) classification by Oppelt, and European Society of Human Reproduction and Embryology/European Society of Gynaecological Endoscopy (ESHRE/ESGE) classification **(Table 1)**.[3-5] However, the most commonly used is the AFS classification. The recent American Society for Reproductive Medicine (ASRM) classification of 2021 has been developed by updating the simple AFS classification, focusing on including the wide spectrum of uterine, cervical, and vaginal anomalies and variants, to standardize the terminology, foster easy

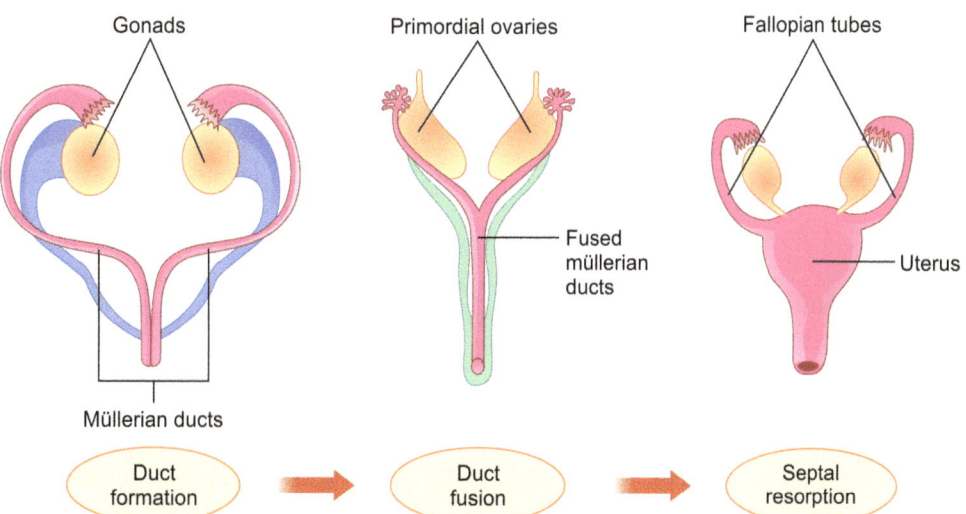

Fig. 1: Process of embryogenesis of the müllerian duct derivatives in the female genital system.

TABLE 1: The most common classifications of müllerian anomalies.

AFS classifications, 1988	ESHRE/ESGE, 2013			ASRM, 2021
• Segmental hypoplasia/agenesis • Unicornuate • Didelphys • Bicornuate • Septate • Arcuate • Diethylstilbestrol drug related	U0—normal uterus	C0—normal cervix	V0—normal vagina	• Müllerian agenesis • Cervical agenesis • Unicornuate uterus • Uterus didelphys • Bicornuate uterus • Septate uterus • Longitudinal vaginal septum • Transverse vaginal septum • Complex anomalies
	U1—dysmorphic uterus	C1—septate cervix	V1—longitudinal nonobstructing vaginal septum	
	U2—septate uterus	C2—double normal cervix	V2—longitudinal obstructing vaginal septum	
	U3—bicorporeal uterus	C3—unilateral cervical aplasia	V3—transverse vaginal septum/imperforate hymen	
	U4—hemiuterus	C4—cervical aplasia	V4—vaginal aplasia	
	U5—aplastic			
	U6—unclassified malformations			

(AFS: American Fertility Society; ASRM: American Society for Reproductive Medicine; ESGE: European Society of Gynaecological Endoscopy; ESHRE: European Society of Human Reproduction and Embryology)

communication and search ability, provide educational information to providers and patients regarding clinical, diagnosis, management and advocacy information, along with information on variants and similar lesions.[4] It is available as an interactive educational tool which has been can be accessed online. It classifies the anomalies into nine categories: müllerian agenesis, cervical agenesis, unicornuate uterus, uterus didelphys, bicornuate uterus, septate uterus, longitudinal vaginal septum, transverse vaginal septum, and complex anomalies.

■ PRESENTATION

Most müllerian anomalies are asymptomatic till puberty. Most common presentations include amenorrhea, abdominal bulge and pain, dyspareunia/apareunia, infertility/subfertility, or recurrent pregnancy losses.[1,4,6] Renal tract abnormalities and renal dysfunction may be seen in a quarter of the women, especially with unicornuate uterus.[6] Diethylstilbestrol (DES)-related anomalies have been associated with carcinomas of the vagina and lower genital tract.

■ INVESTIGATIONS

Local genital examination is of paramount significance, especially for primary amenorrhea with pain to examine for anomalies of the lower genital tract like imperforate hymen or transverse vaginal septum.[6] Radiological imaging is also of great importance in the diagnosis of müllerian anomalies. 2D ultrasound is the initial and most commonly used imaging modality which lacks radiation exposure.[1,2,6] It is simple, easily available but operator dependent and limited by large patient profile and overlying bowel gas. The 3D ultrasound provides more reliable and detailed information with more interobserver reproducibility. However, it is more expensive, needs expert training and is not easily available.

Magnetic resonance imaging (MRI) is considered the best diagnostic imaging with higher sensitivity and reliability.[1,2,6] It is radiation free and provides most accurate information on external and internal profile of genital malformations including obstructive lesions, though tubal anomalies may not be clearly elucidated. Moreover, it is expensive, takes more time, and requires trained personnel.

Sonohysterosalpingography has also used to study uterine and cervical anomalies, it is operator dependent and uterine expansion may change the internal uterine contour and create false-negative images.[6] X-ray hysterosalpingography can provide useful information on the internal contour of the uterine cavity and tubal patency. But, it provides little information on the external contour of the uterus like the presence of noncommunicating rudimentary horn, or differentiates between septate and bicornuate uterus. Moreover, it is a painful and invasive procedure.

Hysteroscopy is a minimally invasive surgical procedure which provides a detailed actual internal examination of the uterus, cervix, and vagina. However, laparoscopy may be needed to evaluate the external contour of the uterus and cervix.

■ MANAGEMENT

Management of the uterine anomalies is tailored individually to the requirements and presentation of the woman, age, and fertility concerns.[7] **Flowchart 1** provides a symptom based

Flowchart 1: A symptom-based algorithm for the management of müllerian anomalies.

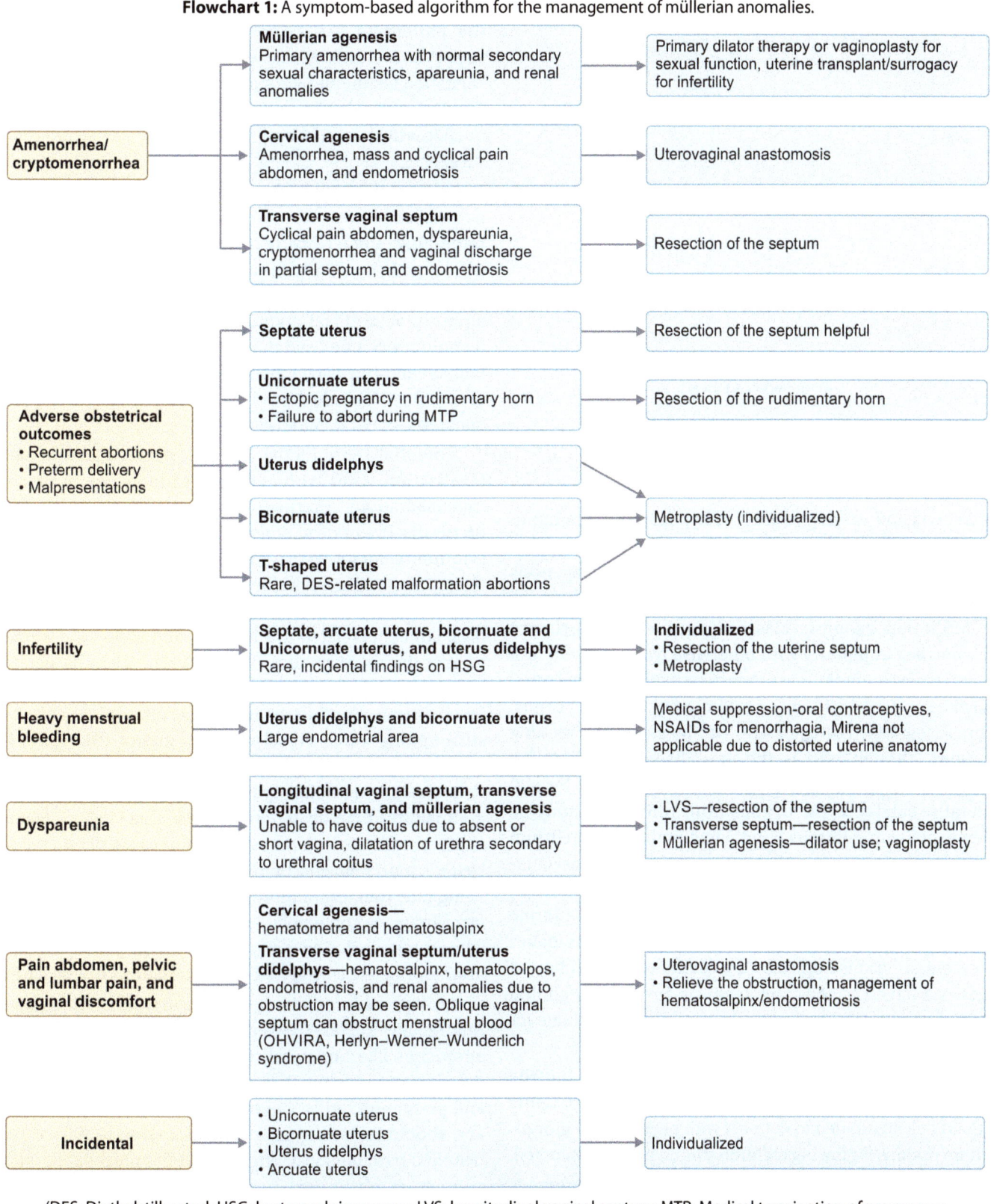

(DES: Diethylstilbestrol; HSG: hysterosalpingogram; LVS: longitudinal vaginal septum; MTP: Medical termination of pregnancy; NSAIDs: Nonsteroidal anti-inflammatory drugs; OHVIRA: obstructed hemivagina and ipsilateral renal anomaly)

algorithm for the management of müllerian anomalies. The women, especially with müllerian and cervical agenesis should be carefully and empathetically counseled and encouraged to connect with peer groups of similar anomalies, as accepting the diagnosis and the comprehending the treatment can be very emotionally challenging for these young women. The primary surgery is the most significant and should be done by experienced surgeons.

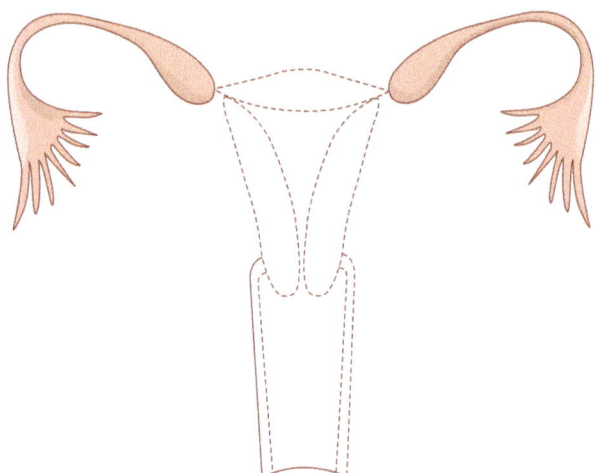

Fig. 2: Absence of uterus cervix and upper vagina seen in müllerian agenesis.

Müllerian Agenesis

This müllerian anomaly is characterized by absence of uterus and cervix and varying degrees of hypoplasia of the upper vagina **(Fig. 2)**. Its variants may present with hypoplasia of unilateral of bilateral uterine remnants. Müllerian agenesis is reported in 1:4,500–1:5,000 women.[8]

Müllerian agenesis classically presents as primary amenorrhea at puberty with otherwise typical growth and pubertal development.[9] On pelvic examination, vaginal canal may be shortened with no or rudimentary uterus of cervix. Ultrasonography (USG) or MRI can be used for screening imaging, though MRI is the nest diagnostic modality. Rudimentary uterine remnants are seen in 75–95%, located laterally, caudal to the ovaries from which they may be connected with a fibrous band. Functioning endometrium is infrequently seen in unilateral rudimentary horns. One-third women may have unilateral or bilateral ectopic ovaries in the inguinal canal or iliac fossa with associated uterine remnants.[4] Evaluation for associated congenital anomalies is essential because up to 53% of patients with müllerian agenesis have concomitant renal or skeletal congenital malformations. USG abdomen must be done to evaluate for aplastic or ectopic kidneys.[4]

Management is directed to the presentation and the patient's needs after adequate counseling. All patients should be encouraged to connect with peer support groups. Future options for having children should be also discussed.

For creation of neovagina, dilators and surgical methods can be used. Primary vaginal elongation by dilation is the appropriate first-line approach in most patients because it is patient-controlled, more cost-effective, and avoids the complications of surgery. Progressive dilators are used at vaginal introitus, typically for 15–20 minutes one to two times a day, for a period of months.[6] The commonly used techniques include Frank technique, Ingram technique, or with dilators attached to cycle seat.[6] These can be taught to the patient to use as self-practice, with intermittent supervision and assessment for proper technique. Dilatation techniques are successful for >90–96% of women. Thus, surgery should be used for the rare patient who is unsuccessful with primary dilator therapy or who prefers surgery.[4]

Surgical treatment, when indicated, includes creation of neovagina between the urethra/bladder and the rectum posteriorly. The reconstruction may be done with insertion of inlay graft, i.e., McIndoe vaginoplasty—split thickness skin graft, full thickness skin graft, buccal mucosa, peritoneum, amnion, or artificial grafts. Alternately, surgical traction techniques can be used that include Vecchietti procedure, Balloon and vulvovaginoplasty (William's procedure). Other techniques include bowel vaginoplasty and Wharton-Sheares-George vaginoplasty.

Potential reproductive options may include in vitro fertilization (IVF) with surrogacy and IVF with uterine transplantation.[10] Uterine transplant is a surgery in which uterus of a live or dead donor is harvested and transplanted into the recipient. Ever since the first transplant in 2000, about 70 procedures have been performed resulting in about 23 live births.[10] Albeit it circumferents the religious and legal concerns related to surrogacy and allows the woman to experience pregnancy, it comes with risks associated with surgery and immunosuppression. Uterine transplant involves transplanting the uterus, cervix, vaginal cuff, and surrounding blood vessels and ligaments. Presence of a functionally normal vagina helps in providing innate immune response. Living donor grafts have been related to fewer graft failures than dead donor transplants (75% vs. 56%).[10] Graft thrombosis is the most common cause of emergency hysterectomy following uterine transplantation, other causes being infection. Commonly used immunosuppressants are tacrolimus, mycophenolate mofetil, and steroids. However, when contemplating pregnancy, tacrolimus along with azathioprine are considered safer alternatives for the fetus.

Most procedures have been done in women with Mayer-Rokitansky-Küster-Hauser (MRKH).[10] Associated renal anomalies like unilateral renal agenesis may predispose the woman to higher chances of developing preeclampsia and premature births. Counseling is of utmost importance and should including extensive discussion of risks versus benefits; psychological, ethical, and financial deliberation apart from obstetrical considerations such as need for cesarean section, chances of successful pregnancy, risks to fetus due to immunosuppressant, and prematurity related to preeclampsia and multiple gestation. Pregnancy is usually planned using IVF and embryos frozen prior to the transplantation. Embryo transfer is usually done about 6 months after the surgery to allow for healing and graft stabilization. Hysterectomy is done after the pregnancy to avoid need for prolonged immunosuppression and its side effects. Though the number of live births is still few, the scientific research looks forward to bioengineered uterine grafts that would potentially minimize the risks to both donors and recipients.

Cervical Agenesis

This developmental disorder manifests with the absence of cervix.[4] Variations include less developed nonfunctional cervix termed cervical dysgenesis or cervical atresia. Congenital cervical atresia occurs in 1:80,000–1:100,000 women.[6] Typically, pubertal age women may present with primary amenorrhea, cyclical regular, or episodic pelvic pain due to uterine distension during menstruation. The lower abdomen may be tender and vagina may be normal or shortened. Cervix is not visualized **(Fig. 3)**.

This entity needs to be differentiated from transverse vaginal septum, MRKH with uterine remnants, and imperforate hymen. MRI T2-weighted images are most useful to ascertain absence of cervix with or without fibrous remnant and to determine the distance between endometrial canal and apex of blind vagina. Hematometra may be seen with functional uterine endometrium. USG may show discontinuity between uterus and normal trilaminar vagina. Treatment incorporates medical suppression with continuous combined contraceptives for pain due to obstructed uterus. Medical therapy may be helpful while confirming the diagnosis, counseling, and planning management. This is followed by surgery for canalizing the vaginal outflow tract. In case of associated vaginal agenesis, vaginal dilatation techniques or surgery needs to be done first for neovaginal reconstruction followed by uterovaginal anastomosis. Surgical expertise of specialist is important for the outcome. Alternately, hysterectomy may be done if the patient does not desire pregnancy, after proper counseling.

Unicornuate Uterus

This congenital maldevelopmental disorder presents with single hemiuterus, cervix, and vagina, developing from one side, while other side müllerian duct derivatives do not develop or are hypoplastic as a rudimentary horn with or without functional endometrium **(Figs. 4A to C)**. It is seen in 1;5,400 women, constituting 0.3–4% of müllerian anomalies.[6]

The women with unicornuate uterus have normal menstruation, but may have lateralized cyclical pelvic pain from obstructed rudimentary horn with functional endometrium. This condition is associated with pregnancy concerns such as preterm labor, malpresentation, and pregnancy loss or may be an incidental finding. Pregnancy in rudimentary horn is rare, but reported in literature. Examination reveals a normal cervix and vagina. Functional uterus is deviated to one side and contralateral uterine remnant may present as adnexal mass. The contralateral ovary may also be at abnormal location.

Three-dimensional (3D) ultrasound and MRI are helpful. MRI is the best diagnostic imaging using T2-weighted oblique images along the long axis of the endometrium, axial, and coronal obliques to assess for rudimentary horn.[4] The uterus is seen as elliptical, small, deviated to one side, and tapering into single cornua. Associated rudimentary horn is seen in 70%, with no endometrial tissue or noncommunicating horn with functional endometrium, close or away from uterus with a fibrous remnant connection. Ectopic or absent kidney may be seen in 40% of cases.

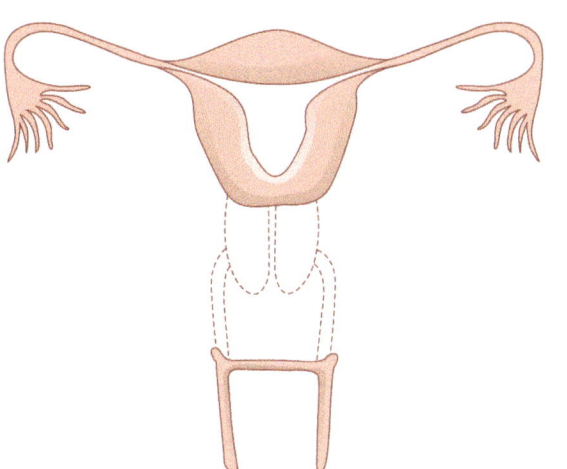

Fig. 3: Cervical agenesis.

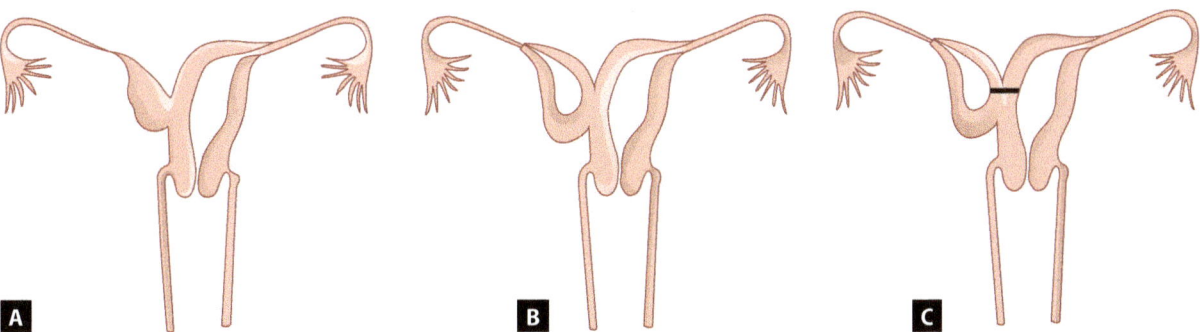

Figs. 4A to C: Unicornuate uterus. (A) R/L unicornuate uterus with R/L associated atrophic uterine remnant; (B) R/L unicornuate uterus with R/L associated atrophic uterine remnant with functional endometrium; (C) R/L unicornuate uterus with R/L uterine body communicating cavities.

Surgical management includes resection of non-communicating uterine remnant with functional endometrium or resection of communicating uterine remnant with functional endometrium for pain relief and to prevent ectopic pregnancy in the horn. Ipsilateral salpingectomy is also recommended in literature.[11] Medical suppression may be useful as adjuvant therapy in individual patients.

Uterus Didelphys

Nonfusion of embryonic müllerian ducts results in this maldevelopment entity of female genital system. It is characterized with two separate uterine bodies, two separate cervices, and may even have a two vaginal cavities separated by a longitudinal vaginal septum **(Fig. 5)**.[6] It comprises 11% of müllerian anomalies.[12]

It is usually asymptomatic, often identified due to obstetrical problems such as preterm labor, malpresentation, and pregnancy loss or due to longitudinal vaginal septum when it presents as dyspareunia, menstrual leakage with tampon use, vaginal discharge, or lateralized pain due to obstructed vaginal septum.[4] On examination, the uterus is widely splayed, there may be two symmetrical or asymmetrical vaginas, cervices, and there may be renal anomalies. USG and MRI are useful imaging modalities which may show two uterus and cervix with and without duplicated vagina. The vaginal septum may be oblique and cause menstrual blood obstruction hematometrocolpos, hematosalpinx, endometriosis, and collection in vagina [e.g., in obstructed hemivagina and ipsilateral renal anomaly (OHVIRA) syndrome] may be seen. When also associated with ipsilateral renal agenesis, it is termed Herlyn–Werner–Wunderlich syndrome.[6] Obstetrical complications like preterm labor may occur but overall prognosis is good.[6] Management may include medical uterine suppression, resection of obstructing vaginal septum, and resection of hemiuterus if associated with obstructed cervix.

Bicornuate Uterus

This developmental anomaly presents as two partially separate uterine bodies, with external fundal indentation of >1 cm, some unification of lower uterine aspect with single cervix and vagina **(Fig. 6)**. It occurs because the upper portions of the müllerian ducts fail to fuse while the caudal portion fuses and develops normally into the lower uterine segment, cervix, and vagina. It constitutes 10% of müllerian anomalies.[6,13]

The entity may be asymptomatic or present with preterm labor, malpresentations, and pregnancy loss. Duplicated cervix and vagina may be associated. The uterine fundus is wide and fundal indentation may be palpable. Ultrasounds, MRI, saline infusion sonography, and hysteroscopy combined with imaging are helpful for diagnosis.[13] Septate uterus should be differentiated from bicornuate uterus, the former being seven times more common.

Surgical options may include reunification in rare cases using Strassman metroplasty, Jones metroplasty, or Tompkins metroplasty. Resection of associated vaginal septum may also be required.[4]

Septate Uterus

Septate uterus includes a single uterine body externally along with single cervix and vagina **(Figs. 7A to E)**. The internal cavity is divided by a fibromuscular septum from the fundus extending to the internal cervical os or further. This anomaly develops due to the failure of resorption of the uterine septum.[4] It represents 55% of müllerian malformations.[6]

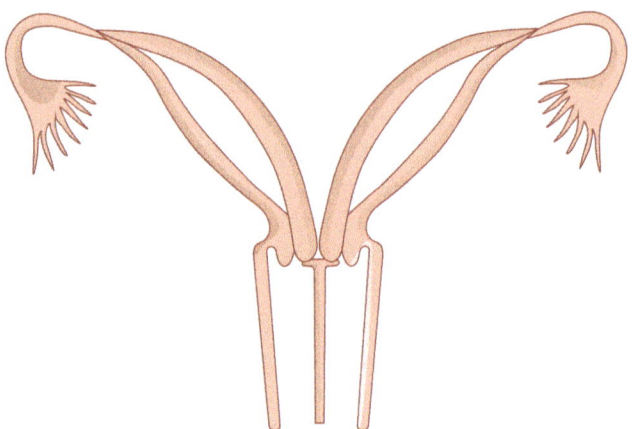

Fig. 5: Uterus didelphys with two uterine cavities, cervix, and septate vagina.

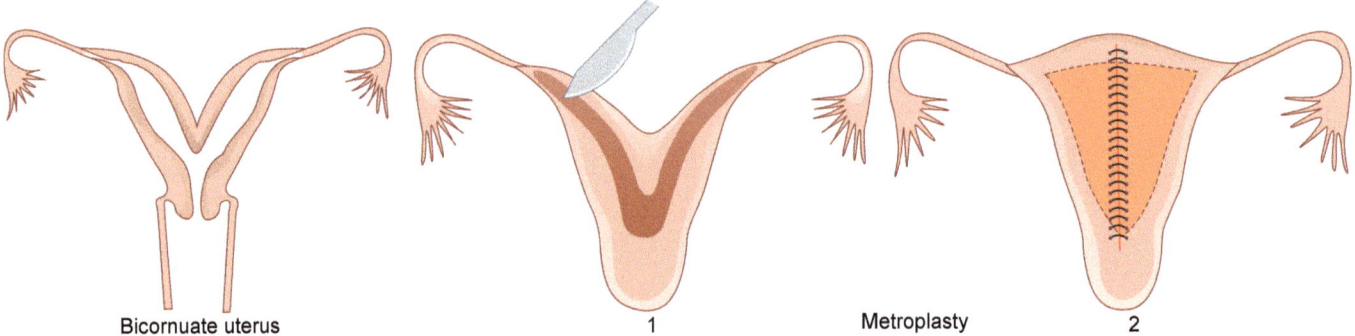

Fig. 6: Bicornuate uterus with two cavities and indentation at the fundus of >1 cm. Metroplasty has been described but its role is controversial.

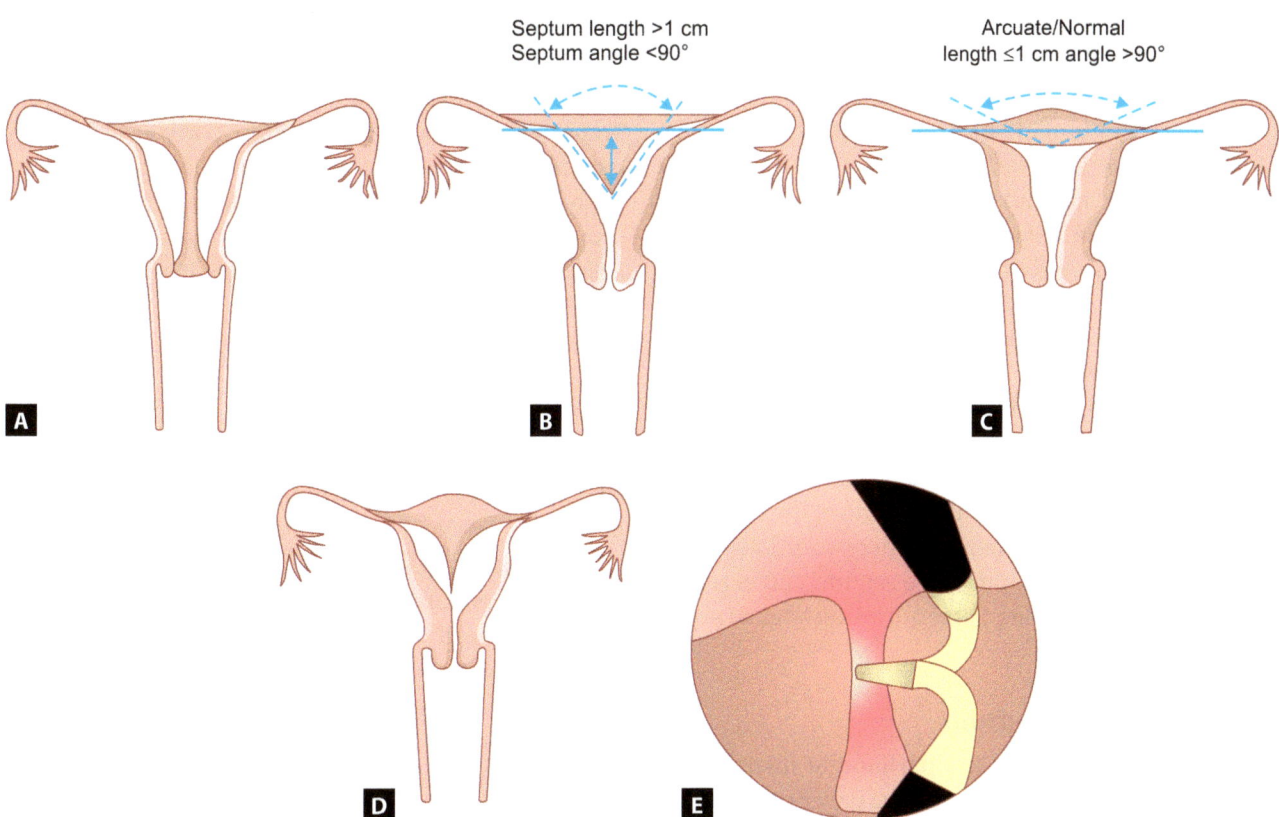

Figs. 7A to E: Septate uterus has two cavities separated by a muscular or fibrous septum from the fundus and extending into the uterine cavity to variable lengths of the uterus (A) to the cervical os in complete septate uterus, (B) short of the cervical os in partial septum (C) of <1 cm in arcuate uterus, (D) Robert's uterus with single external uterine body with wide fundus, external midline fundal indentation of <1 cm and endometrial cavity divided into two—one side occluded above external os and other side has patent outflow tract, and (E) hysteroscopic septal resection with resectoscope.

The septum is defined as having a depth of >1 cm with a <90° or acute angle of leading edge of the septum.[4] Variants include, among others, partial septate uterus, arcuate uterus with fundal indentation of <1 cm and angle of leading edge of >90° between the two uterine cavities, Robert's uterus with single external uterine body with wide fundus, external midline fundal indentation of <1 cm, and endometrial cavity divided into two—one side occluded above external os and other side has patent outflow tract.

They are usually asymptomatic, but may present with severe dysmenorrhea in obstructed Robert's uterus. Septate uterus is associated with the worst adverse pregnancy prognosis with complications such as pregnancy loss, preterm labor, and malpresentations. Pelvic examination may reveal a normal vagina, cervix, and uterine contour or may have duplicated/septate cervix or longitudinal vaginal septum. Ultrasounds, MRI, sonosalpingography, hysterosalpingogram (HSG), and hystseroscopy are useful for identification. 3D US and 3D T2-weighted MRI use helps identify better the long axis of the uterus.[4] Surgical treatment may involve hysteroscopic resection of the uterine septum with or without cervical septum with or without vaginal septal resection, as required. Other surgical procedures that find mention include hysteroscopy metroplasty.[14] Arcuate uterus does not require surgical correction.

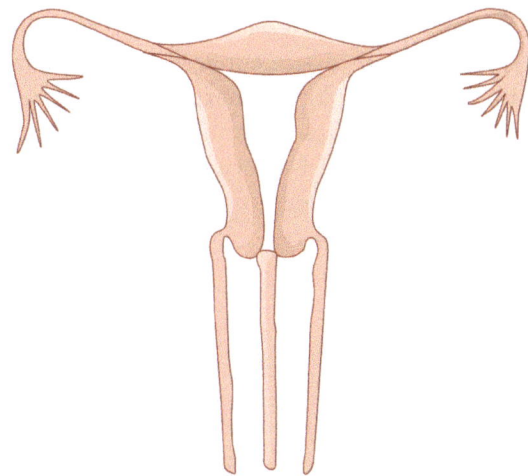

Fig. 8: A longitudinal vaginal septum.

Longitudinal Vaginal Septumv

Longitudinal vaginal septum or double/duplicate vagina manifests with a partition along the long axis, creating two vaginal canals, the septum being partial or extending in full vaginal length, creating two vaginal canals **(Fig. 8)**. This anomaly results due to the incomplete fusion of the lower parts of the müllerian ducts. Its variants include obstructed unilateral hemivagina and uterus bicornuate bicollis and bicornuate bicollis uterus with obstructed unilateral hemivagina.

Without causing obstruction to menstrual flow, they may remain asymptomatic or present with dyspareunia, menstrual leakage with tampon use, or laceration with intercourse. However, with obstruction, the woman may experience lateralized pelvic pain from hematometrocolpos, cyclical or chronic pelvic pain, or abnormal uterine bleeding from microperforate vaginal obstruction.[4] Vaginal septum with or without pelvic mass may be seen on pelvic examination. It should be differentiated from incomplete transverse vaginal septum and vaginal adhesions.

Ultrasound and MRI can be useful though MRI T2-weighted images in axial plane are best. Application of aqueous vaginal gel to distend at least one of the cavities is helpful. Fibrous vaginal septum in upper two-thirds vagina may be seen with inferior transverse septum and cervical/uterine septa or duplications. Surgery involves vaginal septal resection.

Transverse Vaginal Septum

A transverse vaginal septum is a partition or interruption across the vagina in the upper, mid, or lower part formed when the müllerian ducts do not fuse normally to the urogenital sinus **(Fig. 9)**. It may be thin or thick, complete or partial, and results in outflow obstruction. Its reported prevalence is 1:2,100–1:72,000 women.[6]

Complete septum presents at puberty with primary amenorrhea, cyclical or intermittent pelvic pain due to hematometrocolpos. Partial septum may be asymptomatic or may present with dyspareunia, difficulty in tampon use, abnormal vaginal discharge, and intermittent pain from hematocolpos in cases of microperforations. On examination, vagina is shortened, cervix is not seen, and hematocolpos pelvic mass may be seen. Partial vaginal opening may range from pinpoint to vaginal band. This condition should be differentiated from imperforate hymen, distal vaginal atresia, and vaginal malignancy, among others. Transabdominal sonography (TAS) may show discontinuity between the uterine corpus and normal trilaminar vaginal appearance. MRI T2-weighted sagittal images are best to find distance between endocervical canal and vaginal apex while axial images to assess for presence of fibrous remnant and associated vaginal agenesis. Treatment involves resection of septum, pre- and postoperative use of dilators.

Complex Müllerian Anomalies

This category that finds its mention in the ASRM classification 2021 is not well defined and represents unusual combinations of uterine, cervical, and vaginal anomalies. These include uterus isthmus agenesis, bicornuate uterus with bilateral obstructed endometrial cavities, obstructed hemivagina, hemiuterus and single cervix and separate contralateral patent hemiuterus, cervix and vagina, etc. Diagnosis may involve examination under anesthesia (EUA), additional imaging, and interaction of experienced radiologists and clinicians. Surgery should be performed by experienced surgeons.

CONCLUSION

Müllerian anomalies are rare developmental anomalies of female genital system that may present with recurrent pregnancy losses, prematurity and rarely infertility. MRI is most useful for diagnosis. Management is tailored according to the manifestations.

ACKNOWLEDGMENTS

We are thankful to Mr Dharamjit Singh, Senior Artist, PGIMER for contributing the illustrations.

Key Learning Points

- Müllerian anomalies are rare developmental anomalies of the female genital system with a reported prevalence of 0.5–6.7%.
- Various classification systems have been proposed of which the most used include the AFS system, ESHRE/ESGE classification and the recent ASRM 2021 classification.
- They can be asymptomatic, though common symptoms include adverse pregnancy outcomes i.e. recurrent pregnancy losses, prematurity and malpresentations or even infertility.
- MRI is the most useful imaging investigation.
- Treatment is individualized and surgery should be done by skilled professional with expertise.

REFERENCES

1. Saravelos SH, Cocksedge KA, Li TC. Prevalence and diagnosis of congenital uterine anomalies in women with reproductive failure: a critical appraisal. Human reproduction update. 2008;14(5):415-29.

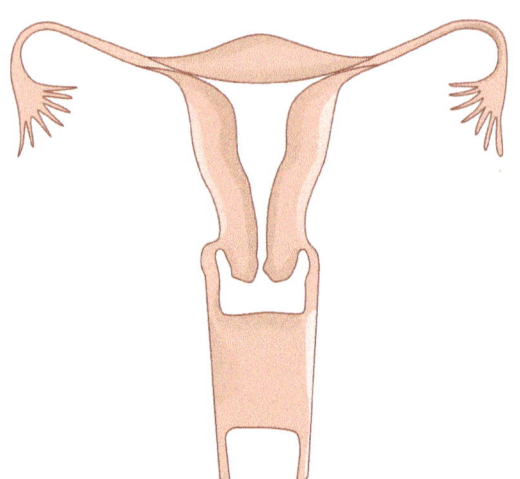

Fig. 9: A transverse vaginal septum is a partition, complete, or perforated, with variable thickness across the vagina in the upper, mid, or lower part.

2. Chandler TM, Machan LS, Cooperberg PL, Harris AC, Chang SD. Mullerian duct anomalies: from diagnosis to intervention. Br J Radiol. 2009;82(984):1034-42.
3. Grimbizis GF, Di Spiezio Sardo A, Saravelos SH, Gordts S, Exacoustos C, Van Schoubroeck D, et al. The Thessaloniki ESHRE/ESGE consensus on diagnosis of female genital anomalies. Gynecol Surg. 2016;13:1-16.
4. Pfeifer SM, Attaran M, Goldstein J, Lindheim SR, Petrozza JC, Rackow BW, et al. ASRM müllerian anomalies classification 2021. Fertil Steril. 2021;116(5):1238-52.
5. Detti L, Peregrin-Alvarez I, Roman RA, Levi D'Ancona R, Gordon JC, Christiansen ME. A comparison of four systems for uterine septum diagnosis and indication for surgical correction. Minerva Obstet Gynecol. 2021;73(3):376-83.
6. Passos I, Britto RL. Diagnosis and treatment of müllerian malformations. Taiwan J Obstet Gynecol. 2020;59(2):183-8.
7. Theodoridis TD, Pappas PD, Grimbizis GF. Surgical management of congenital uterine anomalies (including indications and surgical techniques). Best Pract Res Clin Obstet Gynaecol. 2019;59:66-76.
8. ACOG Committee Opinion No. 728: Müllerian Agenesis: Diagnosis, Management, And Treatment. Obstet Gynecol. 2018;131(1):e35-42.
9. Kaur J, Walia R, Jain V, Bhansali A, Vatsa R, Siwatch S. Clinical indicators to define etiology in patients with primary amenorrhea: Lessons from a decade of experience. J Family Med Prim Care. 2020;9(8):3986-90.
10. Jones BP, Saso S, Yazbek J, Thum MY, Quiroga I, Ghaem-Maghami S, et al. Uterine Transplantation: Scientific Impact Paper No. 65 April 2021. BJOG. 2021;128(10):e51-66.
11. Siwatch S, Mehra R, Pandher DK, Huria A. Rudimentary horn pregnancy: a 10-year experience and review of literature. Arch Gynecol Obstet. 2013;287(4):687-95.
12. Khaladkar SM, Kamal V, Kamal A, Kondapavuluri SK. The Herlyn-Werner-Wunderlich Syndrome—A Case Report with Radiological Review. Pol J Radiol. 2016;81:395-400.
13. Yoo RE, Cho JY, Kim SY, Kim SH. A systematic approach to the magnetic resonance imaging-based differential diagnosis of congenital Müllerian duct anomalies and their mimics. Abdom Imaging. 2015;40(1):192-206.
14. Valle RF, Ekpo GE. Hysteroscopic metroplasty for the septate uterus: review and meta-analysis. J Minim Invasive Gynecol. 2013;20(1):22-42.

CHAPTER 11

Pelvic TB—Work-up and Management

JB Sharma, Mansi Deoghare, Sona Dharmendra

INTRODUCTION

Female genital tuberculosis (FGTB) is a chronic infectious disease of female genital tract due to *Mycobacterium tuberculosis* (rarely *Mycobacterium bovis* from unpasteurized infected milk).[1] It causes significant morbidity, like irregular menstruation, pelvic pain, tubo-ovarian mass, and infertility particularly in Southeast Asia and Africa.[2,3] FGTB usually occurs secondary to pulmonary tuberculosis (TB) through hematogenous route or lymphatic route. It can also occur through spread from adjacent ileocecal TB and rarely through infected semen from tuberculous orchitis in males.[4] In FGTB, fallopian tubes are mostly commonly affected (90–100%) followed by uterus (70%), ovaries (30%), cervix (10%), and rarely vulva and vagina (1% each).[1] FGTB can cause permanent damage to female genital tract in advanced stages. Hence, early diagnosis and treatment in subclinical stage can prevent permanent damage and sequelae of female genital tract with successful pregnancy outcome.[5]

The prevalence of FGTB in infertility patients varies from country to country, and is around 6–25% in India being more in tertiary referral centers and in assisted reproduction centers.[6]

CLINICAL FEATURES OF FEMALE GENITAL TUBERCULOSIS

Female genital tuberculosis is asymptomatic in 10–12% cases. The clinical features of FGTB are listed in **Box 1**.

DIAGNOSIS OF FEMALE GENITAL TUBERCULOSIS

As FGTB can be asymptomatic and may mimic many other diseases, its diagnosis may be missed in many women, especially in early stages. Hence, a high index of suspicion is needed. A detailed history and examination should be done. Investigations are as follows:

- Complete blood count (CBC) with erythrocyte sedimentation rate (ESR), blood sugar fasting and postprandial (PP), renal function test (RFT), and liver function test (LFT)

BOX 1: Clinical features of female genital tuberculosis (FGTB).

Symptoms
- Asymptomatic (10–12%)
- Menstrual disorders:
  - Abnormal uterine bleeding (in early stages)
  - Postmenopausal bleeding
  - Oligomenorrhea
  - Hypomenorrhea
  - Amenorrhea
  - Dysmenorrhea
- Lower abdominal pain
- Chronic pelvic pain
- Abdominal distension
- Infertility (common)
- Abnormal vaginal discharge
- Constitutional symptoms (not always present):
  - Pyrexia
  - Weight loss
  - Loss of appetite
  - Malaise
  - Night sweats
- Symptoms of tuberculosis (TB) of other sites:
  - Cough
  - Expectoration
  - Hemoptysis
  - Chest pain

Signs
- No obvious signs (10–12%)
- Pallor
- Signs of other sites of TB like rhonchi, crepitations, lymphadenopathy, arthritis, etc.
- Adnexal mass and tenderness (unilateral or bilateral)
- Cervical/vaginal/vulvar growth
- Abnormal vaginal discharge, pus coming out of cervix, uterine enlargement in case of pyometra
- Unusual features like vesicovaginal or rectovaginal fistula

- Human immunodeficiency virus serology
- *Mantoux test:* A value of >10 mm may give some clue but is not reliable
- Interferon gamma release assay (IGRA), available as QuantiFERON-TB Gold done on whole blood
- *Serum CA-125:* A level of >35 IU/L may be seen in FGTB
- X-ray chest for any active or old healed pulmonary TB

- *Endometrial aspirate or biopsy:* It is the most important test. Various tests can be done on it as follows:[7]
  - Acid-fast bacilli (AFB) microscopy using Ziehl–Neelsen (ZN) staining. It is a traditional method and lacks sensitivity
  - *AFB culture:* It is gold standard, but takes long time up to 6 weeks to grow. The various medias used are traditional egg-based media like Lowenstein–Jensen (LJ) media, BACTEC 460 radiometric culture system, BACTEC-MGIT 960 system, and Versa TREK liquid based culture system.
  - *Cartridge-based nucleic acid amplification (CB-NAAT) or GeneXpert:* It can detect as low as 133 colony-forming units (CFU)/mL of specimen and is used to diagnose TB and can detect rifampicin resistance within 2 hours. It has sensitivity of 30% and specificity of almost 100% in diagnosing FGTB. Xpert Ultra is a newer test with higher sensitivity.[8]
  - *Polymerase chain reaction (PCR):* It is sensitive and specific test to diagnose TB, but it has a drawback that it remains positive in cases of treated TB and while on antituberculosis treatment (ATT). It is used as a supportive evidence to investigate further for diagnosis of TB.[9]
  - *Loop-mediated isothermal amplification (LAMP):* It has higher sensitivity of about 40% for detecting FGTB but cannot detect drug resistance.[10]
  - *Molecular line probe assays (LPA):* They have been recommended by the WHO for rapid diagnosis of multidrug-resistant TB including FGTB and can detect drug sensitivity also.
  - *Histopathology:* Endometrial aspirate sample is fixed in 10% formalin for detection of epithelioid granulomas. It has almost 100% specificity, though sensitivity is less.[9] As endometrium is shed during menstruation, typical caseation is rare in FGTB.
- *Newer molecular methods:*
  - Next-generation sequencing (NGS) technology can allow acute and rapid sequencing of entire genome of *Mycobacterium* and thus can help in diagnosis and treatment of TB. But it is not routinely available yet.
  - *Nuclear receptors:* They can be used as a biomarker for early detection of FGTB, as nuclear receptors have important role in maintenance of uterine receptivity and immune modulation, especially latent FGTB but they are still in experimental stage.[11]
- *Radiological tests:*
  - *Hysterosalpingography (HSG):* To avoid flare-up of TB, it should be avoided in acute disease. On HSG, various signs of FGTB can be blocked tubes, beaded tubes, tobacco-pouch appearance of tubes, and filling defects in uterine cavity can be seen.
  - *Ultrasound:* Hydrosalpinx can be seen which is visualized as tubal dilatation with septae due to tubal mucosal thickening (cogwheel appearance). Endometritis due to TB, if present may be seen as thin, diffuse endometrial image with irregular borders with fluid accumulation in uterine cavity.
  - *CT, MRI, and positron emission tomography (PET):* One of the three modalities can be used for tuberculous tubo-ovarian masses.
- *Endoscopic techniques:*
  - *Diagnostic laparoscopy:* Considered as gold standard method and is used to detect FGTB by direct visualization of TB lesions. The various new signs that can be seen in TB are perihepatic adhesions and Sharma's hanging gallbladder sign, Sharma's ascending colonic adhesion, Sharma's sigmoid colonic adhesive band, Sharma's parachute sign (adhesions of ascending colon to abdominal wall), and Sharma's compartmentalization sign (multiple compartments are formed by omental adhesions to contain infection).[12-16] Distended fallopian tubes with alternate constrictions and dilatations can also be seen and on dye test tubes can be seen resembling blue python in FGTB cases (Sharma's blue python sign).[17] There can also be fusion of both fallopian tubes due to FGTB (Sharma's kissing fallopian tubes sign).
  - *Hysteroscopy:* It is usually done concomitantly with laparoscopy. It is direct visualization of endometrial cavity. The various TB lesions on hysteroscopy are pale endometrium, caseous nodules, chronic endometritis, edema, micropolyps, varying grades of intrauterine adhesions and distorted and shrunken uterine cavity with obliterated ostia.

MANAGEMENT

Treatment of FGTB is similar to pulmonary TB and is given for total 6 months. It consists of four drugs regimen with rifampicin (r), isoniazid (h), pyrazinamide (z), and ethambutol (E) daily orally for first 2 months of intensive phase.[1] In the continuation phase, three-drug regimen (unlike two drugs in past) is given using rifampicin (R), isoniazid (I), and ethambutol (E) orally daily for next 4 months.[1] Even patients with irregular treatment or defaulters are treated with the earlier mentioned regimen in the case of drug-sensitive TB. The weight wise doses of drugs are as in **Table 1**. All women should be carefully monitored for adherence to treatment and any side effects, especially hepatotoxicity with rifampicin, isoniazid, pyrazinamide, ocular toxicity with ethambutol or peripheral neuritis (with isoniazid). Pyridoxine can be given for any neuritis, and liver function tests should be performed after 3 months of ATT on suspicion of hepatotoxicity. Treatment should preferably

TABLE 1: Drug sensitive female genital tuberculosis (FGTB), dosage of drugs in terms of number of tablets to be taken per day as per weight bands.

Weight category	Intensive phase HRZE 75 mg/150 mg/400 mg/275 mg per FDC tablet (2 months) oral daily treatment	Continuation-phase HRE 75 mg/150 mg/275 mg per FDC tablet (4 months) oral daily treatment	Streptomycin* (g)
25–39 kg	2	2	0.5
40–54 kg	3	3	0.75
55–69 kg	4	4	1
≥70 kg	5	5	1

*Streptomycin is given only for adverse drug reaction to first-line drugs like drug-induced hepatitis when HRZ are withheld and streptomycin, ethambutol, and levofloxacin are given till liver function tests (LFT) return to normal, when RHZ are added sequentially under LFT monitoring.

be directly observed treatment short-course (DOTS) with quality assured free medicines from government DOTS centers present all over India under National TB Elimination Program (previously called Revised National TB Control Program).

CONCLUSION

Female genital tuberculosis is one of the important cause of infertility, especially in developing countries. As there is no single test which is sensitive and specific for the diagnosis of FGTB, a combination of tests should be used to increase the detection rate of FGTB. A high index of suspicion should be kept, especially for women having hypomenorrhea, infertility, and women having past or family history of TB. Treatment of drug sensitivity FGTB is essentially medical using four drugs (RHZE) daily orally for 2 months followed by three drugs (HRE) daily orally for next 4 months (total 6 months).

Key Learning Points

- Female genital TB affects the tubes, uterus, ovaries, and other organs.
- Advanced stages can lead to permanent damage to genital organs leading to infertility.
- There is no single diagnostic test, so a combination of tests can be used to increase the detection rate.
- Treatment comprises of a 6 months course of ATT (four drugs RHZE for 2 months followed by three drugs HRE for the next 4 months) through DOTS.
- Monitoring is important to ensure adherence to drugs and to detect any side effects caused if any.

REFERENCES

1. Sharma JB, Sharma E, Sharma S, Singh J, Chopra N. Genital TB-diagnostic algorithm and treatment. Indian J Tuberc. 2020;67(4S):S111-8.
2. Sharma JB, Sharma E, Sharma S, Dharmendra S. Female genital tuberculosis: revisited. Indian J Med Res. 2018;148(Suppl 1):S71-S83.
3. Grace A, Devaleenal B, Natarajan M. Genital tuberculosis in females. Indian J Med Res. 2017;145(4):425-36.
4. Sharma JB. Current diagnosis and management of female genital tuberculosis. J Obstet Gynaecol India. 2015;65:362-71.
5. Mahajan N, Naidu P, Kaur SD. Insight into the diagnosis and management of subclinical genital tuberculosis in women with infertility. J Hum Reprod Sci. 2016;9(3):135-44.
6. Zahoor D, Bhat MM, Kanth F, Farhana A. Prevalence of genital tuberculosis in infertile women; a study from a Tertiary Care Center in North India. Int J Contemp Med Res. 2019;6(6):F1-3.
7. Munne KR, Tandon D, Chauhan SL, Patil AD. Female genital tuberculosis in light of newer laboratory tests: a narrative review. Indian J Tuberc. 2020;67(1):112-20.
8. Sharma JB, Dharmendra S, Jain S, Sharma SK, Singh UB, Soneja M, et al. Evaluation of Gene Xpert as compared to conventional methods in diagnosis of female genital tuberculosis. Eur J Obstet Gynecol Reprod Biol. 2020;255:247-52.
9. Meenu S, Ramalingam S, Sairam T, Appinabhavi A, Panicker S, Oommen S, et al. Comparison of polymerase chain reaction (PCR), microbiological and histopathological observations in the diagnosis of endometrial tuberculosis. J Obstet Gynaecol India. 2020;70(6):510-5.
10. Sethi S, Dhaliwal L, Dey P, Kaur H, Yadav R, Sethi S. Loop-mediated isothermal amplification assay for detection of Mycobacterium tuberculosis complex in infertile women. Indian J Med Microbiol. 2016;34(3):322-7.
11. Gupta S, Gupta P. Etiopathogenesis, challenges and remedies associated with female genital tuberculosis: potential role of nuclear receptors. Front Immunol. 2020;11:02161.
12. Sharma JB. Sharma's hanging gall bladder sign: a new sign for abdomino-pelvic tuberculosis: an observational study. IVF Lite. 2015;2:94-8.
13. Sharma JB. Sharma's ascending colonic adhesion: a new sign in abdomino-pelvic tuberculosis with infertility. IVF Lite. 2016;3:18-22.
14. Sharma JB. Sharma's sigmoid colonic adhesive band—a new laparoscopic sign in female genital tuberculosis. Indian J Tuberc. 2020;67(3):327-32.
15. Sharma JB. Sharma's abdominal compartmentalization sign: a new laparoscopic sign for abdomino-pelvic tuberculosis. Indian J Tuberc. 2020;67(4):578-85.
16. Sharma JB. Sharma's parachute sign a new laparoscopic sign in abdomino pelvic tuberculosis. Indian J Tubercul. 2021;68(3):389-95.
17. Sharma JB. Sharma's python sign: a new tubal sign in female genital tuberculosis. J Lab Phys. 2016;8(2):120-2.

CHAPTER 12

Asherman's Syndrome

Saloni Kamboj, Neena Malhotra

INTRODUCTION

Asherman's syndrome (AS) is characterized by intrauterine (IU) or intracervical adhesions presenting along with symptoms of menstrual disturbances, infertility, abnormal placentation, and recurrent pregnancy loss. Fritsch in 1894, first described intrauterine adhesions (IUAs) after curettage that caused amenorrhea.[1] More than 50 years later, in 1948, Asherman came out with a series of 29 patients with similar condition.[2] Those 29 patients presented with amenorrhea along with stenosis of internal cervical os. This manifestation was the result of trauma to endometrium according to the author. The author published another series of cases 2 years later wherein IUAs involved uterine cavity which were characterized by filling defects during hysterography.[2] Reported in literature are many cases where IUAs are not associated with any symptoms, perhaps being detected accidentally at diagnostic hysteroscopy, with minor adhesions which may be clinically irrelevant. In these circumstances, the term AS should be better avoided.[2] The term should strictly be reserved for adhesions that are symptomatic. While the entity has been described and understood for long, evidence on the best methods of prevention and treatment to improve fertility are still limited. In this chapter, we deliberate upon the etiology, diagnosis, classification, treatment, and prevention as available through current evidence.

RISK FACTORS AND ETIOPATHOGENESIS

The endometrium has two layers namely basal layer, a layer touching the myometrium, and a superficial functional layer, which is responsive to the recurrent changes that happen upon sex hormones secretion by the ovaries. In the proliferative phase of menstrual cycle, the increased hormone production catalyzes endometrial growth. The decrease in the production of hormones in the late luteal phase causes menstruation and endometrial shedding. The basal layer keeps intact during the menstrual cycle and provides the basis for renewal of functional layer. This new functional layer is completed without development of adhesions. IUAs are formed when there is endometrial injury sufficient enough to cause loss of stroma which is replaced by fibrous tissue. Under such circumstances, there is loss of separation between functional and basal layers of endometrium and an atrophic epithelial mono-layer that is nonresponsive to hormonal stimulation is formed **(Fig. 1)**.[3] This layer replaces both the functional and the basal layers of endometrium.

Early gravid uterus is susceptible to trauma resulting from surgical interventions, most commonly by endometrium's basal layer curettage. Any procedure done in postpartum period causes more severe adhesions as compared to procedures done in first trimester.[2] This happens in postpartum period, due to decline in estrogen levels from loss of placental estrogen superimposed by the antagonistic effects of elevated prolactin levels consequent to breast feeding. An incidence of 15% was noted post spontaneous abortion followed by suction dilation and curettage (D&C) by Gilman et al.[4] A similar study by Hooker et al. reported variable

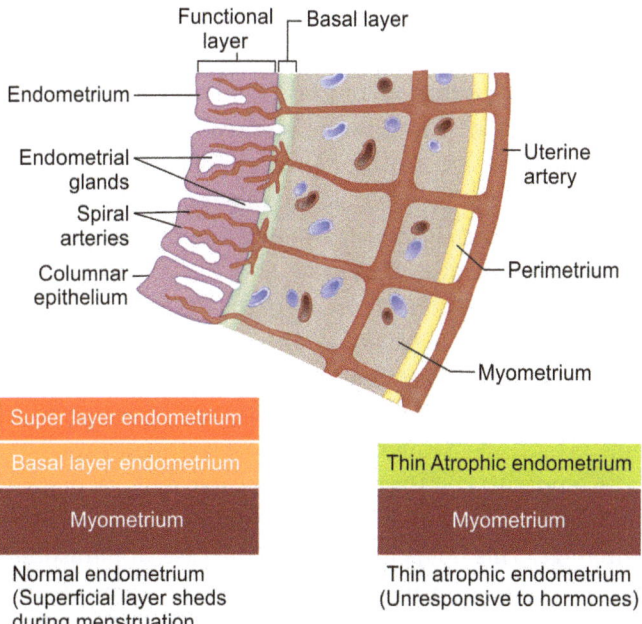

Fig. 1: Endometrial thinning in Asherman's syndrome.

TABLE 1: Summary of risk factors.		
Sr. No.	Risk factors	Incidence (%)
1.	First-trimester curettage	66.7
2.	Postpartum curettage	21.5
3.	Müllerian duct malformation	16
4.	Infection (genital tuberculosis, schistosomiasis)	4
5.	Diagnostic curettage	1.6
6.	Uterine artery embolization	1.4
7.	Hysteroscopic surgeries	06–31
8.	Uterine compressive surgeries for postpartum hemorrhage (PPH)	18.5
9.	Cesarean section	2

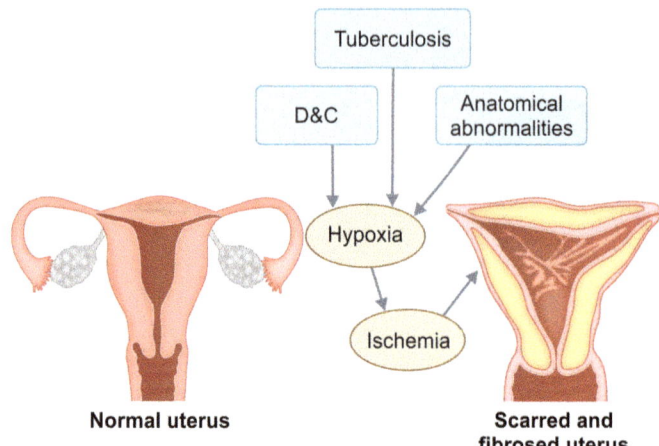

Fig. 2: Risk factors and etiopathogenesis of Asherman's syndrome. (D&C: dilation and curettage)

incidence depending on the type of pregnancy loss; 19% post spontaneous abortion, 21% post medical termination of pregnancy followed by suction D&C, and 30% after suction D&C for retained products of conception (RPOC).[5]

Other surgical interventions such as cesarean section, evacuation of hydatidiform mole, B-lynch sutures, abdominal myomectomy, hysteroscopic myomectomy, and surgical treatment of Müllerian anomalies may also lead to the trauma of the uterine cavity thereby implicated in development of AS.[6] Bhandari et al. reported an incidence of 22% postabdominal myomectomy for fibroids.[7] Yu et al. in his prospective study stated an incidence of 24% posthysteroscopic septum resection even with the use of bipolar current.[8]

Furthermore, infections like *Mycobacterium tuberculosis* and *Schistosoma* have been implicated in causing the AS.[9,10] Besides, genital tuberculosis is apparently associated with recurrent adhesions which are less responsive to treatment. Conditions that result in diminished uterine flow and hypoxia such as uterine artery embolization, also increase the propensity for formation of IUAs. Therefore, it is imperative to counsel patients prior to surgical interventions on the risks of IUAs and the long-term implications. Although data is limited, possible genetic factors could link and explain why certain patients show more prone to develop adhesions without any trigger.

Nevertheless, curettage remains the major factor causing IUAs. Moreover, the number of curettages has also been directly linked with the odds of developing adhesions; a 10% incidence of IUAs was noted after one curettage, which spiked to 30.6% in women with at least two curettages.[11,12]

Comparing curettage to hysteroscopic removal of RPOC postdelivery or miscarriage, more adhesions were noted after curettage. This holds true even in the case of ultrasound-guided curettage, when compared to hysteroscopic removal of RPOC.[13] A summary of risk factors is provided in **Table 1** and **Figure 2**.

There are limited studies available, as regards pathophysiology of AS, with data from Chen Y et al., where evaluation of endometrial cells of patients with AS under electron microscope revealed significant subcellular modifications such as loss of ribosomes, mitochondrial swelling, and hypoxic cellular modifications.[14] In addition, vascular endothelial growth factor (VEGF) and density of micro vessels are significantly raised in patients who responded to treatment. This confirms that in the endometrial regeneration, angiogenesis and revascularization play an important role.[14] In a recent prospective study, Doppler studies of the endometrium suggested high impedance of spiral artery, which explains the reduction in endometrial receptivity and regeneration in patients with AS.[15] A possible association of adhesion-related cytokines, viz. fibroblast growth factor, platelet-derived growth factor, transforming growth factor-type 1, is also suggested in the pathogenesis of AS.[16]

CLINICAL FEATURES

Amenorrhea is present in approximately two-thirds of patients while about one-third of patients present with reduced menstrual flow. The severity of adhesions does not always correlate with the menstrual pattern. About 2–3% of patients who have severe disease might present with menstruation with average flow and duration. Complaint of cyclical dysmenorrhea is present in approximately 3.5% of patients. IUAs are also associated with infertility (7%), recurrent pregnancy loss, and abnormal placentation (**Fig. 3**).[2]

DIAGNOSIS

Early diagnosis of AS is vital in infertile women to achieve good reproductive outcome. However, simple bimanual pelvic examination cannot diagnose AS.[2] With the advent of newer imaging modalities and endoscopic techniques,

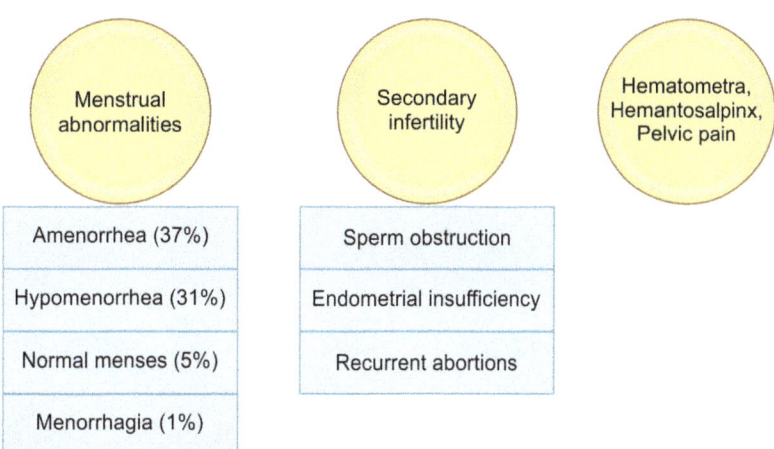

Fig. 3: Spectrum of clinical features.

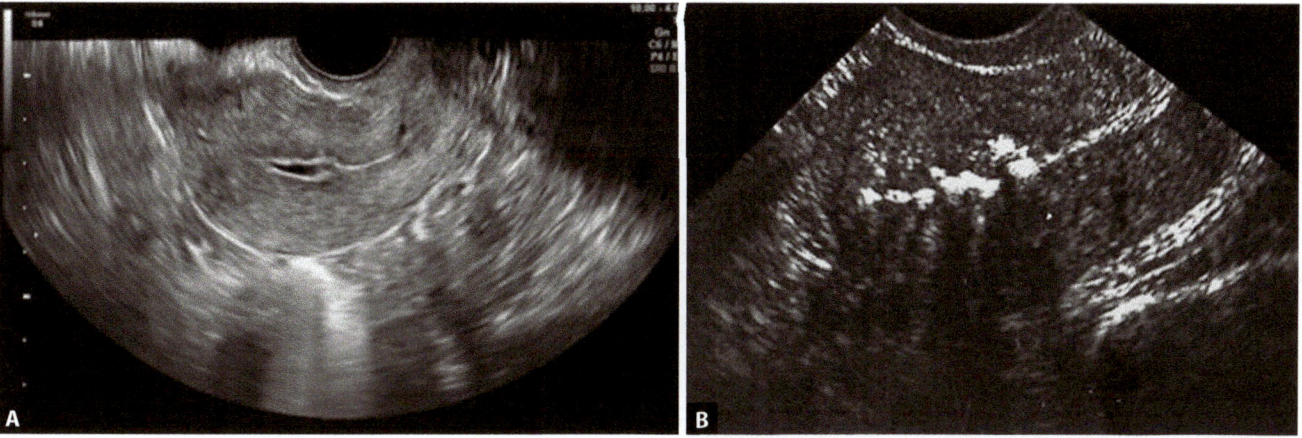

Figs. 4A and B: (A) 2D ultrasonography (USG) showing skip lesions; (B) 2D USG showing calcifications.

diagnosis of AS has become easier. Noninvasiveness, low cost, safety, and applicability to a large scale of population are the characteristics of an ideal diagnostic test.

Ultrasound

Two-dimensional ultrasound is considered as the first-line modality because of its wide availability and low cost. Salient findings on 2D ultrasound are adhesion bands running inside the endometrial cavity, thin atrophic endometrium, hypoechoic patches with interruption of endometrium known as "skip lesions" **(Figs. 4A and B)**, fluid in the endometrial cavity, etc.[17] When compared with gold standard procedure (hysteroscopy), 2D ultrasound has a sensitivity of 52% and specificity of 11%.[17]

Three-dimensional ultrasound enables the real-time assessment of endometrial cavity providing a clear picture of endomyometrial junction **(Fig. 5)**. 3D ultrasound also has a higher sensitivity and specificity as compared to 3D sonohystography.[18] In a recent study, it was found that preoperative 3D transvaginal ultrasound could help in making decisions prior to hysteroscopic adhesiolysis. Patients who underwent preoperative 3D ultrasound had a better surgical success rate.[19] However, because of

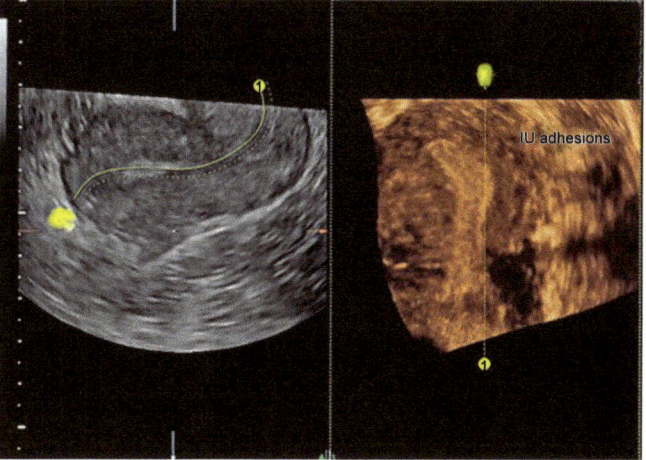

Fig. 5: 3D ultrasonography (USG) showing intrauterine (IU) adhesions obliterating one cornua.

inadequate studies on 3D ultrasound and high cost, its use in clinical practice is limited.

Hysterosalpingography

Hysterosalpingography (HSG) was used as the most widespread diagnostic tool few years back because of its cost effectiveness and it can also assess tubal patency

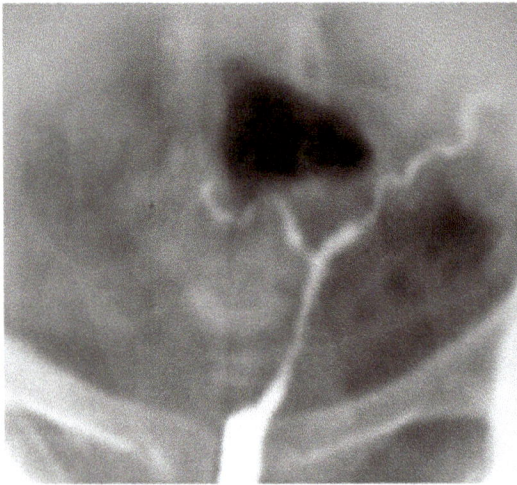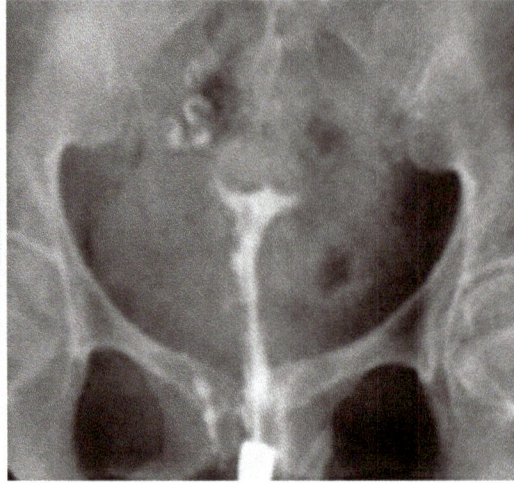

Fig. 6: Hysterosalpingography (HSG) showing shrunken and irregular cavities.

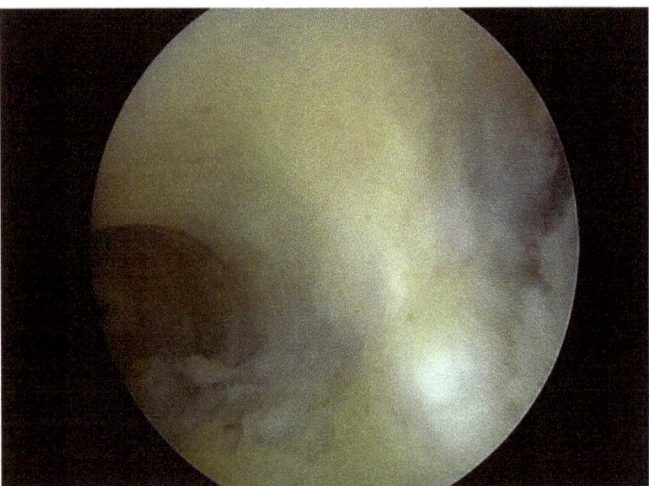

Fig. 7: Hysteroscopic appearance of intrauterine adhesions with pale endometrium.

simultaneously. HSG can be suitable for outlining the endometrial cavity, evaluating the extent and location of adhesions and filling defects **(Fig. 6)**. When compared with hysteroscopy, HSG along with the use of contrast dye has a sensitivity of 75–81% and specificity of 80%.[20] When HSG was compared with sonohysterography (SHG used with saline infusion during the ultrasound scan), a plausible difference was noted in general accuracy (50% in HSG group and 82% in SHG group).[21] Another newer technique that combines 3D ultrasound and SHG has recently been proposed. A few studies stated that this technique showed comparable diagnostic efficacy with hysteroscopy.[22] MRI can also be a useful supplementary diagnostic tool specifically in the case of adhesions in endocervix or when the cavity is completely obliterated.[11] Hysteroscopy remains the gold standard despite the above developments. Hysteroscopy allows assessment of type, extent, character of adhesions, and simultaneously allows treatment in the same setting in favorable cases **(Fig. 7)**.[23]

TABLE 2: Comparison of various techniques used for diagnosis of Asherman's syndrome.

	Advantages	Disadvantages
2D ultrasound	• Low cost • Noninvasive • Easily available	• Difficult to differentiate between adhesions and fibrosis • Influenced by the phase of menstrual cycle
3D ultrasound	• Quantification of the size of cavity • Clear picture of endomyometrial junction	• Costlier • Limited studies available
HSG (hysterosalpingography)	• Tubal patency can be evaluated • Delineates any filling defects	• Expensive • Radiation and contrast exposure • Ovaries and endometrial thickness not evaluated
SHG (sonohysterography)	• Easy • 3D scan can be done simultaneously to evaluate tubal patency	Slow learning curve
Hysteroscopy	• Endometrial cavity can be directly evaluated • Treatment in the same setting	• Expensive • Interobserver variation

Table 2 compares the various techniques used for diagnosis.

CLASSIFICATION

The ideal classification system should have a description of adhesions, severity of adhesions, and should guide clinicians

TABLE 3: Classification of Asherman's syndrome based on hysterosalpingography (HSG) (Toeff and Ballas).

Classification	Condition
Type 1	Atresia of the internal ostium, without concomitant corporal adhesions
Type 2	Stenosis of internal ostium, causing almost complete occlusion without concomitant corporal adhesions
Type 3	Multiple small adhesions in the internal ostium isthmic region
Type 4	Supra-isthmic diaphragm causing complete separation of the main cavity from its lower segment
Type 5	Atresia of the internal ostium with concomitant corporeal adhesions

TABLE 4: American Fertility Society (AFS) classification of Asherman's syndrome based on clinical findings, hysterosalpingography (HSG), and hysteroscopy.

	Characteristics		
Extent of cavity involved	<1/3 1	1/3–2/3 2	>2–3 4
Type of adhesions	1 Flimsy 1	2 Filmy and dense 2	4 Dense 4
Menstrual pattern	Normal 0	Decreased 2	Amenorrhea 4
Prognostic classification		HSG score	Hysteroscopy score
Stage I (Mild)	1–4		
Stage II (Moderate)	5–8		
Stage III (Severe)	9–12		

TABLE 5: European Society for Gynecological Endoscopy (ESGE) classification of intrauterine adhesions (IUAs).

Grade	Extent of intrauterine adhesions
I	*Thin or filmy adhesions:* • Easily ruptured by hysteroscope sheath alone • Cornual areas normal
II	*Singular dense adhesion:* • Connecting separate areas of uterine cavity • Visualization of both tubal ostia possible • Cannot be ruptured by hysteroscope sheath alone
IIa	*Occluding adhesions only in the region of the internal cervical os:* • Upper uterine cavity normal
III	*Multiple dense adhesions:* • Connection separate areas of uterine cavity • Unilateral obliteration of ostial areas of the tubes
IV	*Extensive dense adhesions with (partial) occlusion of the uterine cavity:* • Both tubal ostial areas (partially) occluded
Va	*Extensive endometrial scarring and fibrosis in combination with grade I or grade II adhesions:* • With amenorrhea or pronounced hypomenorrhea
Vb	*Extensive endometrial scarring and fibrosis:* • In combination with grade III or grade IV adhesions • With amenorrhea

for further treatment and outcomes. Toeff and Ballas were the first to classify AS on the basis of HSG findings.[24] The classification is still used for its simplicity **(Table 3)**. Thereafter, American Fertility Society (AFS) devised a classification based on the extent of disease, menstrual pattern, morphological features, and hysteroscopy and HSG findings **(Table 4)**.[25]

European Society for Gynecological Endoscopy (ESGE) also devised a classification system in 1995 based on extent of IUAs from findings at hysteroscopy, hysterography, and during hysteroscopic treatment **(Table 5)**. The American Association of Gynecologic Laparoscopists (AAGL) and the ESGE), in the 2017 Guidelines for Classification of AS, stated that a classification system of IUAs was needed because the prognosis is affected by the severity of this condition (level B recommendation) and each of the classification systems suffers from inherent deficiencies. Therefore, no specific system of classification can be endorsed currently.[11]

MANAGEMENT

Treatment of IUAs is recommended only if the patient is present with clinical symptoms or infertility issues. Goals of any treatment strategy should be restoration of normal uterine shape, volume, endometrial function, normal communication between endometrial cavity, cervical canal and tubal ostia, and prevention of readhesion formation. **Flowchart 1** summarizes principles of management and **Flowchart 2** explains approach to a patient with AS.

Dilation and Curettage

Because of high risk of perforation and advent of hysteroscopy, blind D&C is considered obsolete these days and may be of historical relevance in the present time.[3,9]

Hysteroscopic Surgery

Introduction of hysteroscopy has revolutionized the treatment of AS.[26,27] There has been significant improvement in fertility outcomes and success rates. Hysteroscopic adhesiolysis can be performed using rigid hysteroscope and blunt-tipped 5-Fr scissors. Mechanical transection of adhesions, as they come across, is performed with the scissors or needle **(Fig. 8)**. Filmy adhesions can be dissected bluntly using the tip of hysteroscope. After initial hysteroscopic adhesiolysis performed in the hands of expert surgeons results in the restoration of a normal uterine cavity

Flowchart 1: Summary of principles of management.

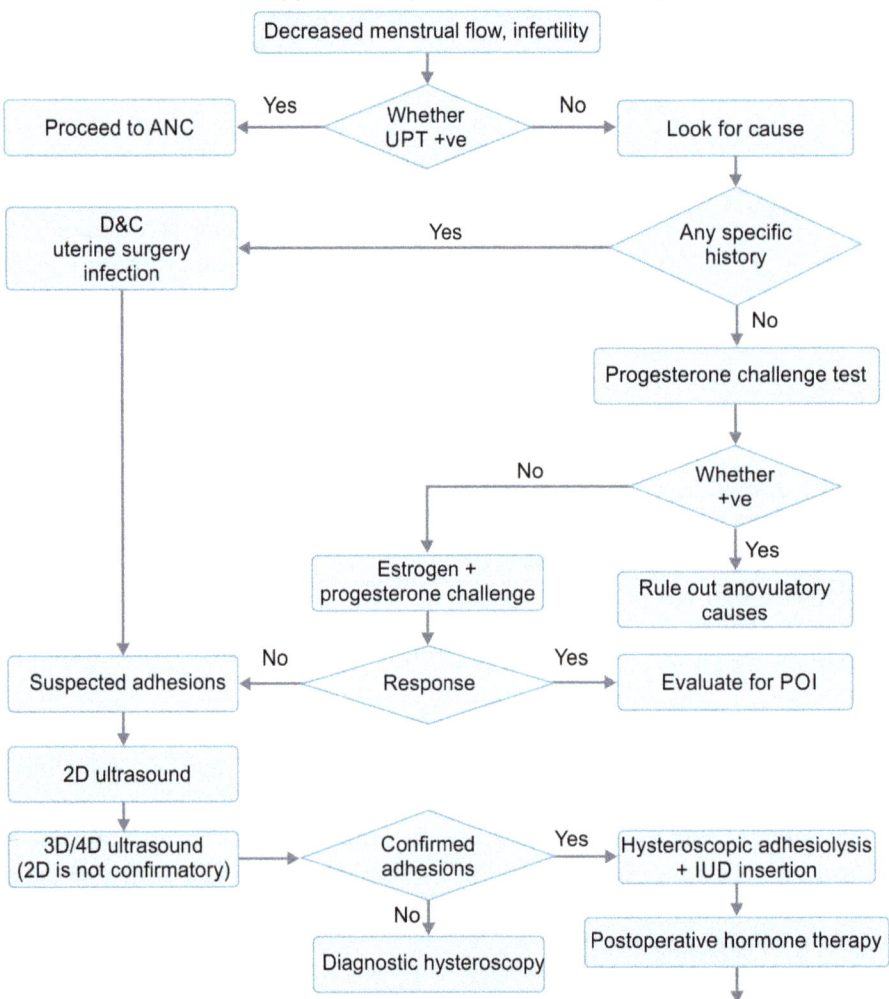

(HSG: hysterosalpingography; IUD: intrauterine device; PRP: platelet-rich plasma)

Flowchart 2: Approach to a patient with Asherman's syndrome.

(ANC: antenatal care; UPT: urine pregnancy test; D&C: dilation and curettage; IUD: intrauterine device; POI: primary ovarian insufficiency)

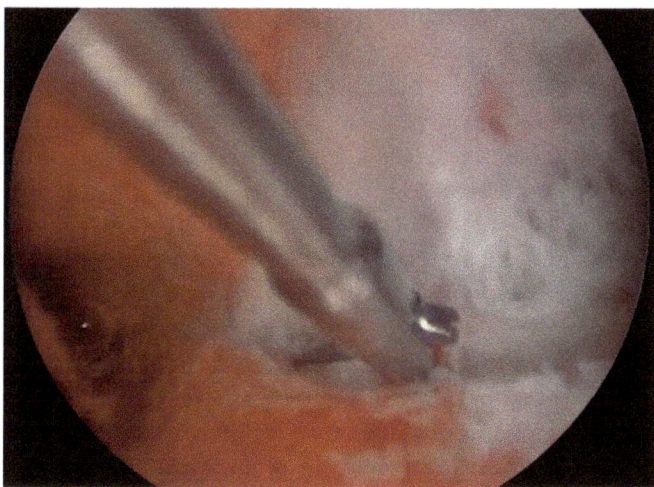

Fig. 8: Hysteroscopic adhesiolysis of intrauterine adhesions (IUAs).

in about 80% of patients.[26] In another technique for lysis of adhesions using energy source, loop/laser electrosurgery (monopolar, bipolar) and Nd: YAG laser is used. It offers easy and precise division of adhesions and better hemostasis. No comparison in these techniques has been made so far among one other. No evidence suggests that one method is superior to another. Nevertheless, adhesiolysis with electrocautery has disadvantage that a healthy endometrium is susceptible to risk of trauma and recurrent adhesive disease can be caused. Surgery with electrosurgical techniques is associated with a statistically significant cumulative negative impact on pregnancy outcomes.[28]

Majority of patients can be offered office-based hysteroscopy using preoperative nonsteroidal anti-inflammatory drugs (NSAIDs) alone for analgesia.[29] Risks associated with intravenous sedation or anesthesia can be avoided using this technique. Candidate selection for this is very important; those with slight to moderate adhesions, having no cervical stenosis have a favorable outcome.

When upper cervix or lower uterine segment is obliterated, there is increased chance of perforation while attempting surgery. In such cases, guidance with transabdominal ultrasound can be used. Advantages of techniques include availability and noninvasive nature of ultrasound. However, uterine perforation is still reported in some cases. Laparoscopic guidance is reported to help in hysteroscopic surgical division of adhesions particularly in severe grade obliterating the entire cavity, allowing concurrent inspection of pelvic organs; however, there is not enough evidence of use of this combined laparoscopic approach.[30,31]

PREVENTION OF RECURRENCE

Treatment of AS is challenging because of high rates of recurrence (30%).[2,32] This is particularly high in severe AS and needs to be informed to patients preoperatively. There are several methods for secondary prevention which are described here.

Mechanical Methods

Literature documents the use of intrauterine device (IUD) to be one of the first attempts in order to prevent adhesion recurrence. By separating the anterior and posterior uterine walls, physiological endometrial regeneration could be feasible with the use of IUD. Although good results have been reported in many studies, uncertainty still remains about what kind of IUD and of what size to be used.[33,34] Some authors nonetheless believe that endometrial injury could be aggravated by the inflammatory factors released by copper device.[35] The IUD that releases levonorgestrel should not be used because of its suppressing effect on the endometrium. A stable separation between the uterine walls is not guaranteed by the T-shaped IUD. Because of its shape, lippes loop was considered to be the most adequate device to prevent adhesion. Although the IUD can be placed in uterine cavity for different durations (1, 2, 3 months), the placement for 3 months has been considered the standard method of maintaining the uterine cavity after intervention.

Other mechanical barriers have also been suggested for the prevention of secondary adhesions. One of the first mechanical devices used for separating uterine walls to prevent the recurrence of the IUAs was the Foley catheter. The use of Foley catheter has also been compared with IUD as an adjunctive therapy. There was a higher conception rate in Foley group compared with the IUD group. In addition, normal menstrual pattern was restored in 81% women.[36] Still, there are no randomized controlled trials attesting the Foley catheter efficacy in the prevention of IUA because of main concerns like uterine perforation, ascending infection from vagina, and the discomfort.

Medical Therapy

The use of estrogen alone and as ancillary treatment with IUD or Foley catheter has been studied. Estrogen helps in rapid growth of residual endometrium immediately after surgery with the twin purpose of preventing new scar formation and restoration of normal uterine environment. When estrogen was used as ancillary treatment, increased menstrual flow was recorded, except in one study on genital tuberculosis.[37] Pregnancy rates were also higher with ancillary use of estrogen. Different regimes of estrogen have been used in the studies thereby being inconclusive on ideal dosage, timing of estrogen, or route of administration (vaginal or oral).[3,35] However, most commonly used regime is with micronized estradiol/estradiol valerate, 2 mg twice daily for 30–60 days and adding progesterone (medroxyprogesterone acetate 10 mg once daily) for the last 10 days of estrogen therapy.

Hyaluronic Acid and Other Adhesion Barriers

The mechanism by which these products act is not completely understood. Hyaluronic acid mechanically obstacles adhesions formation by creating a temporary barrier amongst organs; in addition, these products increase the proliferation rate of mesothelial cells thus influence peritoneal tissue repair. Autocross-linked hyaluronic acid (Hyalobarrier©) is a new mechanical barrier found to be capable of avoiding adhesion formation post gynecological surgery.[38-43] Another antiadhesion barrier which was used for prevention of IUA is characterized by chemically modified hyaluronic acid (sodium hyaluronate) and carboxymethylcellulose (Seprafilm©).[44] A prospective randomized trial including 187 cases evaluated a brand new hyaluronic acid derived (alginate carboxymethylcellulose hyaluronic acid). In the said trial, it was noted that IUAs were significantly lower compared with carboxymethylcellulose hyaluronic acid, 4 weeks after surgery.

Which one of the antiadhesive should be recommended is still not finalized as the choice depends on the local availability and the choice of the surgeon.

TECHNIQUES TO INCREASE VASCULAR FLOW TO ENDOMETRIUM

Various studies have shown the use of medications which can be used to increase vascular perfusion to the endometrium and help in pregnancy such as aspirin, nitroglycerine, and sildenafil citrate.[45,46] However, the numbers of women treated using these therapies are small, and most of the treatments are off-label, and therefore such medications cannot be recommended outside of rigorous research protocols. A new IU stent (silicon made, triangular shape by Cook medical) is also prescribed as a mechanical method to prevent recurrence of adhesions.

Antibiotic Therapy

The use of antibiotic therapy before, during, or after surgical treatment of AS is not supported by data. The American College of Obstetricians and Gynecologists guidelines do not recommend the use of antibiotics for diagnostic or therapeutic hysteroscopy in gynecological procedures.[47] Antibiotics are recommended only in situations when there is a clinical suspicion of infection.

Stem Cells Treatment

In both animal models as well as in small experimental human studies, regeneration of endometrium through stem cell treatment has been evaluated. Bone marrow-derived stem cells, mesenchymal stem cells, and autologous menstrual blood-derived stromal cells have been used in the recent past. Growth factors and cytokines that promote enhanced migration of endometrial epithelial cells and proliferation of endometrial stromal and mesenchymal cells, which are crucial for endometrial regeneration, are contained in platelet-rich plasma (PRP). These are mediated by growth factor receptors, as shown by the upregulation of some of them in cells treated with PRP. Various application methods have been used, e.g., infusion in spiral arterioles through catheters, transmyometrial administration to the subendometrial area, and direct installation of stromal cells in uterine cavity after endometrial scratching.[48,49] Recent experiments on animal as well as human subjects involving transplanting autologous and allogeneic stem cells to treat AS have been performed. Fertility outcomes in mice with iatrogenic AS improved after the administration of a bone marrow-derived stem cell transplant.[50] Autologous bone marrow stem cell transplant in humans has been reported in treatment for patients with refractory AS.[51-53] However, stem cell transplantation for the treatment of AS is far from becoming common as there are limited studies and the procedure needs standardization. Studies on benefits of PRP in AS are also limited.[54] Future bigger studies and randomized trials are needed to conclude whether stem cell treatment has a clinical role in AS.

FERTILITY AND PREGNANCY OUTCOMES

Hysteroscopic adhesiolysis improves the overall conception rate in affected patients. The conception rate after adhesiolysis is higher in mild disease (58%) as compared to moderate and severe cases (30%). Also, likelihood of conception was higher in patients who resumed normal menstrual cycle after adhesiolysis. Pregnancy rate in properly treated cases is about 30–75%.[35] However, these pregnancies are more likely to be complicated by premature delivery, sequelae of abnormal placentations.[55] Other less known complications include spontaneous abortion, ectopic pregnancy, cervical incompetence, and fetal growth restriction.[35]

CONCLUSION

Asherman's syndrome highly impacts female reproduction affecting menstruation and fertility in women in reproductive years. In view of the highest reported incidence of AS after curettage for miscarriage, a major reduction can be achieved if such procedures are limited and judiciously practiced. The success rate both for resumption of menses and fertility outcome has been significantly improved with the introduction of hysteroscopy. Considering the high recurrence rates after surgical corrections, techniques that limit the formation of new adhesions should be considered. Despite the need for more comparative trials, IUD, uterine stent, adhesions barriers, and hormonal treatment have proven efficiency. In situations when the cavity regains its volume and size and yet no clinical improvement in menses and reproduction, the use of stem cell may be an alternative.

A novel approach, based on endometrial stem cells, is an area for research and could be of use in future once ongoing trials may give more evidence.

Key Learning Points

- Intra uterine adhesions are formed when there is endometrial injury sufficient enough to cause loss of stroma which is replaced by fibrous tissue.
- Curettage remains the major factor causing intra-uterine adhesions and number of curettages has been directly linked with the odds of developing adhesions.
- Amenorrhea is present in approximately two-third of patients. Intra uterine adhesions are also associated with reduced blood flow, cyclical dysmenorrhea, infertility, recurrent pregnancy loss and abnormal placentation.
- Hysteroscopy remains the gold standard, other investigations like 3D-USG, HSG can be used as adjuncts.
- Hysteroscopic adhesiolysis remains the first line treatment, it has got high rates of recurrence.
- There are several methods for secondary prevention which include mechanical barriers, estrogen therapy, hyaluronic acid etc.
- Stem cells and PRP treatment could be of use in future once ongoing trials may give more evidence.

REFERENCES

1. Al-Inany H. Intrauterine adhesions. An update. Acta Obstet Gynecol Scand. 2001;80(11):986-93.
2. Conforti A, Alviggi C, Mollo A, De Placido G, Magos A. The management of Asherman syndrome: a review of literature. Reprod Biol Endocrinol. 2013;11:118.
3. Yu D, Wong YM, Cheong Y, Xia E, Li TC. Asherman syndrome-one century later. Fertil Steril. 2008;89(4):759-79.
4. Gilman AR, Dewar KM, Rhone SA, Fluker MR. Intrauterine Adhesions Following Miscarriage: Look and Learn. J Obstet Gynaecol Can. 2016;38(5):453-7.
5. Hooker AB, Lemmers M, Thurkow AL, Heymans MW, Opmeer BC, Brölmann HAM, et al. Systematic review and meta-analysis of intrauterine adhesions after miscarriage: prevalence, risk factors and long-term reproductive outcome. Hum Reprod Update. 2014;20(2):262-78.
6. Deans R, Abbott J. Review of intrauterine adhesions. J Minim Invasive Gynecol. 2010;17(5):555-69.
7. Bhandari S, Ganguly I, Agarwal P, Singh A, Gupta N. Effect of myomectomy on endometrial cavity: A prospective study of 51 cases. J Hum Reprod Sci. 2016;9(2):107-11.
8. Yu X, Yuhan L, Dongmei S, Enlan X, Tinchiu L. The incidence of post-operative adhesion following transection of uterine septum: a cohort study comparing three different adjuvant therapies. Eur J Obstet Gynecol Reprod Biol. 2016;201:61-4.
9. Schenker JG, Margalioth EJ. Intrauterine adhesions: an updated appraisal. Fertil Steril. 1982;37(5):593-610.
10. Krolikowski A, Janowski K, Larsen JV. Asherman syndrome caused by schistosomiasis. Obstet Gynecol. 1995;85(5 Pt 2):898-9.
11. Dreisler E, Kjer JJ. Asherman's syndrome: current perspectives on diagnosis and management. Int J Womens Health. 2019;11:191-8.
12. Hooker AB, de Leeuw R, van de Ven PM, Bakkum EA, Thurkow AL, Vogel NEA, et al. Prevalence of intrauterine adhesions after the application of hyaluronic acid gel after dilatation and curettage in women with at least one previous curettage: short-term outcomes of a multicenter, prospective randomized controlled trial. Fertil Steril. 2017;107(5):1223-31.
13. Rein DT, Schmidt T, Hess AP, Volkmer A, Schöndorf T, Breidenbach M. Hysteroscopic management of residual trophoblastic tissue is superior to ultrasound-guided curettage. J Minim Invasive Gynecol. 2011;18(6):774-8.
14. Chen Y, Chang Y, Yao S. Role of angiogenesis in endometrial repair of patients with severe intrauterine adhesion. Int J Clin Exp Pathol. 2013;6(7):1343-50.
15. Malhotra N, Bahadur A, Kalaivani M, Mittal S. Changes in endometrial receptivity in women with Asherman's syndrome undergoing hysteroscopic adhesiolysis. Arch Gynecol Obstet. 2012;286(2):525-30.
16. Tao Z, Duan H. [Expression of adhesion-related cytokines in the uterine fluid after transcervical resection of adhesion]. Zhonghua Fu Chan Ke Za Zhi. 2012;47(10):734-7.
17. Amin TN, Saridogan E, Jurkovic D. Ultrasound and intrauterine adhesions: a novel structured approach to diagnosis and management. Ultrasound Obstet Gynecol. 2015;46(2):131-9.
18. Salim R, Woelfer B, Backos M, Regan L, Jurkovic D. Reproducibility of three-dimensional ultrasound diagnosis of congenital uterine anomalies. Ultrasound Obstet Gynecol. 2003;21(6):578-82.
19. Knopman J, Copperman AB. Value of 3D ultrasound in the management of suspected Asherman's syndrome. J Reprod Med. 2007;52(11):1016-22.
20. Salazar CA, Isaacson K, Morris S. A comprehensive review of Asherman's syndrome: causes, symptoms and treatment options. Curr Opin Obstet Gynecol. 2017;29(4):249-56.
21. Berridge DL, Winter TC. Saline infusion sonohysterography: technique, indications, and imaging findings. J Ultrasound Med. 2004;23(1):97-112.
22. Salim R, Lee C, Davies A, Jolaoso B, Ofuasia E, Jurkovic D. A comparative study of three-dimensional saline infusion sonohysterography and diagnostic hysteroscopy for the classification of submucous fibroids. Hum Reprod. 2005;20(1):253-7.
23. Soares SR, Barbosa dos Reis MM, Camargos AF. Diagnostic accuracy of sonohysterography, transvaginal sonography, and hysterosalpingography in patients with uterine cavity diseases. Fertil Steril. 2000;11:406-11.
24. Toaff R, Ballas S. Traumatic hypomenorrhea-amenorrhea (Asherman's syndrome). Fertil Steril. 1978;30(4):379-87.
25. The American Fertility Society. Classifications of adnexal adhesions, distal tubal occlusion, tubal occlusion secondary to tubal ligation, tubal pregnancies, Mullerian anomalies and intrauterine adhesions. Fertil Steril. 1988;11:944-55.
26. Valle RF, Sciarra JJ. Intrauterine adhesions: hysteroscopic diagnosis, classification, treatment, and reproductive outcome. Am J Obstet Gynecol. 1988;158(6 Pt 1):1459-70.
27. Pabuçcu R, Atay V, Orhon E, Urman B, Ergün A. Hysteroscopic treatment of intrauterine adhesions is safe and effective in the restoration of normal menstruation and fertility. Fertil Steril. 1997;68(6):1141-3.
28. Cararach M, Panella J, Ubeda A, Labastida R. Hysteroscopic incision of the septate uterus: scissors versus resectoscope. Hum Reprod. 1994;9:87-9.

29. Sugimoto O. Diagnostic and therapeutic hysteroscopy for traumatic intrauterine adhesions. Am J Obstet Gynecol. 1978;11:539-47.
30. Protopapas A, Shushan A, Magos A. Myometrial scoring: a new technique for the management of severe Asherman's syndrome. Fertil Steril. 1998;69:860-4.
31. McComb PF, Wagner BL. Simplified therapy for Asherman's syndrome. Fertil Steril. 1997;68:1047-50.
32. Yang JH, Chen CD, Chen SU, Yang YS, Chen MJ. The influence of the location and extent of intrauterine adhesions on recurrence after hysteroscopic adhesiolysis. BJOG. 2016;123(4):618-23.
33. Polishuk WZ, Weinstein D. The Soichet intrauterine device in the treatment of intrauterine adhesions. Acta Eur Fertil. 1976;11:215-8.
34. Vesce F, Jorizzo G, Bianciotto A, Gotti G. Use of the copper intrauterine device in the management of secondary amenorrhea. Fertil Steril. 2000;11:162-5.
35. March CM. Intrauterine adhesions. Obstet Gynecol Clin North Am. 1995;11:491-505.
36. Orhue AA, Aziken ME, Igbefoh JO. A comparison of two adjunctive treatments for intrauterine adhesions following lysis. Int J Gynaecol Obstet. 2003;11:49-56.
37. Roy KK, Baruah J, Sharma JB, Kumar S, Kachawa G, Singh N. Reproductive outcome following hysteroscopic adhesiolysis in patients with infertility due to Asherman's syndrome. Arch Gynecol Obstet. 2010;11:355-61.
38. Pellicano M, Bramante S, Cirillo D, Palomba S, Bifulco G, Zullo F, et al. Effectiveness of autocrosslinked hyaluronic acid gel after laparoscopic myomectomy in infertile patients: a prospective, randomized, controlled study. Fertil Steril. 2003;11:441-4.
39. Guida M, Acunzo G, Di Spiezio Sardo A, Bifulco G, Piccoli R, Pellicano M, et al. Effectiveness of auto-crosslinked hyaluronic acid gel in the prevention of intrauterine adhesions after hysteroscopic surgery: a prospective, randomized, controlled study. Hum Reprod. 2004;11:1461-4.
40. Metwally M, Watson A, Lilford R, Vandekerckhove P. Fluid and pharmacological agents for adhesion prevention after gynaecological surgery. Cochrane Database Syst Rev. 2006;11:CD001298.
41. Reijnen MM, Falk P, van Goor H, Holmdahl L. The anti-adhesive agent sodium hyaluronate increases the proliferation rate of human peritoneal mesothelial cells. Fertil Steril. 2000;11:146-51.
42. Carta G, Cerrone L, Iovenitti P. Postoperative adhesion prevention in gynecologic surgery with hyaluronic acid. Clin Exp Obstet Gynecol. 2004;11:39-41.
43. Mais V, Cironis MG, Peiretti M, Ferrucci G, Cossu E, Melis GB. Efficacy of auto-crosslinked hyaluronan gel for adhesion prevention in laparoscopy and hysteroscopy: a systematic review and meta-analysis of randomized controlled trials. Eur J Obstet Gynecol Reprod Biol. 2012;11:1-5.
44. Tsapanos VS, Stathopoulou LP, Papathanassopoulou VS, Tzingounis VA. The role of Seprafilm bioresorbable membrane in the prevention and therapy of endometrial synechiae. J Biomed Mater Res. 2002;11:10-14.
45. Sher G, Fisch JD. Vaginal sildenafil (Viagra): a preliminary report of a novel method to improve uterine artery blood flow and endometrial development in patients undergoing IVF. Hum Reprod. 2000;11:806-9.
46. Takasaki A, Tamura H, Miwa I, Taketani T, Shimamura K, Sugino N. Endometrial growth and uterine blood flow: a pilot study for improving endometrial thickness in the patients with a thin endometrium. Fertil Steril. 2010;11:1851-8.
47. ACOG Committee on Practice Bulletins ACOG Practice Bulletin No. 74. Antibiotic prophylaxis for gynecologic procedures. Obstet Gynecol. 2006;108:225-34.
48. Gargett CE, Nguyen HP, Ye L. Endometrial regeneration and endometrial stem/progenitor cells. Rev Endocr Metab Disord. 2012;11:235-51.
49. Nagori CB, Panchal SY, Patel H. Endometrial regeneration using autologous adult stem cells followed by conception by in vitro fertilization in a patient of severe Asherman's syndrome. J Hum Reprod Sci. 2011;11:43-8.
50. Alawadhi F, Du H, Cakmak H, Taylor HS. Bone marrow-derived stem cell (BMDSC) transplantation improves fertility in a murine model of Asherman's syndrome. PLoS One. 2014;9(5):e96662.
51. Singh N, Mohanty S, Seth T, Shankar M, Bhaskaran S, Dharmendra S. Autologous stem cell transplantation in refractory Asherman's syndrome: a novel cell based therapy. J Hum Reprod Sci. 2014;7(2):93-8.
52. Santamaria X, Cabanillas S, Cervello I, Arbona C, Raga F, Ferro J, et al. Autologous cell therapy with CD133+ bone marrow-derived stem cells for refractory Asherman's syndrome and endometrial atrophy: a pilot cohort study. Hum Reprod. 2016;31(5):1087-96.
53. Tan J, Li P, Wang Q, Li Y, Li X, Zhao D, et al. Autologous menstrual blood-derived stromal cells transplantation for severe Asherman's syndrome. Hum Reprod. 2016;31(12):2723-9.
54. Zhang S, Li P, Yuan Z, Tan J. Platelet-rich plasma improves therapeutic effects of menstrual blood-derived stromal cells in rat model of intrauterine adhesion. Stem Cell Res Ther. 2019;10(1):61.
55. Deans R, Vancaillie T, Ledger W, Liu J, Abbott JA. Live birth rate and obstetric complications following the hysteroscopic management of intrauterine adhesions including Asherman syndrome. Hum Reprod. 2018;33(10):1847-53.

13. Management of Endometriosis

Mamta Dighe, Pallavi Kalghatgi

INTRODUCTION

- Endometriosis is defined as the presence of endometrial glands and stroma like lesions outside of the uterus.[1] The lesions detected could vary from being peritoneal lesions, superficial implants or cysts on the ovary, or deep infiltrating disease.[2]
- Endometriosis is a chronic inflammatory, estrogen-dependent disease that gives rise to pain and infertility and occurs primarily in women of reproductive age. Hence, it is crucial to take into account patients' fertility when treating endometriosis. Previous studies have suggested that roughly 25-50% of infertile women have endometriosis, and about 30-50% of women with endometriosis are infertile. In comparison the incidence of endometriosis in the general population is 2-10%.[3,4]

CAUSES OF INFERTILITY IN ENDOMETRIOSIS (FIG. 1)

Factors affecting infertility is depicted in **Figure 1**.

WORK-UP IN ENDOMETRIOSIS

Work-up in endometriosis is depicted in **Flowchart 1**.

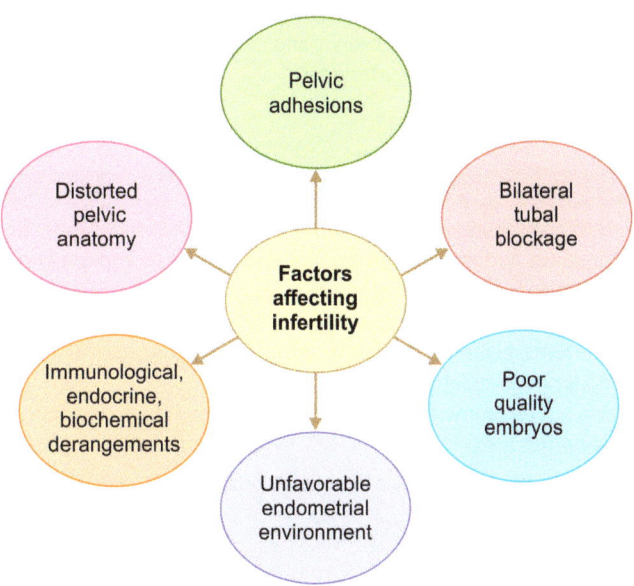

Fig. 1: Factors affecting infertility.[5]

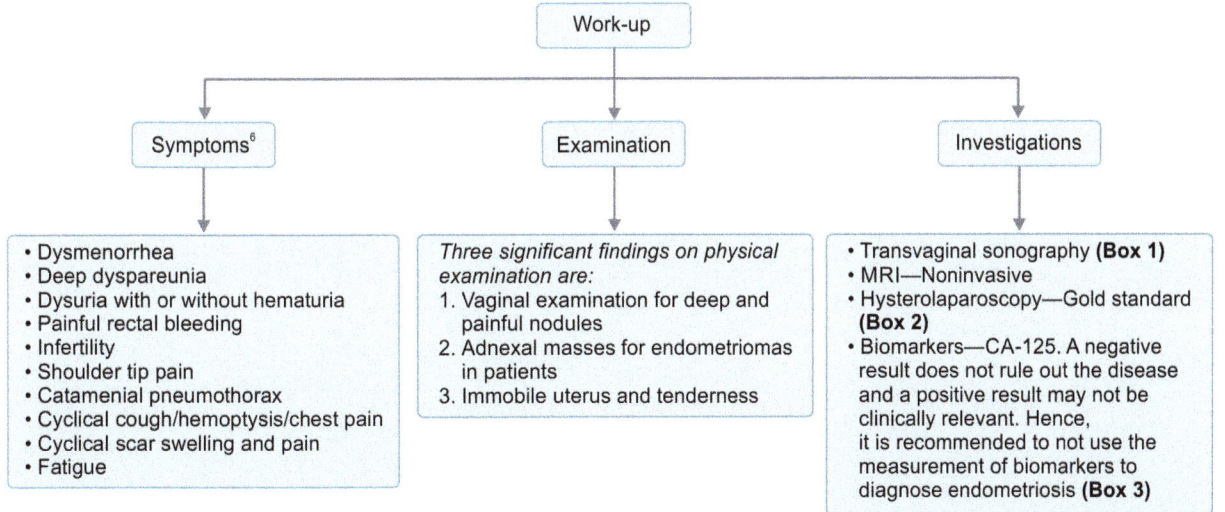

Flowchart 1: Work-up in endometriosis.

Symptoms[6]
- Dysmenorrhea
- Deep dyspareunia
- Dysuria with or without hematuria
- Painful rectal bleeding
- Infertility
- Shoulder tip pain
- Catamenial pneumothorax
- Cyclical cough/hemoptysis/chest pain
- Cyclical scar swelling and pain
- Fatigue

Examination

Three significant findings on physical examination are:
1. Vaginal examination for deep and painful nodules
2. Adnexal masses for endometriomas in patients
3. Immobile uterus and tenderness

Investigations
- Transvaginal sonography (**Box 1**)
- MRI—Noninvasive
- Hysterolaparoscopy—Gold standard (**Box 2**)
- Biomarkers—CA-125. A negative result does not rule out the disease and a positive result may not be clinically relevant. Hence, it is recommended to not use the measurement of biomarkers to diagnose endometriosis (**Box 3**)

> **BOX 1:** Features of endometrioma on ultrasound.
> - Unilocular cyst with acoustic enhancement
> - Diffuse homogeneous ground-glass echoes due to hemorrhagic debris[7]
> - Round/oval mass
> - Hyperechogenic cyst wall
> - Hypoechoic content
> - Absence of papillae

> **BOX 2:** Features on hysterolaparoscopy.
> - Number, location, and size of the endometriotic plaques, implants, lesions, and cysts are determined and confirmed by histology although negative histology does not entirely rule out the disease
> - Ovarian endometrioma is confirmed by histology or by presence of following features:
>   – Adhesions to pelvic side wall and/or broad ligament
>   – Endometriotic spots on ovarian surface
>   – Thick, tarry, and chocolate colored fluid inside the cyst
> - Morphology of peritoneal and ovarian implants are characterized as follows:
>   – Red (red, red-pink, and clear lesions)
>   – White (white, yellow-brown, and peritoneal defects)
>   – Black (black and blue lesions)

> **BOX 3:** Guidelines for investigations in endometriosis (ESHRE).
> - It is recommended to use imaging (US or MRI) in the diagnostic work-up for endometriosis, but it is important to understand that a negative finding does not exclude endometriosis, especially superficial peritoneal disease
> - In patients with negative imaging results or where empirical treatment was unsuccessful or inappropriate, the GDG recommends that clinicians consider offering laparoscopy for the diagnosis and treatment of suspected endometriosis
> - The GDG recommends that laparoscopic identification of endometriotic lesions is confirmed by histology although negative histology does not completely rule out the disease
> - It is not recommended to use measurement of biomarkers in endometrial tissue, blood, menstrual, or uterine fluids to diagnose endometriosis
>
> (ESHRE: European Society of Human Reproduction and Embryology; GDG: Guideline Development Group; MRI: magnetic resonance imaging; US: ultrasound)

ENDOMETRIOSIS STAGING

Staging systems used are:
- American Society for Reproductive Medicine (ASRM) **(Fig. 2)**
- ENZIAN **(Fig. 3)**
- Endometriosis fertility index (EFI) (used for fertility management) **(Fig. 4)**

AMERICAN SOCIETY FOR REPRODUCTIVE MEDICINE REVISED CLASSIFICATION OF ENDOMETRIOSIS

Patient's Name ______________________________ Date ______________

Stage I (Minimal) - 1–50
Stage II (Mild) - 6–15
Stage III (Moderate) - 16–40
Stage IV (Severe) - >40
Total ______________

Laparoscopy ______ Laparotomy ______ Photography ________
Recommended treatment ______________________________
____

Prognosis ______________________________

Peritoneum	**Endometriosis**	<1 cm	1.3 cm	>3 cm
Peritoneum	Superficial	1	2	4
Peritoneum	Deep	2	4	6
Ovary	R superficial	1	2	4
Ovary	Deep	4	16	20
Ovary	L superficial	1	2	4
Ovary	Deep	4	16	20
	Posterior cul-de-sac obliteration	Partial	Complete	
		4	40	
Ovary	**Adhesions**	<1/3 Enclosure	1/3–2/3 Enclosure	>2/3 Enclosure
Ovary	R Filmy	1	2	4
Ovary	Dense	4	8	16
Ovary	L Filmy	1	2	4
Ovary	Dense	4	8	16
Tube	R Filmy	1	2	4
Tube	Dense	4*	8*	16
Tube	L Filmy	1	2	4
Tube	Dense	4*	8*	16

***If the fimbriated end of the fallopian tube is completely enclosed, change the point assignment to 16.**

Denote appearance of superficial implant types as red [(R), red, red-pink, flamelike, vesicular blobs, clear vesicles], white [(W), opacifications, peritoneal defects, yellow-brown], or black [(B) black, hemosiderin deposits, blue]. Denote percent of total described as R___%, W___%, and B___%. Total should equal 100%.

Additional endometriosis: ______________________________

Associated pathology: ______________________________

To be used with normal tubes and ovaries

L R

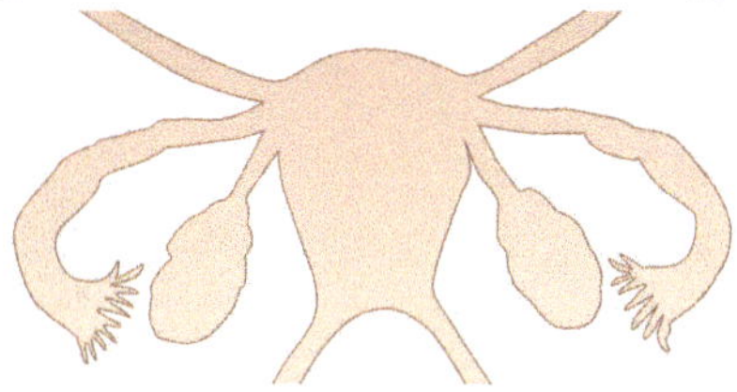

To be used with abnormal tubes and/or ovaries

L R

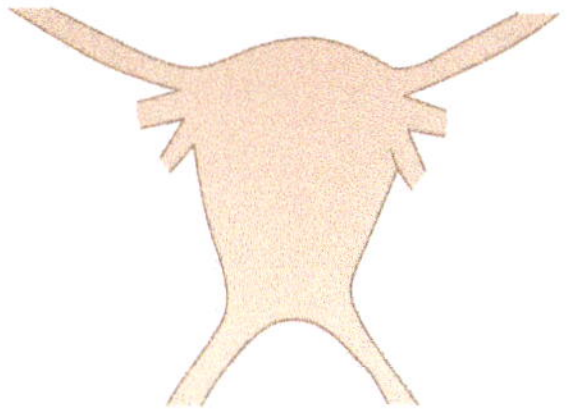

Fig. 2: American Society for Reproductive Medicine classification system.[8]

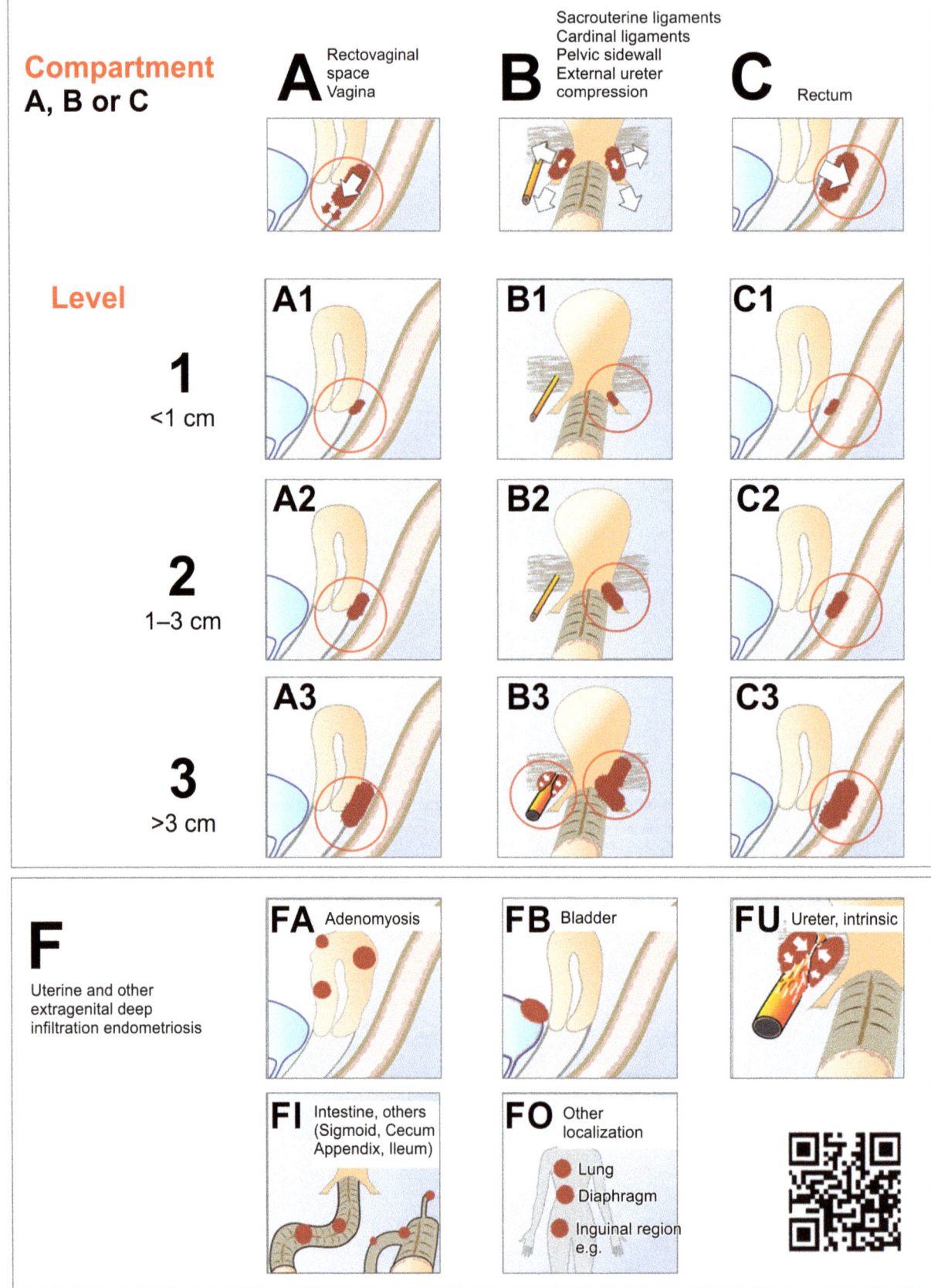

Fig. 3: Detection and localization of deep endometriosis by means of MRI and correlation with the ENZIAN score.[9]

Least function (LF) score at conclusion of surgery

Score		Description
4	=	Normal
3	=	Mild dysfunction
2	=	Moderate dysfunction
1	=	Severe dysfunction
0	=	Absent or nonfuctional

	Left	Right
Fallopian tube		
Fimbria		
Ovary		

To calculate the LF score, add together the lowest score for the left side and the lowest score for the right side. If an ovary is absent on one side, the LF score is obtained by doubling the lowest score on the side with the ovary

Lowest score: Left + Right = LF score

Endometriosis fertility index (EFI)

Historical factors				Surgical factors		
Factor	Description	Points	Factor	Description		Points
Age			LF score			
	If age is <35 years	2		If LF score = 7 to 8 (high score)		3
	If age is 36 to 39 years	1		If LF score = 4 to 6 (moderate score)		2
	If age is ³40 years	0		If LF score = 1 to 3 (low score)		0
Years infertile			AFS endometriosis score			
	If years infertile is £3	2		If AFS endometriosis lesion score is <16		1
	If years infertile is >3	0		If AFS endometriosis lesion score is ³16		0
Prior pregnancy			AFS Total score			
	If there is a history of a prior pregnancy	2		If AFS total score is <71		1
	If there is no history of a prior pregnancy	0		If AFS total score is ³71		0
Total historical factors			**Total surgical factors**			

EFI = Total historical factors + Total surgical factors:

Historical + Surgical = EFI score

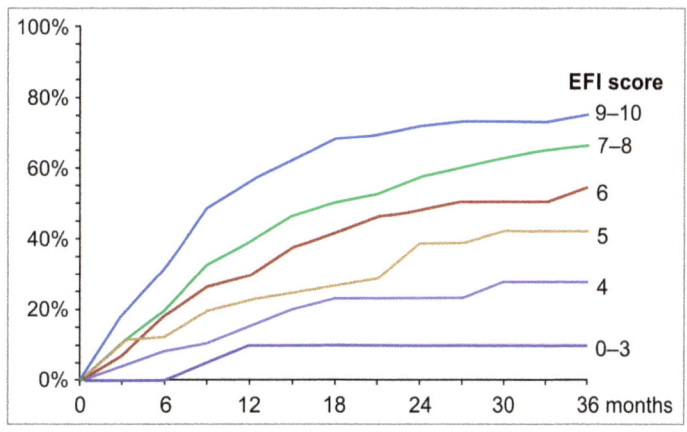

Fig. 4: Endometriosis fertility index.[10]

■ MANAGEMENT

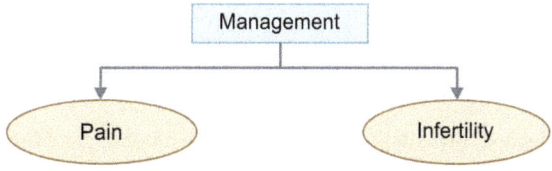

Management of Pain Associated with Endometriosis

Management for pain is depicted in **Flowchart 2**.

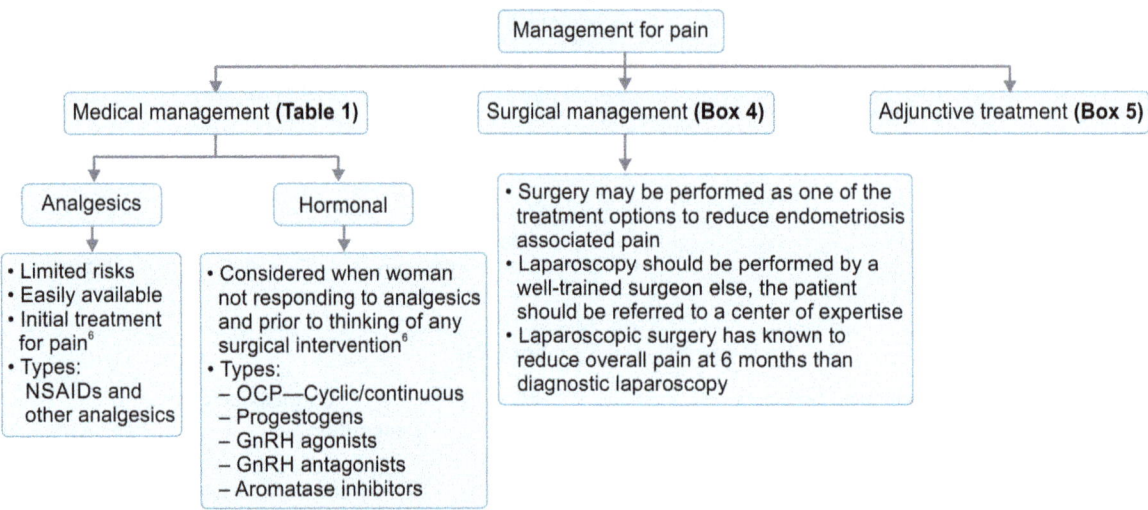

Flowchart 2: Management for pain.

(GnRH: gonadotrophin-releasing hormone; NSAIDs: nonsteroidal anti-inflammatory drugs; OCP: oral contraceptive pill)

TABLE 1: Recommendations for medical management of pain in endometriosis (ESHRE).

	Type of treatment	Recommendation
1.	Analgesics	NSAIDs or other analgesics may be offered for the treatment of endometriosis-associated pain
2.	Oral contraceptives	• Recommended to prescribe women a combined hormonal contraceptive (oral, vaginal ring, or transdermal) • Continuous use of a combined hormonal contraceptive pill can be recommended
3.	Progestins, depot medroxyprogesterone acetate, cytoproterone acetate, medroxyprogesterone acetate, norethindrone/norethisterone acetate, desogestrel, and dienogest	• Recommended to prescribe women progestogens to reduce endometriosis associated pain after taking side effects of each into account • First-line therapy equally effective as oral contraceptives
4.	GnRH agonist	• Recommended if hormonal contraceptives or progestogens have been ineffective • For long-term use consider combined hormonal add-back therapy alongside GnRH agonist therapy to prevent bone loss and hypoestrogenic symptoms
5.	GnRH antagonist	• Evidence is very limited regarding dosage and duration • Prescribed only as second line (e.g., if hormonal contraceptives or progestogens have been ineffective)
6.	Aromatase inhibitors	• Recommended if refractory to other medical or surgical treatment • May be prescribed in combination with oral contraceptives, progestogens, GnRH agonists or GnRH antagonists

(ESHRE: European Society of Human Reproduction and Embryology; GnRH: gonadotrophin-releasing hormone; NSAIDs: nonsteroidal anti-inflammatory drugs)

BOX 4: Recommendations for surgical management of pain in endometriosis (ESHRE).

- Excision of endometriosis instead of ablation may be considered to reduce endometriosis-associated pain
- In case of ovarian endometrioma, while performing surgery, cystectomy should be performed instead of drainage and coagulation. It is seen that cystectomy lowers the recurrence of endometrioma and endometriosis-associated pain
- Both cystectomy and CO_2 laser vaporization can be considered in a case of ovarian endometrioma, as both techniques seem to have similar recurrence rates in the first year after surgery. Early postsurgical recurrence rates may be lower after cystectomy
- When performing surgery for ovarian endometrioma, specific precaution should be taken to minimize ovarian damage
- Clinicians can consider performing surgical removal of deep endometriosis, as it may reduce endometriosis-associated pain and improves quality of life
- The GDG recommends that women with deep endometriosis are referred to a center of expertise
- The GDG recommends that patients undergoing surgery particularly for deep endometriosis are informed on potential risks, benefits, and long-term effect on quality of life

(ESHRE: European Society of Human Reproduction and Embryology; GDG: Guideline Development Group)

> **BOX 5:** Recommendations for adjunctive treatment of pain in endometriosis (ESHRE).
> - Prescribing preoperative hormone treatment to improve the immediate outcome of surgery for pain in women with endometriosis is not recommended
> - Postoperative hormone treatment can be advised to improve the outcome of surgery for pain in women with endometriosis if not desiring immediate pregnancy
> - With no proven harm, postoperative hormone therapy may be prescribed for other indications, such as contraception or secondary prevention (weak recommendation)

(ESHRE: European Society of Human Reproduction and Embryology)

The Guideline Development Group (GDG) recommends that a shared decision-making approach be taken by the clinician and to take individual preferences, side effects, individual efficacy, costs, and availability into consideration when choosing hormone treatments for endometriosis-associated pain.

Empirical Management of Pain Suspected from Endometriosis

- In patients suspected to have endometriosis and not planning conception, especially in the primary care setting, if show negative imaging results [transvaginal sonography (TVS)] but are symptomatic, usually are offered hormonal treatment mostly in the form of the oral contraceptive pill or progestogens as a first-line treatment (Kuznetsov et al., 2017).
- If symptoms improve, endometriosis is presumed the main underlying condition, although other clinical causes can (co-)exist. This "blinded" approach is widely known as *empirical treatment*.[11,12]

Medical versus Surgical Management for Pain Associated with Endometriosis

- Clinicians must take a shared decision-making approach and take individual preferences, side effects, individual efficacy, costs, and availability into consideration when choosing between hormone treatments and surgical treatments for endometriosis-associated pain.
- There is no accurate evidence to make any definitive recommendation on whether medical therapies or surgery are more effective for relieving pain in women with endometriosis.
- Surgery may be a potential "instant" treatment, but surgical complications may occur and often give only temporary pain relief with a considerable risk of recurrence.
- Patients with endometriosis managed medically can be associated with short and long-term side effects.

Management of Infertility Associated with Endometriosis

Management of infertility is depicted in **Flowchart 3**.

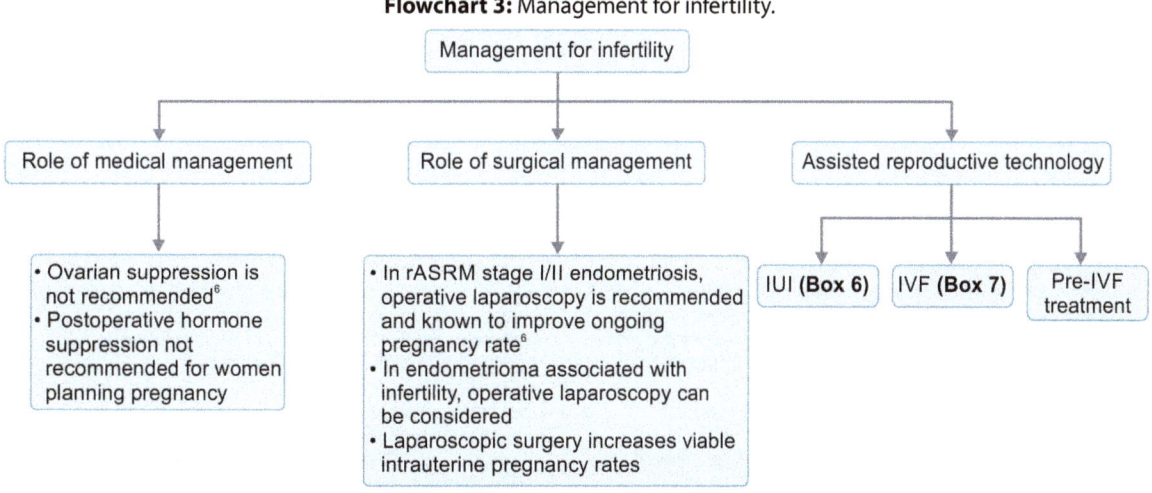

Flowchart 3: Management for infertility.

(IUI: intrauterine insemination; IVF: in vitro fertilization; rASRM: revised American Society for Reproductive Medicine)

Assisted Reproduction

Factors determining treatment options:
- Age of the woman
- Period of infertility
- Ovarian reserve
- Stage of endometriosis
- Previous H/O surgery i/v/o endometriosis
- Tubal patency
- Male factor.

BOX 6: Intrauterine insemination recommendations (ESHRE).

- In infertile women with rASRM stage I/II endometriosis, intrauterine insemination (IUI) with ovarian stimulation is the treatment of choice
- Expectant management or IUI alone show reduced pregnancy rates when compared with IUI with ovarian stimulation
- In these women, it is ideal to perform intrauterine insemination with ovarian stimulation within 6 months after surgical treatment
- The use of IUI with ovarian stimulation could be considered in infertile women with rASRM stage III/IV endometriosis with tubal patency, though with uncertain value[8]

(ESHRE: European Society of Human Reproduction and Embryology; rASRM: revised American Society for Reproductive Medicine)

Assisted Reproductive Technology

BOX 7: Recommendations for ART (ESHRE).

- In women with infertility associated with endometriosis with compromised tubal function, if there is male factor infertility, in case of low EFI and/or if other treatments have failed, ART should be considered
- A specific protocol for ART in women with endometriosis cannot be recommended. Both GnRH antagonist and agonist protocols show no difference in pregnancy or live birth rate and so can be offered based on patients' and physicians' preferences
- Women with endometriosis can be reassured regarding the safety of ART since the recurrence rates are not increased compared to those women not undergoing ART
- In women with endometrioma, use of antibiotic prophylaxis at the time of oocyte retrieval can be considered, although the risk of ovarian abscess formation following follicle aspiration is low

(ART: assisted reproductive technology; EFI: endometriosis fertility index; ESHRE: European Society of Human Reproduction and Embryology; GnRH: gonadotrophin-releasing hormone)

Role of Pre-in Vitro Fertilization Treatment in Endometriosis

Pre-in vitro fertilization treatment is depicted in **Flowchart 4**.

Flowchart 4: Pre-in vitro fertilization treatment.

```
                      Pre-IVF treatment
                      /               \
            Medical treatment      Surgical treatment
```

Medical treatment:
- Medical treatment of endometriosis like GnRH agonists, prior to ART has some evidence to improve outcome, either because of improving oocyte quality or endometrial receptivity
- As per previous ESHRE guideline prolonged downregulation for 3–6 months with a GnRH agonist in women with endometriosis increases the odds of clinical pregnancy by more than fourfold
- In contrast, the updated version of this Cochrane review concluded that the effect of GnRH agonist pretreatment (for at least 3 months) was very uncertain, both on clinical pregnancy rate and live birth rate
- Using continuous combined oral contraceptive (OCP) for 6–8 weeks prior to treatment of ART has shown no evidence of improvement when compared with no pretreatment before ART
- Administration of dienogest (DNG) 12 weeks before IVF not found to be useful

Surgical treatment:
- Routinely performing surgery prior to ART to improve live birth rates in women with rASRM stage I/II endometriosis is not recommended as the potential benefits are unclear
- No evidence to show benefit of routinely performing surgery for ovarian endometrioma prior to ART to improve live birth rates, and is likely to have a negative impact on ovarian reserve
- Surgery for endometrioma prior to ART may help to improve pain associated with endometriosis or accessibility of follicles
- The decision to offer surgical excision of deep endometriosis lesions prior to ART should be guided mainly by pain symptoms and patient preference as its effectiveness on reproductive outcome is uncertain due to lack of randomized studies

Based on the mentioned recommendations, an algorithm can be formulated for treatment of endometriosis associated infertility **(Fig. 5)**.
- After detailed imaging studies, endometriosis can be confirmed and the stage can be determined.
- Treatment for infertility depends on multiple factors and can be deduced with the help of algorithm depicted in **Flowchart 5**.

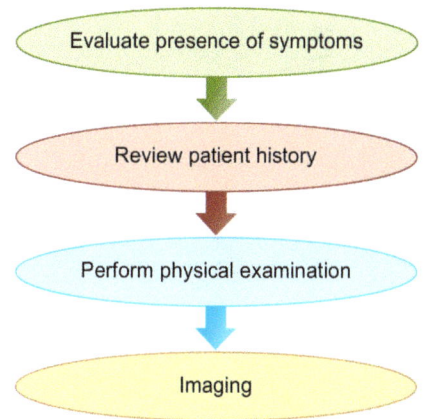

Fig. 5: Overview of management of Infertility associated with endometriosis.

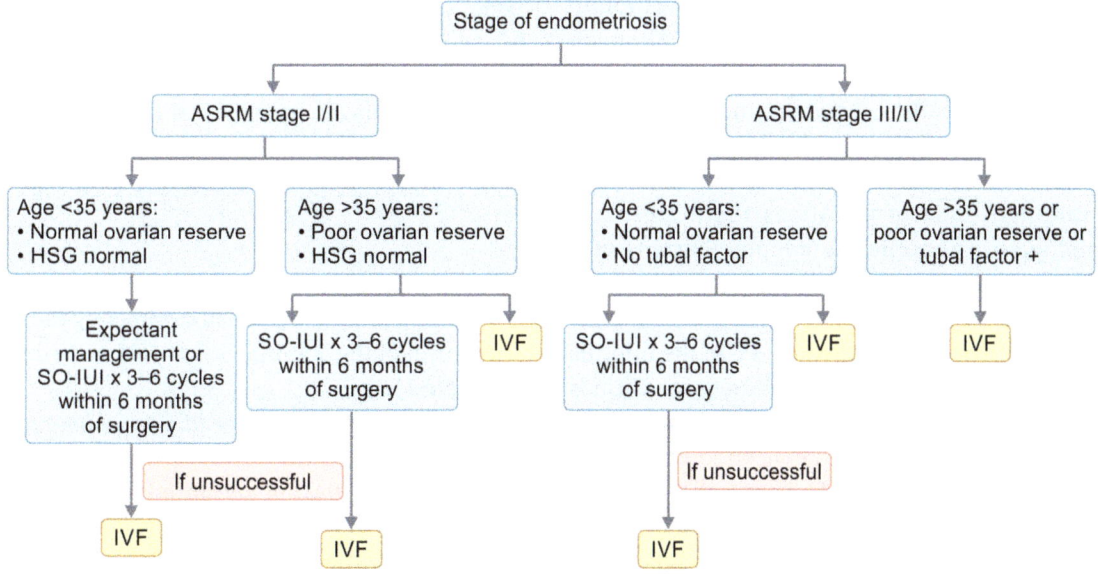

Flowchart 5: Treatment of infertility depending on stage of endometriosis.

(ASRM: American Society for Reproductive Medicine; HSG: hysterosalpingogram; IUI: intrauterine insemination; IVF: in vitro fertilization)

REFERENCES

1. Giudice LC, Kao LC. Endometriosis. Lancet. 2004;364(9447):1789-99.
2. Nisolle M, Donnez J. Peritoneal endometriosis, ovarian endometriosis, and adenomyotic nodules of the rectovaginal septum are three different entities. Fertil Steril. 1997;68(4):585-96.
3. Missmer SA, Hankinson SE, Spiegelman D, Barbieri RL, Marshall LM, Hunter DJ. Incidence of laparoscopically confirmed endometriosis by demographic, anthropometric, and lifestyle factors. Am J Epidemiol. 2004;160:784-96.
4. Practice Committee of the American Society for Reproductive Medicine Endometriosis and infertility: a committee opinion. Fertil Steril. 2012;98:591-8.
5. Miller JE, Ahn SH, Monsanto SP, Khalaj K, Koti M, Tayade C. Implications of immune dysfunction on endometriosis associated infertility. Oncotarget. 2017;8:7138-47.
6. Dunselman GA, Vermeulen N, Becker C, Calhaz-Jorge C, D'Hooghe T, De Bie B, et al. ESHRE guideline: management of women with endometriosis. Hum Reprod. 2014;29(3):400-12.
7. Moore J, Copley S, Morris J, Lindsell D, Golding S, Kennedy S. A systematic review of the accuracy of ultrasound in the diagnosis of endometriosis. Ultrasound Obstet Gynecol. 2002;20(6):630-4.
8. Revised American Society for Reproductive Medicine classification of endometriosis: 1996. Fertil Steril. 1997;67(5):817-21.
9. Di Paola V, Manfredi R, Castelli F, Negrelli R, Mehrabi S, Pozzi Mucelli R. Detection and localization of deep endometriosis by means of MRI and correlation with the ENZIAN score. Eur J Radiol. 2015;84(4):568-74.
10. Ibrjam I, Veleva G, Karagjozova G, Ivanov S. Endometriosis fertility index. Akush Ginekol (Sofiia). 2016;55 Suppl 1 Pt 2:5-10.
11. Kuznetsov L, Dworzynski K, Davies M, Overton C. Diagnosis and management of endometriosis: summary of NICE guidance. BMJ. 2017;358:j3935.
12. NICE. (2017). Endometriosis: diagnosis and management. [online] Available from nice.org.uk/ng73. [Last accessed February, 2023].

14 Management of Fibroids and Adenomyosis in Infertility

Sangita Sharma

■ INTRODUCTION

Uterine fibroids or leiomyomas are the most common benign gynecological tumors, the prevalence being around 20–40% in the women of reproductive age group. Although most of the fibroids are asymptomatic, others may present as abnormal uterine bleeding, pelvic pain, dyspareunia, pressure symptoms, constipation, and increased frequency of micturition. Fibroids have also been associated with infertility, although most of the times there are other causative etiologies in the infertile couple. Fibroids may coincidentally be present in around 25% of infertility cases, but when all other causes are ruled out, it is seen that fibroids are responsible for decreased fertility in <5% of the infertile couples.[1,2] It is now a known fact that submucosal fibroids and intramural fibroids with submucosal components do negatively affect natural and assisted conception rates, and are also responsible for increased risk of miscarriage.[1,3-7] The role of noncavity-distorting intramural myomas in infertility is still controversial with conflicting data.[8,9] In some studies, such intramural fibroids, especially if >4–5 cm have been found to reduce pregnancy rates significantly.[10,11]

In this chapter we shall discuss the practical approach to an infertile couple with fibroids and adenomyosis. We shall discuss the classification of fibroids, types of adenomyosis, evidence on their role in infertility, different treatment options available, and most importantly when to decide for myomectomy. Ruling out other causes of infertility, addressing previous treatment taken for infertility [intrauterine insemination/assisted reproductive technology (IUI/ART) cycles] and a detailed fibroid mapping are extremely important in deciding the further management of the fibroid in an infertile woman.

■ CLASSIFICATION OF FIBROIDS (LEIOMYOMA)

- *European Society for Gynaecological Endoscopy (ESGE) Classification:* This classification of submucosal fibroids was proposed by Wamsteker et al. in 1993 and has been adopted by the ESGE.[12] It is a simple and clinically relevant classification, therefore has been commonly used

TABLE 1: Wamsteker and ESGE classification of submucous fibroids.

Type	Degree of intramural extension
0	No intramural extension. Fibroid is attached to the cavity by a narrow pedicle
1	Intramural extension <50%
2	Intramural extension >50%

(ESGE: European Society for Gynaecological Endoscopy)

worldwide. This classification helps the gynecologists in predicting the likelihood of completing the hysteroscopic removal of the submucosal fibroid in a single procedure **(Table 1)**.

- *International Federation of Gynecology and Obstetrics (FIGO) classification:* The most popular classification of leiomyoma is the one proposed by the FIGO.[13] There are eight types of leiomyomas according to this classification along with the hybrid types. This classification gives a better understanding of the topographical "fibroid mapping" and helps in planning the approach to management further. The hybrid fibroids are given two numbers, e.g., 2–5 and 2–6, the first number tells the relation of the fibroid with the endometrium and the second tells the relation to the uterine serosa **(Table 2 and Fig. 1)**.
- *Lasmar's size, topography, extension, penetration, and wall (STEPW) classification of submucous fibroids:* Discussed in the section "Surgical Management" (vide infra).

■ DIAGNOSIS OF FIBROIDS

Diagnosis of fibroids is incomplete till proper mapping is done. To prognosticate the chances of conception and to plan further management of the fibroids, a detailed description is recommended including the following points:
- Number of fibroids
- Size of each one of them
- Type of fibroid (FIGO classification)

TABLE 2: Classification of leiomyoma according to the International Federation of Obstetrics and Gynecology (FIGO).		
	Type	Location
Submucosal	0	Pedunculated intracavitary
	1	<50% intramural
	2	>50% intramural
Others	3	Contacts endometrium, 100% intramural
	4	Intramural
	5	Subserous >50% intramural
	6	Subserous <50% Intramural
	7	Subserous pedunculated
	8	Others (specify, e.g., cervical and parasitic)
Hybrid leiomyomas	e.g., 2–5 and 2–6	Impact both endometrium and serosa

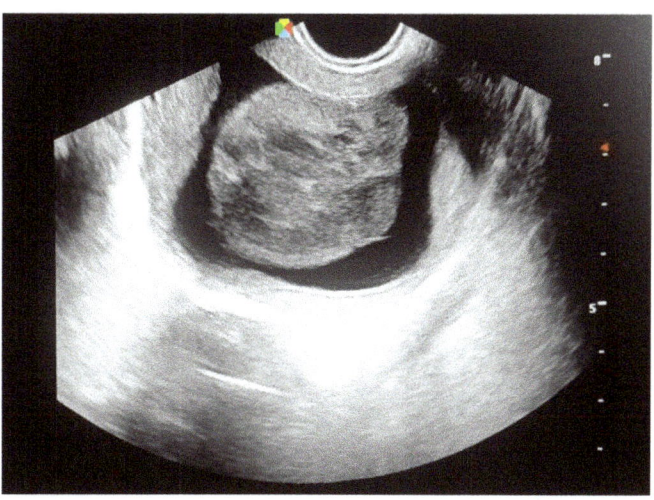

Fig. 2: Type 0 Submucosal fibroid delineated on saline infusion sonography (SIS).
(*Courtesy:* Dr Anita Sharma, IVF Centre, SMS Medical College, Jaipur).

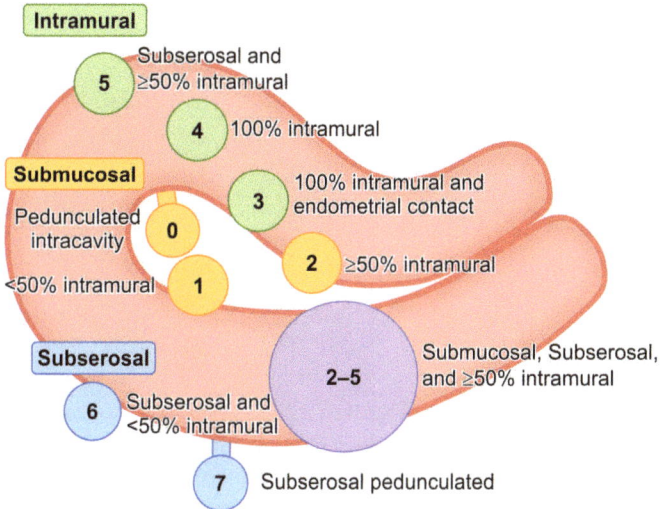

Fig. 1: FIGO classification of fibroids.
(*Courtesy:* Dr Sachintha Hapugoda, Radiopaedia.org, rID: 62908).

- Distance from the junctional zone (JZ) myometrium
- Nature of the fibroid (e.g., any degeneration, calcification, and vascularity pattern).

Modalities for Diagnosing Fibroids

- *2D ultrasound:* Most of the fibroids are diagnosed by a 2D ultrasound, preferably by a transvaginal probe.
- Saline infusion sonography (SIS) or hysterosalpingo-contrast sonography (HyCoSy) scan be used to demarcate any submucosal component of the fibroids **(Fig. 2)**.
- 3D ultrasound helps in better assessment of the uterine cavity and topographical study and might be more informative for fibroid mapping in case of multiple fibroids.
- MRI is limited by its cost and is indicated in case of complex masses, to differentiate between adenomyoma and fibroids and when the diagnosis remains doubtful on ultrasound **(Fig. 3)**.

- *Hysteroscopy:* It is minimally invasive. It has the advantage of diagnosing and simultaneously performing myomectomy, but only for type L0 to L2 fibroids (those with submucosal component) **(Figs. 4 and 5)**.

■ EFFECTS OF FIBROIDS ON FERTILITY

Uterine leiomyomas are associated as sole factor for infertility in <5-10% of infertility cases.[14] The different theories proposed to explain how fibroids can cause infertility are:
- Anatomical disruption of the uterine architecture and distortion of the uterine cavity[15]
- Abnormal uterine contractility which can adversely affect sperm transport[16]
- Greater distance for sperm travel
- Encroachment and sometimes occlusion of the tubal ostia
- Vascular changes
- Submucosal leiomyomas in particular may interfere with embryo implantation[6]
- Aberrant expression of endometrial growth factors and other biomarkers of endometrial receptivity, e.g., leukemia inhibitory factor (LIF), glycodelin, cytokines [interleukin-1 (IL-1) and IL-11][16]
- Decreased expression of HOXA-10 in the endometrium.[17]

Due to heterogeneity in studies, different patient characteristics contributing to the pregnancy rates and diversity in the number, location, and size of fibroids, it is difficult to study the exact role of fibroids in impairing implantation and pregnancy rates.

- However, the literature is clear that *submucosal fibroids and intramural fibroids distorting the uterine cavity (FIGO type L0, L1, and L2)* negatively affect implantation, pregnancy and live birth rates in both natural and assisted conception. Removal of these types of fibroids improves

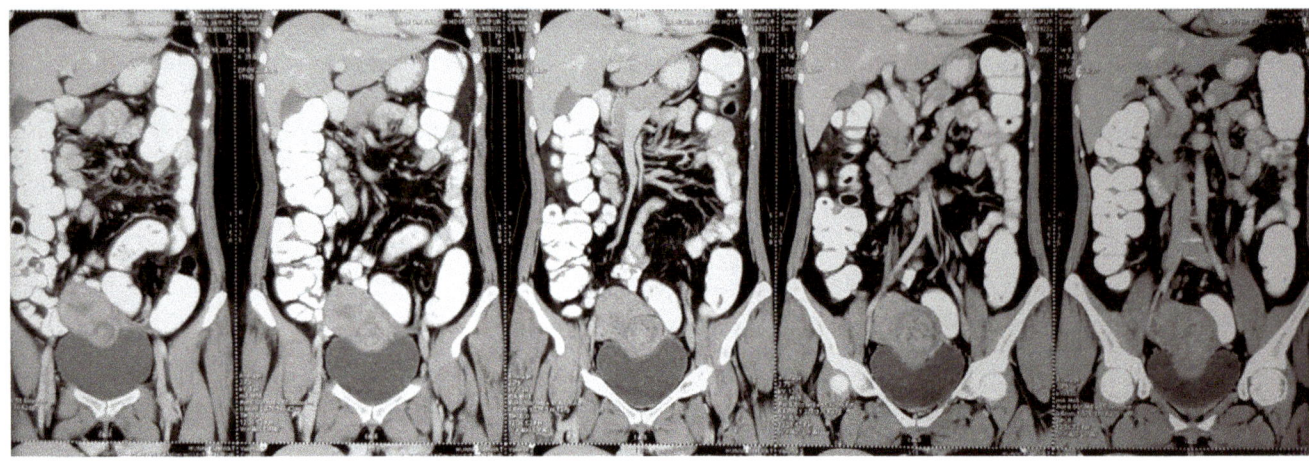

Fig. 3: MRI view of hybrid myomas (Type 2–6)
(*Courtesy:* Dr Vijay Nahata, Mahatma Gandhi Hospital, Jaipur)

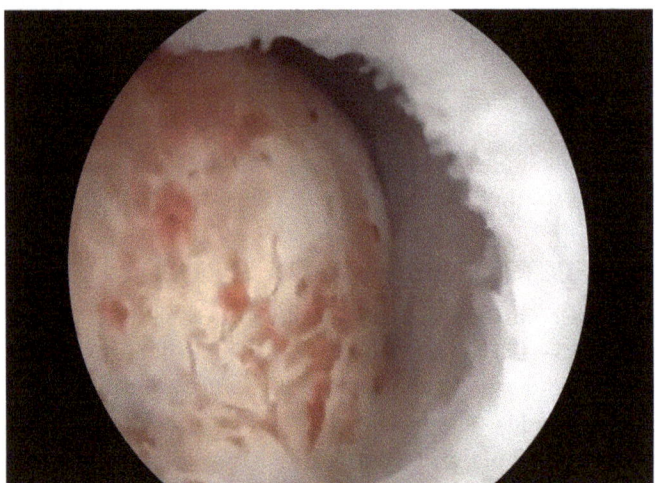

Fig. 4: Type 0 submucous fibroid.
(*Courtesy:* Dr Vijay Nahata, Mahatma Gandhi Hospital, Jaipur)

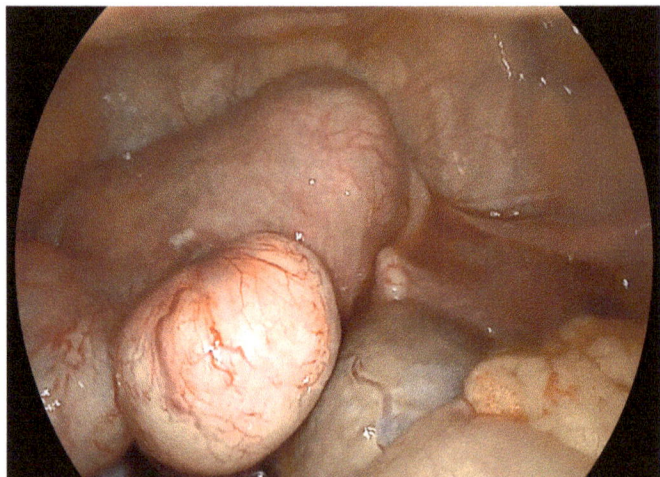

Fig. 6: Laparoscopic view of multiple subserosal fibroids.
(*Courtesy:* Dr Vijay Nahata, Mahatma Gandhi Hospital, Jaipur)

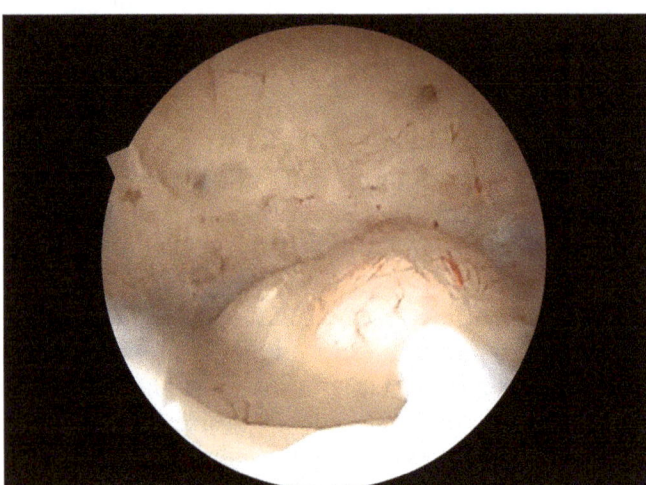

Fig. 5: Type 2 submucous fibroid.
(*Courtesy:* Dr Vijay Nahata, Mahatma Gandhi Hospital, Jaipur)

the implantation and pregnancy rates and reduces the risk of early miscarriage.[4-7]

- Although, in a recent Cochrane systematic review, it was reported that there is uncertainty whether hysteroscopic removal of submucous fibroids improves the clinical pregnancy rates in women with otherwise unexplained subfertility.[18]
- The American Society for Reproductive Medicine (ASRM) guidelines published in 2017 conclude that there is fair evidence that hysteroscopic myomectomy for cavity-distorting myomas improves clinical pregnancy rates but insufficient evidence regarding the impact of this procedure on the likelihood of live birth or early pregnancy loss. However, they summarize that in women with asymptomatic cavity-distorting myomas, myomectomy may be considered to optimize pregnancy outcomes.[6]
- *Subserosal fibroids* have no effect on reproductive outcome and their removal is not indicated for infertility **(Fig. 6)**.
- The controversy is only regarding the effect of *noncavity-distorting intramural fibroids* on reproductive outcomes.

- Although data is conflicting, yet most of the meta-analyses have concluded that this kind of fibroids decrease the implantation, clinical pregnancy, and live birth rates significantly, whereas the miscarriage rate is significantly increased.[4,9] This includes a recent meta-analysis of 28 studies and 9,189 in vitro fertilization (IVF) cycles.[19]
- One randomized controlled trial (RCT) studied the effect of myomectomy for a solitary intramural or subserosal myoma <4 cm, and concluded that myomectomy was not associated with improvement in pregnancy rates.[20]
- Oliviera et al., in a retrospective analysis, found that patients with intramural fibroids >4.0 cm had lower pregnancy rates in IVF-intracytoplasmic sperm injection (ICSI) cycles compared to patients with intramural fibroids ≤4.0 cm.[10]
- In a nonrandomized comparative study, Bulletti et al. found higher cumulative clinical pregnancy (33% vs. 15%) and delivery (25% vs. 12%) rates after one to three cycles of IVF treatment in women who underwent laparoscopic myomectomy for intramural fibroids >5 cm compared to those who decided against myomectomy.[11]
- Hart et al. performed a large prospective controlled study, evaluating the effect of the fibroids on the outcome of assisted reproduction. They concluded that even small intramural fibroids reduced the implantation rate by half. They also found that the ongoing pregnancy rates after ART are significantly affected by the presence or absence of an intramural fibroid.[21]
- A recent retrospective case control study reported that type 3 fibroids ≥30 mm might negatively impact implantation, clinical pregnancy, and live birth rates of IVF cycles.[22]

Despite so much evidence on the noncavity-distorting intramural fibroids having adverse impacts on IVF outcomes, there is still no definite evidence suggesting routine myomectomy for this kind of fibroid. Most of the earlier mentioned studies and meta-analyses have concluded that it is still unclear whether the removal of such fibroids will reverse the process and normalize fertility or even be beneficial to the patient. Thus, a large well-designed randomized control trial is needed to see whether myomectomy for noncavity-distorting intramural fibroids would improve the efficacy of IVF-embryo transfer (ET) treatment or not. The decision can be individualized based on previous reproductive outcome, duration of infertility, any pregnancy losses, or treatment taken in past.

INDICATIONS OF MYOMECTOMY

To summarize and extrapolate from the available evidence, the indications of myomectomy in women with infertility and fibroids are (after ruling out all other causes of infertility; vide infra)[4,5,9-11,19]

- Submucosal fibroids (L0, L1, and L2)
- Intramural fibroids >4–5 cm
- Intramural fibroids <4–5 cm with
  - Heavy vaginal bleeding
  - Pressure symptoms
  - Multiple failed cycles of IUI/IVF after optimizing all other factors
- Subserosal fibroids
  - Not much role in infertility
  - For pressure symptoms.

MANAGEMENT OF FIBROIDS WITH INFERTILITY

When fibroids are diagnosed in couples facing infertility, further decision to manage the fibroid is based on three important factors:

1. Any other factors responsible for infertility in the couple
2. The probability of achieving a pregnancy with the coexisting fibroid, based on its location (FIGO type), size, and number
3. Treatment taken in past for infertility, e.g., number of attempts taken with IUI or IVF in past.

The management of fibroids in an infertile couple is outlined in **Flowchart 1**.

Before considering the fibroid as a causative factor for infertility in a couple, it is extremely important to rule out other causative etiologies of infertility by preliminary investigations viz;

- Anovulation
  - Day 21 serum progesterone levels
  - Serial follicular study scans
  - Evaluation of the baseline serum gonadotropin levels where indicated
  - Thyroid profile
  - Serum prolactin levels
- Tubal factor
  - Hysterosalpingography (HSG)/HyCoSy (might not be accurate in presence of large fibroids or fibroids at specific locations, e.g., cornual or submucosal near the tubal ostia)
  - Laparoscopy might be considered when HSG/HyCoSy are showing tubal block or are inconclusive or in the earlier mentioned situations where HSG/HyCoSy might be inaccurate. The added advantage is simultaneous assessment of the pelvis and myomectomy, if required.
- Male factor
  - Basic semen analysis
  - Other investigations (hormonal evaluation, scrotal ultrasound, and genetic testing where required)
- Ovarian reserve
  - Antral follicle count
  - Anti-müllerian hormone levels.

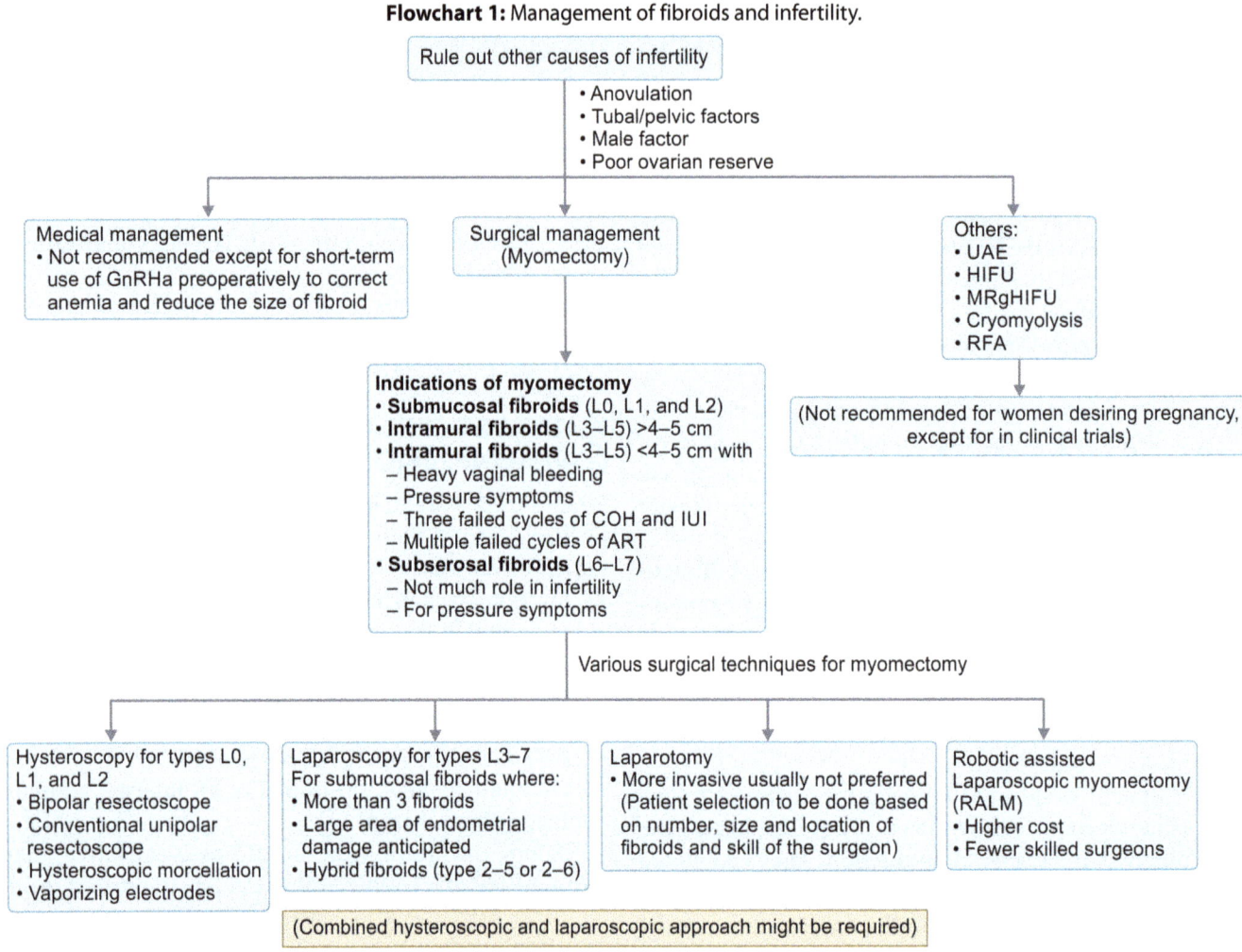

Flowchart 1: Management of fibroids and infertility.

(ART: assisted reproductive technology; COH: controlled ovarian hyperstimulation; GnRHa: gonadotropin-releasing hormone agonist; HIFU: high-intensity focused ultrasound; IUI: intrauterine insemination; MRgHIFU: magnetic resonance-guided high-intensity focused ultrasound; RALM: robotic-assisted laparoscopic myomectomy; RFA: radiofrequency ablation; UAE: uterine artery embolization)

If the fibroids are coexisting with other causative factors of infertility, it is difficult to assess the exact contribution of the fibroid to the failure of conception. Thus it is advisable to correct or treat other causative factors and then to proceed with myomectomy (more relevant for noncavity-distorting myomas). Whereas, in otherwise unexplained infertility where other treatment modalities have been unsuccessful, myomectomy might be considered.

Management Options for Fibroids and Infertility

Medical Management

Medical management of fibroids usually comprises of the drugs such as oral contraceptive pills (OCPs), progestins, levonorgestrel intrauterine system (LNG-IUS), and gonadotropin-releasing hormone (GnRH) analogs, which are effective in symptoms of pain and pressure, but have no role in fibroids with infertility as they inhibit ovulation. Short-term preoperative therapy with GnRH analogs might be useful in reducing blood loss, correcting anemia and reducing the volume of the fibroid, thus letting us choose a more optimal route and technique of myomectomy. Some studies have come up on role of ulipristal acetate (UPA) in fibroids. UPA is a selective progesterone receptor modulator (SPRM) with antiproliferative effect on cells of myoma. It is not recommended in females with fibroid and infertility due to limited data and adverse side effects.[5,7,23]

Surgical Management (Myomectomy)

Myomectomy can be done through the following techniques, depending on the location, size and number of fibroids, available equipment, surgical expertise and skill of the surgeon, and any comorbidities in the patient.

Hysteroscopy: This is the standard procedure for removing submucous fibroids (L0, L1, and L2). It is a minimally invasive procedure which can be done as an office procedure for small submucous fibroids, whereas others might require anesthesia. The different surgical techniques available are:

- *Bipolar resectoscope:* It is safer as compared to the conventional monopolar resectoscope as it requires isotonic electrolyte-containing distension media like normal saline **(Fig. 7)**.
- *Monopolar resectoscope:* This requires nonelectrolyte hypotonic distension media, e.g., glycine and sorbitol. Excessive absorption of such media can lead to symptoms such as hyponatremia, pulmonary edema, hypertension, and cardiac failure. One should try to minimize damage to endometrium and myometrium.
- *Hysteroscopic morcellator:* This has an integrated system of morcellation and suction of the myoma. The procedure is faster and reduces the risk of perforation as compares to resectoscopes. Moreover, as electric current is not used and damage to endometrium is minimal, the subsequent implantation rates may be better.
- *Vaporizing electrodes:* Electrosurgical vaporization of the myoma is performed. The disadvantage is that due to vaporization, tissue is not available for histopathological examination.

According to a recent review, no single hysteroscopic myomectomy technique is superior to the other. Gynecologists should use them judiciously based on the type, number, size, and location of the myomas.[24] Although rare, the complications of hysteroscopic myomectomy include uterine perforation, injury to pelvic viscera, fluid intravasation, metabolic complications, and postoperative adhesion formation.[18]

Seeing the different level of complexities and complications being faced during hysteroscopic myomectomies, Lasmar et al. proposed a new preoperative classification of submucous fibroids, the STEPW classification which considers the **S**ize, **T**opography, **E**xtension of the base, **P**enetration of the fibroid into myometrium, and involvement of lateral **W**all.[25] The authors found that this new scoring system had a better correlation with completeness of the myomectomy in a single sitting, time spent in surgery, fluid deficit, and other peroperative and postoperative complications. Thus, as compared to the ESGE classification, it contributed better in preoperative prognostication, patient counseling, preoperative preparations, and sometimes resorting to alternatives to hysteroscopic myomectomy **(Table 3)**.[26]

Laparoscopy: This is the preferred minimally invasive method for the removal of all other myomas except FIGO type L0, L1, and L2 (where hysteroscopic removal is preferred). The other indications where a laparoscopic approach should be preferred are:[27]

- When damage to a large area of endometrial surface is anticipated by the hysteroscopic route
- Multiple submucous myomas
- Hybrid myomas (FIGO type 2-5 and 2-6).

In these cases, sometimes a combined laparoscopic and hysteroscopic approach might be required.

Laparotomy: In the era of laparoscopy, open surgery is usually not preferred nowadays. It is performed only when laparoscopy is contraindicated in the patient, there are multiple or large fibroids or the surgeon does not have experience or skill in laparoscopy. In infertile couples, cumulative pregnancy rates are similar by the laparoscopic

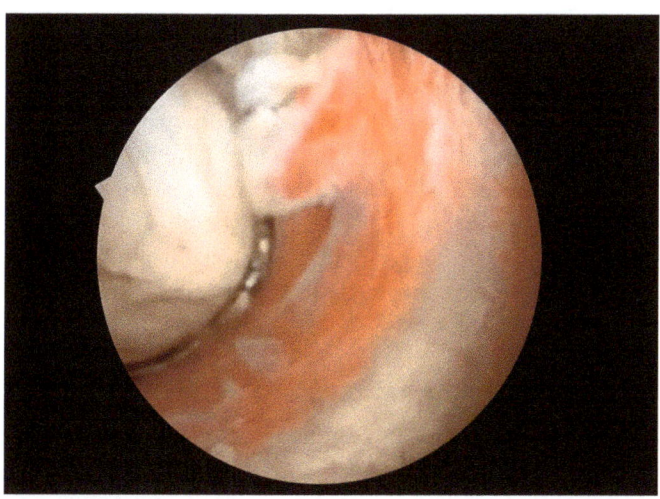

Fig. 7: Type 1 submucous fibroid with resectoscope loop. (*Courtesy:* Dr Vijay Nahata, Mahatma Gandhi Hospital, Jaipur)

TABLE 3: Lasmar's STEPW preoperative classification of submucous myomas.

Points	Size (cm)	Topography	Extension of the base	Penetration	Lateral wall
0	<2	Lower	<1/3	0	+1 additional point
1	>2–5	Middle	1/3 to 2/3	<50%	
2	>5	Upper	>2/3	>50%	
Score	+	+	+	+	+
Total score	Group	Level of complexity anticipated in hysteroscopic myomectomy			
0–4	I	Low complexity hysteroscopic myomectomy			
5–6	II	Complex hysteroscopic myomectomy Consider preparing with gonadotropin-releasing hormone (GnRH) analog and/or two stage surgery			
7–9	III	Recommend an alternative nonhysteroscopic technique			

and minilaparotomy approaches. A recent Cochrane systematic review concluded that evidence is uncertain whether laparoscopic myomectomy compared to laparotomy or minilaparotomy improves live birth rate.[28] The only differences are a quicker recovery, less postoperative pain, and less febrile morbidity in the laparoscopic approach.[29]

The microsurgical principles should be followed including atraumatic tissue handling, good hemostasis, minimal and judicious use of electrocautery, continuous moistening of the tissue, meticulous approximation of the dissected tissue planes, and minimum exposed suture and knots.[30] Preferably, anterior wall incision should be given and adhesion barriers (e.g., *Interceed* and *Gore-Tex*) can be used to prevent postoperative adhesions.

Robotic-assisted laparoscopic myomectomy (RALM): This is also an advanced abdominal method of myomectomy, the added advantages being the articulation of instruments by 540° and easier intracorporeal suturing. But the limitations are cost, lesser skilled surgeons, and not so easy availability.

It is advisable to wait for 3–6 months after myomectomy before planning a pregnancy either naturally or by IVF. This allows the healing of the uterine tissue. In women with poor ovarian reserve or older age, an IVF cycle can be planned earlier with cryopreservation of the resulting embryos, to be transferred later after adequate uterine healing.

Other Methods

Uterine artery embolization (UAE), high-intensity focused ultrasound (HIFU), magnetic resonance-guided focused ultrasound surgery (MRgFUS), myolysis/cryomyolysis, and radiofrequency ablation (RFA) should not be routinely offered to women who wish to maintain or improve their fertility due to lack of data on their safety and effectiveness. These methods can only be used in the setting of approved clinical trials on the management of fibroids in women with infertility.[5,7,23]

ADENOMYOSIS AND INFERTILITY

Adenomyosis as defined by Bird in 1972 is "the benign invasion of endometrium into the myometrium, producing a diffusely enlarged uterus which microscopically exhibits ectopic non-neoplastic, endometrial glands, and stroma surrounded by the hypertrophic and hyperplastic myometrium".[31]

Due to lack of any standardized definition and diagnostic criteria, it is difficult to know the exact prevalence of adenomyosis. In women younger than 40 years of age, adenomyosis affects around 20% of the women, whereas its incidence increases to around 80% between 40 and 50 years of age.[32]

Symptoms

One-third of the women with adenomyosis are asymptomatic, whereas others might present with the following symptoms:
- Menorrhagia (in up to 50% patients)
- Intermenstrual bleeding
- Metrorrhagia
- Dysmenorrhea and pelvic pain
- Infertility.

Diagnosis

In the absence of clear pathognomonic clinical or laparoscopic diagnostic criteria, the diagnosis of adenomyosis is mainly based on ultrasound and MRI.

Ultrasound

Usually ultrasound is the first-line imaging done in women with infertility. A transvaginal scan (TVS) is recommended for better accuracy. It has been shown to have a sensitivity of 80–86%, specificity of 50–96%, and an overall accuracy of 68–86% in diagnosing diffuse adenomyosis.[33]

The *ultrasound* features of adenomyosis are as follows:[34,35]
- *Diffuse adenomyosis:*
  - Globally enlarged uterus
  - Asymmetric thickness of anterior and posterior wall (pseudo-widening sign)
  - Cystic anechoic spaces in the myometrium
  - JZ not clearly visible, thickening of the JZ
  - Heterogeneous echogenicity of the myometrium
- *Focal adenomyosis:*
  - Focal disturbances in myometrium layer
  - Sometimes confused with intramural myoma
  - Anechoic cysts.

Magnetic Resonance Imaging

Magnetic resonance imaging is considered to be gold standard imaging tool for assessing the JZ in the evaluation of adenomyosis.[36] The common features of adenomyosis on MRI include:
- Thickening of the JZ, JZ thickness ≥12 mm, or irregular junctional thickness with a difference of >5 mm between the maximum thickness and the minimum thickness,
- An ill-defined area of low signal intensity in the myometrium on T2-weighted MR images, and
- Islands of ectopic endometrial tissue identified as punctate foci of high signal intensity on T1-weighted image.[37]

An MRI is limited by its cost and is not easily available in every setup. In a systematic review, it has been concluded that both TVS and MRI show high levels of accuracy for the noninvasive diagnosis of adenomyosis.[37] MRI is particularly useful in differentiating a myoma from a focal adenomyoma and planning surgery accordingly.

Effect of Adenomyosis on Fertility

Adenomyosis is considered to be more common in multiparous uteri, but evidence has also shown an association between infertility and adenomyosis.[38] The different mechanisms proposed are:
- Altered uterotubal transport, impairment of sperm transport
- Aberrant uterine contractility
- Reduced expression of implantation markers, inadequate decidual reaction
- Alterations in cell proliferation, apoptosis, and free radical metabolism.

Its effect on reproductive outcomes has been studied better in IVF cycles, and has been found to result in:[39]
- Decreased implantation and clinical pregnancy rates
- Higher miscarriage rates
- Lower live birth rates
- Recurrent implantation failure (RIF) in IVF cycles.

Management

The management of women with adenomyosis and infertility is shown in **Flowchart 2**.

Medical Management

Medical management for adenomyosis has been used for the relief of symptoms such as menorrhagia and dysmenorrhea, but most of the options available for medical management, viz., OCPs, progestins, LNG-IUS, GnRH agonist, etc., also inhibit ovulation and are not practically beneficial in women with adenomyosis and infertility. Role of aromatase inhibitors and ulipristal in adenomyosis associated infertility requires to be studied more. Use of GnRH agonist has been shown to improve the outcomes in IVF cycles (vide infra).[40]

Surgical Management

- Adenomyomectomy (laparoscopic or robotic assisted) has been found to improve the clinical pregnancy rates following IVF. However a balance is required and optimum resection and reconstruction is of utmost importance to avoid obstetric complication, e.g., uterine rupture in the subsequent pregnancies.
- Hysteroscopic resection might be done for subendometriotic adenomyotic implants.
- Hysterectomy—not indicated in women desiring conception.

Other Modalities

Other modalities such as UAE, HIFU, and magnetic resonance-guided high-intensity focused ultrasound (MRgHIFU) are not yet recommended in women desiring pregnancy and more evidence is required.

Assisted Reproductive Technology

- Lower implantation, clinical pregnancy, and live birth rates have been observed in women with adenomyosis during IVF cycles.
- *Prolonged pretreatment with GnRH agonist* has been tried before IVF, although the results are conflicting.[40,41]
- In cases where prolonged suppression with GnRH agonist is not done, *GnRH agonist long protocol* is found to be associated with increased pregnancy and decreased miscarriage rates as compared to GnRH antagonist protocol.[42]
- *Frozen embryo transfer (FET)* cycles have been tried and results are encouraging. IVF cycle is completed, oocytes are retrieved, embryos created and vitrified. Later after prolonged suppression with GnRH agonist, FET is performed.[40] More robust evidence is required before recommending FET in all women with adenomyosis.
- *Surrogacy* can be offered to women with diffuse adenomyosis and enlarged uterus after multiple cycles of unsuccessful IVF cycles.

There is no optimum recommended treatment for women with adenomyosis and infertility. It has to be an individualized approach and a combination of different

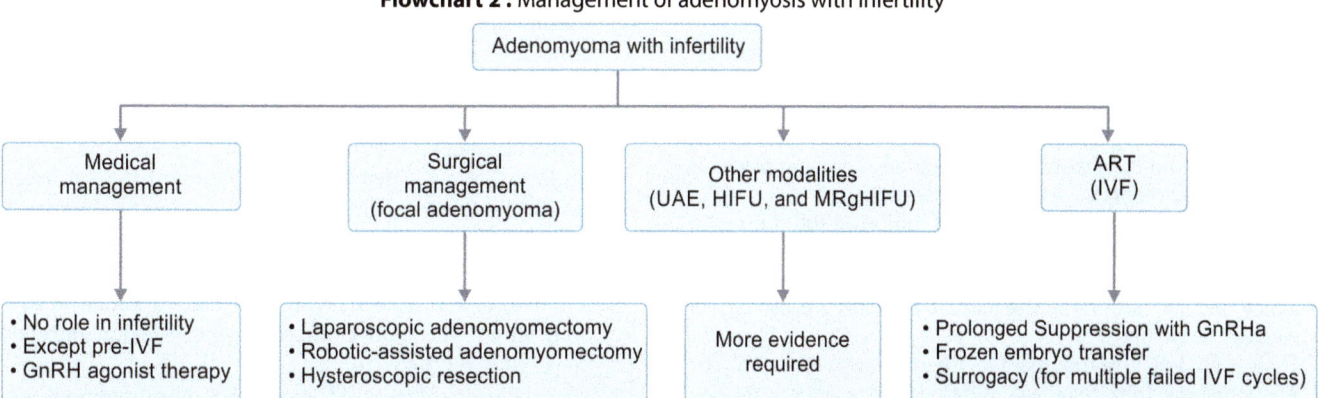

Flowchart 2: Management of adenomyosis with infertility

(ART: assisted reproductive technology; GnRHa: gonadotropin-releasing hormone agonist; HIFU: high-intensity focused ultrasound; IVF: in vitro fertilization; MRgHIFU: magnetic resonance-guided high-intensity focused ultrasound; UAE: uterine artery embolization)

strategies might be required, e.g., laparoscopic adenomyomectomy followed by IVF, prolonged suppression with GnRH agonist, and a FET later.

CONCLUSION

Uterine fibroids with infertility still remain a dilemma for the clinician, given the fact that fibroids are the most common benign gynecological tumors in the reproductive age group and evidence on their role in infertility is still conflicting. The management will depend on certain important factors, viz., any associated symptoms, other causes of infertility in the couple, location, size and number of the fibroids, and previous treatment taken in past for infertility. A proper mapping of the fibroids by ultrasound is essential to decide the further management and surgical approach for removal, if it is required. Evidence is clear that submucosal and cavity-distorting intramural fibroids have a negative impact on the reproductive outcome. Hysteroscopic myomectomy should be the procedure of choice for type L0, L1, and L2 fibroids. Role of noncavity-distorting intramural fibroids is less clear, but there is some evidence showing decreased clinical pregnancy and live birth rates in ART, especially when the size of the intramural noncavity-distorting myoma is >4 cm. Laparoscopic myomectomy can be considered in such cases, particularly when there is history of previous unsuccessful IVF cycles. Subserosal fibroids do not affect fertility and their removal is not required to improve pregnancy or live birth rates. Adenomyosis impairs the implantation, clinical pregnancy, and live birth rates, both in natural and IVF conception. Adenomyosis is challenging, where probably a combined approach will have to be implemented, including prior laparoscopic adenomyomectomy in selected cases, followed by prolonged suppression by a GnRH agonist in conjunction with IVF.

Key Learning Points

- While managing fibroids with infertility, all other causes of infertility should be evaluated and ruled out, before considering the fibroids as the causative factor.
- There is no role of the medical management of fibroids with infertility.
- The decision of myomectomy depends on the size, location, number of fibroids, and IUI/ART cycles taken in past.
- Hysteroscopic myomectomy should be considered for types L0, L1, and L2, as these fibroids are known to reduce implantation and pregnancy rates significantly.
- Role of noncavity-distorting myomas is controversial, but removal can be considered if the size is >4–5 cm and previous infertility treatments have been unsuccessful.
- Removal of subserous fibroids is not indicated for improving reproductive outcomes.
- Adenomyosis is known to reduce implantation, clinical pregnancy, and live birth rates. The miscarriage rates are also higher with adenomyosis.
- There is no definitive treatment for infertility with adenomyosis.
- Adenomyomectomy may be considered for focal adenomyomas.
- Pretreatment with GnRH agonists and IVF might be considered, but the outcomes still remains suboptimal.

REFERENCES

1. Klatsky PC, Tran ND, Caughey AB, Fujimoto VY. Fibroids and reproductive outcomes: a systematic literature review from conception to delivery. Am J Obstet Gynecol. 2008;198:357-66.
2. Buttram VC Jr, Reiter RC. Uterine Leiomyomata: etiology, symptomatology and management. Fertil Steril. 1981;36:433-45.
3. Falcone T, Parker WH. Surgical Management of Leiomyomas for fertility or uterine preservation. Obstet Gynecol. 2013;121:856-68.
4. Pritts EA, Parker WH, Olive DL. Fibroids and infertility: an updated systematic review of the evidence. Fertil Steril. 2009;91(4):1215-23.
5. RANZCOG. (2018). Fibroids in Infertility. [online] Available from https://ranzcog.edu.au/wp-content/uploads/2022/05/Fibroids-in-infertility.pdf. [Last accessed November, 2022].
6. Practice Committee of the American Society of Reproductive Medicine. Removal of Myomas in asymptomatic patients to improve fertility and/or reduce miscarriage rate: a guideline. Fertil Steril. 2017;108:416-25.
7. SOGC Clinical Practice Guidelines. The Management of Uterine Fibroids in Women with Otherwise Unexplained Infertility. J Obstet Gynaecol Can. 2015;37(3):277-85.
8. Metwally M, Farquhar CM, Li TC. Is another meta-analysis on the effects of intramural fibroids on reproductive outcomes needed? Reprod Biomed Online. 2011;23(1):2-14.
9. Sunkara SK, Khairy M, El-Toukhy T, Khalaf Y, Coomarasamy A. The effect of intramural fibroids without uterine cavity involvement on the outcome of IVF treatment: a systematic review and meta-analysis. Hum Reprod. 2010;25(2):418-29.
10. Oliveira FG, Abdelmassih VG, Diamond MP, Dozortsev D, Melo NR, Abdelmassih R. Impact of subserosal and intramural uterine fibroids that do not distort the endometrial cavity on the outcome of in vitro fertilization–intracytoplasmic sperm injection. Fertil Steril. 2004;81(3):582-7.
11. Bulletti C, De Ziegler D, Levi Setti P, Cicinelli E, Polli V, Stefanetti M. Myomas, Pregnancy Outcome, and In Vitro Fertilization. Ann N Y Acad Sci. 2004;1034(1):84-92.
12. Wamsteker K, Emanuel MH, de Kruif JH. Transcervical hysteroscopic resection of submucosal fibroids for abnormal uterine bleeding: results regarding the degree of intramural extension. Obstet Gynecol. 1993;82(5):736-40.
13. Munro MG, Critchley HO, Fraser IS, FIGO Menstrual Disorders Committee. The two FIGO systems for normal and abnormal uterine bleeding symptoms and classification of causes of abnormal uterine bleeding in the reproductive years: 2018 revisions. Int J Gynecol Obstet. 2018;143:393-408.
14. Bajekal N. Fibroids, infertility and pregnancy wastage. Hum Reprod Update. 2000;6(6):614-20.
15. Bulletti C, De Ziegler D, Polli V, Flamigni C. The Role of Leiomyomas in Infertility. J Am Assoc Gynecol Laparoscopists. 1999;6(4):441-5.
16. Surrey ES, Lietz AK, Schoolcraft WB. Impact of intramural leiomyomata in patients with a normal endometrial cavity on in vitro fertilization–embryo transfer cycle outcome. Fertil Steril. 2001;75(2):405-10.
17. Lisiecki M, Paszkowski M, Woźniak S. Fertility impairment associated with uterine fibroids—a review of literature. Menopausal Rev. 2017;16(4):137-40.

18. Bosteels J, van Wessel S, Weyers S, Broekmans FJ, D'Hooghe TM, Bongers MY, et al. Hysteroscopy for treating subfertility associated with suspected major uterine cavity abnormalities. Cochrane Database Syst Rev. 2018;12(12):CD009461.
19. Wang X, Chen L, Wang H, Li Q, Liu X, Qi H. The Impact of Noncavity-Distorting Intramural Fibroids on the Efficacy of In Vitro Fertilization-Embryo Transfer: An Updated Meta-Analysis. Bio Med Res Int. 2018;2018:1-13.
20. Casini ML, Rossi F, Agostini R, Unfer V. Effects of the position of fibroids on fertility. Gynecol Endocrinol. 2006;22(2):106-9.
21. Hart R, Khalaf Y, Yeong C-T, Seed P, Taylor A, Braude P. A prospective controlled study of the effect of intramural uterine fibroids on the outcome of assisted conception. Hum Reprod. 2001;16(11):2411-7.
22. Bai X, Lin Y, Chen Y, Ma C. The impact of FIGO type 3 fibroids on in-vitro fertilization outcomes: A nested retrospective case-control study. Eur J Obstet Gynecol Reprod Biol. 2020; 247:176-80.
23. Purohit P, Vigneswaran K. Fibroids and Infertility. Curr Obstet Gynecol Rep. 2016;5:81-8.
24. Friedman JA, Wong JMK, Chaudhari A, Tsai S, Milad MP. Hysteroscopic myomectomy: a comparison of techniques and review of current evidence in the management of abnormal uterine bleeding. Curr Opin Obstet Gynecol. 2018;30(4):243-51.
25. Lasmar RB, Lasme BP, Celeste RK, da Rosa DB, de Batista Depes D, Coelho Lopes RG. A new system to classify submucous myomas: a Brazilian multicenter study. J Minim Invasive Gynecol. 2012;19(5):575-80.
26. Lasmar RB, Xinmei Z, Indman PD, Celeste RK, Spiezio Sardo AD. Feasibility of a new system of classification of submucous myomas: a multicenter study. Fertl Steril. 2011;95(6)2073-7.
27. American Association of Gynecology Laparoscopists (AAGL), Advancing Minimally Invasive Gynecology Worldwide. AAGL practice report: practice guidelines for the diagnosis and management of submucous leiomyomas. J Minim Invasive Gynecol. 2012;19(2):152-71.
28. Metwally M, Raybould G, Cheong YC, Horne AW. Surgical treatment of fibroids for subfertility. Cochrane Database Syst Rev. 2020;(1):CD003857.
29. Vilos GA, Allaire C, Laberge P-Y, Leyland N, Vilos AG, Murji A, et al. The Management of Uterine Leiomyomas. J Obstet Gynaecol Can. 2015;37(2):157-78.
20. Munro MG. Uterine leiomyomas, current concepts: pathogenesis, impact on reproductive health, and medical, procedural, and surgical management. Obstet Gynecol Clin N Am. 2011;38:703-31.
31. Bird CC, McElin TW, Manalo-Estrella P. The elusive adenomyosis of the uterus-revisited. Am J ObstetGynecol. 1972; 112(5):583-93.
32. Harada T, Khine YM, Kaponis A, Nikellis T, Decavalas G, Taniguchi F. The Impact of Adenomyosis on Women's Fertility. Obstet Gynecol Surv. 2016;71:557-68.
33. Reinhold C, Atri M, Mehio A, Zakarian R, Aldis AE, Bret PM. Diffuse uterine adenomyosis: morphologic criteria and diagnostic accuracy of endovaginal sonography. Radiology. 1995;197(3):609-14.
34. Dueholm M, Lundorf E. Transvaginal ultrasound or MRI for diagnosis of adenomyosis. Curr Opin Obstet Gynecol. 2007;19(6):505-12.
35. Szubert M, Koziróg E, Olszak O, Krygier-Kurz K, Kazmierczak J, Wilczynski J. Adenomyosis and Infertility—Review of Medical and Surgical Approaches. Int J Environ Res Public Health. 2021;18:1235.
36. Reinhold C, Tafazoli F, Mehio A, Wang L, Atri M, Siegelman ES, et al. Uterine adenomyosis: Endovaginal US and MR imaging features with histopathologic correlation. Radiographics. 1999;19:S147-60.
37. Champaneria R, Abedin P, Daniels J, Balogun M, Khan KS. Ultrasound scan and magnetic resonance imaging for the diagnosis of adenomyosis: Systematic review comparing test accuracy. Acta Obstet Gynecol Scand. 2010;89(11):1374-84.
38. Li JJ, Chung JPW, Wang S, Li TC, Duan H. The Investigation and Management of Adenomyosis in Women Who Wish to Improve or Preserve Fertility. Biomed Res Int. 2018;2018:6832685.
39. Squillace ALA, Simonian DS, Allegro MC, Borges E Jr, Bianchi PHM, Bibancos M. Adenomyosis and in vitro fertilization impacts—a literature review. JBRA Assist Reprod. 2021;25(2):303-9.
40. Park CW, Choi MH, Yang KM, Song IO. Pregnancy rate in women with adenomyosis undergoing fresh or frozen embryo transfer cycles following gonadotropin-releasing hormone agonist treatment. Clin Exp Reprod Med. 2016;43:169-73.
41. Zhou L-M, Zheng J, Sun Y-T, Zhao Y-Y, Xia A-L. Study on leuprorelin acetate in treatment of uterine adenomyosis with infertility. Zhonghua Fu Chan Ke Za Zhi. 2013;48(5):334-7.
42. Tao T, Chen S, Chen X, Ye D, Xu L, Tian X, et al. Effects of uterine adenomyosis on clinical outcomes of infertility patients treated with in vitro fertilization/intracytoplasmic sperm injection-embryo transfer (IVF/ICSI-ET). Nan Fang Yi Ke Da Xue Xue Bao. 2015;35(2):248-51.

CHAPTER 15: Management of PCOS: Infertility and Long-term Management

Devi R, G Rani Aishwarya

INTRODUCTION

Polycystic ovarian syndrome (PCOS) is the most common endocrine disorder seen in women of reproductive age. The prevalence of PCOS is 10–15%.[1] This multifaceted disorder has a complex pathophysiology and a wide variety of presenting symptoms. Diagnostic criteria for the same are evolving. Management of PCOS requires a multidisciplinary approach, while the pillars of management lie in a good, guided lifestyle modification; and pharmacological approaches are often needed for the infertile population. Sensitizing and screening for long-term complications of this endocrine disorder are gaining lots of momentum.

PATHOPHYSIOLOGY OF PCOS (FLOWCHARTS 1 AND 2; FIGS. 1 AND 2)

Barker's hypothesis[1,2]	• Fetal origin of adult disease • In utero program
LH hypothesis[3,4]	Neuroendocrine defect
Ovarian hypothesis[5]	• Alteration in both theca and granulosa cell function • Disordered folliculogenesis
Adrenal hypothesis[4]	Alteration in cortisol metabolism
Insulin hypothesis[6,7]	• Insulin resistance • Hyperinsulinemia
Altered sympathetic tone[8]	High sympathetic activity

Source: Bremer AA. Polycystic ovary syndrome in the pediatric population. Metab Syndr Relat Disord. 2010;8(5):375-94.

Flowchart 1: LH hypothesis-neuroendocrine defect.

(GnRH: gonadotropin-releasing hormone; LH: luteinizing hormone)
Source: Bremer AA. Polycystic ovary syndrome in the pediatric population. Metab Syndr Relat Disord. 2010;8(5):375-94.

Flowchart 2: Etiopathogenesis of PCOS.

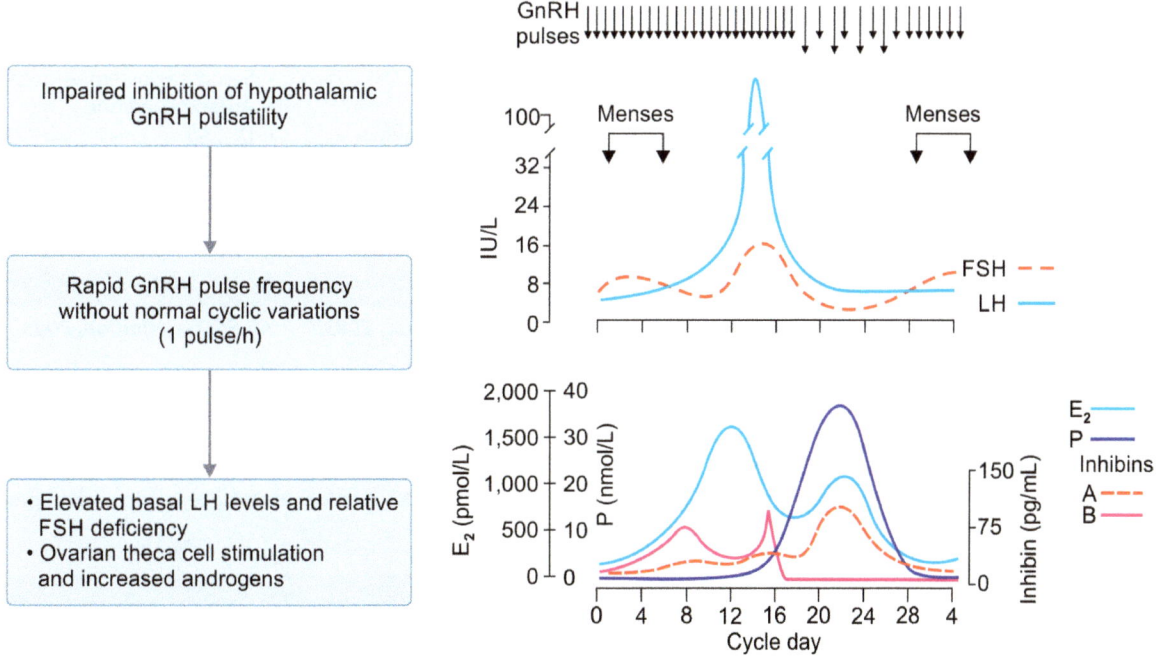

(AMH: anti-Mullerian hormone; HPO: hypothalamic-pituitary-ovarian; LH: luteinizing hormone; PCOS: polycystic ovarian syndrome)
Source: Speroff L, Fritz MA. Anovulation and the polycystic ovary. In: Speroff L, Fritz MA, editors. Clinical Gynecologic Endocrinology and Infertility, 8th edn. Philadelphia (PA): Lippincott Williams and Wilkins.

Fig. 1: FSH and LH surge at ovulation, estradiol peak before the LH surge and peak progesterone in the midluteal phase.
(FSH: follicle-stimulating hormone; GnRH: gonadotropin-releasing hormone; LH: luteinizing hormone)
Source: Speroff L, Fritz MA. Anovulation and the polycystic ovary. In: Speroff L, Fritz MA, editors. Clinical Gynecologic Endocrinology and Infertility, 8th edn. Philadelphia (PA): Lippincott Williams and Wilkins.

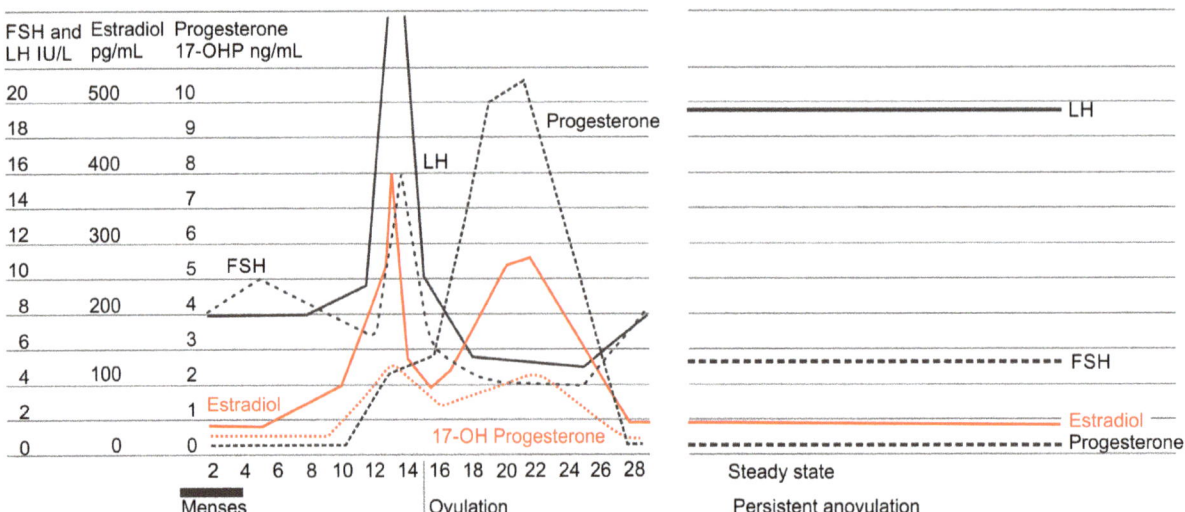

Fig. 2: Persistent anovulation due to tonic LH in PCOS. (FSH: follicle-stimulating hormone; LH: luteinizing hormone).
Source: Adapted from Marshall JC, Dalkin AC, Haisenleder DJ, Paul SJ, Ortolano GA, Kelch RP. Gonadotropin-releasing hormone pulses: regulators of gonadotropin synthesis and ovulatory cycles. Recent Prog Horm Res. 1991;47:155-87.

DIAGNOSIS OF PCOS

Clinical features of PCOS are as follows:

- Hyperandrogenism
- Ovulatory dysfunction
- PCOM on ultrasound

Based on the presence of these clinical features there are many diagnostic criteria which are listed in **Table 1**.

NIH 2012 extension of the European Society of Human Reproduction and Embryology (ESHRE)/American Society for Reproductive Medicine (ASRM) 2003[12]

(Two of three criteria required)
1. Hyperandrogenism **(Table 2)**
2. Ovulatory dysfunction **(Table 3)**
3. Polycystic ovarian morphology

1. *Hyperandrogenism:*

Clinical	Biochemical
• Hirsutism	• Serum testosterone-(total/free)
• Acne	• Androstenedione
• Androgenic alopecia	• DHEAS
	• SHBG

(DHEAS: dehydroepiandrosterone sulfate; SHBG: sex hormone-binding globulin)

TABLE 1: Various diagnostic criteria of PCOS based on the clinical features.

Clinical features	NIH Consensus, 1990[9]	Rotterdam Consensus, 2003[10]	AE-PCOS definition, 2006[11]
Clinical/Biochemical HA	+	+/–	+
Oligo/amenorrhea, anovulation/OD	+	+/–	+/–
PCOM on USG		+/–	+/–
	All Required	2 out of 3 required	Androgen excess + one other criteria

(AE PCOS: Androgen Excess and PCOS society HA: hyperandrogenism; OD: ovulatory dysfunction; PCOM: polycystic ovarian morphology; NIH: National institute of Health)

TABLE 2: Biochemical markers of hyperandrogenism.

Marker	Normal range	Remarks
Total testosterone	8–60 ng/mL	Exclude androgen secreting neoplasm
Free testosterone	0.3–1.9 pg/mL	Most sensitive to establish diagnosis
DHEA	600–3400 ng/mL	Exclude androgen secreting neoplasm
Androstenedione	0.4–2.7 ng/mL	Establish diagnosis
17 alpha hydroxyprogesterone	<2 µg/L (follicular phase)	Exclude NCAH[13]

(DHEA: dehydroepiandrosterone; NCAH: non-classical congenital adrenal hyperplasia)
Source: Azziz R, Carmina E, Dewailly D, Diamanti-Kandarakis E, Escobar-Morreale HF, Futterweit W, et al; Task Force on the Phenotype of the Polycystic Ovary Syndrome of the Androgen Excess and PCOS Society. The Androgen Excess and PCOS Society criteria for the polycystic ovary syndrome: the complete task force report. Fertil Steril. 2009;91(2):456-88.

Total testosterone in PCOS: >60 ng/mL and ≤150 ng/mL
(>2.5-/= 5 nmol/L) Free testosterone: >0.75 ng/dL

Free androgen index (FAI) in PCOS: >8.5
FAI = Total testosterone × 100/SHBG

SHBG in PCOS: <5 nmol/L

Hirsutism: Presence of terminal hair on the face and/or body in a male type of pattern in a female.

Each of the nine body areas is rated from 0 (absence of terminal hairs) to 4 (extensive terminal hair growth).
- mFG score with a level ≥6 is used as a cutoff for hirsutism **(Fig. 3)**
  Hirsutism has been graded as:
  • *Mild:* up to a score of 15
  • *Moderate:* for a score of 16–25
  • *Severe:* above the score of 25
2. *Ovulatory dysfunction:*

Assessment of ovulation is done by:
- History of menstrual cycles
- Mid luteal phase serum progesterone levels and
- Ultrasound

History:
Ovulatory dysfunction[15] manifests as an irregular menstrual cycle—the most common being oligo/amenorrhea.

Reason/pathophysiology of ovulatory dysfunction	Manifestation/menstrual irregularity
Anovulation	Oligo/amenorrhea
Chronic anovulation and/or unopposed exposure to estrogen	Menorrhagia/menometrorrhagia
Irregular ripening/irregular shedding	Metrorrhagia

mFG score in PCOS is mild to moderate as compared to androgen-secreting tumors in which it is severe.

Irregular menstrual cycle[16] can be normal in the first year post menarche. What is abnormal is: Ovulatory dysfunction can occur even with regular cycles, day 22–24 serum progesterone levels (P) can be measured to confirm anovulation

- >1 to <3 years post menarche :<21 or >45 days
- >3 years post menarche to perimenopause:<21 or >35 days or <8 cycles per year
- >1 year post menarche >90 days for any one cycle

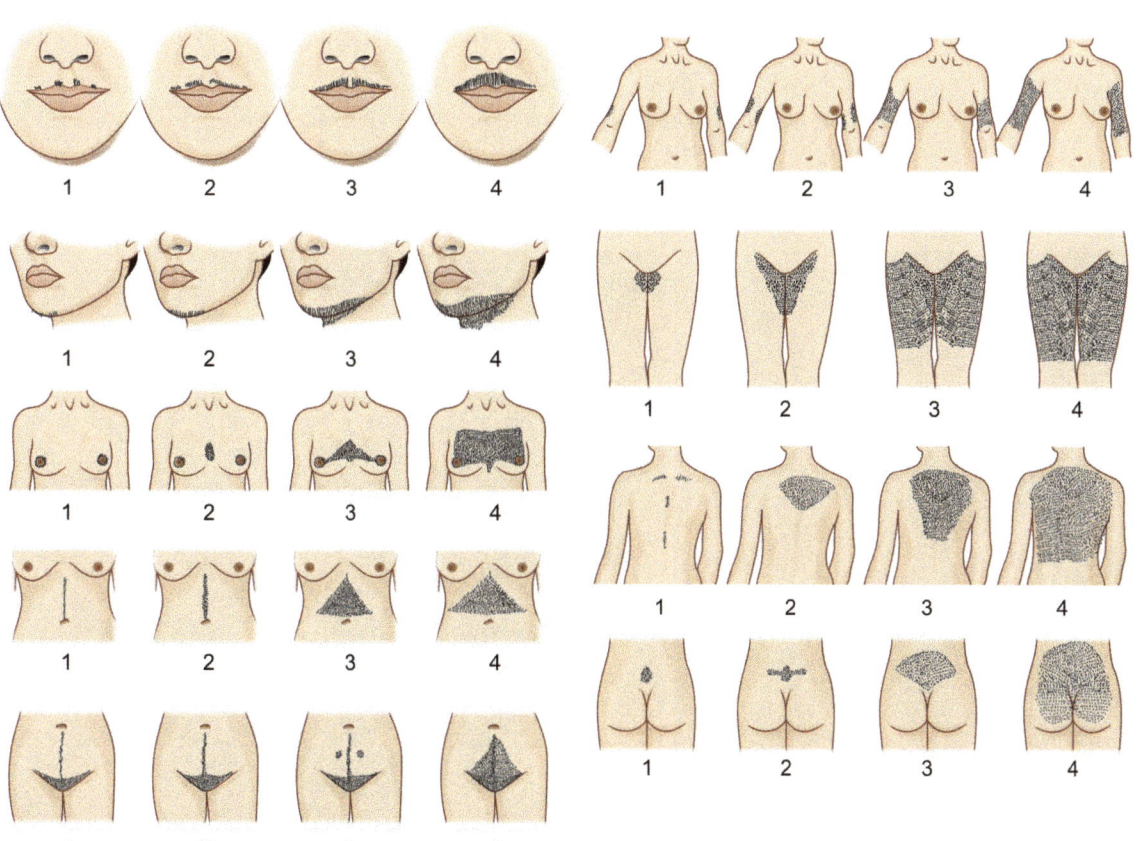

Fig. 3: Modified Ferriman and Gallway score (mFG score).[14]
Source: Adapted from Ferriman D, Gallwey JD. Clinical assessment of body hair growth in women. J Clin Endocrinol Metab. 1961 Nov;21: 1440-7.

TABLE 3: Tests for ovulatory dysfunction.

Test	PCOS	Remarks
Serum progesterone	Mid luteal phase P levels are measured 7 days before the anticipated menses in two consecutive cycles	A single mid-luteal phase (day 21) P >10 ng/mL or 30 nmol/L confirms ovulation *Limitation:* Peak P levels remain only for a short time and so, samples not taken in appropriate time might result in a low value
Ultrasound[17]	No evidence of ovulation	No dominant follicle, no cyclical changes in endometrial pattern, no free fluid in POD, no corpus luteum

(PCOS: polycystic ovarian syndrome; POD: pouch of Douglas)
Source: Balen AH, Morley LC, Misso M, Franks S, Legro RS, Wijeyaratne CN, et al. The management of anovulatory infertility in women with polycystic ovary syndrome: an analysis of the evidence to support the development of global WHO guidance. Hum Reprod Update. 2016;22(6):687-708.

3. *Polycystic ovarian morphology* **(Fig. 4)**.

| Pelvic ultrasound | *B mode ultrasound:* To assess:
• Polycystic ovarian morphology (PCOM)
  – FNPO as per criteria
  – and/or ovarian volume ≥10 cc
• Stromal echogenicity-hyperechoic, more than the echogenicity of the myometrium
• Stromal/ovarian area >0.32, in HA (Hypothalamic amenorrhea) PCOS[18]
• Endometrial thickness
Doppler: Stromal vascularity is increased with a raised stromal Peak systolic velocity due to LH and vascular endothelial growth factor (VEGF)-induced angiogenesis | • As per Rotterdam criteria, follicular number per ovary (FNPO) for the definition of PCOM is ≥12, follicles measuring 2–9 mm
• The Androgen Excess and PCOS Society (AEPCOS) task force recommends FNPO with a threshold of ≥25, but only when using maximal resolution with transducer frequency ≥8 MHz[18] |

Note: Ultrasound should not be used for the diagnosis of PCOS in those patients who present <8 years after menarche, due to high incidence of multi follicular ovaries.

Twenty or more follicles per ovary (AEPCOS) and 12 or more follicles per ovary (Rotterdam criteria); size 2–9 mm (endovaginal ultrasound transducers with a frequency bandwidth that includes 8 MHz)

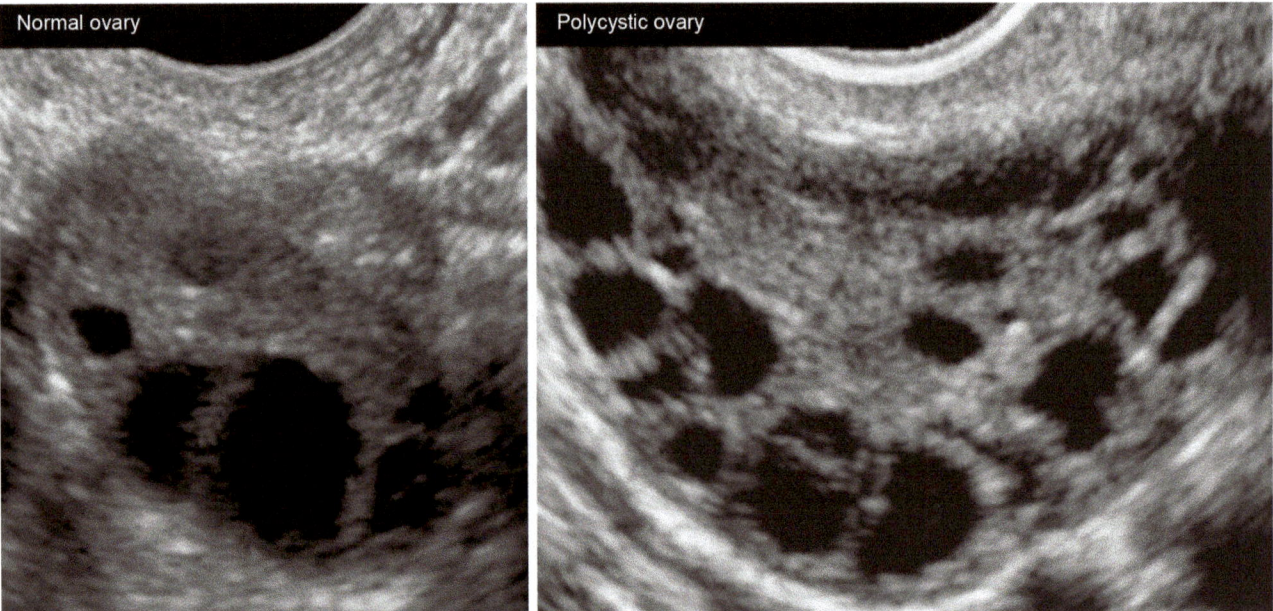

Fig. 4: Normal and polycystic ovaries.
Source: Taylor HS, Fritz MA, Pal L, Seli E. Speroff's Clinical Gynecologic Endocrinology and Infertility, 9th edn. Philadelphia PA: Wolters Kluwer; 2020.

APPROACH TO INFERTILITY IN PCOS

Evaluation

Patient history	Any predisposing factors to PCOS such as low birth weight with excessive catch-up growth, history of large for gestation baby or premature adrenarche/pubarche
Family history	35% of mothers and 40% of sisters of women with PCOS are affected
Menstrual history	• Menarche and nature of menstrual cycles to be enquired • Irregular cycles (>35 or <21 days) continuing for more than 2 years after the onset of menarche are likely to reflect oligoovulation or anovulation
Evaluation of HA	• Hirsutism, acne and/or alopecia • *Biochemical assessment of HA:* Total testosterone is more markedly elevated in PCOS and is a good screening tool to exclude other causes of androgen excess
• Physical examination • Blood pressure (BP) • Body mass index (BMI)	25–30 kg/m² (overweight) >30 kg/m² (obese) • Class 1: BMI of 30 to <35 • Class 2: BMI of 35 to <40 • Class 3: BMI of 40 or higher[19]
• Waist circumference • Waist-hip ratio	≥88 cm >0.85 is suggestive of visceral adiposity[15,19]
Stigmata of insulin resistance (IR)	• Acanthosis nigricans • Central obesity/adiposity

Laboratory

Investigations Indicated

Insulin resistance

Test	Normal value (N) and value in PCOS	Remarks
OGTT[20]	2-hour 75 g glucose	• Fasting values • N: <100 mg/dL • Impaired: 100–125 mg/dL • Type 2 DM: >126 mg/dL • 2-hour glucose values • N: <140 mg/dL • Impaired: 140–199 mg/dL • Type 2 DM: >200 mg/dL20, 21

Metabolic disorder

Test	Normal value
Lipid Profile	Triglycerides ≥150 mg/dL HDL cholesterol ≤40 mg/dL

Fertility evaluation

Test	Normal value (N) and value in PCOS	Remarks
AMH	N: 2–3.5 ng/mL or 5–15 pmol/L	It acts as a surrogate marker, as a substitute of AFC in PCOS diagnosis *Note:* Lack of standardization of AMH assay makes it unreliable.
• FSH • LH • Estradiol	• N: 2–8 IU/L • N: 2–10 IU/L • N: 50–80 pg/mL	Measured on day 2/day 3 of the cycle
LH:FSH ratio	–	• LH:FSH ratio (>2:1) has been regarded as the marker of PCOS, more so in lean PCOS than in obese[10,11] • Ratio varies with assays used to measure, hence not a reliable diagnostic criterion

Investigations to rule out other reasons for anovulation

Test	Normal Value (N) and value in PCOS	Remarks
Prolactin	N: 25–30 ng/mL	To rule out hyperprolactinemia-induced anovulation
Thyroid-stimulating hormone (TSH)	N: 0.5–2.5 mIU/mL	To rule out thyroid disorders causing ovulatory disturbances

Investigations not routinely indicated

Test	Normal Value (N) and value in PCOS	Remarks
17-Hydroxyprogesterone (17-OHP)	17-OHP >200 ng/mL: To do corticotropin stimulation test 17-OHP >800 ng/mL establishes diagnosis of late-onset congenital adrenal hyperplasia	To rule out nonclassical/late-onset congenital adrenal hyperplasia
a. 24-hour urine free cortisol b. Overnight dexamethasone suppression test		a and b to rule out Cushing's Syndrome
a. Fasting insulin (FI)	FI (N): <30 mIU/mL IR: >20–30 mIU/mL	Not routine; measured due to lack of standardized insulin assay
b. 2-hour postprandial insulin (PPI)	PPI(N): <80–100 mIU/mL IR: >100 mIU/mL	Instead oral glucose tolerance test (OGTT) is done
c. Fasting glucose/insulin (FG/FI) ratio	FG/FI(N) >4.5; IR <4.5	
Others: a. Serum homocysteine (SH) b. Endometrial sampling	a. SH(N): 5–11 µmol/L PCOS: >11 µmol/L	b. Endometrial sampling is done in women with potential long-term exposure to unopposed estrogen stimulation, to rule out endometrial hyperplasia

■ TREATMENT OPTIONS IN PCOS-RELATED INFERTILITY

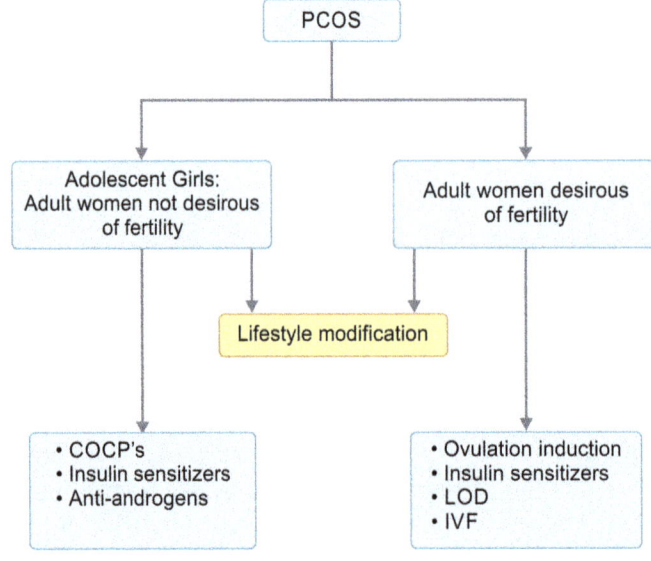

(COCPs: combined oral contraceptive pills; IVF: in vitro fertilization; LOD: laparoscopic ovarian drilling)

Lifestyle Modifications

Dietary modifications	Exercise	Behavioral Strategies
Atkins diet:[22] Intake of low glycemic index such as vegetables, fruit, fiber, whole grain foods and high protein from vegetable sources. To avoid refined carbohydrates and trans-fat-containing hydrogenated oils. • A low-calorie diet of 1,000–2,000 kcal/day with calorie Restriction of 500 kcal/day restriction typically reduces the total body weight by 10% over 6 months.	• Aerobic exercises of 3–4 times /week for 20–30 minutes burns 100–200 kcal with 40% improvement in insulin resistance in 48 hours. • A minimum of 150 min/week of moderate-intensity physical activity or 75 min/week of vigorous intensities or an equivalent Combination of both including muscle strengthening activities on 2 nonconsecutive days/week.[23]	Reduction of psychosocial stressors

Foods to eat:
- Meats: beef, pork, lamb, chicken, bacon, and others
- Fatty fish and seafood: salmon, trout, sardines, and mackerel
- Eggs: Omega-3-enriched or pastured—most nutrient-dense
- Low-carb vegetables: kale, spinach, broccoli, asparagus, and others
- Full-fat dairy: butter, cheese, cream, full fat yogurt
- Nuts and seeds: almonds, macadamia nuts, walnuts, sunflower seeds

Foods to limit:
- Sugar: Found in soft drinks, fruit juices, cakes, candy, ice cream, and similar products
- Grains: Wheat, spelt, rye, barley, rice
- "Diet" and "low-fat" foods are sometimes very high in sugar
- High-carb vegetables: carrots, turnips, etc.
- High carb fruits: bananas, apples, oranges, pears, grapes
- Starches: potatoes, sweet potatoes
- Legumes: lentils, beans, chickpeas, etc.

■ Weight loss should be encouraged prior to ovulation induction treatments, preferably to a BMI <30 kg/m^2

A modest loss of 5–10% of total body weight can achieve a 30% reduction of central fat, improvement in insulin sensitivity and restore ovulation[15,18,20,24-28]

Metabolic approach	Reproductive approach
• Lifestyle modification • Insulin sensitizers • Metformin • Inositols • Bariatric surgery	• Oral ovulogens • Gonadotropins • Lap ovarian drilling • Antiretroviral therapy (ART)/in vitro fertilization (IVF)

Treatment Options in PCOS-related Infertility

Algorithm for Management of Infertility[29]

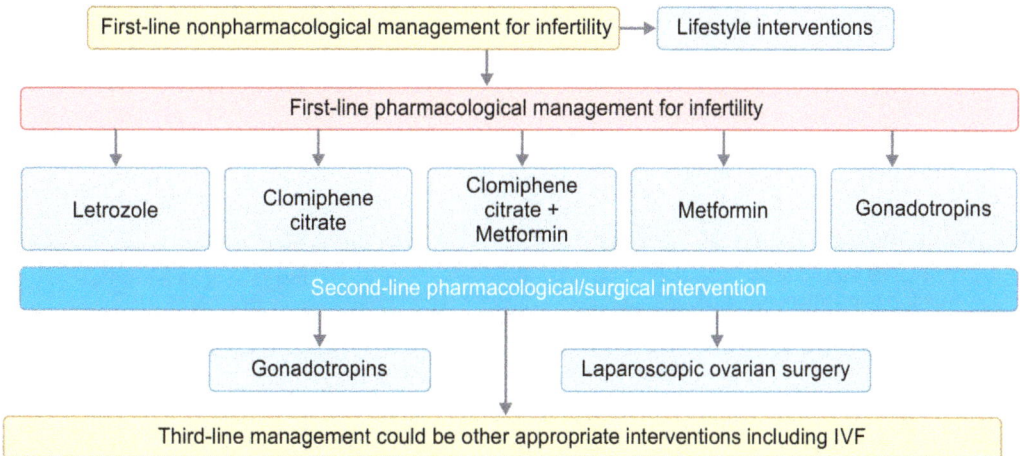

First-line pharmacological management for infertility in PCOS: Oral ovulogens

- SERM-clomiphene citrate and tamoxifen
  - Clomiphene citrate: 50/100/150 mg/day for 5 days
  - Tamoxifen: 40–80 mg/day as twice a day dose for 5 days
- Aromatase inhibitors: Letrozole, anastrozole
  - Letrozole: 2.5 mg, 5 mg, 7.5 mg/day for 5 days

Start any within the first 5 days of the menstrual cycle

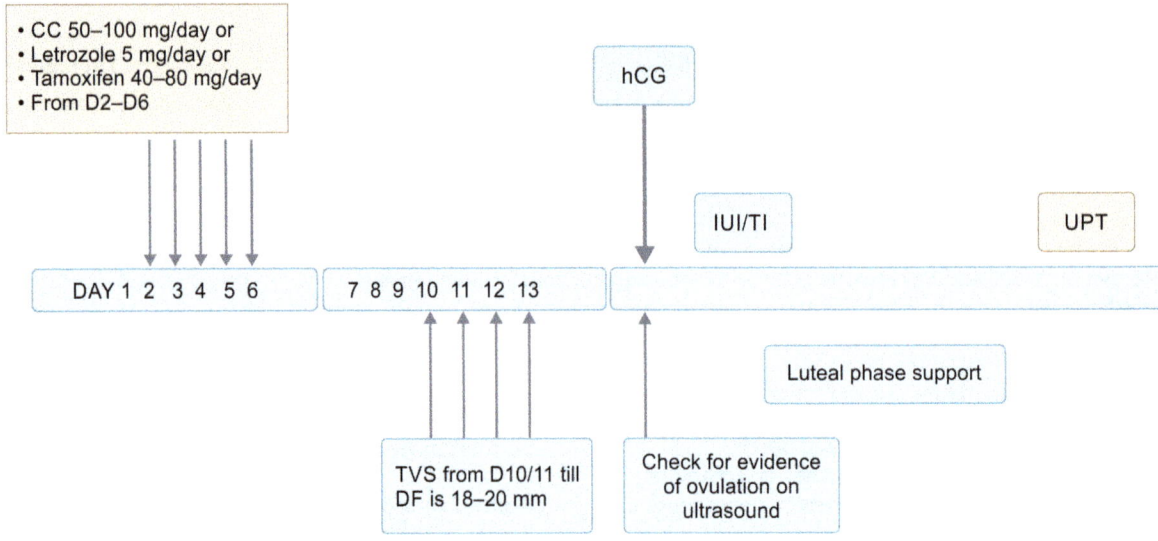

(hCG: human chorionic gonadotropin; IUI: intrauterine insemination; TI: timed intercourse; TVS: transvaginal ultrasound; UPT: urine pregnancy test)

Second-line ovulation induction agent: Gonadotropins

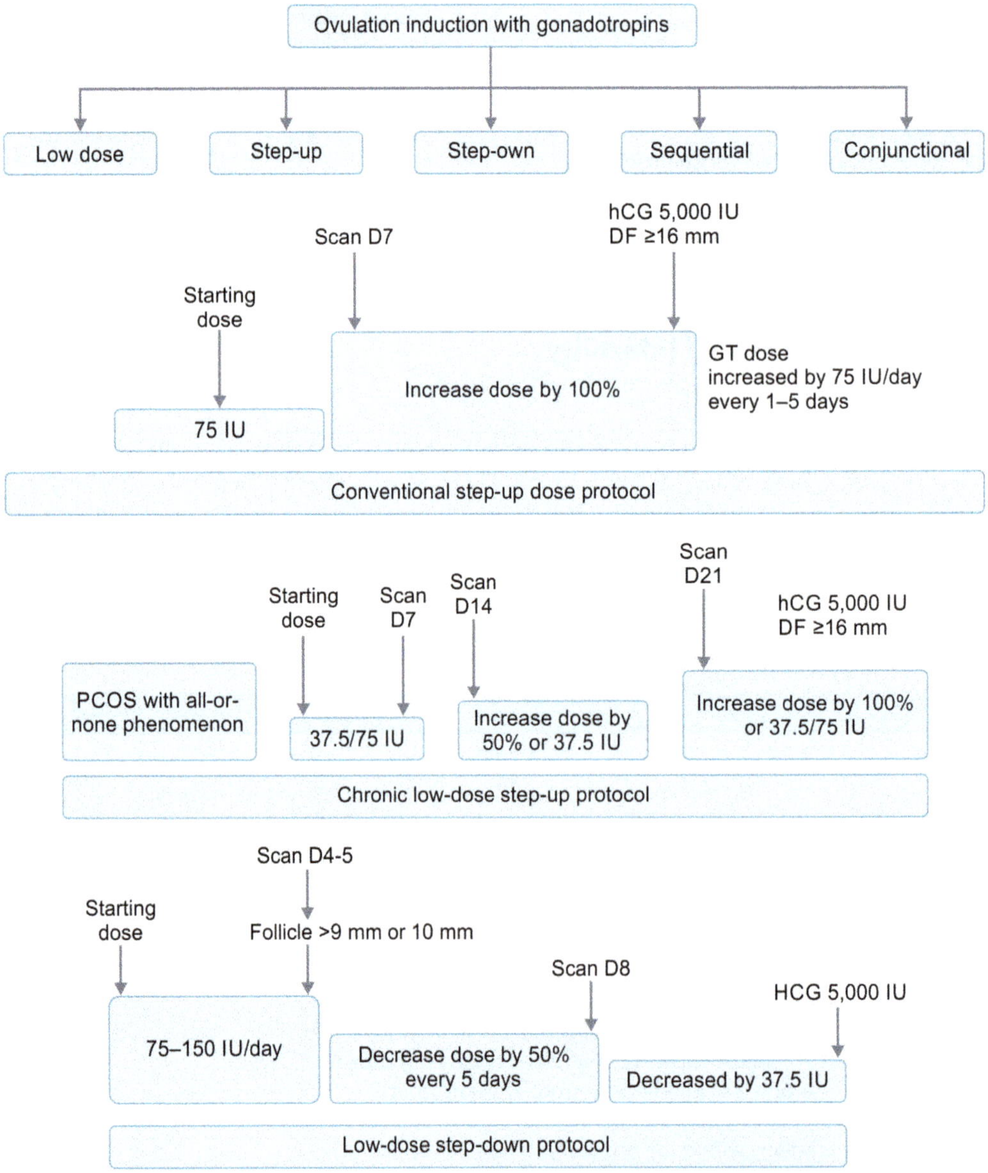

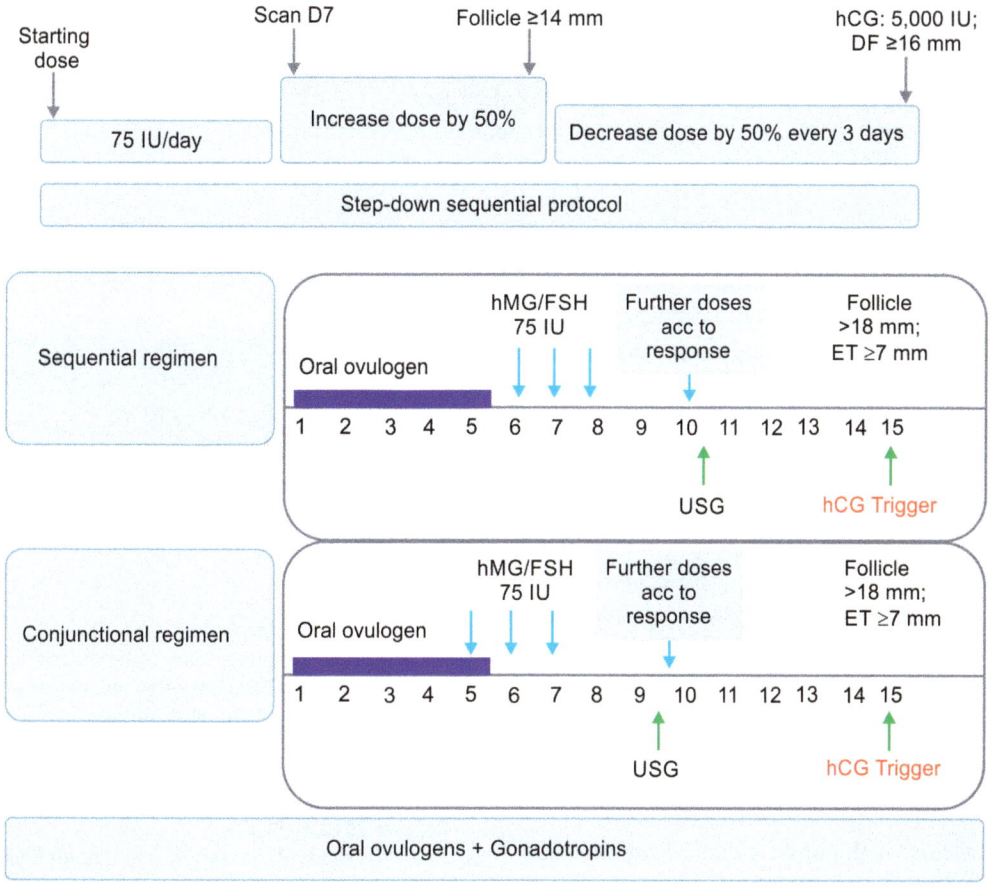

Laparoscopic Ovarian Drilling

Second-line therapy for anovulatory infertility when no other factor

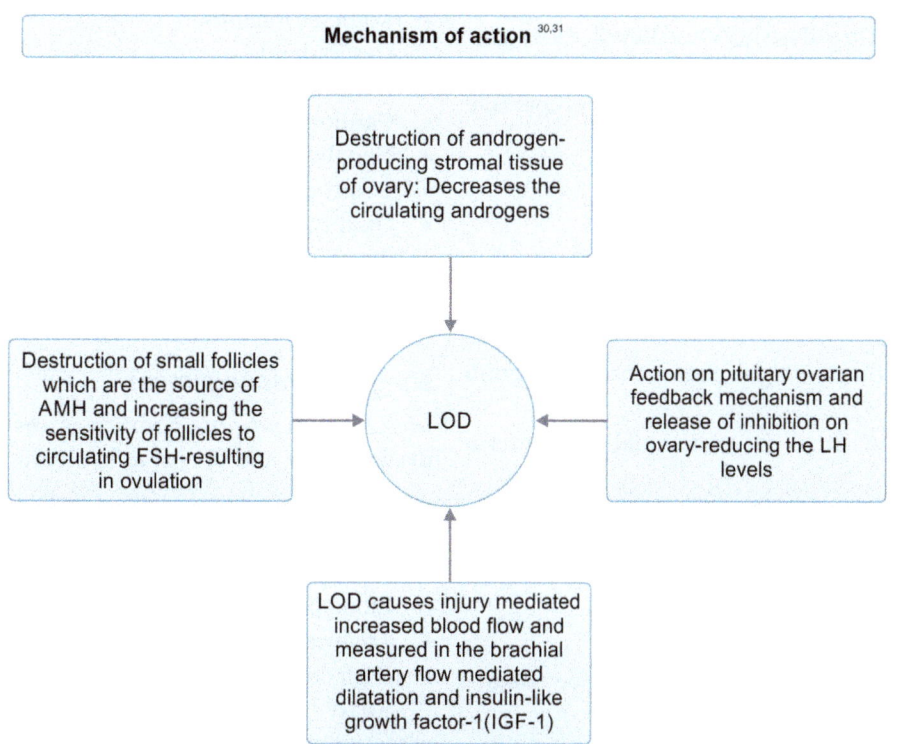

(LH: luteinizing hormone; LOD: laparoscopic ovarian drilling)

Indications Of LOD[15,17,22]

Beneficial	Adverse effects
Persistent high LH (>10 IU/L)	Risk of surgery
High AMH (>7–8 ng/mL)	Periadnexal adhesions
Lean PCOS	Risk of decreased ovarian reserve due to overzealous drilling

Antiretroviral Therapy Indications

- Third-line option for the management of infertility
- Coexisting indications for ART (tubal damage/endometriosis/male factor infertility/long history of infertility)
- Reduced risk of multiple pregnancies
- Advanced age.

Principles of IVF in PCOS Patients

- CC/Letrozole-resistant PCOS
- Requiring high-dose gonadotropins for ovulation induction
- Requiring intensive monitoring during gonadotropin therapy (uncontrollable response to gonadotropin, all-or-none phenomenon)
- Previous ovarian hyperstimulation syndrome (OHSS)
- Requiring laparoscopic assessment of pelvis for other indications
- Anovulatory lean PCOS with tonic elevated LH (>10 IU/L) levels.

- *Preferred protocols:* Antagonist cycles, Progesterone-primed ovarian stimulation (PPOS)
- Lowest and the most effective use of gonadotropins
- Compartmentalization of IVF by using agonist protocol and freeze-all strategy followed by frozen embryo transfer. The purpose of this approach is to eliminate OHSS **(Fig. 5)**.[32]
- Agonist trigger with fresh embryo transfer and modified luteal support (low-dose hCG and double-dose progesterone) can be tried in suitable cases. This approach keeps OHSS rates reduced while maintaining comparable pregnancy and live birth rates.[33-35]

Indications of Bariatric Surgery[36,37]

It is an experimental therapy in women with PCOS.

Following considerations have to be made:
- Comparative Costs
- Need for a structured weight management program postoperatively
- *Perinatal morbidity:* Small-for-gestational age, preterm labor
- Avoidance of pregnancy for 12 months post surgery
- Preventive management of nutritional deficiencies.

Long-term Sequelae Of PCOS[25]

- BMI >35 kg/m²: One or more severe complications expected to improve with weight loss
- BMI >40 kg/m²: Failure of nonsurgical treatment
- BMI >50 kg/m²: First line

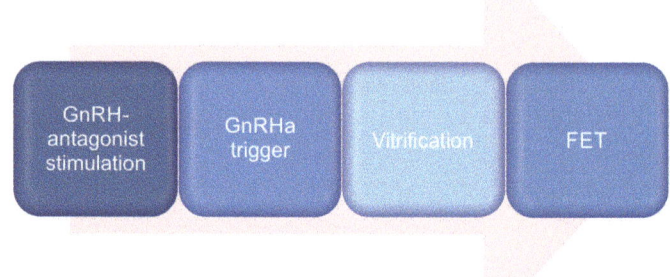

Fig. 5: The "freeze-all" protocol.[32,33]
(GnRHa: gonadotropin-releasing hormone agonist; FET: frozen embryo transfer; SWOT: (strengths, weaknesses, opportunities, and threats) analysis of a freeze-all strategy)
Source:
1. Blockeel C, Drakopoulos P, Santos-Ribeiro S, Polyzos NP, Tournaye H. A fresh look at the freeze-all protocol: a SWOT analysis. Hum Reprod. 2016;31(3):491-7.
2. Haahr T, Roque M, Esteves SC, Humaidan P. GnRH agonist trigger and LH Activity luteal phase support versus hCG trigger and conventional luteal phase support in fresh embryo transfer IVF/ICSI cycles—A systematic PRISMA review and meta-analysis. Front Endocrinol.

- Impaired glucose tolerance
- Diabetes mellitus
- Dyslipidemia
- Hypertension
- Cardiovascular disease
- Nonalcoholic fatty liver disease
- Obstructive sleep apnea
- Quality of life affected with manifestations of anxiety, depression, and psychological and behavioral disorders
- Endometrial hyperplasia
- Ovarian cancer and breast cancer.

Long-term Management

Metabolic syndrome comprises insulin resistance (IR), dyslipidemia, and obesity as key features.

Any three or more of the following: Diagnostic criteria
- Waist circumference >88 cm
- Impaired glucose tolerance/ fasting glucose ≥110 mg/dL
- Blood pressure >130/85 mm Hg
- Triglycerides >150 mg/dL
- High density lipoprotein <50 mg/dL.

Apart from detailed history and examination, initial assessment of all PCOS patients should also aim to determine risk factors for long-term complications.

Investigations at first visit should include:

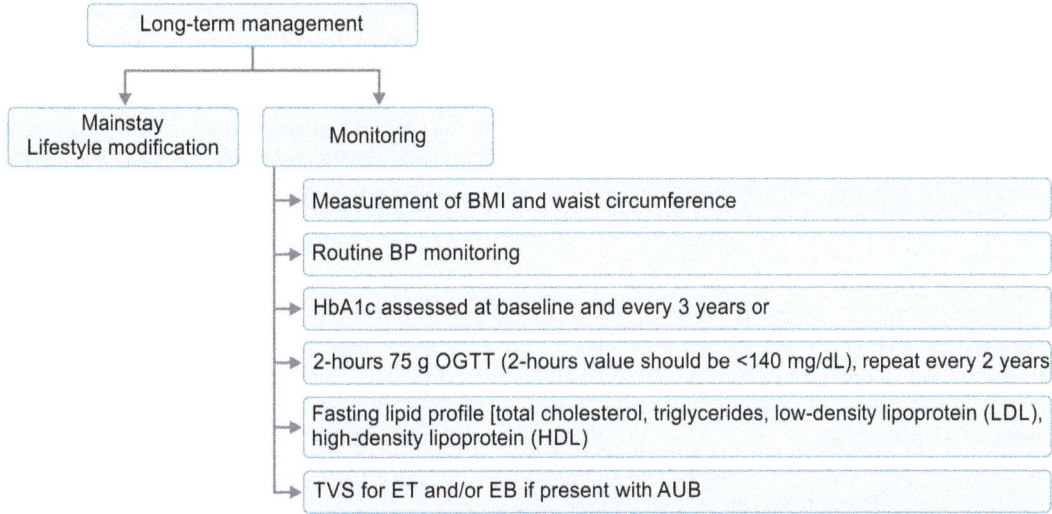

The ESHRE/ASRM Consensus group has recommended a proper endometrial surveillance with ultrasound and/or biopsy to assess endometrial thickening in PCOS women who experience extended periods of amenorrhea.

To minimize this risk, in these women periodic progesterone withdrawal is also recommended at least four episodes per year.

Regular withdrawal bleeding with monthly progesterone or oral contraceptive pills ensures cyclicity in menstruation and prevent endometrial buildup ultimately reducing the risk of endometrial cancer

Key Learning Points

- Polycystic ovary syndrome is an endocrine, metabolic, and chronic inflammatory disorder with hyperandrogenemia, insulin resistance, and obesity being the key factors.
- First-line therapy for all PCOS women is lifestyle modifications targeting weight loss in obese and overweight women while it is prevention of weight gain in lean women.
- Clomiphene citrate or letrozole should be the first-line pharmacological therapy to improve the fertility outcomes in PCOS.
- Exogenous gonadotropins or laparoscopic ovarian drilling are the second-line interventions recommended if the first line fails to result in pregnancy.
- Great care must be taken during induction of ovulation to avoid adverse consequences such as OHSS and multiple pregnancies particularly with gonadotropins.
- Women with PCOS have an increased prevalence of metabolic dysfunctions, impaired glucose intolerance and type 2 diabetes mellitus.
- Metabolic syndrome is a cluster of risk factors, predisposing to both cardiovascular disease and type 2 diabetes mellitus.
- Metabolic syndrome assessment: Blood pressure, HbA1c, lipid profile (LDL, HDL, triglycerides, cholesterol), waist circumference, waist-hip ratio are assessed.
- PCOS women should be closely followed as they may be at increased risk for the development of GDM, gestational hypertension and neonatal complications. This may be exacerbated by obesity and/or insulin resistance.
- Women with PCOS have an increased risk for endometrial carcinoma. Most endometrial cancers are well differentiated and have a good prognosis.

REFERENCES

1. Abbott DH, Barnett DK, Bruns CM, Dumesic DA. Androgen excess fetal programming of female reproduction: a developmental aetiology for polycystic ovary syndrome? Hum Reprod Update. 2005;11(4):357-74.
2. Homburg R. Androgen circle of polycystic ovary syndrome. Hum Reprod. 2009;24(7):1548-55.
3. Blank SK, McCartney CR, Helm KD, Marshall JC. Neuroendocrine effects of androgens in adult polycystic ovary syndrome and female puberty. Semin Reprod Med. 2007;25(5):352-9.
4. Bremer AA. Polycystic ovary syndrome in the pediatric population. Metab Syndr Relat Disord. 2010;8(5):375-94.
5. Diamanti-Kandarakis E. Polycystic ovarian syndrome: pathophysiology, molecular aspects and clinical implications. Expert Rev Mol Med. 2008;10:e3.
6. Fritz MA, Speroff L. Clinical Gynecologic Endocrinology and Infertility, 9th edition. Philadelphia: Lippincott Williams and Wilkins; 2011.
7. Practice Committee of the American Society for Reproductive Medicine. Role of metformin for ovulation induction in infertile patients with polycystic ovary syndrome (PCOS): A guideline. Fertil Steril. 2017;109:426-41.
8. Tekin G, Tekin A, Kiliçarslan EB, Haydardedeoğlu B, Katircibaşi T, Koçum T, et al. Altered autonomic neural control of the cardiovascular system in patients with polycystic ovary syndrome. Int J Cardiol. 2008;130(1):49-55.
9. Zawadski JK Dunaif A. Diagnostic Criteria for Polycystic Ovary Syndrome: Towards a Rational Approach. In: Dunaif A, Givens JR, Haseltine F (Eds). Polycystic Ovary Syndrome. Boston: Blackwell Scientific; 1992. pp. 377-84.
10. Rotterdam ESHRE/ASRM-Sponsored PCOS Consensus Workshop Group. Revised 2003 consensus on diagnostic criteria and long-term health risks related to polycystic ovary syndrome. Fertil Steril. 200;81(1):19-25.
11. Azziz R, Carmina E, Dewailly D, Diamanti-Kandarakis E, Escobar-Morreale HF, Futterweit W, et al; Task Force on the Phenotype of the Polycystic Ovary Syndrome of The Androgen Excess and PCOS Society. The Androgen Excess and PCOS Society criteria for the polycystic ovary syndrome: the complete task force report. Fertil Steril. 2009;91(2):456-88.

12. National Institutes of Health. (2012). Evidence-based methodology workshop on polycystic ovary syndrome (PCOS). [online] Available from https://prevention.nih.gov/research-priorities/research-needs-and-gaps/pathways-prevention/evidence-based-methodology-workshop-polycystic-ovary-syndrome-pcos. [Last accessed March, 2023].
13. Escobar-Morreale HF, Sanchón R, San Millán JL. A prospective study of the prevalence of nonclassical congenital adrenal hyperplasia among women presenting with hyperandrogenic symptoms and signs. J Clin Endocrinol Metab. 2008;93(2):527-33.
14. Yildiz BO, Bolour S, Woods K, Moore A, Azziz R. Visually scoring hirsutism. Hum Reprod Update. 2010;16(1):51-64.
15. ESHRE Capri Workshop Group. Health and fertility in World Health Organization group 2 anovulatory women. Hum Reprod Update. 2012;18(5):586-99.
16. Teede HJ, Misso ML, Costello MF, Dokras A, Laven J, Moran L, et al; International PCOS Network. Recommendations from the international evidence-based guideline for the assessment and management of polycystic ovary syndrome. Hum Reprod. 201;33(9):1602-18.
17. Balen AH, Morley LC, Misso M, Franks S, Legro RS, Wijeyaratne CN, et al. The management of anovulatory infertility in women with polycystic ovary syndrome: an analysis of the evidence to support the development of global WHO guidance. Hum Reprod Update. 2016;22(6):687-708.
18. Dewailly D, Lujan ME, Carmina E, Cedars MI, Laven J, Norman RJ, et al. Definition and significance of polycystic ovarian morphology: a task force report from the Androgen Excess and Polycystic Ovary Syndrome Society. Hum Reprod Update. 2014;20(3):334-52.
19. National Institute of Health and Care Excellence. (2022). NICE guidelines. [online] Available from https://www.nice.org.uk/terms-andconditions#notice-of-rights. [Last accessed March, 2023].
20. Royal College of Obstetricians and Gynecologists. (2014). Long-term Consequences of Polycystic Ovary Syndrome. (Green-top Guideline No. 33). [online] Available from https://www.rcog.org.uk/guidance/browse-all-guidance/green-top-guidelines/long-term-consequences-of-polycystic-ovary-syndrome-green-top-guideline-no-33/. [Last accessed March, 2023].
21. American Diabetes Association Professional Practice Committee; American Diabetes Association Professional Practice Committee: Draznin B, Aroda VR, Bakris G, Benson G, Brown FM, Freeman R, et al. Diabetes Care in the Hospital: Standards of Medical Care in Diabetes-2022. Diabetes Care. 2022;45(Suppl 1):S244-53.
22. Thessaloniki ESHRE/ASRM-Sponsored PCOS Consensus Workshop Group Hum Reprod. 2008;23(3):462-77.
23. U.S. Department of Health and Human Services (DHSS). (2018). Physical activity and health: a report of the Surgeon General. Atlanta: DHSS, Centers for Disease Control and Prevention, National Center for Chronic Disease Prevention and Health Promotion. [online] Available from http://www.cdc.gov/nccdphd/sgr/pdf/sgr full.pdf. [Last accessed March, 2023].
24. American Diabetes Association. Standards of Medical Care in Diabetes—2015 Abridged for Primary Care Providers. Clin Diabetes. 2015;33(2):97-111.
25. Fauser BCJM, Tarlatzis BCM, Rebar RW. Consensus on women's health aspects of polycystic ovary syndrome (PCOS): the Amsterdam ESHRE/ASRM-Sponsored 3rd PCOS Consensus Workshop Group. Fertil Steril. 2012;97(1):28-38.
26. Carmina E. Ovarian and adrenal hyperandrogenism. Ann N Y Acad Sci. 2006;1092:130-7.
27. Dewailly D. Diagnosis of polycystic ovary syndrome (PCOS): Revisiting the threshold values of follicle count on ultrasound and of the serum AMH level for the definition of polycystic ovaries. Hum Reprod. 2011;26(11):3123-9.
28. Berker B, Kaya C, Aytac R, Satiroglu H. Homocysteine concentrations in follicular fluid are associated with poor oocyte and embryo qualities in polycystic ovary syndrome patients undergoing assisted reproduction. Hum Reprod. 2009;24(9):2293-302.
29. Monash Centre for Health Research and Implementation (MCHRI). (2018). International evidence-based guideline for the assessment and management of polycystic ovary syndrome. [online] Available from https://www.monash.edu/medicine/sphpm/mchri/pcos/guideline. [Last accessed March, 2022].
30. Fernandez H, Morin-Surruca M, Torre A, Faivre E, Deffieux X, Gervaise A, Ovarian drilling for surgical treatment of polycystic ovarian syndrome: a comprehensive review. Reprod Biomed Online. 2011;22(6):556-68.
31. Amer SA, Li TC, Ledger WL. The value of measuring anti-Müllerian hormone in women with anovulatory polycystic ovary syndrome undergoing laparoscopic ovarian diathermy. Hum Reprod. 2009;24(11):2760-6.
32. Blockeel C, Drakopoulos P, Santos-Ribeiro S, Polyzos NP, Tournaye H. A fresh look at the freeze-all protocol: a SWOT analysis. Hum Reprod. 2016;31(3):491-7.
33. Haahr T, Roque M, Esteves SC, Humaidan P. GnRH agonist trigger and LH Activity luteal phase support versus hCG trigger and conventional luteal phase support in fresh embryo transfer IVF/ICSI cycles—A systematic PRISMA review and meta-analysis. Front Endocrinol.
34. Castillo JC, Haahr T, Martínez-Moya M, Humaidan P. Gonadotropin-releasing hormone agonist for ovulation trigger–OHSS prevention and use of modified luteal phase support for fresh embryo transfer. Ups J Med Sci. 2020;125(2):131-7.
35. Aflatoonian A, Mansoori-Torshizi M, Farid Mojtahedi M, Aflatoonian B, Khalili MA, Amir-Arjmand MH, et al. Fresh versus frozen embryo transfer after gonadotropin-releasing hormone agonist trigger in gonadotropin-releasing hormone antagonist cycles among high responder women: A randomized, multi-center study. Int J Reprod Biomed. 2018;16(1):9-18.
36. Hu L, Ma L, Xia X, Ying T, Zhou M, Zou S, et al. Efficacy of bariatric surgery in the treatment of women with obesity and polycystic ovary syndrome. J Clin Endocrinol Metab. 202214;107(8):e3217-29.
37. Lee R, Joy Mathew C, Jose M, O Elshaikh A, Shah L, Cancarevic I. A review of the impact of bariatric surgery in women with polycystic ovary syndrome. Cureus. 2022;12(10):e10811.

CHAPTER 16

Management of Hirsutism

Chaitra Nayak

■ INTRODUCTION
Hirsutism has widespread physical, social and psychological impact, and is one of the important reasons for dermatological/gynecologist consultation. It is essential to understand steps for evaluation/management of Hirsutism.

■ DEFINITION
- Hirsutism is a condition wherein a woman develops excessive coarse, rough, and dark hair (terminal hair) in an adult male distribution.[1,2]
- Visible increase in terminal hair over the face, sternum, lower abdomen, back, and thigh in women.

■ INCIDENCE[1]
- 5–10% of women of reproductive age suffer from hirsutism.
- It is the most common manifestation of hyperandrogenemia (HA).
- The most common cause of hyperandrogenism in women is polycystic ovary syndrome (PCOS) (70-80%).

■ DIAGNOSIS
- Any patient who comes with complaints of hirsutism needs evaluation.[1,2]
- The gold standard for evaluation clinically is *modified Ferriman–Gallwey score* (**Fig. 1**).[3]
- *Nine* most androgen-sensitive areas are scored individually for density and pattern of hair distribution from zero (0) which indicates no hair to 4 which indicates virile hair.
- The total score of ≥8 is hirsutism and needs further evaluation.
- Serum testosterone (free and total) are initial blood tests done.

■ DIFFERENTIAL DIAGNOSIS FOR HIRSUTISM[4]
Differential diagnosis of hirsutism is given in **Table 1**.

■ SIGNS OF HYPERANDROGENISM
- Hirsutism
- Acne
- Alopecia.

■ SIGNS OF INSULIN RESISTANCE
- Acanthosis nigricans
- Skin tags
- Hypertension
- Hyperandrogenism.

■ SOURCE OF ANDROGEN IN WOMEN
- Ovarian theca
- Adrenal cortex
- End-organ peripheral conversion.

■ MAJOR ANDROGENS IN WOMEN
- Dehydroepiandrosterone (DHEA)
- Dehydroepiandrosterone sulfate (DHEA-S)
- Androstenedione
- Testosterone ⎫ Potent and
- Dihydrotestosterone. ⎭ high affinity

■ RED FLAGS OF HIRSUTISM
- Virilization
- Acute/rapid symptom progression
- Pelvic/abdominal mass.

■ EVALUATION OF HIRSUTISM/HYPERANDROGENISM (FLOWCHART 1)[1,2]

History Taking[1,2]
A targeted history focused on:
- Age of thelarche, adrenarche, and menarche
- Menstrual history—frequency and duration
- Symptoms of hyperandrogenism (HA)
- Onset and progression of symptoms—HA

Management of Hirsutism

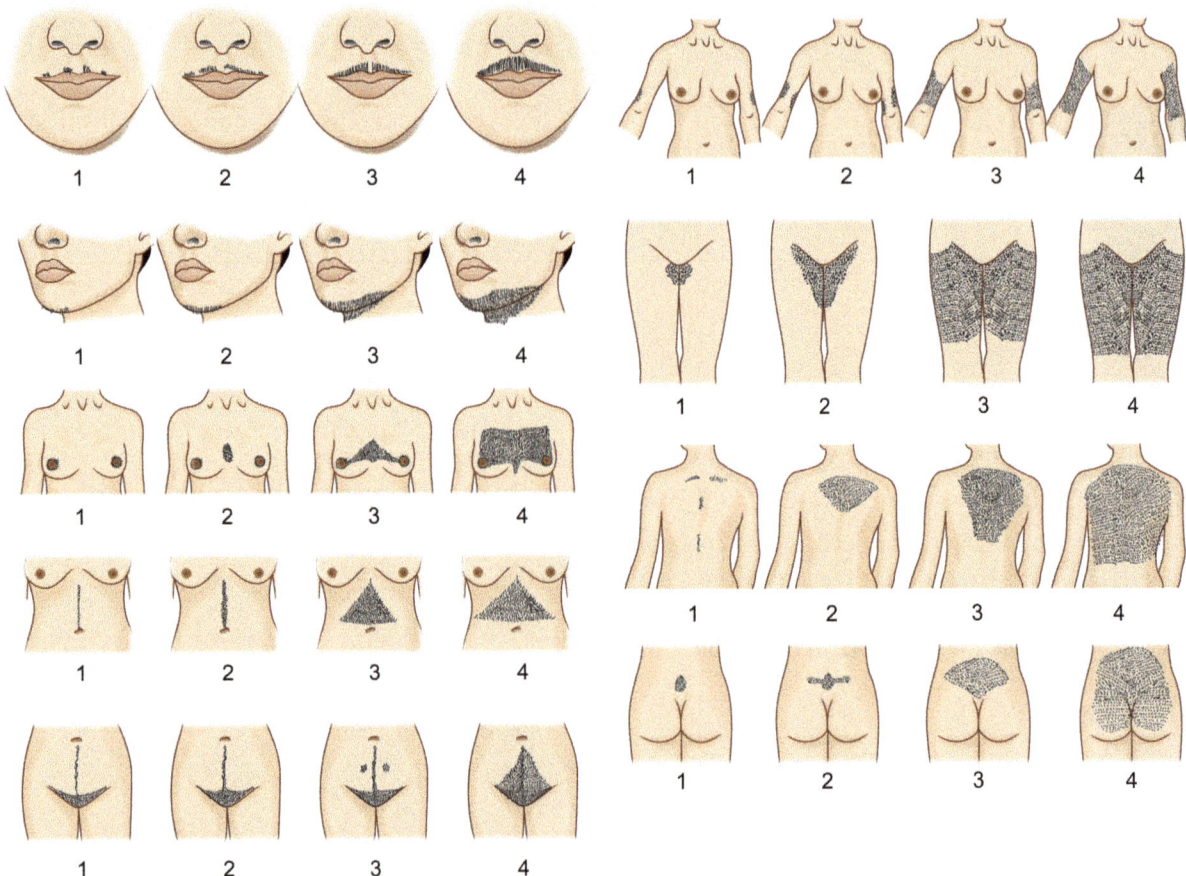

Fig. 1: Modified Ferriman–Gallwey chart for measuring hirsutism.

TABLE 1: Differential diagnosis for hirsutism.	
Common causes	**Rare causes**
• PCOS • Idiopathic hirsutism • Physiological HA of puberty • Idiopathic HA	• NCCAH • Hypothyroidism • Cushing disease • Androgen-secreting tumor • Severe hyperprolactinemia
(HA: hyperandrogenemia; NCCAH: nonclassical congenital adrenal hyperplasia; PCOS: polycystic ovarian syndrome)	

- Family history—PCOS, HA, and obesity
- Past treatment—laser, epilation, and shaving
- Medications—steroids/testosterone supplements.

Examination

Need to look for:
- Blood pressure
- Body mass index (BMI)
- Ferriman-Gallwey score
- Other signs of HA
- Signs of insulin resistance
- External genitalia—Clitoromegaly.

Investigations

- Total testosterone
- Free testosterone
- 17-hydroxyprogesterone (17-OHP)—if there is strong family history or ethnicity.

MANAGEMENT

- Multimodal therapy is best
- Counseling[1,5,6] plays an important role. It is vital to explain about:
  • Discuss expectations from proposed treatment measures.
  • Terminal hair has a lifespan of 6 months.
  • Any therapy will take 6 months to show an effect.
  • Lifestyle modification is an essential part of treatment.
  • Psychosocial effects of HA need to be addressed.
  • Lifelong treatment may be required in a few individuals.

Flowchart 1: Work-up of patient with Hirsutism.

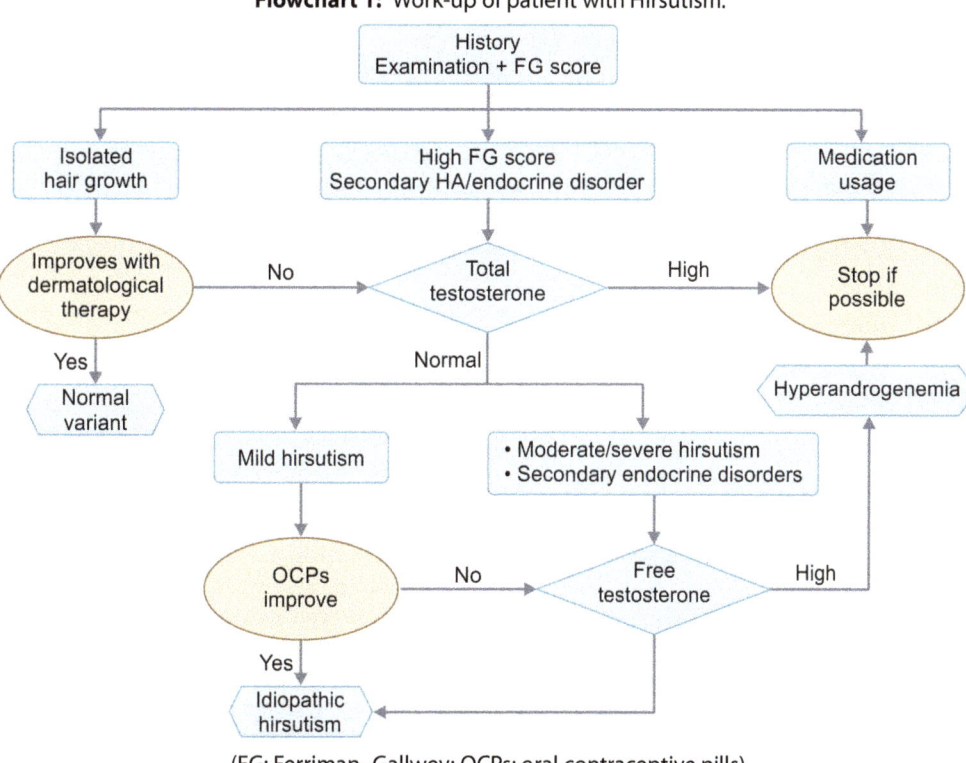

(FG: Ferriman–Gallwey; OCPs: oral contraceptive pills)

- *Lifestyle modification:*
  - Weight loss is beneficial in PCOS/obese women.
  - Glycemic control is beneficial to reduce HA.
- *Medication therapy:* Principle of treatment:
  - Third-generation oral contraceptive pills (OCPs) are the best initial therapy.
  - OCP needs to be continued for 6 months to show adequate effect.
  - Any class of OCP can be used for treatment, as they are equally effective with low risk.
  - In obese/older (>39 years) women, low dose OCP is preferred to avoid risk of venous thromboembolism (VTE).
  - Hormonal therapy must be avoided before menarche.
  - OCP increase sex hormone-binding globulin (SHBG) production and reduce free testosterone.
  - Contraceptive vaginal rings/patch has shown similar effects.
  - OCP has no effect on existing hair but helps in controlling new hair growth.
  - Avoid antiandrogen monotherapy as the first line.
  - Use adequate contraception if antiandrogens are being added. Additional antiandrogens may be added after 6 months if treatment is unsatisfactory.
  - Antiandrogen therapy as a first line can be give only if patient is not sexually active, has had permanent sterilization, or on long-acting reversible contraception.
- Avoid flutamide as it has hepatotoxicity.
- Avoid insulin lowering agents for solely treating hirsutism in BMI <25 kg/m^2.
- Combination of OCP + metformin may be beneficial for overweight/obese women with hirsutism.[7]
- Avoid using gonadotropin releasing hormone (GnRH) agonist for hirsutism treatment
- Severe distressing hirsutism—start both anti-androgens and OCP together.
- Older women with hirsutism—start with low dose third-generation OCP.
- *Physical methods:*
  - Shaving, bleaching, waxing, and chemical depilation are temporary measures.
  - Electrolysis and laser hair removal are permanent measures.
  - Photoepilation is better for women with black, brown, and auburn hair.
  - Electrolysis is recommended for blonde or white hair.
  - Long wave long-pulse laser line neodymium-doped yttrium aluminum garnet (Nd:YAG) or diode laser with adequate cooling is recommended.
  - Eflornithine can be added to photoepilation for rapid response.
  - Eflornithine cream is used for facial hirsutism to thin hair growth.

- *Laser therapy in hirsutism:*[8]
  - Most women with hirsutism will benefit from photoepilation.
  - Sources of photoepilation—four types of laser (ruby, alexandrite, diode, and Nd:YAG) and intense pulsed light (IPL) sources (wavelength of 500–1,200 nm).
  - Recommended for women with black, auburn, and auburn hair.
  - Avoid photoepilation in Mediterranean and Middle Eastern women due to risk of paradoxical hypertrichosis.
  - Photoepilation is quicker than electrolysis with fewer sittings required.

Mild Hirsutism

- Either direct hair removal or pharmacological therapy can be used as first line of therapy.

Patient-important Hirsutism

- Pharmacological therapy is stated first, for 6 months and if no benefit occurs, physical methods are added upon.

Idiopathic Hirsutism

- Hirsutism in eumenorrheic women with no evidence of hyperandrogenism or PCOS on evaluation.
- Seen in 5–20% of hirsute women.
- Most will present with mild hirsutism.
- These women may have polycystic ovarian morphology on ultrasound.

Note: The work-up of hyperandrogenism is beyond the scope of this chapter and will be covered elsewhere.

Key Learning Points

- Hirsutism affects 5–10% of reproductive age women.
- All women with patient-important hirsutism are evaluated by Ferriman–Gallwey scoring.
- Sudden/severe/progressive hirsutism/virilization needs immediate evaluation.
- Counseling and lifestyle modification are important components of treatment, especially in women with PCOS.
- Treatment modalities range from OCP, epilation, and depilation to additional androgens.

REFERENCES

1. Screening and Management of the Hyperandrogenic Adolescent: ACOG Committee Opinion, Number 789. Obstet Gynecol. 2019;134(4):e106-14.
2. Mimoto MS, Oyler JL, Davis AM. Evaluation and Treatment of Hirsutism in Premenopausal Women. JAMA. 2018; 319(15):1613-4.
3. Wild RA, Vesely S, Beebe L, Whitsett T, Owen W. Ferriman Gallwey self-scoring I: performance assessment in women with polycystic ovary syndrome. J Clin Endocrinol Metab. 2005;90(7):4112-4.
4. Matheson E, Bain J. Hirsutism in women. Am Fam Physician. 2019;100(3):168-75.
5. Zehravi M, Maqbool M, Ara I. Depression and anxiety in women with polycystic ovarian syndrome: a literature survey. Int J Adolesc Med Health. 2021;33(6):367-73.
6. Pate C. Issues Faced by Women with Hirsutism: State of the Science. Health Care Women Int. 2016;37(6):636-45.
7. Fraison E, Kostova E, Moran LJ, Bilal S, Ee CC, Venetis C, et al. Metformin versus the combined oral contraceptive pill for hirsutism, acne, and menstrual pattern in polycystic ovary syndrome. Cochrane Database Syst Rev. 2020;8(8): CD005552.
8. Lee CM. Laser-assisted hair removal for facial hirsutism in women: A review of evidence. J Cosmet Laser Ther. 2018; 20(3):140-4.

Ovulation Induction Protocols for Intrauterine Insemination

Shivani Singh Kapoor, Shalu Gupta

■ AIM OF OVULATION INDUCTION

Development of one or more mature follicle/s leads to ovulation and release of one or more mature oocytes capable of fertilization and embryo formation.

Goal: Mono-ovulation in polycystic ovarian syndrome (PCOS) anovulatory patients and no more than three follicles in ovulatory subfertile patients.

■ INDICATIONS OF OVULATION INDUCTION

- Formation of single/more follicles in anovulatory women
- Formation of more than one follicle in an ovulating woman with unexplained infertility, mild male factor infertility, or donor insemination. This is also called superovulation.

■ PREREQUISITE FOR OVULATION INDUCTION

- *History and physical examination of the couple:* Make sure couple is in optimal health before starting OI.
- Optimize weight and body mass index (BMI)
- Stop smoking, check rubella immunization status, and advise periconceptional use of folic acid.
- At least one tube should be patent.
- Uterine causes of infertility should be ruled out.
- Severe male factor infertility should be ruled out—semen analysis.
- Baseline hormonal evaluation [thyroid-stimulating hormone (TSH), prolactin, etc.] should be normal.
- Thorough counseling regarding various treatment options available, their success rate and complications, and obtaining informed consent.

Figure 1 shows classification of anovulation by World Health Organization (WHO).

■ METHODS OF OVULATION INDUCTION

- *Oral agents:*
  - Selective estrogen receptor modulators (SERM), e.g., clomiphene citrate (CC), tamoxifen
  - Aromatase inhibitors, e.g., letrozole, anastrozole
  - Insulin-sensitizing agents, e.g., metformin, myo-inositol, etc.
- *Injectable agents:*
  - Urinary gonadotropins
  - Recombinant gonadotropins
  - Gonadotropin-releasing hormone (GnRH) analogs in hypogonadotropic-hypogonadism.
- *Ovarian drilling:* Laparoscopic ovarian drilling could be second-line therapy for women with PCOS, who are CC resistant, with anovulatory infertility and no other infertility factors.

Laparoscopic ovarian drilling could potentially be offered as first-line treatment if laparoscopy is indicated for another reason

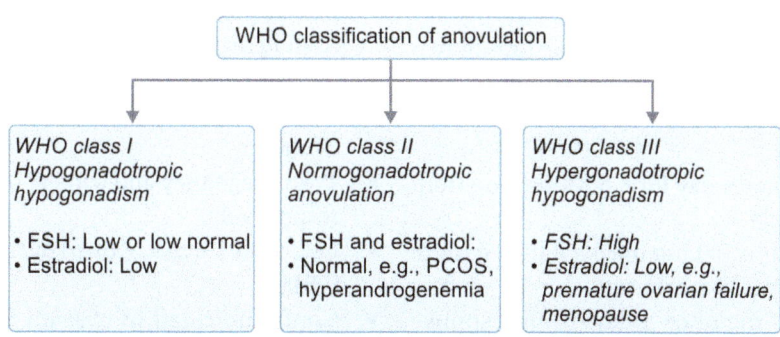

Fig. 1: World Health Organization (WHO) classification of anovulation.
(FSH: follicle-stimulating hormone; PCOS: polycystic ovarian syndrome)

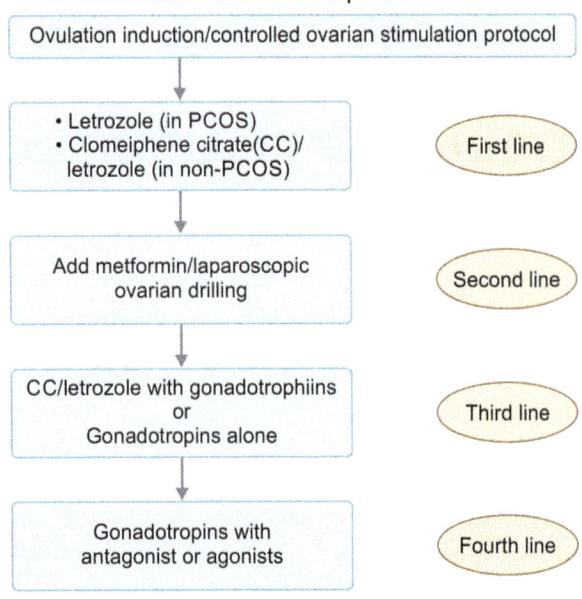

Flowchart 1: Ovulation induction/controlled ovarian stimulation protocol.

(PCOS: polycystic ovarian syndrome)

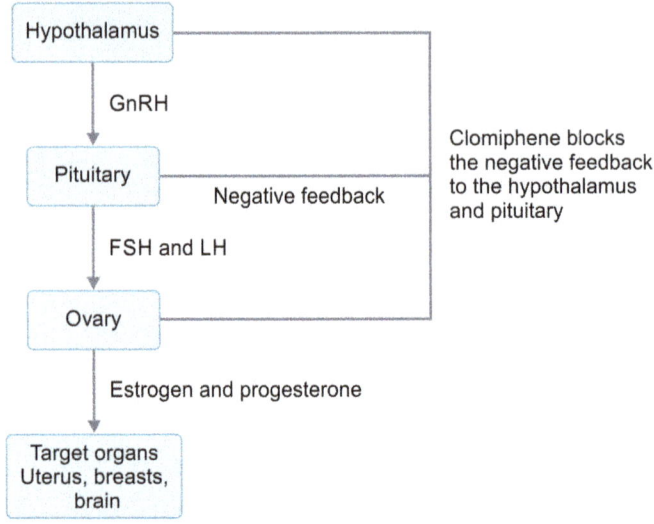

Flowchart 2: Mechanism of action of clomiphene citrate.

(FSH: follicle-stimulating hormone; GnRH: gonadotropin-releasing hormone; LH: luteinizing hormone)

Need to discuss:
- Comparative cost
- Expertise required for use in OI
- Intra- and postoperative risks higher in overweight and obese
- Small associated risk of lower ovarian reserve or loss of ovarian function
- Periadnexal adhesion formation may be an associated risk.

Flowchart 1 shows ovulation induction (OI)/controlled ovarian stimulation protocol.

Clomiphene Citrate

- It was first synthesized in 1956.
- It is a nonsteroidal triphenylethylene derivative, an SERM. It acts as both, an estrogen agonist (at very low estrogen concentrations) as well as a competitive estrogen receptor antagonist.
- Metabolized by the liver and excreted in stools.
- About 85% of the administered dose is eliminated after about 6 days.
- Most commonly used OI agent.
- Commercially available CC is a racemic mixture of two stereoisomers: Enclomiphene and zuclomiphene.
- Enclomiphene is responsible for OI action due to its antiestrogenic effect.
- *Starting dose:* 50 mg once a day for 5 days starting from day 2 to day 5 of the cycle
- Dose can be increased to 100 mg once a day in case of clomiphene failure with a 50 mg dosage.
- Maximum dosage 200 mg once a day. If no response even with this dose, the patient is labeled as clomiphene resistant.

- *Ovulation rate:* 70–80%
- *Pregnancy rate (PR):* Much lower (9–17%). The odds ratio of pregnancy per cycle is 2.5 [95% confidence interval (CI) 1.35–4.62] for unexplained subfertility in women.[1]

Mechanism of action: Competitive estrogen receptor blocker
Competes with endogenous estrogens for the estrogen receptors and blocks them for an extended time period
↓
Prolonged receptor binding leads to downregulation of the estrogen receptors
↓
At the hypothalamic-pituitary level, this receptor downregulation is perceived as low circulating estrogen levels
↓
This reduces the negative feedback of estrogen on the hypothalamus leading to an increase in GnRH secretions
↓
Increase in follicle-stimulating hormone (FSH) and luteinizing hormone (LH) pulse at pituitary levels
↓
Growth of a dominant follicle and its ovulation

- It can only be used in women with intact hypothalamic-pituitary-ovarian (HPO)-axis **(Flowchart 2)**. It cannot be used in hypogonadotropic hypogonadism
- It can result in thin endometrium
- It can result in poor cervical mucus secretions around ovulation
- Twin pregnancy and triplets with CC are 5–7% and 0.3%, respectively.
- Less than 1% risk of ovarian hyperstimulation syndrome (OHSS)
- Contraindicated in ovarian cysts, especially with suspected malignancy, clomiphene failure in the previous cycle, and liver diseases

- *Side effects:* Hot flushes, breast tenderness, vaginal dryness, bloating, nausea, floaters in vision, light flashes, and blurred vision
- *Long-term treatment (>12 months):* Slight-increased risk of ovarian cancers[2] borderline
- *Clomiphene failure:* No pregnancy even after three cycles of clomiphene treatment with documented ovulation.

Tamoxifen

- Tamoxifen also belongs to the class of SERM with a similar mechanism of action as clomiphene.
- *Dosage:* 20–40 mg once a day for 5 days starting from day 2 to 5 of the cycle.
- Weaker ovulation-inducing agent as compared to clomiphene.
- More favorable effect on uterine endometrium as it does not affect estrogen receptors of the endometrium.
- Drug of choice for OI for patients with a previous history of breast carcinoma.

Aromatase Inhibitors

- Competitive inhibitors of aromatase enzymes
- *Mechanism of action*: Aromatase inhibitors inhibit the conversion of androgens to estrogens → significantly lowers serum estradiol and estrone levels → reducing negative feedback of the estrogens on the hypothalamus and anterior pituitary gland → increases GnRH secretions → increases FSH and LH pulsatility → growth of dominant follicle and its ovulation **(Flowchart 3)**.

Letrozole

- It is a third-generation aromatase inhibitor highly specific in inhibiting the aromatase enzyme without significant inhibition of the other steroidogenesis enzymes.

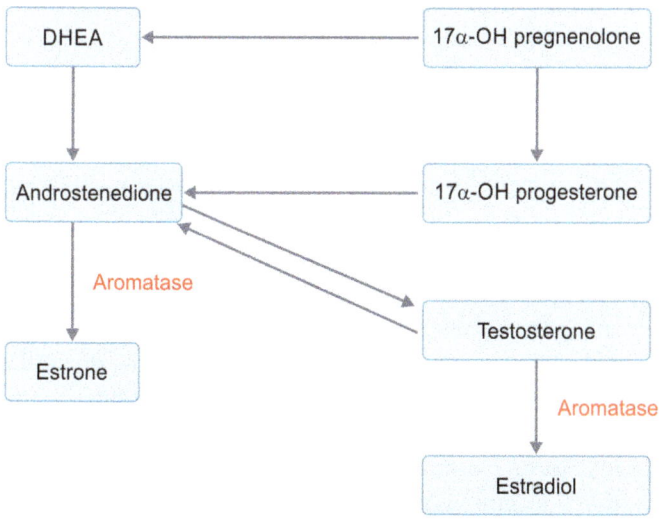

Flowchart 3: Mechanism of action of aromatase inhibitors.

(17α-OH: 17α-hydroxyprogesterone; DHEA: dehydroepiandrosterone)

- Almost 100% bioavailable
- Short half-life of around 48 hours
- Well tolerated with minimal side effects
- Metabolized mainly in the liver and excreted through biliary (85%) and urinary (15%) systems.
- Side effects include bone pain, hot flushes, dry vagina, nausea, acidity, and occasional headache.
- Initially, letrozole was marred with controversy because of some potential teratogenic effects, especially cartilaginous and bone malformation. But later on, a multicentric study by Tulandi et al. refuted these claims.[3]
- In 2018, European Society of Human Reproduction and Embryology (ESHRE), American Society for Reproductive Medicine (ASRM), Centre for Research Excellence in Polycystic Ovary Syndrome (CREPCOS), and Monash University released International evidence-based guidelines for the assessment and management of PCOS. Letrozole was deemed as the first-line OI agent in PCOS.[4]
- *Dosage:* 2.5–5 mg once a day for 5 days starting from day 2 to 5 of the cycle
- Ovulation occurs in 75% of women with PCOS; pregnancy is attained in 15%.
- In PCOS, letrozole was found to be better than clomiphene for ovulation rate per patient, PR per patient, and live birth rate per patient.[4]
- Also, the drug of choice for women for OI with the previous history of ovarian carcinoma or endometrial hyperplasia.
- Lower risk of multiple pregnancies (MPs) as compared to clomiphene as the chances of multiple follicular responses with letrozole is lower.

Insulin-sensitizing Agents

- Insulin resistance is common in PCOS, high insulin levels lower sex hormone-binding globulin (SHBG) and insulin-like growth factor-binding protein (IGFBP), thus increasing the bioavailability of free androgens.
- Insulin also stimulates theca cells to increase the IGF-2 and IGF-1, thereby increasing ovarian androgen biosynthesis and increased bioavailability of free androgens. Excess local ovarian androgen production
- Hyperandrogenemia causes premature follicular atresia and anovulation.
- Insulin-sensitizing agents reduce insulin resistance and thereby reduce overall insulin secretion.
- In the last decade, there has been renewed interest in these drugs as it was noted that PCOS women have high levels of circulating insulin in their blood and often have deranged oral glucose tolerance test (OGTT).
- The biguanide metformin is the most widely used insulin-sensitizing agent.

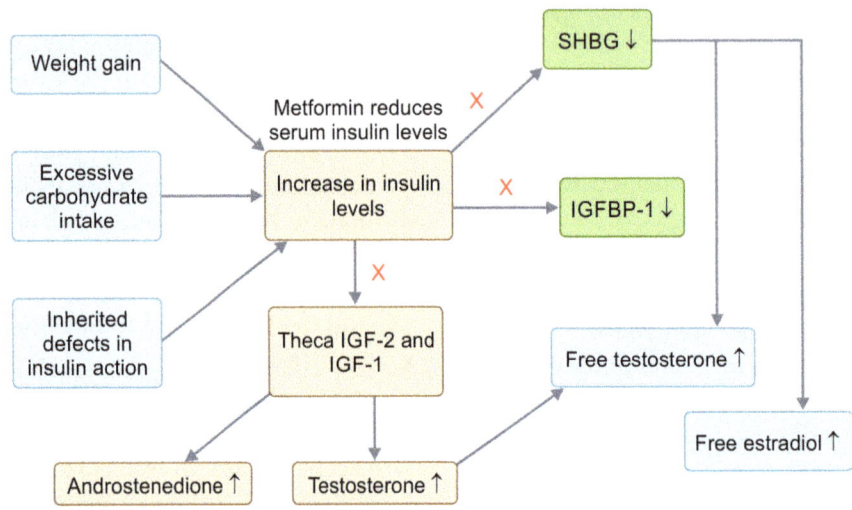

Flowchart 4: Mechanism of action of metformin.

(IGFBP: insulin-like growth factor-binding protein; SHBG: sex hormone-binding globulin)

- *Mechanism of action of metformin* (**Flowchart 4**):
  - Suppress hepatic gluconeogenesis
  - Enhances binding of insulin to its receptors
  - Interfere with mitochondrial respiratory chain
  - Inhibits intestinal absorption of glucose

  ↓
  Increases insulin sensitivity
  ↓
  Decreases serum insulin levels
  ↓
  ↑ SHBG, ↑ IGFBP-1, ↑ Theca IGF-1, and IGF-2
  ↓
  ↓ Free testosterone, ↓ free estradiol, ↓ serum androstenedione
  Reduces hyperandrogenemia and hyperestrogenemia

- Half-life of metformin is 1.5–3 hours
- Duration of action 6–8 hours
- It is excreted in urine
- Starting dose 500 mg twice a day
- Maximum dose 2500 mg/day
- *Side effects:* Anorexia, nausea, gastritis, metallic taste, mild diarrhea, and tiredness.
- Lactic acidosis is the most serious complication.
- It can cause vitamin B12 deficiency due to intestinal malabsorption.
- In a Cochrane systematic review,[5] metformin was concluded to be an effective treatment for anovulation in women with PCOS, as it increases the live birth rates (37 vs. 19%) as compared to the placebo.
- Ovulation rates with metformin alone were around 46% but when it was combined with CC, ovulation rates increased to about 76%. The live birth rate with CC alone is 24% which may change to between 23 and 34% with metformin and clomiphene combined.[5]
- While comparing metformin with CC, there were no statistically significant differences between metformin and clomiphene for live birth rate per pregnancy, MPs per pregnancy, miscarriage rate per pregnancy, PR, or ovulation rate. When subgrouped by BMI, clomiphene was better than metformin for live birth rate, PR, and ovulation rate in BMI >30 kg/m^2; and metformin was better than clomiphene for PR in BMI <30 kg/m^2.[4]
- Metformin + CC was better than metformin alone for ovulation rate, PR, and live birth rate. There was no statistically significant difference between metformin + CC and metformin alone for miscarriage rate or adverse events.[4]
- Clomiphene/letrozole therapy requires specialist care. Costs to the patient of monitoring (tests and specialist visits) and accessibility to specialist care may present barriers. Metformin is low cost, accessible, and can be used alone and/or in combination with clomiphene/letrozole. This at times makes metformin the first line of treatment for anovulatory PCO.

Oral Ovulation Induction Agents in Combination with Gonadotropins

- 2018 ESHRE-ASRM Consensus, while comparing CC versus CC + gonadotropin reached a conclusion that there was insufficient evidence to determine whether one intervention was better than the other.[4]
- In practice, we often combine oral OI agents with gonadotropins to cut down the cost and bring down the dose of gonadotropins, with variable success rates.
- One of the largest randomized controlled trials (RCTs) in 2005 on clomiphene versus gonadotropins concluded that the combination of clomiphene with gonadotropins or gonadotropins only appears to be more effective than clomiphene alone.[6]

Injectable Gonadotropins

Gonadotropins were introduced into clinical practice in 1961, and soon assumed a central role in OI. Gonadotropins are like a double-edged sword—they increase the PR, but also increase risk of MP, high-order multiple pregnancy (HOMP), and OHSS due to multifollicular recruitment.

Choice of Gonadotropin

- Both urinary human menopausal gonadotropin (hMG)/FSH and recombinant FSH (rFSH) are available.
- Equal efficacy of both drugs in terms of PR even in PCOS patients
- Urinary preparations have the advantage of low cost.
- Clinical choice of gonadotropin should depend on availability, cost, personal preference, and convenience.[7]

Physiology

- A certain "threshold" level of FSH is required to initiate follicular recruitment.
- This opens "FSH window" which sustains follicular growth (Fig. 2)
- Wider the FSH window larger (multiple) is the follicular recruitment".[8]
- Large doses of exogenous gonadotropin widen the FSH window.

STIMULATION PROTOCOLS

- Gonadotropins can be used alone or
- Combination protocol
- Along with oral OI agents
- Reduce the physical, financial burden on the patient
- Thought to reduce complication
- Safest is the chronic low-dose protocol.

Gonadotropin-only Protocols

Conventional therapy uses supraphysiological doses of gonadotropins, initiates the development of a large follicular cohort, and rescues follicles destined for atresia.

The dose that initiates follicular development is continued until the criteria for giving the ovulation trigger with human chorionic gonadotropin (hCG) are attained.

Step-down Protocol

- More physiological as it mimics the natural cycle.
- Initial high dose of gonadotropins followed by a drop in the dosage.
- 150 IU/day is started from day 2 of the period and continued until a dominant follicle >10 mm is seen on ultrasound (Fig. 3).
- The dose is then decreased to 37.5 IU every 3 days till minimum dose of 75 IU is reached.
- This is then continued till hCG administration.[9]

Step-up Protocol

- Starting dose of 150 IU/day
- Had very high multiple pregnancy rate (MPR) of 36% and an OHSS rate of 14%. It is no longer used for OI for intrauterine insemination (IUI) (Fig. 4).[8]

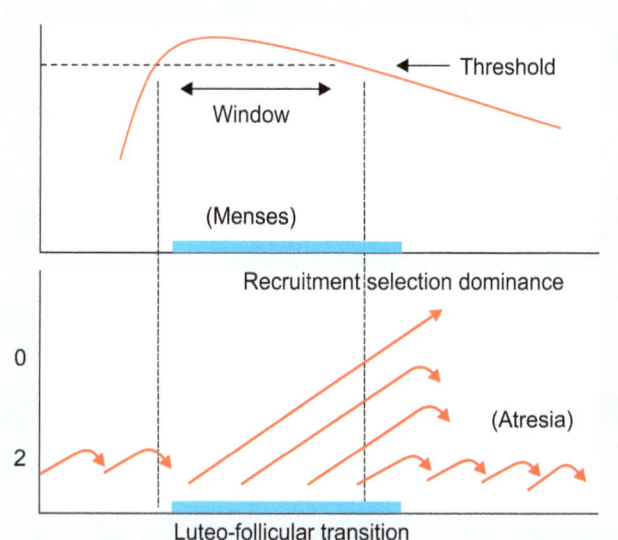

Fig. 2: Luteo-follicular transition in follicle-stimulating hormone (FSH) window.

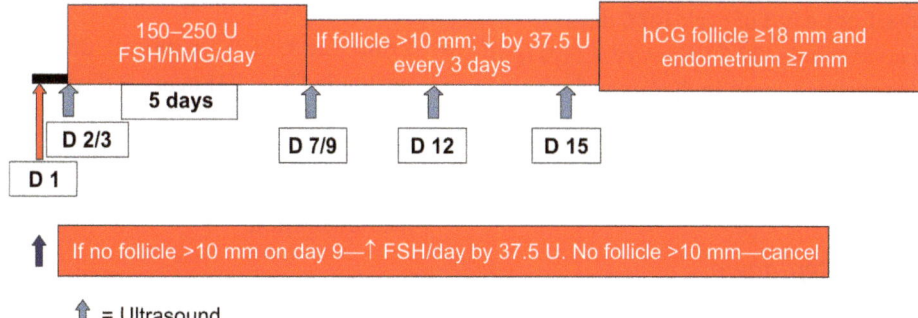

Fig. 3: Step-down protocol.
(D: day; FSH: follicle-stimulating hormone; hCG: human chorionic gonadotropin; hMG: human menopausal gonadotropin)

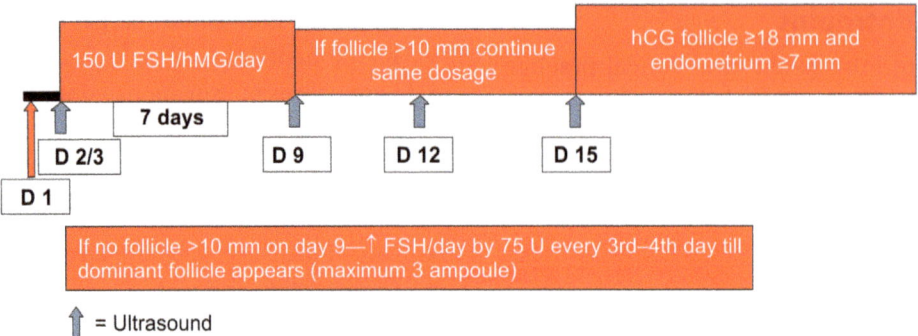

Fig. 4: Step-up protocol.
(D: day; FSH: follicle-stimulating hormone; hCG: human chorionic gonadotropin; hMG: human menopausal gonadotropin)

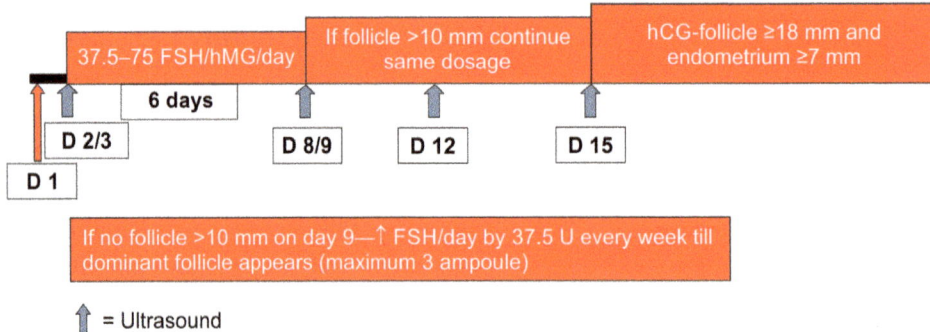

Fig. 5: Low-dose step-up protocol.
(D: day; FSH: follicle-stimulating hormone; hCG: human chorionic gonadotropin; hMG: human menopausal gonadotropin)

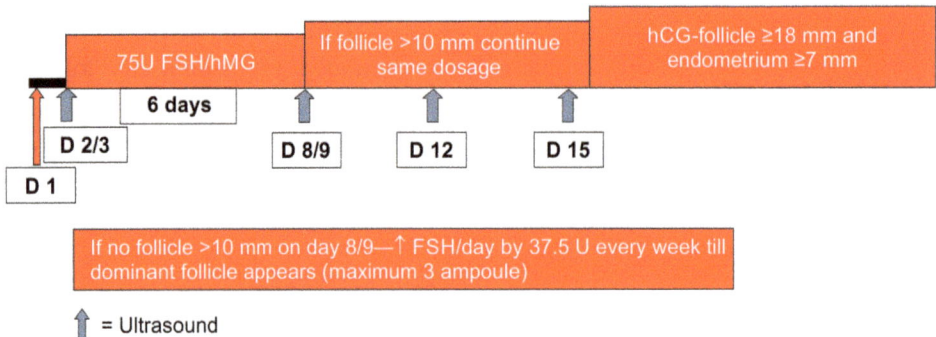

Fig. 6: Sequential step-up and step-down.
(D: day; FSH: follicle-stimulating hormone; hCG: human chorionic gonadotropin; hMG: human menopausal gonadotropin)

Low-dose Step-up Protocol

- 75 IU is stating dose from day 3 of cycle for 6 days.
- Increased by half an ampoule (37.5 IU) every 6 days until the leading follicle reaches 10 mm in diameter.[10]
- This dose (i.e., the threshold dose) is then maintained until the criteria for triggering ovulation is reached (at least one follicle 18 mm in diameter) **(Fig. 5)**.[11]

Sequential Step-up and Step-down

- Combines an initial step-up gonadotropin administration followed by a step-down regimen after follicular selection **(Fig. 6)**

- *Advantage:* Reduces medium-sized follicles and lowers estradiol levels.[12]
- From day 3, 75 IU is started; dose is increased by half an ampoule (37.5 IU) every 6 days until the leading follicle reaches 10 mm in diameter. This dose is maintained till the leading follicle reaches 14 mm in diameter and the FSH dose is reduced by half until the time of hCG administration.

Chronic Low-dose (Step-up) Protocol

- In PCOS for monofollicular development and reduction in MPR, HOMP, and OHSS.

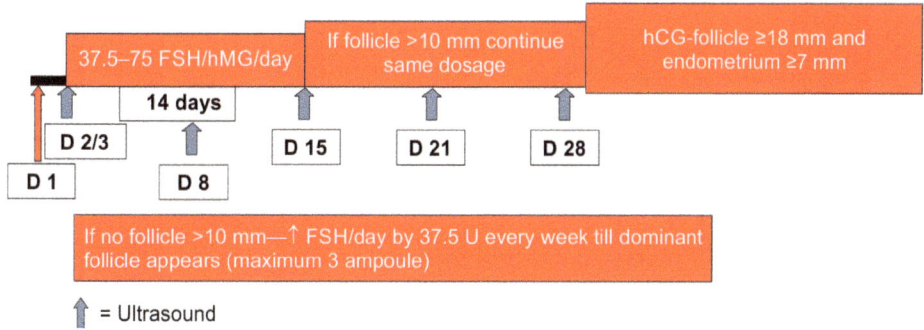

Fig. 7: Chronic low-dose (step-up) protocol.
(D: day; FSH: follicle-stimulating hormone; hCG: human chorionic gonadotropin; hMG: human menopausal gonadotropin)

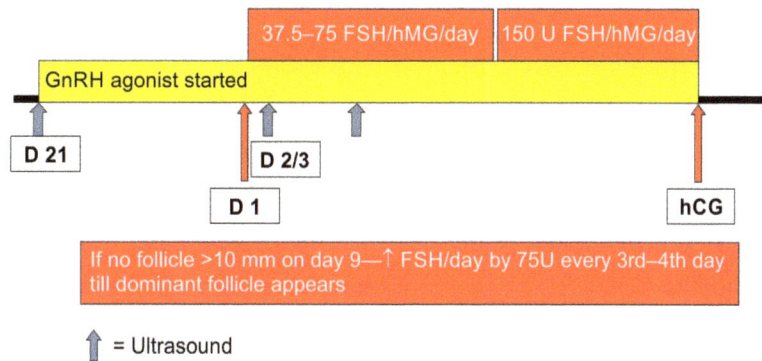

Fig. 8: Agonist regimen.
(D: day; FSH: follicle-stimulating hormone; hCG: human chorionic gonadotropin; hMG: human menopausal gonadotropin)

- A daily dose of 37.5 IU/75 IU of gonadotropin for 14 days from day 2/3.
- If there is no follicle >10 mm after 14 days, then an additional 37.5 IU is added.
- An increase in the dose (37.5 IU) is done every 7 days till the follicle is >10 mm.
- Once the follicle reaches 10 mm, the dose remains unchanged until criteria for hCG administration are reached **(Fig. 7)**.[13]

Modification of Conventional Chronic Low-dose Protocol

- Lower starting doses of 37.5 IU and 50 IU
- Increase in dose to be initiated at 7 days instead of 14 days and subsequent increments to be made at 5 day intervals.

Role of GnRH analogs in OI:

- GnRH analogs are introduced to prevent cycle cancellation due to the premature LH surge.
- A premature LH surge and premature luteinization (PL), reported around 24%, may be responsible for the low PR and high miscarriage rate in IUI cycles. The incidence of PL has been reported to be around 24%.[14]

Agonist Regimen

- Use of GnRH agonists in IUI is not popular.
- Amount and duration of gonadotropins is greatly increased and thereby increasing the cost of treatment **(Fig. 8)**
- An increased risk of multifollicular development, MPs, and OHSS without clear benefits in terms of PR[15]
- GnRH agonist is started from day 21 of previous cycle and continued till date of trigger. Starting dose of FSH 150 U is administered for 7 days, followed by increases (e.g., 75 IU) at intervals of 3–4 days until follicular development is initiated.

Gonadotropin-Releasing Hormone Antagonist[16]

- It can be administered at any time during follicular phase to prevent a premature LH surge.
- Two preparations of GnRH antagonist are available in the market—cetrorelix (0.25 mg or 3 mg) and ganirelix (0.25 mg) **(Fig. 9)**
- Repeated every 24 hours till the hCG trigger is given
- Used as a "fixed protocol"—daily injections started from day 6 of stimulation, or "flexible protocol"—when follicle size is 14 mm or estradiol level >200 pg/mL
- Current evidence does not support the use of antagonist in IUI cycles to improve cycle outcome.

Monitoring during Gonadotropin Stimulation

Following points should be followed while monitoring during gonadotropins stimulation:

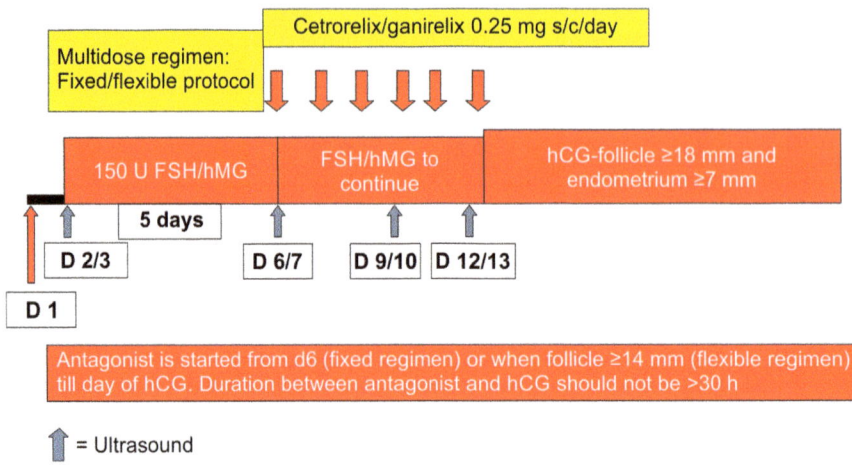

Fig. 9: Antagonist regimen.
(D: day; FSH: follicle-stimulating hormone; hCG: human chorionic gonadotropin; hMG: human menopausal gonadotropin)

- Both ultrasound and estradiol monitoring are essential during gonadotropin stimulation to avoid OHSS and MP.
- Transvaginal scan should be started from day 2/3 onward.
- Day 2/3 should be done as baseline scan to rule out any cyst and note significant findings.

Why Gonadotropins?

In Cochrane, largest review of 43 trials involving 3,957 women, the following conclusions were made:[17]

- Significantly higher PRs with gonadotropins (OR: 1.8; 95% CI: 1.2–2.7) in comparison to oral ovulogens.
- No significant difference between different types of gonadotropins.
- Gonadotropins alone are more effective than with the addition of a GnRH agonist or antagonist
- No significant difference between antiestrogens and aromatase inhibitors (OR: 1.2; 95% CI: 0.64–2.1).
- No evidence of the benefit in doubling the dose of gonadotropins (OR: 1.2; 95% CI: 0.67–1.9), although the multiple PRs and ovarian hyperstimulation rates were increased.

MONOFOLLICULAR VERSUS MULTIFOLLICULAR CYCLES

Multifollicular growth is associated with higher PRs in COS-IUI.

In a meta-analysis, PR was 5% higher with two follicles and 8% higher with three or four follicles. However, the risk of MP was increased by 6, 10, and 14% with two, three, and four follicles, respectively.[18]

A study quoted cumulative PR (CPR) of 19.7% in monofollicular cycles and 29.4% in multifollicular cycles.[19]

CONCLUSION

Gonadotropins in IUI cycles should be used in resistant PCOS cases and where there are three failed IUI cycles with oral OI agents. Gonadotropins should be used in lowest possible dose/minimal stimulation to prevent complication.

In case of multifollicular development, more than three follicles >16 mm cycle patient should be thoroughly counseled. Options like cancellation/converting to in vitro fertilization (IVF) should be discussed.

Key Learning Points

- Mono-ovulation in PCOS anovulatory patients and no more than three follicles in ovulatory subfertile patients.
- Use gonadotropins for OI in IUI only in CC-resistant PCOS cases and in patients who failed to achieve pregnancy after three cycles with oral agents.
- Counsel patients when planning multiple follicle formation about risk of OHSS, MP, HOMP, and cost.
- Start with low-dose gonadotropin to avoid complication.
- Customize treatment.
- Low threshold for cycle cancellation or convert to IVF cycle if development more than three follicles of >16mm size.
- Relook into every failed cycle before starting new one.

REFERENCES

1. Hughes E, Collins J, Vandekerckhove P. Clomiphene citrate for unexplained subfertility in women. Cochrane Database Syst Rev. 2000;(3):CD000057.
2. Rossing MA, Daling JR, Weiss NS. Ovarian tumors in a cohort of infertile women. N Engl J Med. 1994;331:771-6.
3. Tulandi T, Martin J, Al Fadhli R, Kabli N, Forman R, Hitkari J, et al. Congenital malformation among 911 newborns conceived after infertility treatment with letrozole or clomiphene citrate. Fertil Steril. 2006;85:1761-5.
4. Teede HJ, Misso ML, Costello MF, Dokras A, Laven J, Moran L, et al. Recommendations from the international evidence-based guidelines for the assessment and management of polycystic ovary syndrome. Hum Reprod. 2018;33(9):1602-18.
5. Sharpe A, Morley LC, Tang T, Norman RJ, Balen AH. Metformin for ovulation induction in women with a diagnosis of polycystic ovarian syndrome and infertility. Cochrane Database Syst Rev. 2019;12(12):CD013505.

6. Dorn C, Van der van H. Clomiphene citrate versus gonadotrophins for ovulation stimulation. Reprod Biomed Online. 2005;10 Suppl 3:37-43.
7. van Wely M, Kwan I, Burt AL, Thomas J, Vail A, der Veen FV, et al. Recombinant versus urinary gonadotrophin for ovarian stimulation in assisted reproductive technology cycles. Cochrane Database Syst Rev. 2011;(2):CD005354.
8. Fauser BC, Van Heusden AM. Manipulation of human ovarian function: physiological concepts and clinical consequences. Endocr Rev. 1997;18(1):71-106.
9. van Santbrink EJ, Donderwinkel PF, van Dessel TJ, Fauser BC. Gonadotrophin induction of ovulation using a step-down dose regimen: single-centre clinical experience of 82 patients. Hum Reprod. 1995;10(5):1048-53.
10. Brown JB. Pituitary control of ovarian function—concepts derived from gonadotrophin therapy. Aust N Z J Obstet Gynaecol. 1978;18(1):46-54.
11. Wang CF, Gemzell C. The use of human gonadotrophins for induction of ovulation in women with polycystic ovarian disease. Fertil Steril. 1980;33(5):479-86.
12. Hugues JN, Cédrin-Durnerin I, Avril C, Bulwa S, Herve F, Uzan M. Sequential step-up and stepdown dose regimen: an alternative method for ovulation induction with follicle-stimulating hormone in polycystic ovarian syndrome. Hum Reprod. 1996;11(12):2581-4.
13. Homburg R, Howles CM. Low-dose FSH therapy for anovulatory infertility associated with polycystic ovary syndrome: rationale, results, reflections and refinements. Hum Reprod. Update. 1999;5(5):493-9.
14. Cunha-Filho J, Kadoch J, Righini C, Fanchin R, Frydman R, Olivennes F. Premature LH and progesterone rise in intrauterine insemination cycles: analysis of related factors. Reprod Biomed Online. 2003;7(2):194-9.
15. Fleming R, Haxton MJ, Hamilton MP, McCune GS, Black WP, Coutts JR, et al. Successful treatment of infertile women with oligomenorrhoea using a combination of an LHRH agonist and exogenous gonadotrophins. Br J Obstet Gynaecol. 1985;92(4):369-73.
16. Lambalk CB, Leader A, Olivennes F, Fluker MR, Andersen AN, Ingerslev J, et al. Treatment with the GnRH antagonist ganirelix prevents premature LH rises and luteinization in stimulated intrauterine insemination: results of a double-blind, placebo-controlled, multicentre trial. Hum Reprod. 2006;21(3):632-9.
17. Cantineau AEP, Cohlen BJ. Ovarian stimulation protocols (anti-oestrogens, gonadotrophins with and without GnRH agonists/antagonists) for intrauterine insemination (IUI) in women with subfertility. Cochrane Database Syst Rev. 2007;(2):CD005356.
18. Van Rumste MM, Custers IM, van der Veen F, van Wely M, Evers JLH, Mol BWJ. The influence of the number of follicles on pregnancy rates in intrauterine insemination with ovarian stimulation: a meta-analysis. Hum Reprod Update. 2008;14(6):563-70.
19. Jain S, Majumdar A. Impact of gonadotropin-releasing hormone antagonist addition on pregnancy rates in gonadotropin-stimulated intrauterine insemination cycles. J Hum Reprod Sci. 2016;9(3):151-8.

CHAPTER 18

Sperm Selection in IUI and IVF

Mohammed Ashraf C, Ms Lakshmishree BR

■ INTRODUCTION

Around 50% of the infertility cases are due to male factors. Recently, the European Society of Human Reproduction and Embryology (ESHRE) reported that delivery rate per artificial reproductive technique [assisted reproductive technology (ART)] cycle in 2014 and 2016 were 21 and 22%, respectively. The quality of spermatozoa is considered to be the most important reason for this relatively low efficiency, and presence of high percentages of deoxyribonucleic acid (DNA)-damaged spermatozoa in ejaculates is possibly one of the main factors reducing the ART outcomes. To ensure the best quality of spermatozoa used, particularly, in terms of genetic integrity is one of the main challenges in ART.

Currently we lack an effective methodology to separate this specific sperm subpopulation for its use in ARTs. This is especially relevant if we consider that both in vitro fertilization (IVF) and intracytoplasmic sperm injection (ICSI) bypass the sperm selection operating in vivo, increasing the risk of fertilization of oocyte with defective spermatozoa that could lead to developmental failure.

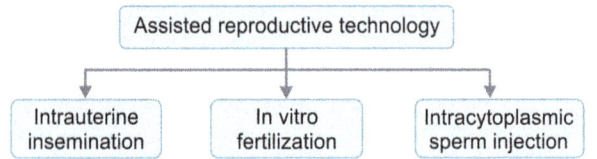

Numerous attempts have been made over years to maximize the sperm recovery through the use of effective intrauterine insemination (IUI) processing techniques and the selection of specific sperm for ICSI. These includes:

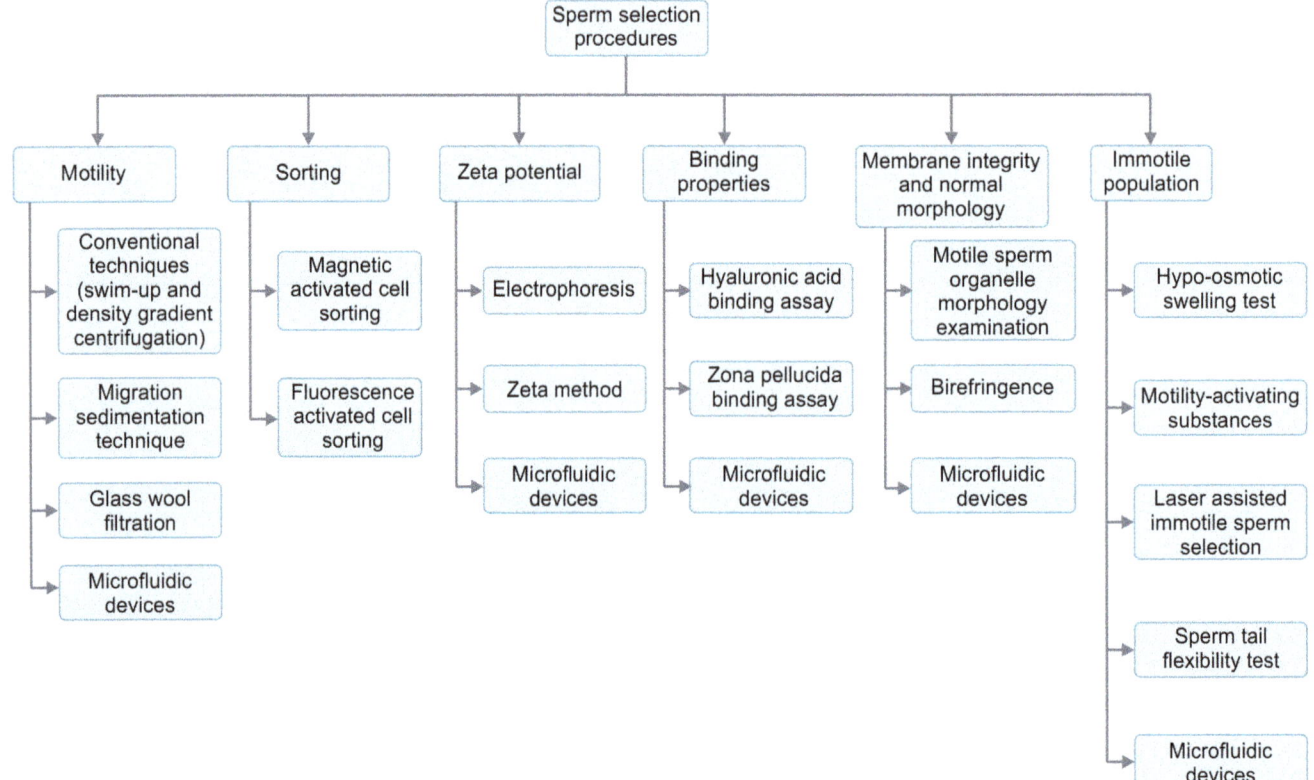

Sperm Selection in IUI and IVF

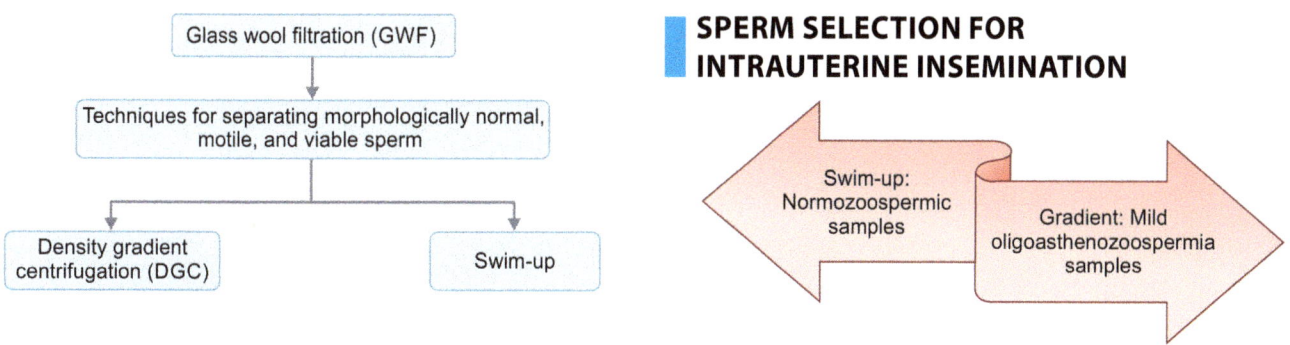

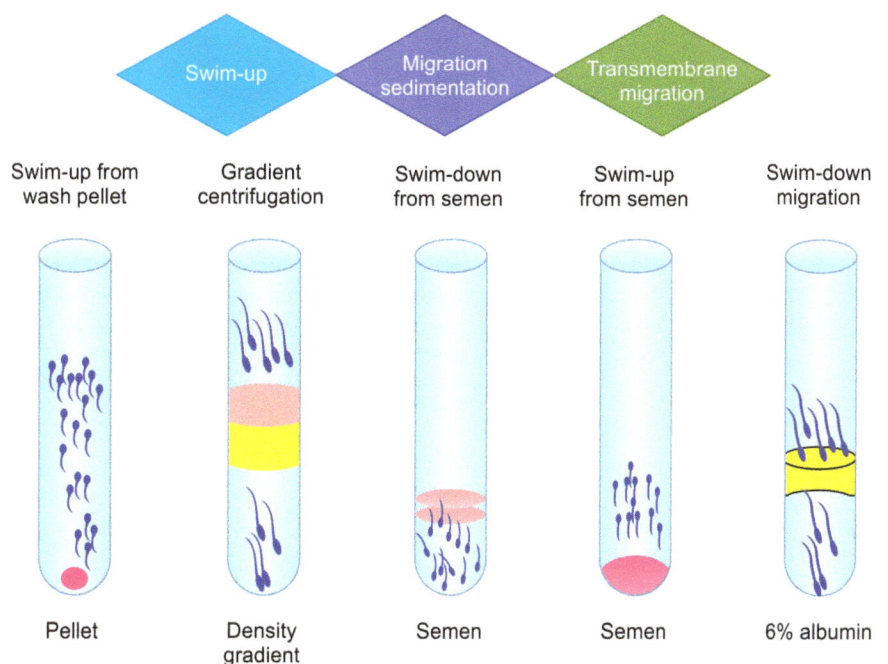

Fig. 1: Migration method.
Source: Tandulwadkar S, Mittal B. Optimizing IUI Results: A Guide to Gynecologists, 1st edition. New Delhi: Jaypee Brothers Medical Publishers (P) Ltd.; 2010.

Swim-up Technique (Fig. 2)

Principle: Recovery of motile spermatozoa that migrate toward a cell free medium usually placed above the sperm sample.[4,5]

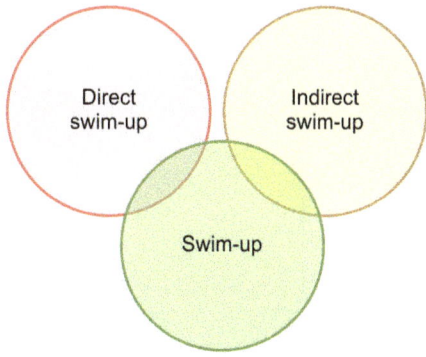

Fig. 2: Swim-up technique.

Direct swim-up **(Fig. 3)**

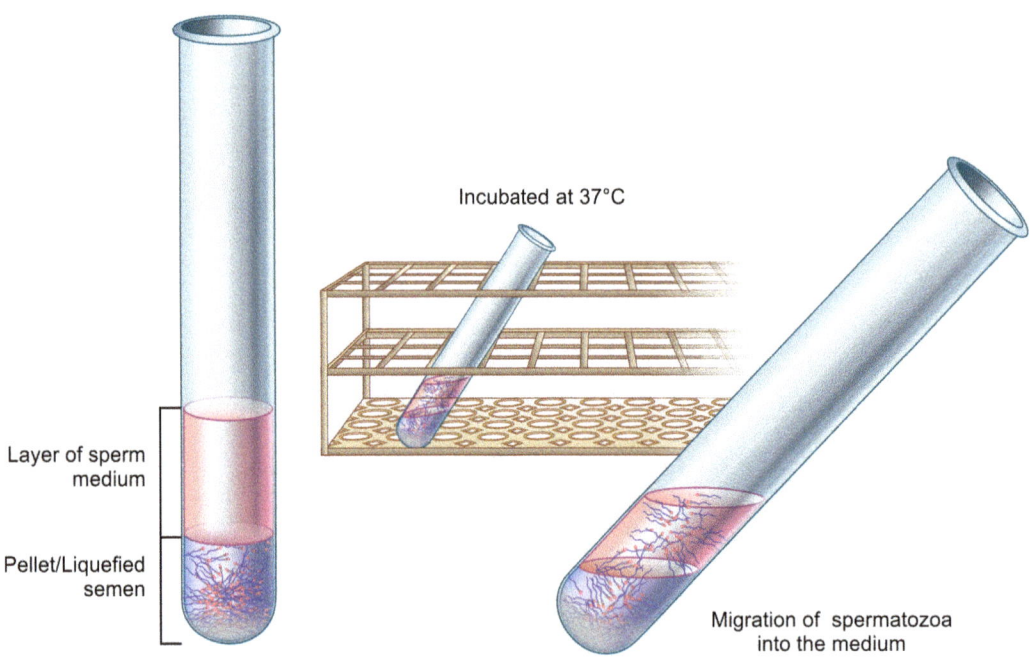

Fig. 3: Direct swim-up.
Source: Beydola T, Sharma RK, Lee W, Agarwal A, Rizk B, Aziz N, Agarwal A. Sperm preparation and selection techniques. In: Rizk B, Aziz N, Agarwal A (Eds). Male Infertility Practice. New Delhi: Jaypee Brothers Medical Publishers (P) Ltd.; 2013. pp. 244-51.

Advantage	This method avoids both the centrifugation process and any toxicity from reactive oxygen species (ROS).
Disadvantage	Possibility of seminal plasma contaminating the fluid cannot be fully ruled out.

Indirect swim-up **(Fig. 4)**

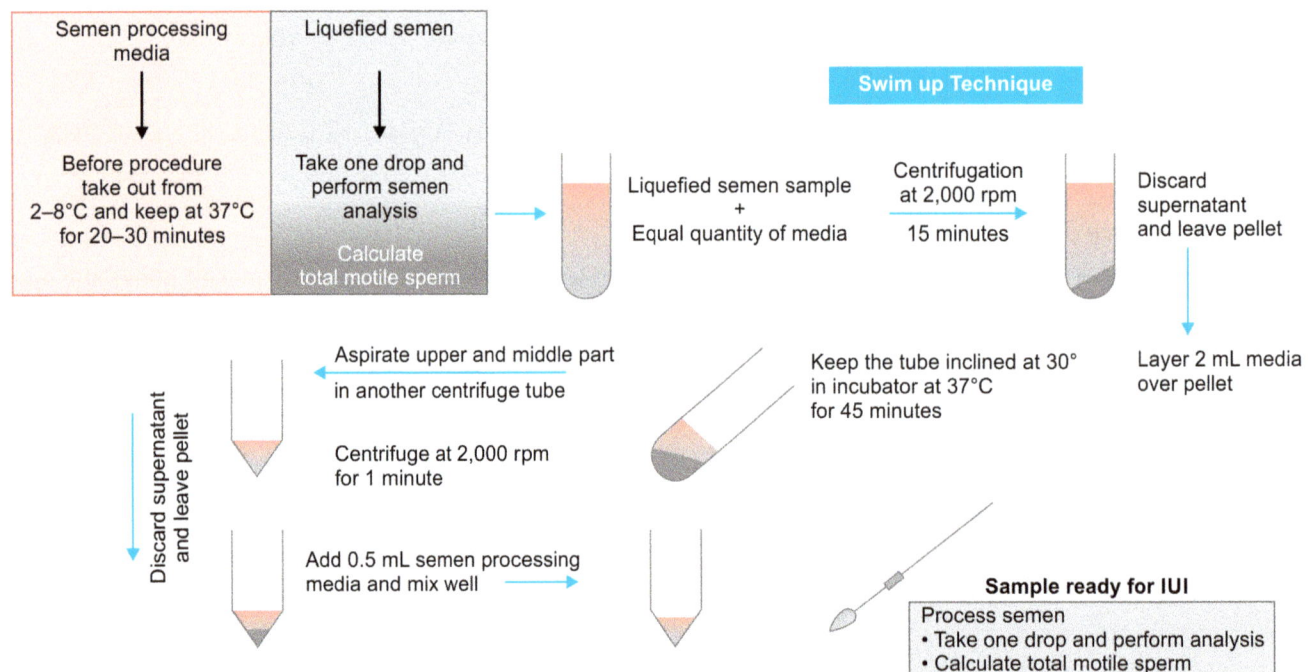

Fig. 4: Indirect swim-up.
Source: Malhotra N, Malhotra J, Malhotra N. Manual on IUI: What, When and Why, 1st edition. New Delhi: Jaypee Brothers Medical Publishers (P) Ltd.; 2013.

Migration Sedimentation

- Low motility samples are treated using this technique **(Fig. 5)**.
- Depends on the gravity-driven environment in which spermatozoa naturally occur **(Fig. 6)**.

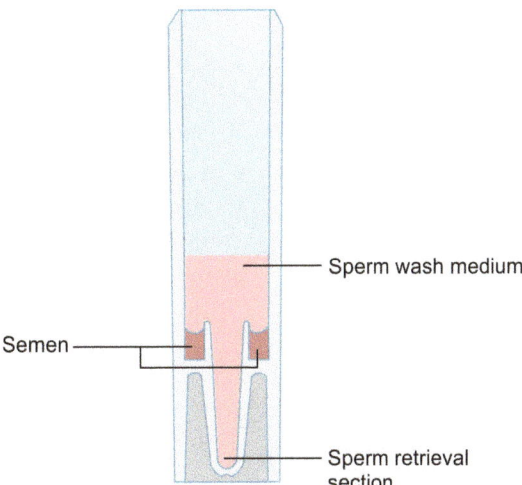

Fig. 5: Migration sedimentation.
Source: Kiratli S, Yuncu M, Kose K, Ozkavukcu S. A comparative evaluation of migration sedimentation method for sperm preparation. Syst Biol Reprod Med. 2018;64(2):122-9.

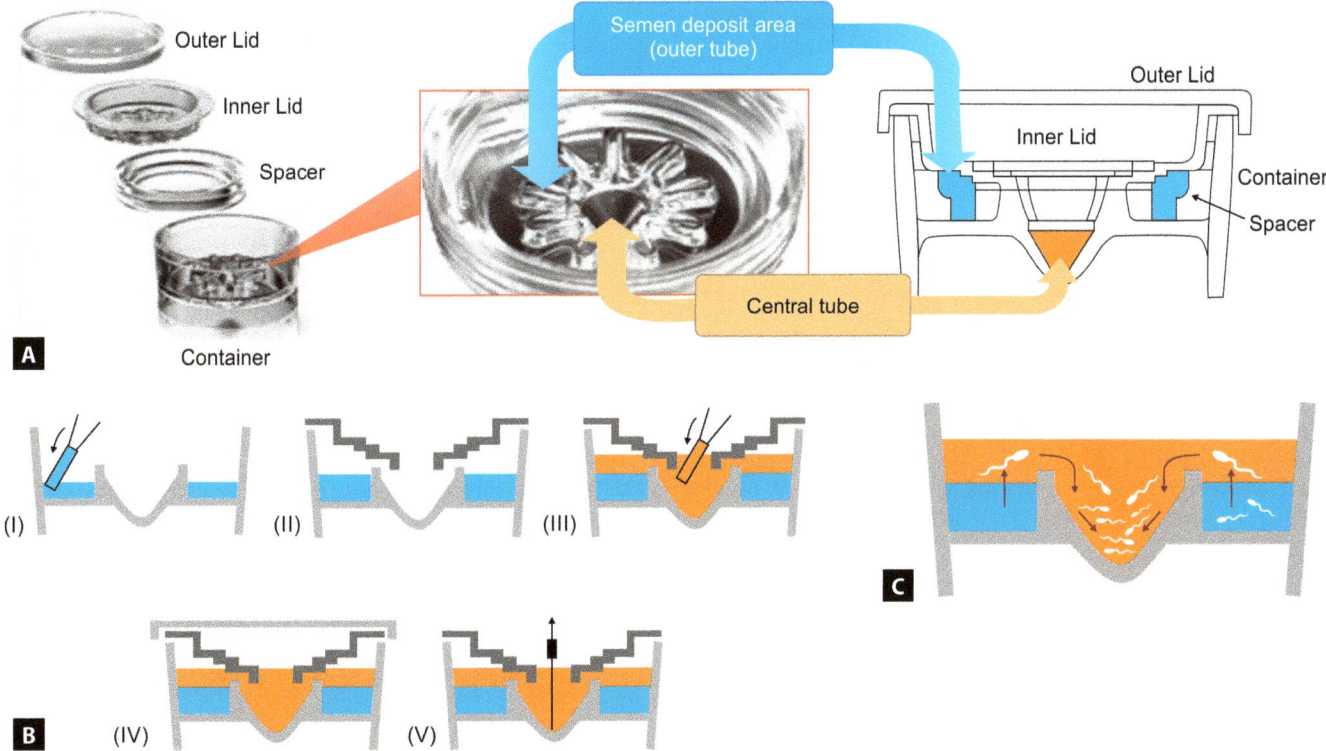

Fig. 6: Transmembrane migration.
Source: Tatsumi K, Tatsumi T, Uchida T, Saito K, Saito H. New device for sperm preparation involving migration-gravity sedimentation without centrifugation compared with density-gradient centrifugation for normozoospermic intrauterine insemination. F S Rep. 2020;1(2):106-12.

- This method's advantage is that it produces less ROS and is mild.
- This method's drawback was its lesser yield and lack of widespread acceptance in ART.

Transmembrane Migration

- This approach is used to examine the motility of sperm populations that had been exposed to various pharmacological substances.

- The transmembrane migration method involves movement via a membrane filter through cylinder-shaped pores that are perpendicular to the membrane's plane.[6]

Density Gradient Method

Density gradient centrifugation (DGC) is based on the capacity of motile spermatozoa to progress through a gradient of density constituted by colloidal particles during centrifugation.

- This separates sperm according to density.
- The density of a mature, morphologically healthy sperm is 1.10 g/mL.
- The density of the immature and morphologically abnormal sperms is 1.06 g/mL and 1.09 g/mL, respectively (**Fig. 7**).
- The preparation method utilized most frequently in ART is a double density gradient.
- Conical bottom tubes with an 80/40 gradient are used in the density gradient centrifugation (DGC) method for sperm preparation (**Fig. 8**).
- Caspase activation, mitochondrial membrane potential disturbance, and externalized phosphatidylserine were all found to be lower in DGC.[7-9]
- To eliminate HIV-1 RNA and proviral DNA, DGC and modified swim-up were advised.[10]

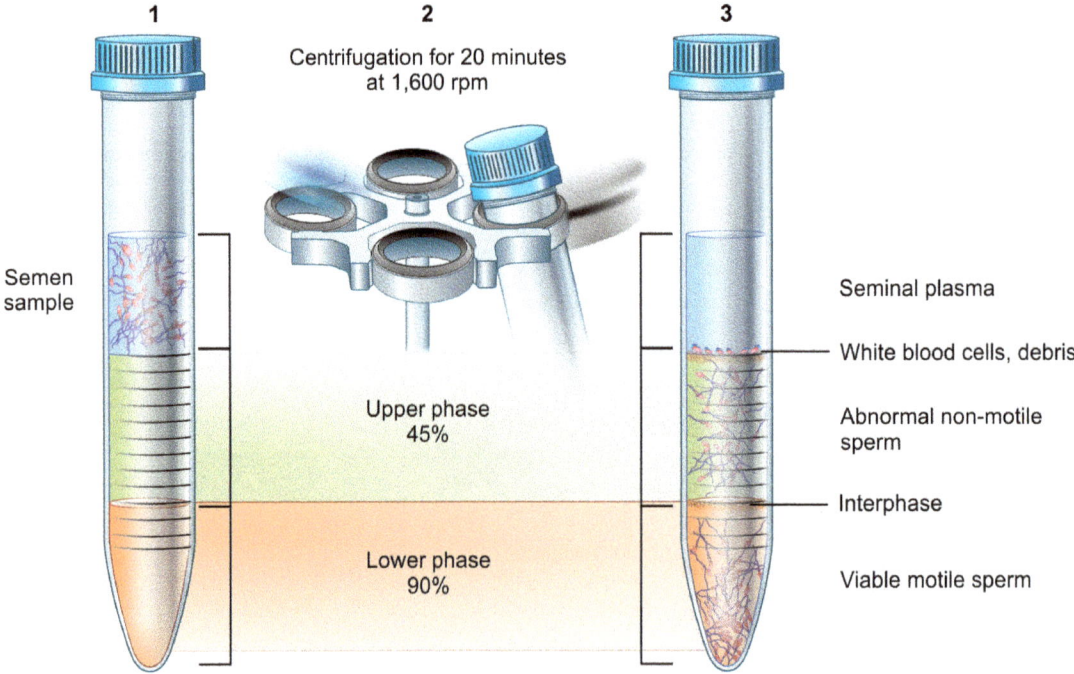

Fig. 7: Density gradient.
Source: Malvezzi H, Sharma R, Agarwal A, Abuzenadah AM, Abu-Elmagd M. Sperm quality after density gradient centrifugation with three commercially available media: a controlled trial. Reprod Biol Endocrinol. 2014;12(1):1-7.

Technique used	Time	Cost	Yield	Quality
Simple wash	Low	Low	High	Low
Direct swim up	Highest	Low	Lowest	Highest
Density gradient	High	Highest	Highest	High

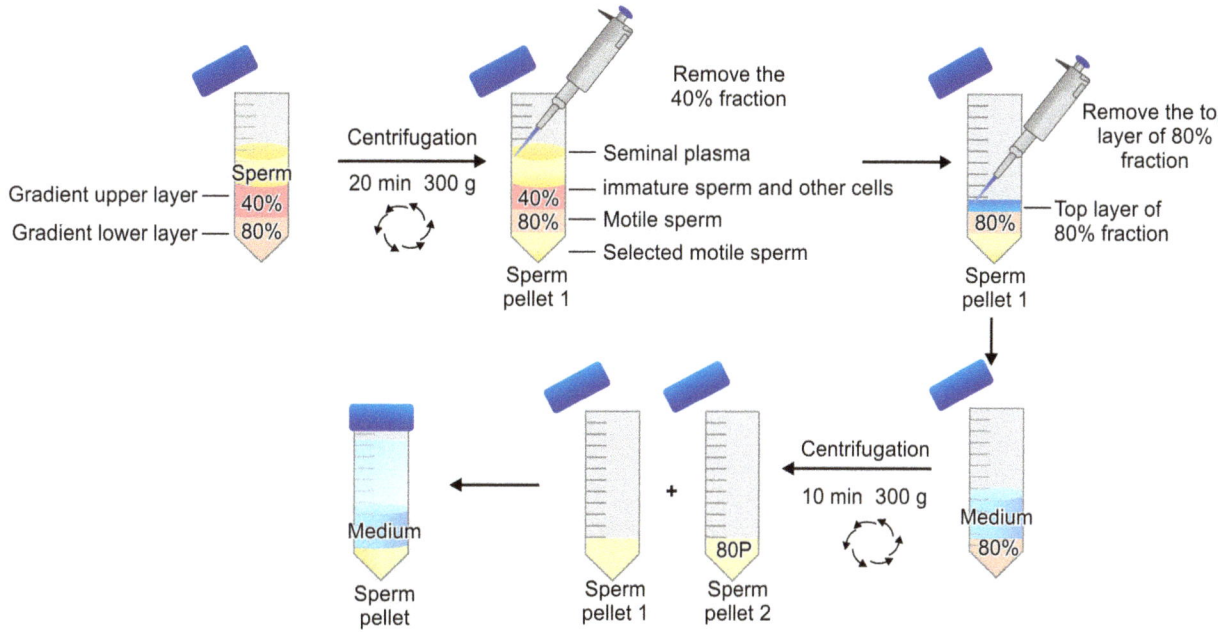

Fig. 8: Density gradient centrifugation.
Source: Aboulmaouahib S, Madkour A, Kaarouch I, Saadani B, Sefrioui O, Louanjli N, et al. Effect of semen preparation technique and its incubation on sperm quality in the Moroccan population. Andrologia. 2017;49(6):e12688.

*Comparison made for the same volume of liquefied sample prepared.

FILTRATION TECHNIQUES[11-13]

*Glass wool
*Glass bead
*Sephadex columns.

Filtration techniques for sperm separation in accordance with the *glass wool filtration*.

- This process divides spermatozoa based on sperm head size and motility.
- This method of sperm preparation is based on the idea that spermatozoa move independently and that glass wool has a filtration effect **(Fig. 9)**.
- This technique effectively separates the leukocytes by up to 90%, preventing ROS-related sperm destruction.
- Motile spermatozoa are separated from one another using gravity force and tightly packed glass wool fibers **(Fig. 10)**.
- Each filtration's effectiveness is influenced by the following:[14,15]

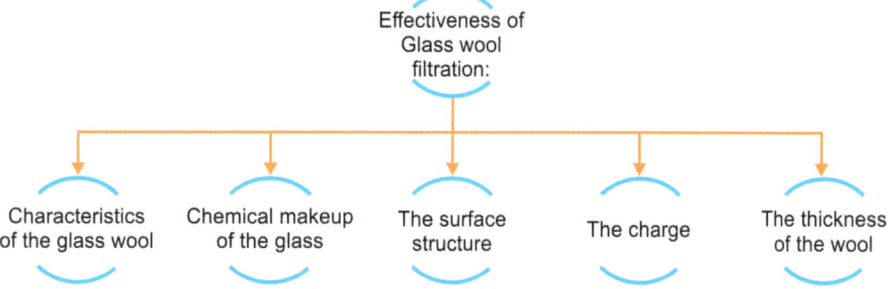

Advantages

- Simple to perform
- Recovery of sperm with good motility
- Leukocytes are eliminated to a large extent
- ROS are significantly reduced
- This method outperforms DGC in terms of functional integrity and offers optimum recovery over the swim-up method.
- Retrograde ejaculation can be used to prepare patient spermatozoa for motility.
- Additionally, this method chooses spermatozoa with proper chromatin condensation, a marker for in vitro fertilization.

Disadvantages

- Introduction of glass particles into the filtration.

- The discovery of sperm with acrosome damage.
- Remnants of debris are still present.

- The limitation of this technique was found to be due to transfer of glass bead into the filtrate. Not widely accepted sperm preparation technique in ART.

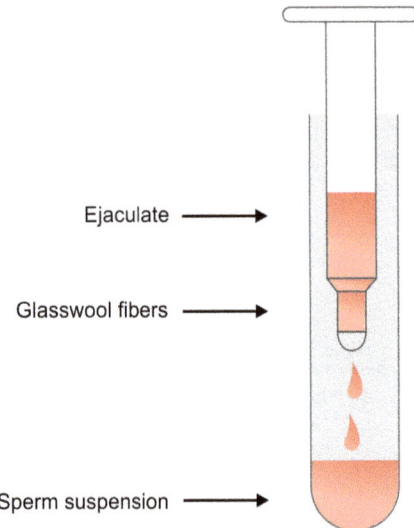

Fig. 9: Glass wool filteration.
Source: Michelmann HW. Intrauterine Insemination, 1st edition. New Delhi: Jaypee Brothers Medical Publishers (P) Ltd.; 2005.

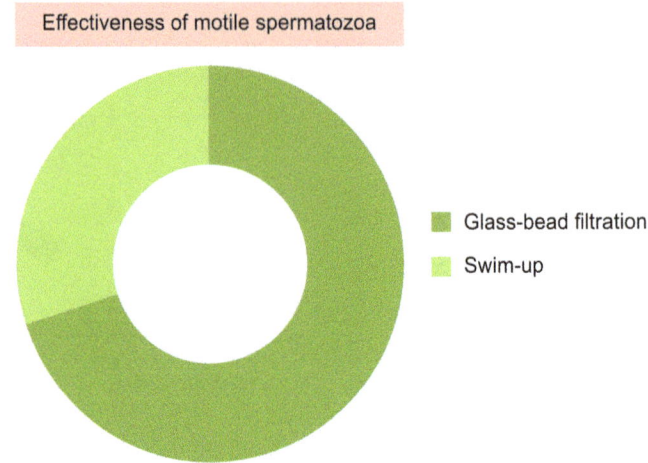

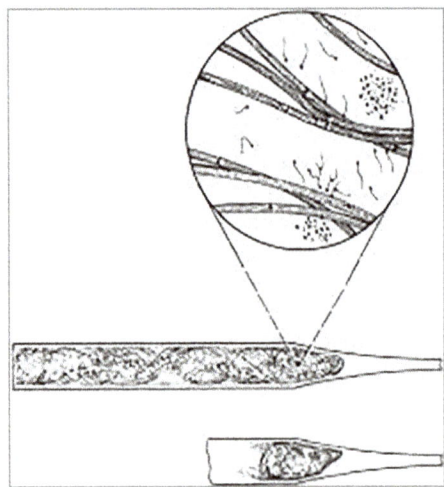

Fig. 10: Glass wool filteration microscopic view.
Source: Paulson JD, Comhaire F, Emperaire JC. Glass wool filtration of human semen. In: Emperaire JC, Audebert A, Hafez ESE (Eds). Homologous Artificial insemination (AIH). New York: Springer; 1980.

Glass Bead Filtration[16]

- This method successfully concentrate human spermatozoa from frozen semen samples was examined.
- This technique can be used clinically to produce motile spermatozoa from subpar semen for in vitro fertilization.
- Spheres of glass bead arranged in a column used to separate highly motile spermatozoa.

Sephadex Columns[17]

- Process of preparing sperm using Sephadex columns first appeared in the early 1990s.
- This method is founded on chromatographic media made up of microscopic beads produced synthetically from polysaccharide dextran.
- A high yield and more mobile spermatozoa separation was reported in comparison to swim-up and DGC.[18]

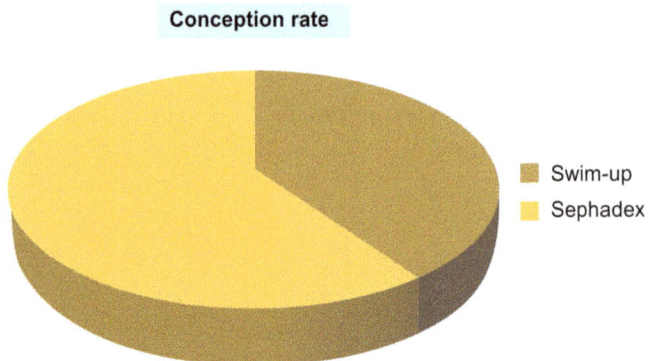

These conventional methods are not efficient methods to select spermatozoa in terms of apoptosis, DNA integrity, membrane maturation, and sperm ultrastructure.[19] Therefore, new sperm selection methods are required that should be based on sperm characteristics that are better connected to fertilization ability and quality of the spermatozoa, as well as on their contribution to support embryo development and improving pregnancy rate and live birth rate.

SPERM SELECTION FOR INTRACYTOPLASMIC SPERM INJECTION

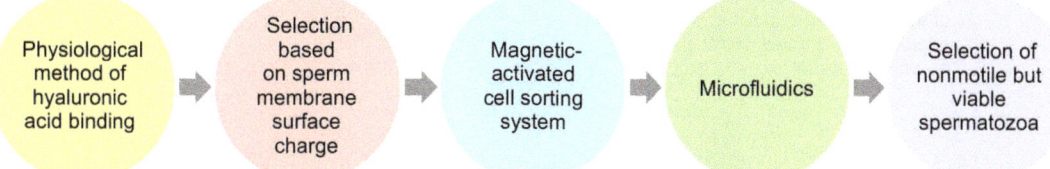

MORPHOLOGICAL ANALYSIS—ULTRASTRUCTURAL EVALUATION

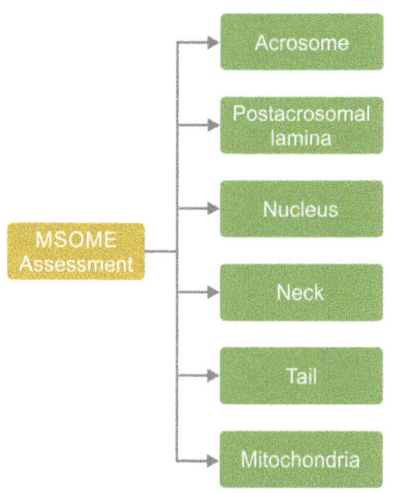

Fig. 11: Morphological evaluation.
Source: Monte GL, Murisier F, Piva I, Germond M, Marci R. Focus on intracytoplasmic morphologically selected sperm injection (IMSI): a mini-review. Asian J Androl. 2013;15(5):608-15.

- There was a positive correlation between motile sperm organelle morphology examination (MSOME) selected with successful ICSI outcomes and prior failures[20-22] **(Figs. 11 and 12).**
- MSOME criteria grade big vacuoles in the nucleus as having the most DNA fragmented spermatozoa.
- The larger size vacuoles range from 4 to 50% of the total volume **(Fig. 13).**

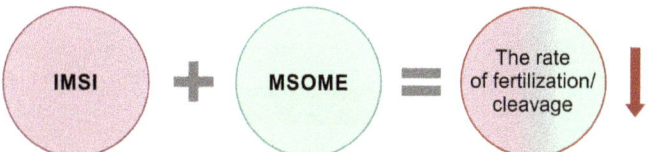

A meta-analysis conducted by Setti et al. and various other studies concluded that IMSI resulted in significantly higher implantation, pregnancy rates, and live birth rates when compared to a previous ICSI cycle performed to the same patients when male factor (oligoasthenoteratozoospermia) was the cause of infertility, suggesting an actual utility of IMSI for these specific cases[23,24]

The use of IMSI has helped to increase the number of ongoing pregnancies while decreasing the number of abortions in patients with recurrent implantation failures[22,25-27]

Many other studies failed to show any benefit with IMSI for improving ART outcome[28,29]

Pregnancy and delivery rates for ICSI and IMSI in the very first ART cycle of a couple shows that conventional ICSI appears to be sufficient for an unselected group[25,26]

Overall, literature do not support the routine use of IMSI, but it seems that IMSI could be indicated for severe cases of male factor and in case of recurrent ICSI failure

Only semen sample with high DNA fragmentation are recommended for using the procedure in a prospective randomized control experiment using frozen spermatozoa

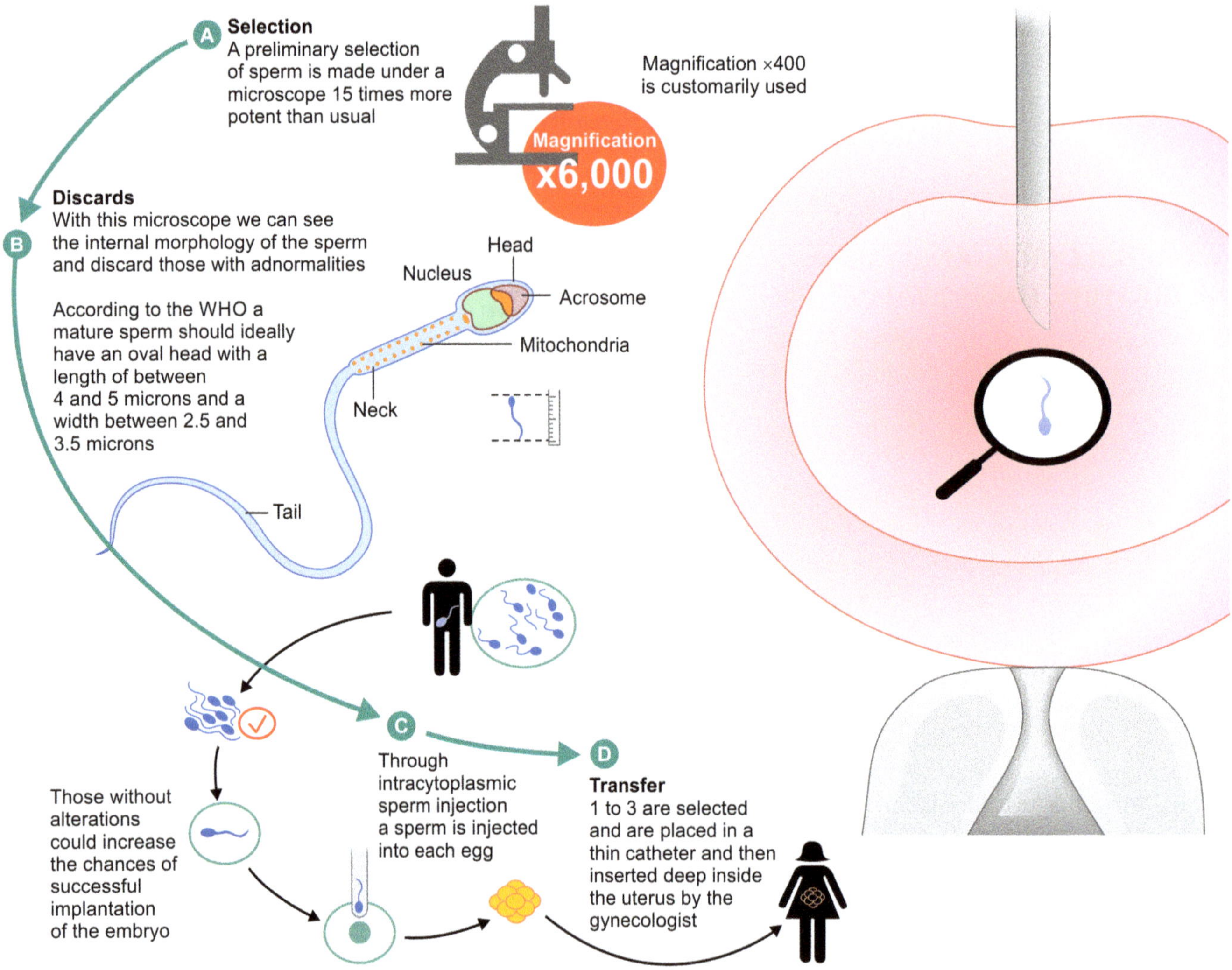

Fig. 12: Intracytoplasmic morphologically selected sperm injection (IMSI).
Source: BridgeClinic. (2019). How Can IMSI used with IVF Help You? [online] Available from https://www.thebridgeclinic.com/blog/how-can-imsi-used-with-ivf-help-you-. [Last accessed February, 2023].

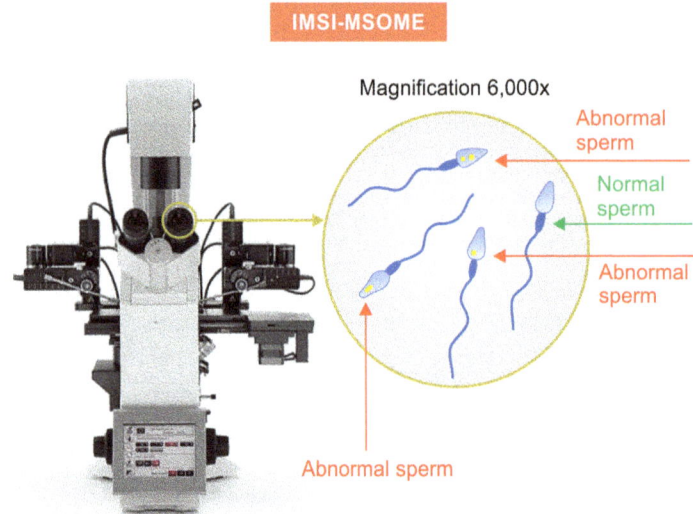

Fig. 13: Intracytoplasmic morphologically selected sperm injection (IMSI)-Motile sperm organelle morphology examination (MSOME).
Source: Baldini D, Ferri D, Baldini GM, Lot D, Catino A, Vizziello D, et al. Sperm Selection for ICSI: Do We Have a Winner? Cells. 2021; 10(12):3566.

MORPHOLOGICAL ANALYSIS—SPERM BIREFRINGENCE

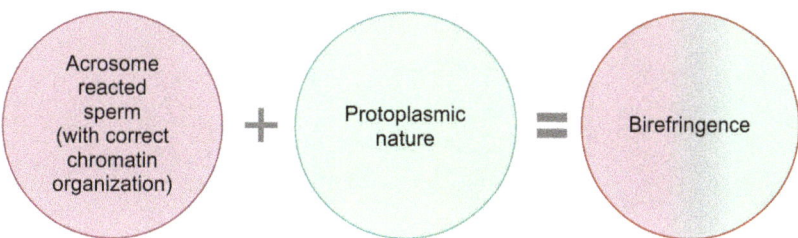

Birefringence properties of human spermatozoa, which represent the condition of internal protoplasmic structures **(Fig. 14)**.

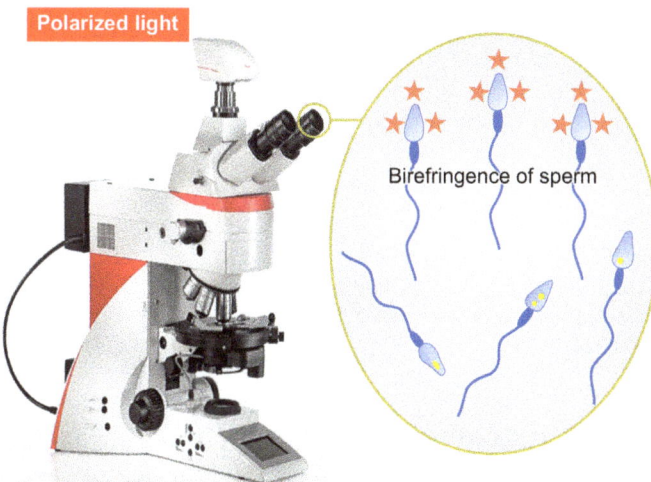

Fig. 14: Sperm birefringence.
Source: Baldini D, Ferri D, Baldini GM, Lot D, Catino A, Vizziello D, et al. Sperm Selection for ICSI: Do We Have a Winner? Cells. 2021;10(12):3566.

PHYSIOLOGICAL METHOD OF HYALURONIC ACID BINDING

- The hyaluronic acid (HA) is one of the main components of the extracellular matrix surrounding the cumulus-oocyte complex (COC), and normal healthy mature spermatozoa exhibit binding sites to it.
- A study conducted by Erberelli et al. concluded that ICSI using HA-coated dishes in patients with various categories of male factor particularly teratozoospermic samples leads to significant improvement in implantation and clinical pregnancy rate.[29]
- In a randomized study by Miller et al. including 2,772 did not find any significant benefit of HA-coated dishes compared to conventional ICSI in terms of ICSI outcomes.[30] These results collectively show a poor capacity of HA binding methods for improving ICSI.
- In this procedure, mature normal spermatozoa that are exclusively capable of adhering to hyaluronic acid are chosen for ICSI **(Fig. 15)**.

- Normal spermatozoa for ICSI can be chosen using petri-dish intracytoplasmic sperm injection (PICSI) dish with hyaluron gel coated as a dot or a solution form of hyaluronic acid.
- Hyaluronic acid binding has been linked to reports of increased rates of fertilization but not of pregnancy,[31] but not of increased rates of fertilization and pregnancy.[32]
- Traditional ICSI has lower clinical pregnancy rates.[33]
- The sperm chosen using this approach were found to have less DNA fragmentation.

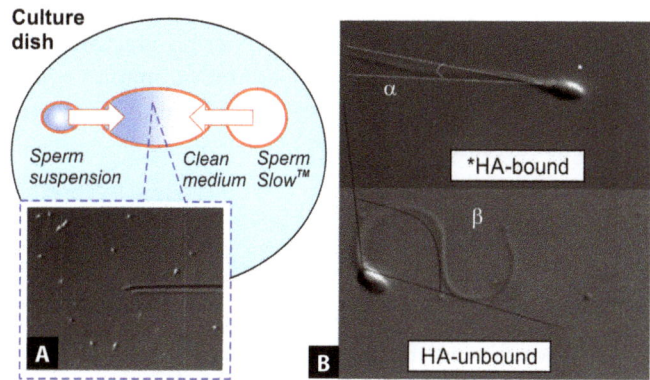

Fig. 15: Physiological method of hyaluronic acid binding.
Source: Parmegiani L, Cognigni GE, Bernardi S, Troilo E, Taraborrelli S, Arnone A, et al. Comparison of two ready-to-use systems designed for sperm–hyaluronic acid binding selection before intracytoplasmic sperm injection: PICSI vs. Sperm Slow: a prospective, randomized trial. Fertil Steril. 2012;98(3):632-7.

SPERM SELECTION BASED ON SURFACE CHARGE

Electrophoretic Method (Fig. 16)

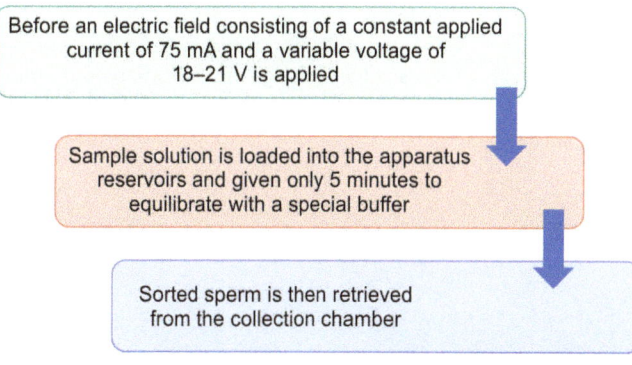

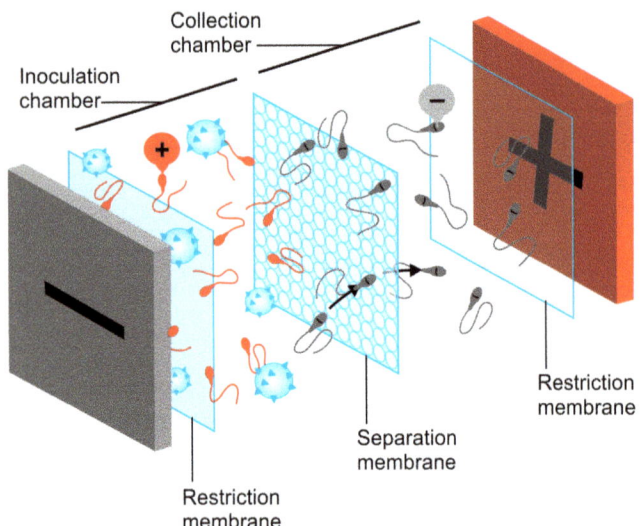

Fig. 16: Sperm selection based on surface charge.
Source: Simon L, Shamsi MB, Carrell DT. Sperm selection techniques and their relevance to ART. In: Schatten H (Ed). Human Reproduction: Updates and New Horizons. New York: Wiley-Blackwell; 2016. pp. 1-43.

Zeta Potential Method

- This technique is based on the sperm's electrokinetic potential, ranges from −16 to −20 mV in mature sperm and is an electric potential between the sperm membrane and its surroundings **(Fig. 17)**.[34,35]

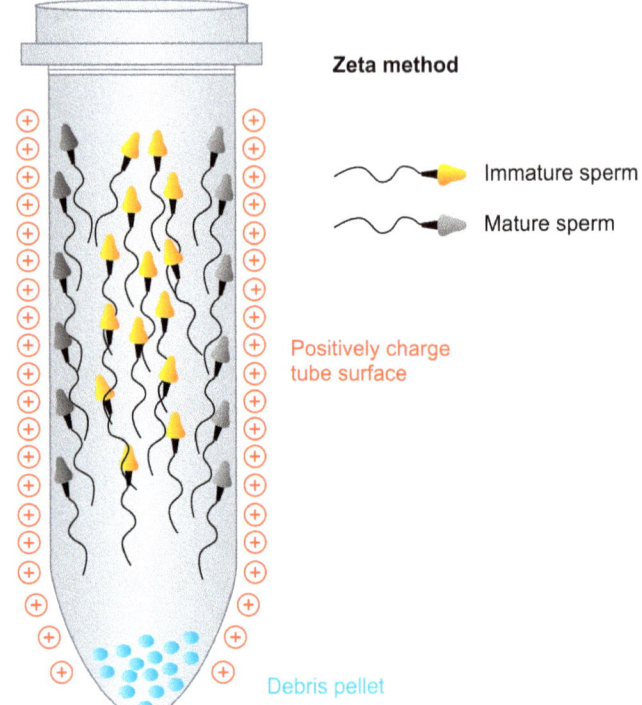

Fig. 17: Zeta potential method.
Source: Baldini D, Ferri D, Baldini GM, Lot D, Catino A, Vizziello D, et al. Sperm Selection for ICSI: Do We Have a Winner? Cells. 2021;10(12):3566.

Magnetic Activated Cell Sorting of Nonapoptotic Spermatozoa

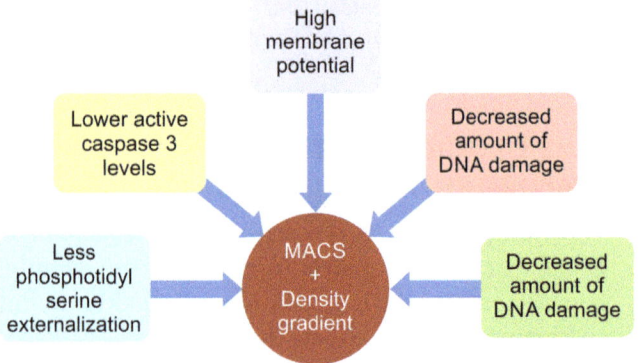

- Prior unsuccessful ICSI cycles with poor fertilization and embryo development were reported with a greater rate of clinical pregnancy with magnetic activated cell sorting (MACS) compared to density gradient with abnormal semen characteristics **(Figs. 18 and 19)**.[36]

It involves rotating a tube twice or three times while wearing a rubber glove and inserting cleaned sperm into positively charged centrifuge tubes

The tube is centrifuged and inverted after 1 minute to get rid nonadhering sperms and other impurities

Rinse the tube with material that has been treated with serum, adherent (negatively charged, mature) sperm can be extracted

Advantages:
- Increased morphology
- Hyperactivation
- DNA integrity
- Mature sperms

Disadvantages:
- Limited recovery for oligoasthenozoospermic samples
- Inapplicability for surgically extracted sperm
- Possibility of charge neutralization nonhumid environments

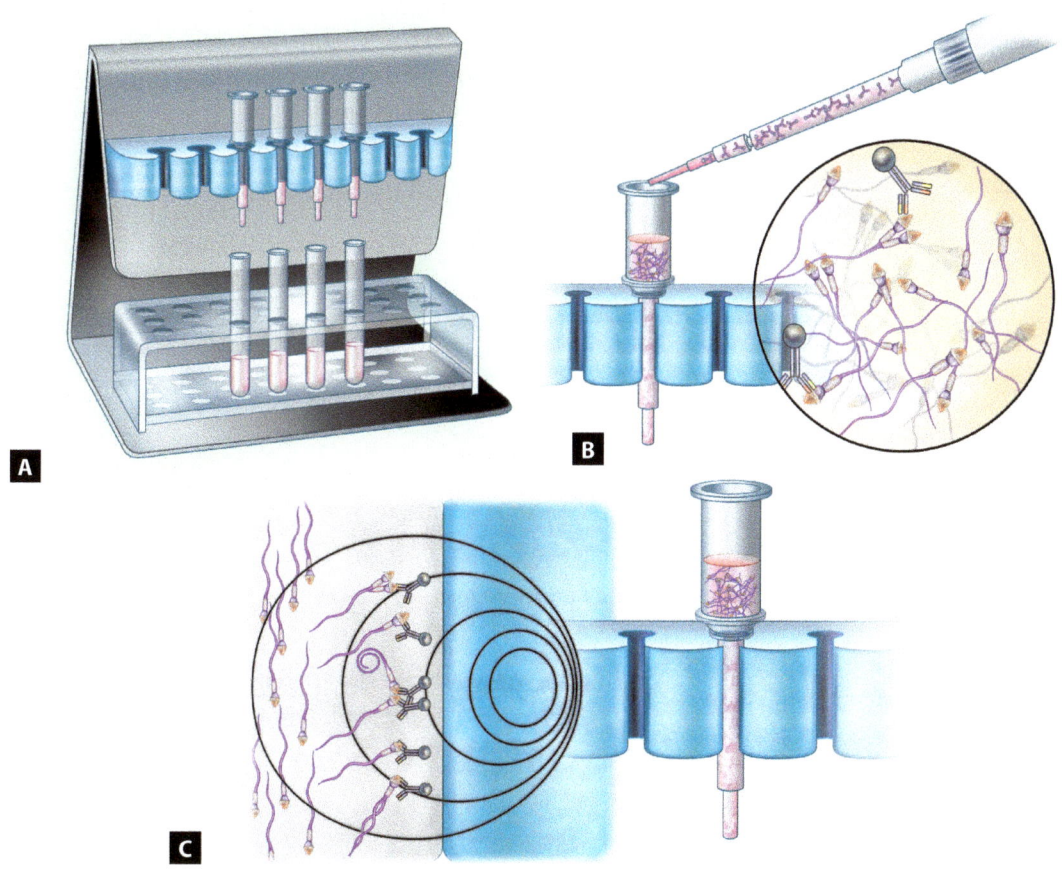

Fig. 18: Magnetic activated cell sorting (MACS).
Source: Beydola T, Sharma RK, Lee W, Agarwal A, Rizk B, Aziz N, et al. Sperm preparation and selection techniques. In: Rizk B, Aziz N, Agarwal A (Eds). Male Infertility Practice. New Delhi: Jaypee Brothers Medical Publishers (P) Ltd.; 2013. pp. 244-51.

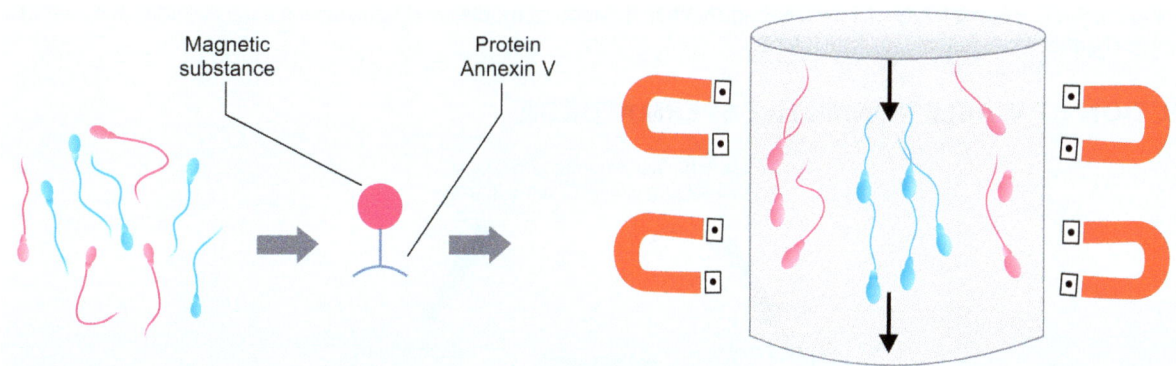

Fig. 19: Magnetic activated cell sorting (MACS).
Source: Lee TH, Liu CH, Shih YT, Tsao HM, Huang CC, Chen HH, et al. Magnetic-activated cell sorting for sperm preparation reduces spermatozoa with apoptotic markers and improves the acrosome reaction in couples with unexplained infertility. Hum Reprod. 2010;25(4):839-46.

MICROFLUIDICS-BASED SPERM SELECTION[37,38]

- It is demonstrated in a pump-less microfluidic system using hydrostatic pressure, in which the sperm swim through laminar flows to collect in a specific location **(Fig. 20)**.
- It distinguishes between motile and immotile sperm, dead sperm or cells, and debris in raw semen.
- Utilizing conventional photolithography and micromolding processes, channel architectures made of polydimethylsiloxane (PDMS) are constructed using microfluidics.
- The bottom surface of the microchannels and the device's foundation were created by plasma bonding these structures to a glass microscope slide.

- The system included a microchannel with a diameter of 250 mm, an input for inserting medium and sperm, and an exit for releasing air as these components are inserted.
- Microfluidic channels had a 3 cm maximum length (**Fig. 21**).
- It is limited to low volume processing of semen sample at rate of 20–40 μs/h.

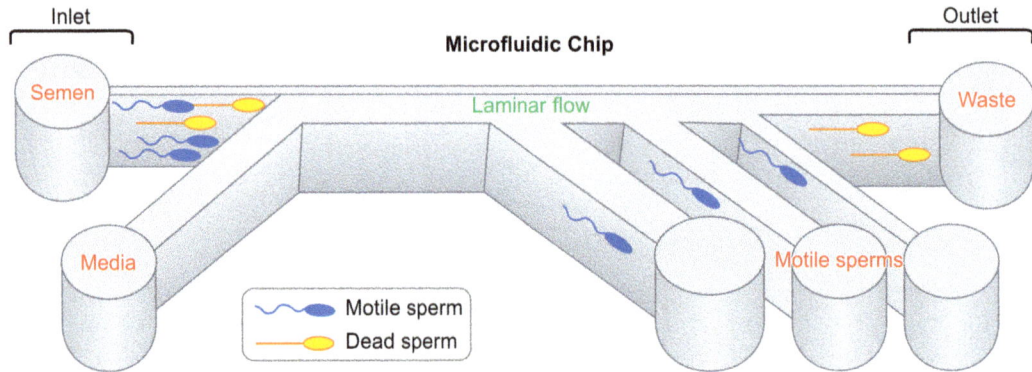

Fig. 20: Microfluidics based sperm selection.
Source: Huang HY, Fu HT, Tsing HY, Huang HJ, Li CJ, Yao DJ. Motile human sperm sorting by an integrated microfluidic system. J Nanomed Nanotechnol. 2014;5(3):1.

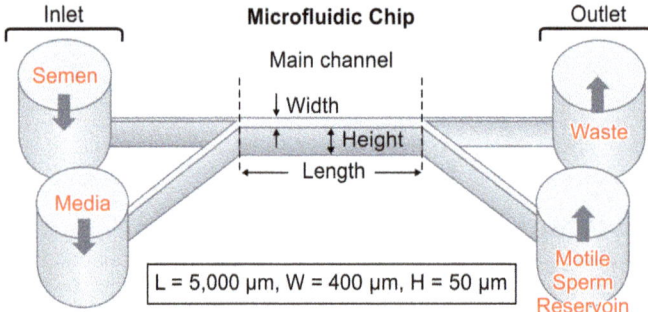

Fig. 21: Microfluidics based sperm selection.
Source: Huang HY, Wu TL, Huang HR, Li CJ, Fu HT, Soong YK, et al. Isolation of motile spermatozoa with a microfluidic chip having a surface-modified microchannel. J Lab Autom. 2014;19(1):91-9.

SELECTION OF VIABLE NONMOTILE SPERMATOZOA

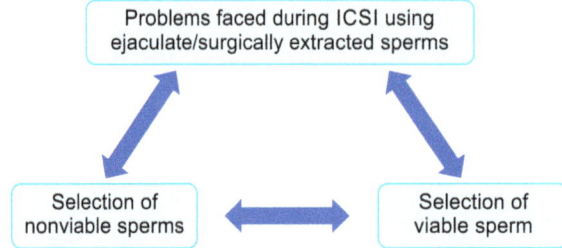

- These challenges can result in further ongoing clinical pregnancy and live birth.
- To choose the viable spermatozoa, various techniques have been described here.

Modified Hypo-osmotic Swelling Test

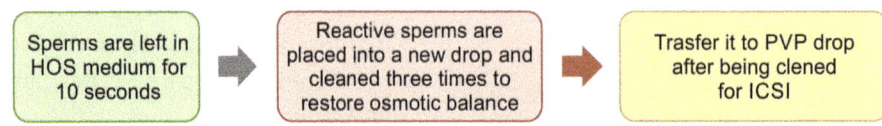

- Viable sperm are selected based on a bent or enlarged tail (**Fig. 22**).
- Immotile testicular sperm from fresh and cryopreserved samples had a greater clinical pregnancy rate in a randomized experiment employing modified hypo-osmotic-based sperm selection compared to no treatment.[39]

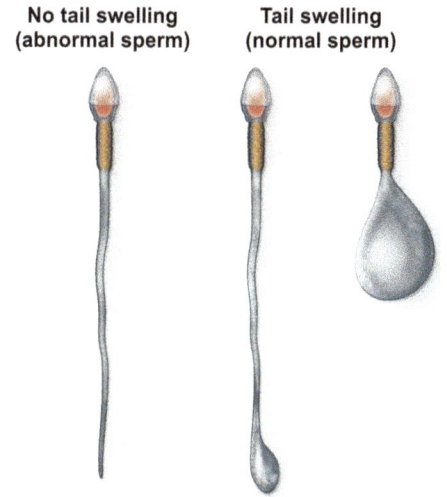

Fig. 22: Hypo-osmotic swelling.
Source: Hypo-osmotic sperm swelling test: sperm with an intact cell membrane are able to exclude the hypo-osmotic media and will not swell.

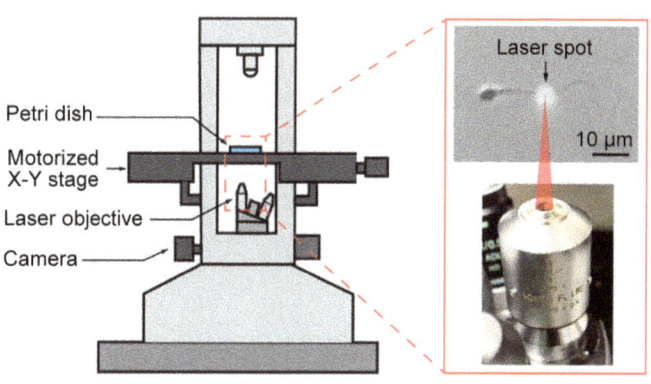

Fig. 23: Laser-assisted sperm selection.
Source: Zhang Z, Dai C, Wang X, Ru C, Abdalla K, Jahangiri S, et al. Automated laser ablation of motile sperm for immobilization. IEEE Robot Autom Lett. 2019;4(2):323-9.

Laser-assisted Sperm Selection[40,41]

- A technique for the identification of viable but immotile spermatozoa.
- A single laser shot of 129 µJ for approximately 1.2 ms being directed to the tip of the flagellum **(Fig. 23)**.
- The successful application of this laser selection was the identification of viable spermatozoa in a patient with primary ciliary dyskinesia that resulted in a pregnancy.
- The method was used on immotile spermatozoa from testicular biopsies and ejaculated asthenozoospermic samples to show that its capacity to count the amount of viable spermatozoa in a sample was comparable to that of the hypo-osmotic swelling (HOS) test (22.0% vs. 21.5%).
- Laser-tested TESE spermatozoa selection under immotile circumstances has been discovered to be a quick, simple, reproducible, and secure method of viability testing.

Interpretation:
- *Viable:* Live but immotile spermatozoa cause a curling or coiling of the tail.
- *Nonviable:* If no such change is observed

Chemical Stimulators Mediated Sperm Selection[42,43]

- The selection of motile sperms from a population of immotile sperms that have viability and can become motile on stimulation was found to be made possible by the use of pentoxifylline and theophylline to induce sperm motility by inhibiting the phosphodiesterase activity and thereby increasing intracellular cyclic adenosine monophosphate (cAMP) levels **(Fig. 24)**.

- In cases of oligozoospermia or asthenozoospermia when failure to fertilize in prior IVF cycles was addressed by incubation with pentoxifylline without affecting the acrosome reaction at various concentrations.
- After only 30 minutes of incubation, the addition of 3.6 mM pentoxifylline was observed to significantly increase motility in testicular samples.
- Before utilizing ICSI, it is advised to carefully cleanse the exposed sperm.
- Pentoxifylline use considerably decreases the time needed to discover and choose motile spermatozoa.
- The compound pentoxifylline is efficient in the selection of spermatozoa with structural defects such as axonemal, enzymatic or functional tail defects, and able to activate ejaculated spermatozoa from a patient with Kartagener's syndrome that resulted in a viable pregnancy.

The benefits of shorter exposure are advised due to worries about the safety of these chemical substances.

FUTURE DIRECTIONS

- Sperm separation from seminal fluid also removes the natural protective antioxidants contained in the seminal fluid.
- To prevent excessive oxidative stress to the sperm, antioxidants like human serum albumin must be added to sperm preparation and incubation media for assisted reproduction.
- Standard sperm selection techniques like DGC are able to reduce oxidative stress by depletion of immature sperm and leukocytes.
- Prolonging the selection methods, sperm selection with enhanced motility may be achieved but at the expense of DNA damage due to oxidative stress.
- Advanced sperm separation techniques focus rather on the depletion of already damaged sperm. In ART,

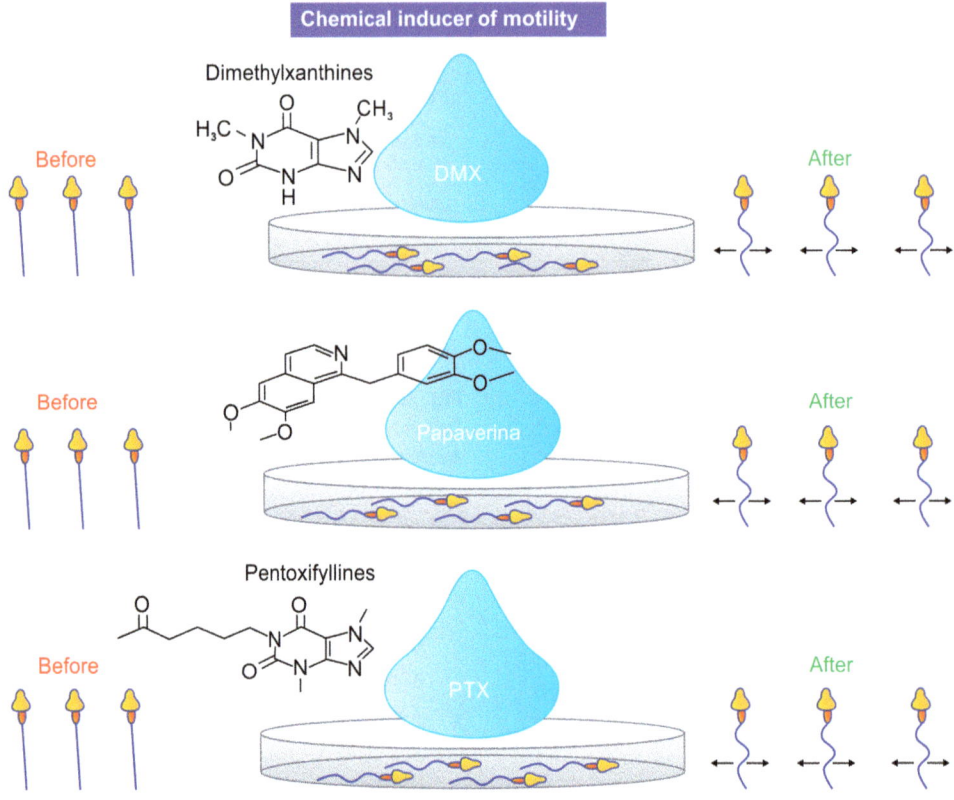

Fig. 24: Chemical stimulators mediated sperm selection.
Source: Baldini D, Ferri D, Baldini GM, Lot D, Catino A, Vizziello D, et al. Sperm Selection for ICSI: Do We Have a Winner? Cells. 2021;10(12):3566.

procedures such as IVF and especially ICSI require fewer spermatozoa, so lower sperm recovery is not an adverse factor, and therefore microfluidic techniques are more versatile. Microfluidics offers new opportunities to better understand human sperm migration and to use this understanding to prepare sperm for IUI, IVF, and ICSI.

- New sperm sorting technologies have been shown to improve DNA integrity, morphology, and motility, but whether these improvements are significant over the conventional centrifuged-based techniques is unclear, and these devices need thorough evaluation.

■ CONCLUSION

In summary, we have described a number of sperm preparation methods that are available to process sperm for use in ART. Each infertile couple must be carefully examined to determine the best sperm preparation method. Future research should seek to improve the efficacy and the safety of the sperm preparation techniques. Advanced sperm selection strategies include selection according to surface charge, sperm birefringence, sperm morphology under ultra-high magnification, ability to bind to HA, sperm apoptosis, and microfluidic separation. These techniques may improve the chances of selecting structurally intact and mature sperm with high DNA integrity for and help improve fertilization and pregnancy.

Key Learning Points

- Clinical implications: A variety of techniques can be used to select sperm for use in ART both IUI and IVF and ICSI.
- Conventional methods such as sperm preparation by swim-up and density gradient are more commonly performed.
- In addition, the introduction of newer techniques such as preparation by MACS alone or in combination with density gradient separation is also being used.
- The goal is to use a method that selects a highly motile sperm population with intact DNA from the raw semen.
- In this context, sperm selection utilizing the microfluidic techniques is important and is gaining popularity.
- It allows the rapid selection of sperm with intact DNA in a one-step process which replaces the previous multistage processes involving centrifugation steps associated with oxidative stress and iatrogenic risks.

■ REFERENCES

1. Paulson JD, Polakoski KL. A glass wool column procedure for removing extraneous material from the human ejaculate. Fertil Steril. 1977;28:178-81.
2. Arcidiacono A, Walt H, Campana A, Balerna M. The use of Percoll gradients for the preparation of subpopulations of human spermatozoa. Int J Androl. 1983;6:433-45.
3. Mahadevan M, Baker G. Assessment and preparation of semen for in vitro fertilization. In: Wood C, Trounson A (Eds). Clinical In Vitro Fertilization. Berlin: Springer-Verlag; 1984. pp. 83-97.

4. Berkovitz A, Eltes F, Lederman H, Peer S, Ellenbogen A, Feldberg B, et al. How to improve IVF-ICSI outcome by sperm selection. Reprod Biomed Online. 2006;12:634-8.
5. Yener C, Mathur S, Parent B. Comparison of two sperm preparation techniques using automated sperm motion analysis: migration sedimentation versus swim-up. Arch Androl. 1990;25:17-20.
6. Chijioke PC, Crocker PR, Gilliam M, Owens MD, Pearson RM. Importance of filter structure for the trans-membrane migration studies of sperm motility. Hum Reprod. 1988; 3:241-4.
7. Larson KL, Brannian JD, Timm BK, Jost LK, Evenson DP. Density gradient centrifugation and glass wool filtration of semen remove spermatozoa with damaged chromatin structure. Hum Reprod. 1999;14:2015-9.
8. Ollero M, Gil-Guzman E, Lopez MC, Sharma RK, Agarwal A, et al. Characterization of subsets of human spermatozoa at different stages of maturation: implications in the diagnosis and treatment of male infertility. Hum Reprod. 2001;16:1912-21.
9. Barroso G, Taylor S, Morshedi M, Manzur F, Gavino F, et al. Mitochondrial membrane potential integrity and plasma membrane translocation of phosphatidylserine as early apoptotic markers: a comparison of two different sperm subpopulations. Fertil Steril. 2006;85:149-54.
10. Kato S, Hanabusa H, Kaneko S, Takakuwa K, Suzuki M, Kuji N, et al. Complete removal of HIV-1 RNA and proviral DNA from semen by the swim-up method: assisted reproduction technique using spermatozoa free from HIV-1. AIDS. 2006;20:967-73.
11. Sanchez R, Concha M, Ichikawa T, Henkel R, Schill WB. Glass wool filtration reduces reactive oxygen species by elimination of leukocytes in oligozoospermic patients with leukocytospermia. J Assist Reprod Genet. 1996;13:489-94.
12. Ford WCL, McLaughlin EA, Prior SM, Rees JM, Wardle PG, Hull MG. The yield, motility and performance in the hamster egg test of human spermatozoa prepared from cryopreserved semen by four different methods. Hum Reprod. 1992; 7:654-9.
13. Daya S, Gwatkin RB, Bissessar H. Separation of motile human spermatozoa by means of a glass bead column. Gamete Res. 1987;17:375-80.
14. Gabriel LK, Vawda AI. Preparation of human sperm for assisted conception: a comparative study. Arch Androl. 1993;30:1-6.
15. Zavos PM, Centola GM. Methods of semen preparation for intrauterine insemination and subsequent pregnancy rates. Tohoku J Exp Med. 1992;168:583-90.
16. Lechtzin N, Garside W, Heyner S, Hillman N. Glass-bead column separation of motile and nonmotile human spermatozoa. J In Vitro Fert Embryo Transf. 1991;8:96-100.
17. Drobnis EZ, Zhong CQ, Overstreet JW. Separation of cryopreserved human semen using Sephadex columns, washing, or Percoll gradients. J Androl. 1991;12:201-8.
18. Hammadeh ME, Zavos PM, Rosenbaum P, Schmidt W. Comparison between the quality and function of sperm after semen processing with two different methods. Asian J Androl. 2001;3:125-30.
19. Said TM, Land JA. Effects of advanced selection methods on sperm quality and ART outcome: a systematic review. Hum Reprod Update. 2011;17(6):719-33.
20. Hazout A, Dumont-Hassan M, Junca A, Cohen Bacrie P, Tesarik J. High-magnification ICSI overcomes paternal effect resistant to conventional ICSI. Reprod Biomed Online. 2006;12:19-25.
21. Antinori M, Licata E, Dani G, Cerusico F, Versaci C, d'Angelo D, et al. Intracytoplasmic morphologically selected sperm injection: a prospective randomized trial. Reprod Biomed Online. 2008;16:835-41.
22. Mauri AL, Petersen CG, Oliveira JB, Massaro FC, Baruffi RL, Franco JG Jr. Comparison of day 2 embryo quality after conventional ICSI versus intracytoplasmic morphologically selected sperm injection (IMSI) using sibling oocytes. Eur J Obstet Gynecol Reprod Biol. 2010;150:42-6.
23. Setti AS, Braga DP, Figueira RC, Iaconelli A Jr, Borges E. Intracytoplasmic morphologically selected sperm injection results in improved clinical outcomes in couples with previous ICSI failures or male factor infertility: a meta-analysis. Eur J Obstet Gynecol Reprod Biol. 2014;183:96-103.
24. Goswami G, Sharma M, Jugga D, Gouri DM. Can intra-cytoplasmic morphologically selected spermatozoa injection be used as first choice of treatment for severe male factor infertility patients? J Hum Reprod Sci. 2018;11(1):40-44.
25. De Vos A, Van de Vede H, Bocken G, Eylenbosch G, Franceus N, Meersdom G, et al. Does intracytoplamic morphologically selected sperm injection improve embryo development? A randomized sibling-oocyte study. Hum Reprod. 2013;28:617-26.
26. Oliveira JB, Cavagna M, Petersen CG, Mauri AL, Massaro FC, Silva LF, et al. Pregnancy outcomes in women with repeated implantation failures after intracytoplasmic morphologically selected sperm injection (IMSI). Reprod Biol Endocrinol. 2011;9:99-105.
27. Klement AH, Koren-Morag N, Itsykson P, Berkovitz A. Intracytoplasmic morphologically selected sperm injection versus intracytoplasmic sperm injection: a step toward a clinical algorithm. Fertil Steril. 2013;99:1290-3.
28. Fortunato A, Boni R, Leo R, Nacchia G, Liguori F, Casale S, et al. Vacuoles in sperm head are not associated with head morphology, DNA damage and reproductive success. Reprod Biomed Online. 2016;32(2):154-61.
29. Leandri RD, Gachet A, Pfeffer J, Celebi C, Rives N, Carre-Pigeon F, et al. Is intracytoplasmic morphologically selected sperm injection (IMSI) beneficial in the first ART cycle? A multicentric randomized controlled trial. Andrology. 2013;1(5):692-7.
30. Erberelli RF, Salgado RM, Pereira DH, Wolff P. Hyaluronan-binding system for sperm selection enhances pregnancy rates in ICSI cycles associated with male factor infertility. JBRA Assist Reprod. 2017;21(1):2-6.
31. Miller D, Pavitt S, Sharma V, Forbes G, Hooper R, Bhattacharya S, et al. Physiological, hyaluronan-selected intracytoplasmic sperm injection for infertility treatment (HABSelect): a parallel, two-group, randomised trial. Lancet. 2019;393(10170):416-22.
32. Nasr-Esfahani MH, Razavi S, Vahdati AA, Fathi F, Tavalaee M. Evaluation of sperm selection procedure based on hyaluronic acid binding ability on ICSI outcome. J Assist Reprod Genet. 2008;25:197-203.
33. Parmegiani L, Cognigni GE, Bernardi S, Troilo E, Ciampaglia W, Filicori M. 'Physiologic ICSI': hyaluronic acid (HA) favors selection of spermatozoa without DNA fragmentation and

with normal nucleus, resulting in improvement of embryo quality. Fertil Steril. 2010;93:598-604.
34. Chan PJ, Jacobson JD, Corselli JU, Patton WC. A simple zeta method for sperm selection based on membrane charge. Fertil Steril. 2006;85:481-6.
35. Kam TL, Jacobson JD, Patton WC, Corselli JU, Chan PJ. Retention of membrane charge attributes by cryopreserved-thawed sperm and zeta selection. J Assist Reprod Genet. 2007;24:429-34.
36. Grunewald S, Paasch U, Said TM, Rasch M, Agarwal A, Glander HJ. Magnetic-activated cell sorting before cryopreservation preserves mitochondrial integrity in human spermatozoa. Cell Tissue Bank. 2006;7:99-104.
37. Zhang B, Yin TL, Yang J. A novel microfluidic device for selecting human sperm to increase the proportion of morphologically normal, motile sperm with uncompromised DNA Integrity. Anal Methods. 2015;7:5981-8.
38. Eravuchira PJ, Mirsky SK, Barnea I, Levi M, Balberg M, Shaked NT. Individual sperm selection by microfluidics integrated with interferometric phase microscopy. Methods. 20018;136:152-9.
39. Sallam HN, Farrag A, Agameya AF, El-Garem Y, Ezzeldin F. The use of the modified hypo-osmotic swelling test for the selection of immotile testicular spermatozoa in patients treated with ICSI: a randomized controlled study. Hum Reprod. 2005;20:3435-40.
40. Aktan TM, Montag M, Duman S, Gorkemli H, Rink K, Yurdakul T. Use of a laser to detect viable but immotile spermatozoa. Andrologia. 2004;36:366-9.
41. Nordhoff V, Schuring AN, Krallmann C, Zitzmann M, Schlatt S, Kiesel L, et al. Optimizing TESE-ICSI by laser-assisted selection of immotile spermatozoa and polarization microscopy for selection of oocytes. Andrology. 2013;1:67-74.
42. De Turner E, Aparicio NJ, Turner D, Schwarzstein L. Effect of two phosphodiesterase inhibitors, cyclic adenosine 3':5'-monophosphate, and a beta-blocking agent on human sperm motility. Fertil Steril. 1978;29:328-31.
43. Griveau JF, Lobel B, Laurent MC, Michardiere L, Le Lannou D. Interest of pentoxifylline in ICSI with frozen-thawed testicular spermatozoa from patients with non-obstructive azoospermia. Reprod Biomed Online. 2006;12:14-8.

Controlled Ovarian Stimulation Protocols for In Vitro Fertilization

Pratibha S Malik

INTRODUCTION

Controlled ovarian hyperstimulation (COH) refers to the use of oral or injectable drugs to recruit several dominant follicles simultaneously to obtain multiple mature oocytes at follicular aspirations in vitro fertilization-intracytoplasmic sperm injection (IVF-ICSI) cycles. This is done to improve chances of conception in addition to compensating for inherent biological limits and imperfect laboratory performance of IVF laboratories.

GOALS

To improve the chances of conception by transfer of best quality embryos, to prevent ovarian hyperstimulation syndrome (OHSS), cycle cancelation, and multiple pregnancies. The predictors of response in vitro fertilization are given in **Table 1**.

Pretreatment options for scheduling the start of stimulation—oral contraceptive pill (OCP),[1] progesterone, luteal estradiol,[1] premenstrual gonadotropin-releasing hormone (GnRH) antagonist (CRASH protocol)[2]

TYPES OF RESPONSE TO STIMULATION

1. High responders—peak estradiol (E2) >3,000 pg/mL and retrieval of >15 oocytes.
2. Normal responders—retrieval of 8–15 oocytes.
3. Poor responders—retrieval of less ≤3 oocytes.

Monitoring: Stimulation is tailored according to the unique characteristics of each patient to maximize the success called as individualized controlled ovarian stimulation (iCOS)[3] **(Fig. 1)**.

PROTOCOLS

Urinary and recombinant gonadotropins are used during ovarian stimulation in IVF-ICSI cycles with almost equal results.[4] In conventional COH protocols, ovarian stimulation is mostly done by using daily injections of gonadotropins, which are typically started on Day 2 or 3 following menses. GnRH analogs (agonists and antagonists) are administered concomitantly in different protocols to avoid premature luteinizing hormone (LH) surge due to the supraphysiological estradiol levels. GnRH agonist protocols can be long or short and cause initial flare by release of endogenous gonadotropins. GnRH antagonists are administered either in fixed or flexible protocols. Final oocyte maturation is triggered by either GnRH agonists or human chorionic gonadotropin (HCG) or both[1] **(Table 2 to 4 and Box 1)**.

The best protocol for IVF in various types of patients is debatable and inconclusive **(Flowchart 1)**.[3]

BATCH IN VITRO FERTILIZATION (FIG. 15)

Oral contraceptive pill pretreatment started on Day 2 of the previous cycle. Day of oocyte pick-up is planned according to the availability of the embryologist (Day 0). Twenty-one days before the planned pick-up date, GnRH agonist is started (Day 21) and 17 days before the planned ovum pick-up date, OCP is stopped for all patients (Day 17). Stimulation with gonadotropins is started 11 or 12 days before the planned pick-up date (Day 11). Trigger with HCG is given 36 hours before oocyte pick-up (Day 2).[12]

TABLE 1: Predictors of response.

Clinical predictors	Investigational predictors
Age	AFC
BMI	Serum AMH
Smoking status	Basal FSH
Previous response to stimulation	Basal estradiol
Previous ovarian surgery, pelvic adhesions	Total ovarian volume
Endometriosis, PCOS	Inhibin B

(AFC: antral follicle count; AMH: anti-Müllerian hormone; BMI: body mass index; FSH: follicle-stimulating hormone; PCOS: polycystic ovary syndrome)

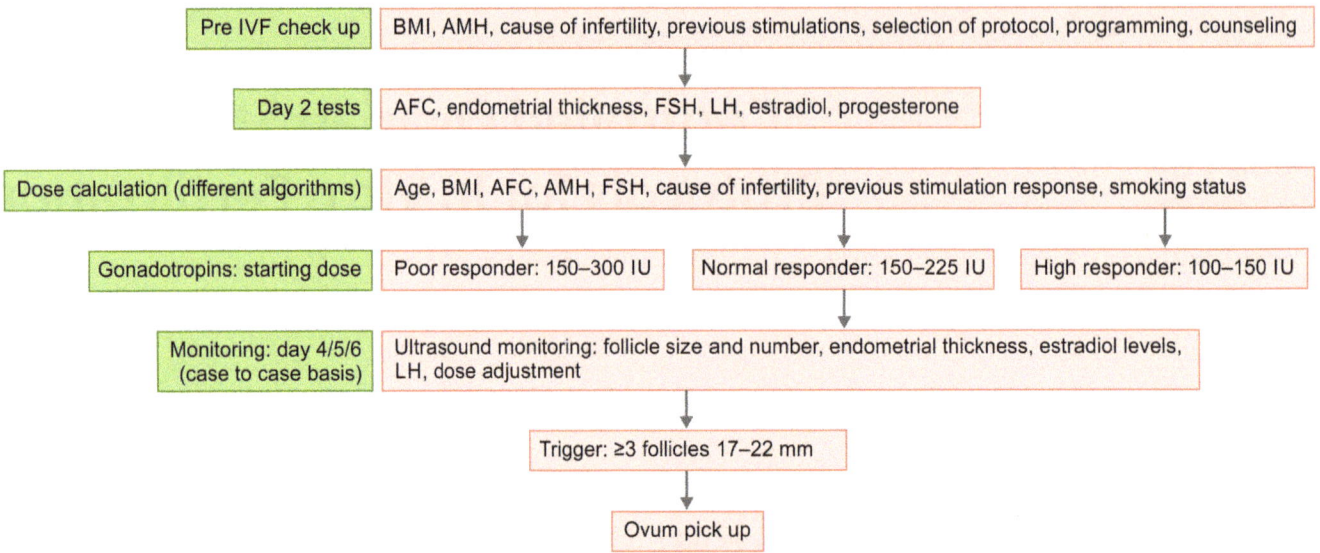

Fig. 1: Individualized controlled ovarian stimulation.

TABLE 2: Types of protocols.

Types	Protocols	Preferred in patient groups with	Rationale, figure, references
Long luteal agonist protocol	Agonist started on Day 21 of previous cycle and continued till day of HCG, dose of agonist may (mini dose long protocol) or may not be halved once gonadotropins are started on day 2	Normal responders, poor responders	**Figure 2**[1]. Maximizes number of oocytes retrieved so more risk of OHSS, more embryos cryopreserved, high pregnancy rate per cycle
Ultra long agonist protocol	GnRH agonist depot (3.75 mg) given monthly once for 3 months followed by gonadotropin stimulation from day 2 up to day of HCG trigger	Endometriosis	**Figure 3**. Giving GnRH agonists before IVF or ICSI could increase the chances of pregnancy in women with endometriosis[5] downregulation of GnRH receptors
Long follicular agonist protocol	Single dose of GnRH Agonist 3.75 mg given in early follicular phase of previous cycle. Gonadotropins started from day 2 of next cycle along with GnRH antagonist till day of trigger	Normal responder	**Figure 4**.[6] Lower incidence of OHSS, decreased LH fluctuations during the course of COH
Short or flare up agonist protocol	Agonist started on Day 1/2 of cycle, gonadotropins started on Day 3 of cycle till day of HCG trigger	Poor responder	**Figure 5**.[1,7] Initial stimulation of GnRH receptors releases endogenous gonadotropins adds to the effect of exogenous gonadotropin
Microcode flare agonist protocol	OCP or progesterone pretreatment for 14–21 days, low-dose agonist given from Day 2, gonadotropins given from Day 3 of cycle till day of trigger	Poor responders	**Figure 6**.[7] Due to the OCP pretreatment, there is no rise in progesterone and androgen concentration at start of withdrawal bleed
Ultra short agonist protocol	Agonist started on cycle day 2/3 and stopped on cycle day 4/5. Gonadotropins started on Day 2 till day of HCG trigger	Poor responders	**Figure 7**[7]. 1. Ovarian suppression is not excessive; 2. Initial stimulation of GnRH receptors releases endogenous gonadotropins adds to the effect of exogenous gonadotropins
Menstrual early cessation agonist protocol	Agonist started on Day 21 of previous cycle till onset of menses, followed by gonadotropins till day of HCG trigger	Poor responders	**Figure 8**[7]. Reduced ovarian suppression. Pituitary recovery after cessation takes around 14 days
Follicular early cessation protocol	Agonist started on Day 21 of the previous cycle till day 5 of stimulation with gonadotropins. Gonadotropins started from Day 2 of menses till day of HCG trigger	Poor responders	**Figure 9**[1,7]. Reduced ovarian suppression. Pituitary recovery after cessation takes around 14 days

Contd...

Contd...

Types	Protocols	Preferred in patient groups with	Rationale, figure, references
Antagonist protocol (multiple doses)	Gonadotropins are started on day 2/3 of cycle and antagonist is started on Day 6 of stimulation in fixed protocol or when lead follicle reaches 12–14 mm or E2 reaches 300–400 pg/mL in flexible protocol till day of trigger (HCG or GnRH agonist)	PCOS, normal responder, poor responders	**Figure 10**[2]. Immediate gonadotropin suppression, shorter duration of stimulation, lesser dose of gonadotropins required, advantageous in hyper responders, lesser risk of OHSS, can be triggered by GnRH agonist, HCG or rLH
Natural cycle	Aim is to obtain single best quality oocyte. Cycle monitored with USG, hormone levels, no medication used	Poor responders, cancer patients	Low cost, high cancelation due to premature ovulation[8]
Modified natural with HCG	Aim is to retrieve single best quality oocyte. Gonadotropin, GnRH antagonist may or may not be used. Cycle is triggered with HCG once follicle reaches >15 mm to reduce premature ovulation	Poor responders	Reduced cancelation rate[8]
Modified natural with addition of GnRH antagonist	Aim is to retrieve single best quality oocyte. Once dominant follicle reaches 13–14 mm, antagonist is given till day of trigger with HCG. Cycle monitored with USG, hormone levels. Gonadotropins as add back may or may not be used	Poor responders	Safe, low cost, patient friendly, reducing complications like premature ovulation[8]
Mild antagonist stimulation protocol	Aim is retrieval of 2–7 good quality oocytes. Oral antiestrogens-CC or letrozole with low dose gonadotropins (≤150 IU/d) are used in an antagonist protocol	Poor responders, poor patients, low-cost IVF	**Figure 11.** Reduced dose, complexity, discomfort, risks, cancelation, drop outs and cost. Beneficial effect on oocyte and embryo quality[8]
Corifollitropin alfa	Single dose of corifollitropin alfa on Day 2 of cycle, additional gonadotropins on cycle day 8, 9 with antagonist on cycle Day 5 up to day of HCG trigger	Normal responders, normal BMI	**Figure 12**[9]. One single s.c. injection of corifollitropin alfa is able to initiate and sustain multiple follicular growth for a week. Risk of OHSS is present
Double stimulation or Shanghai protocol	Follicular stimulation is done with CC, letrozole from Day 3 and HMG from Day 6 in an antagonist protocol followed by oocyte pick-up. Luteal stimulation is done with HMG and letrozole with antagonist and oocyte retrieved. Trigger in both by GnRH analogue	Poor responders, cancer patients	**Figure 13**[10]. Existing antral follicles in the luteal phase can undergo ovarian stimulation. Helpful in fertility preservation in cancer patients and those with low response to stimulation
Progesterone primed ovarian stimulation	Gonadotropins started on Day 2 and MPA 10 mg/d on Day 7 of stimulation or when lead follicle >14 mm and continued till day of trigger	Freeze all, oocyte donor, **PGT-A**, oocyte cryopreservation cycles	**Figure 14**[11]. 1. Progestins can effectively prevent premature ovulation; 2. Reduced cost, complexity

(CC: clomiphene citrate; COH: controlled ovarian hyperstimulation; GnRH: gonadotropin-releasing hormone; HCG: human chorionic gonadotropin; HMG: human menopausal gonadotropin; ICSI: intracytoplasmic sperm injection; IVF: in vitro fertilization; LH: luteinizing hormone; MPA: Medroxyprogesterone; OHSS: ovarian hyperstimulation syndrome; PGT-A: preimplantation genetic testing for aneuploidy; s.c.: subcutaneous; USG: ultrasonogram).

TABLE 3: Agonist protocols.

Salient features	Disadvantages
Protocol starts in previous cycle	Profound pituitary suppression leading to increased dose of gonadotropins
Initial flare up effect for 3–4 days followed by pituitary desensitization and receptor down regulation	Increased costs
Agonist continued till trigger day, ensures prevention of LH surge	Functional cyst formation
Synchronous follicular growth	OHSS as only HCG can be used as trigger
Favors batch IVF	Longer treatment

(HCG: human chorionic gonadotropin; IVF: in vitro fertilization; LH: luteinizing hormone; OHSS: ovarian hyperstimulation syndrome).

TABLE 4: Antagonist protocols.

Advantages	Disadvantages
Physiological, patient friendly, less stressful, shorter, no need for pituitary desensitization before starting	Does not suppress raised LH levels in early phase of stimulation
Safer, lower gonadotropin doses, GnRH agonist as trigger to prevent OHSS	Does not favor batching of cycles
Less costly with use of oral agents	Does not allow flexibility in IVF programming

(IVF: in vitro fertilization; GnRH: gonadotropin-releasing hormone; LH: luteinizing hormone; OHSS: ovarian hyperstimulation syndrome).

BOX 1: Long agonist protocols.

Long and ultra long agonist protocols
Confirmation of down regulation:
- Serum estradiol <50 pg/mL
- Serum LH <5 mIU/mL
- Serum progesterone <0.5 ng/mL
- Endometrial thickness <5 mm

(LH: luteinizing hormone).

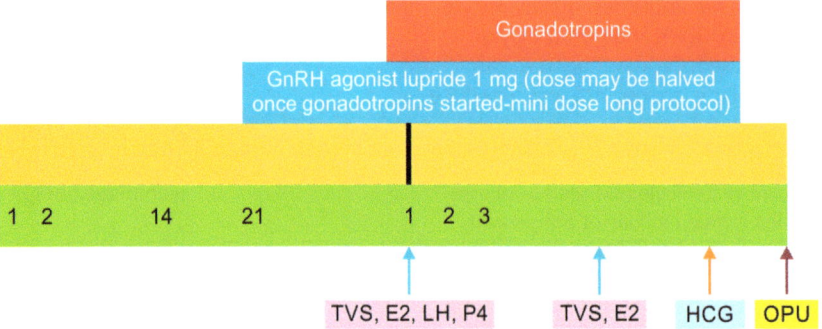

Fig. 2: Long luteal GnRH agonist protocol.

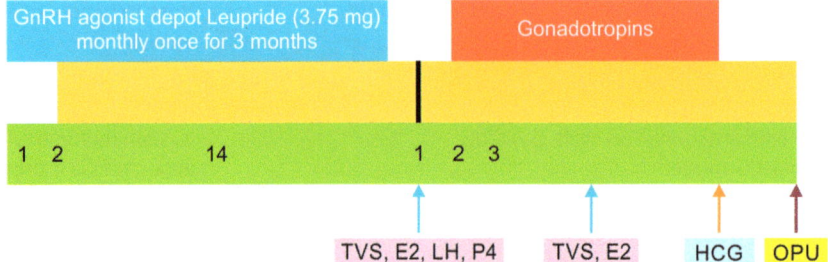

Fig. 3: Ultra long GnRH agonist protocol.

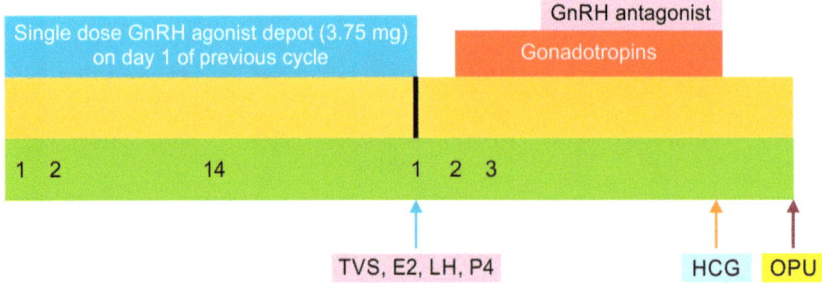

Fig. 4: Long follicular GnRH agonist protocol.

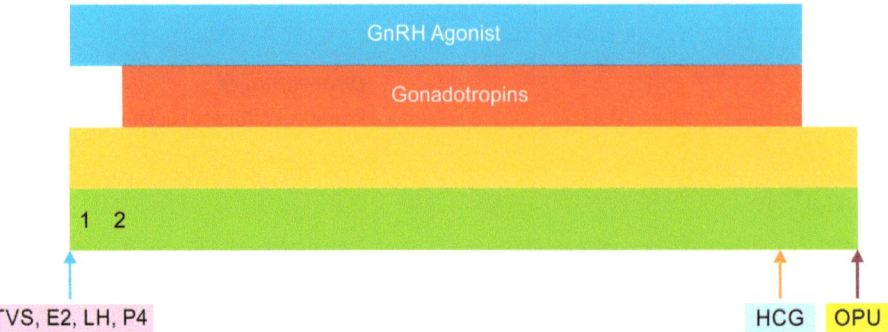

Fig. 5: Short or flare up agonist protocol.

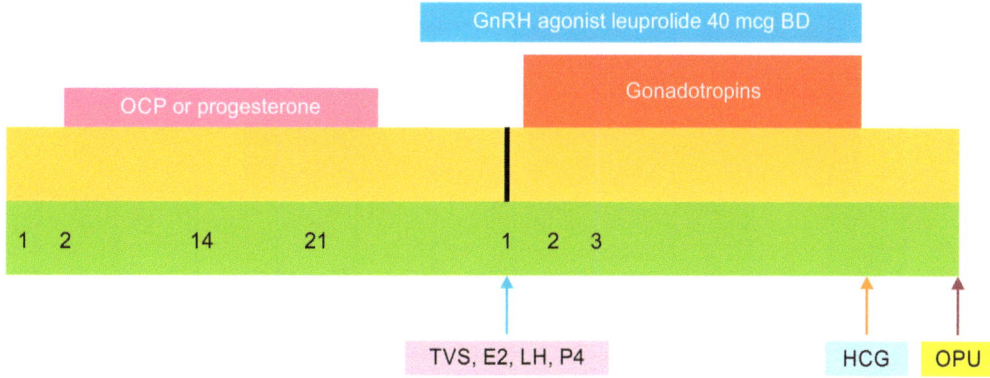

Fig. 6: Micro dose flare protocol.

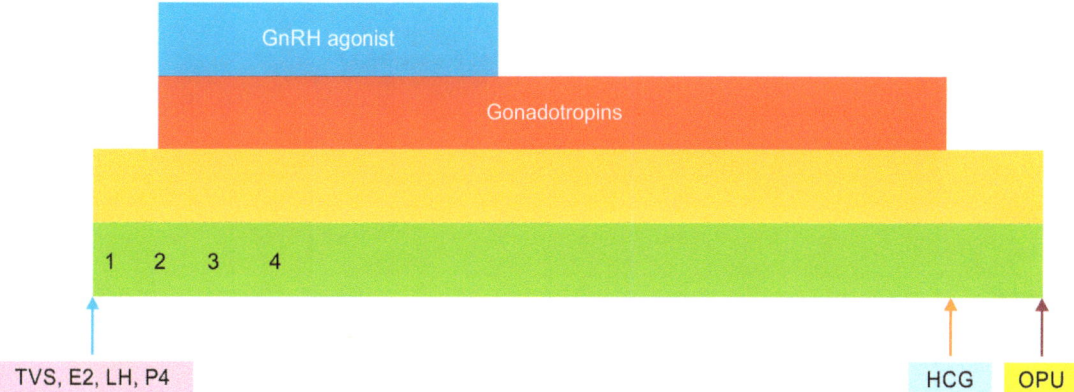

Fig. 7: Ultra short agonist protocol.

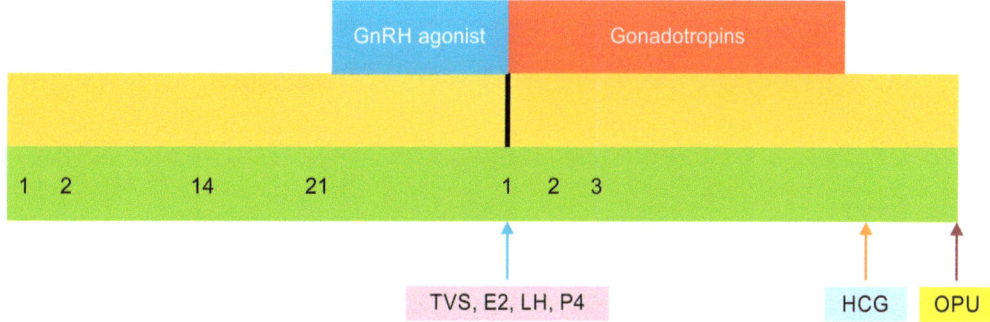

Fig. 8: Menstrual early cessation agonist protocol.

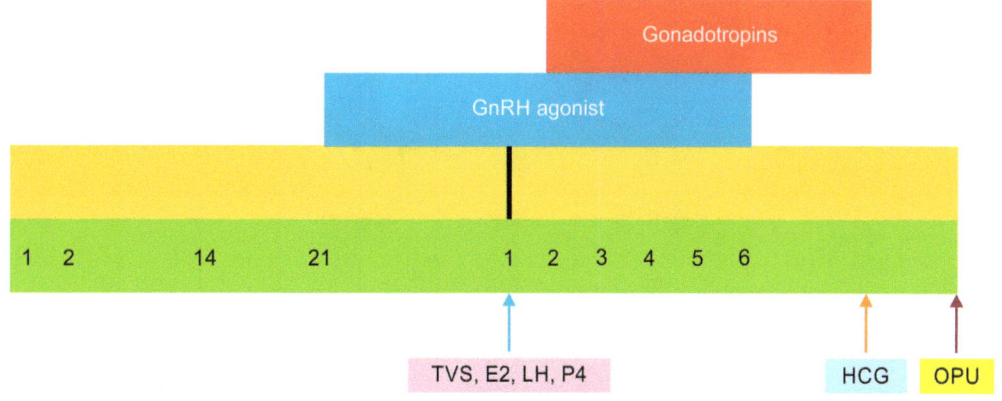

Fig. 9: Follicular early cessation agonist protocol.

166 Controlled Ovarian Stimulation Protocols for In Vitro Fertilization

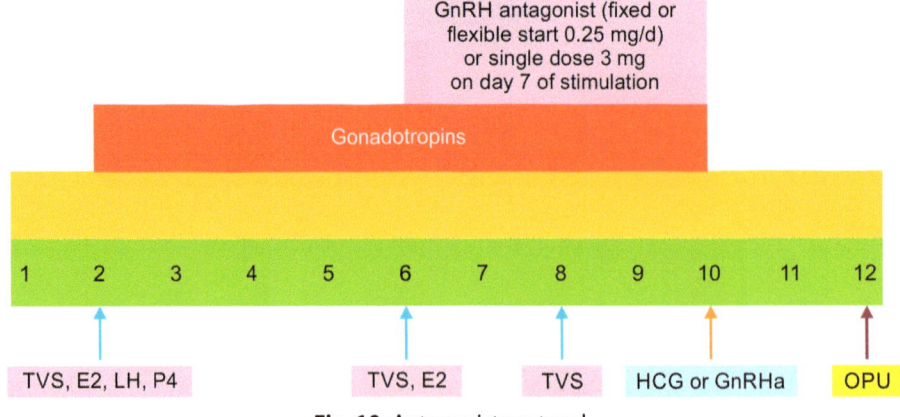

Fig. 10: Antagonist protocol.

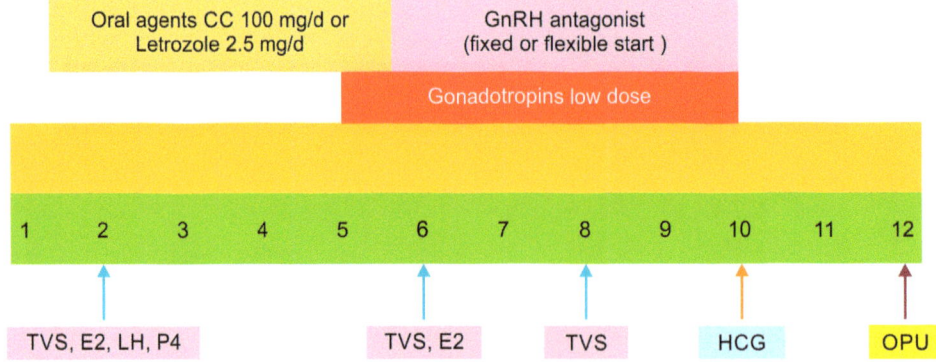

Fig. 11: Mild antagonist protocol.

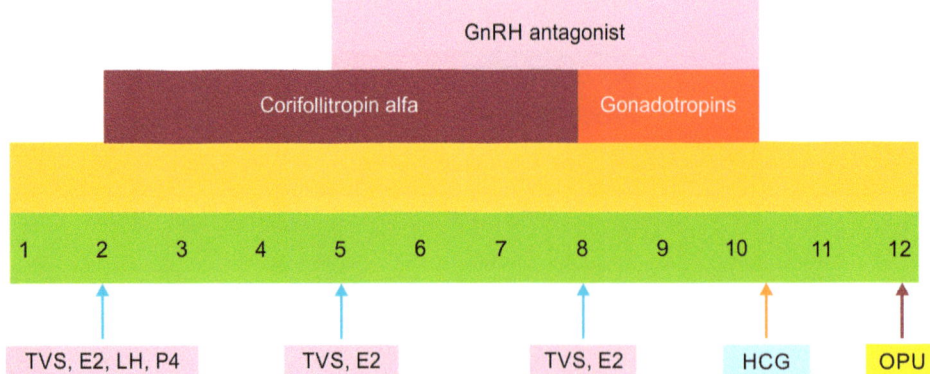

Fig. 12: Corifollitropin alfa.

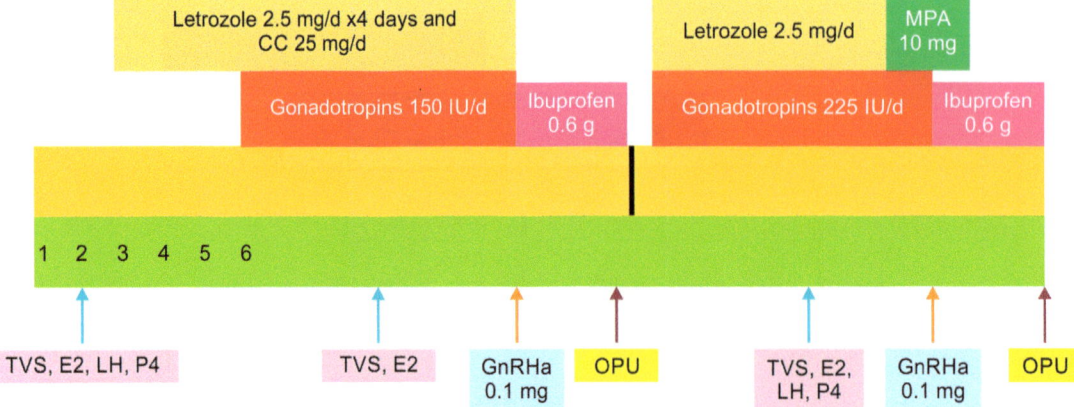

Fig. 13: Double stimulation (Shanghai) protocol.

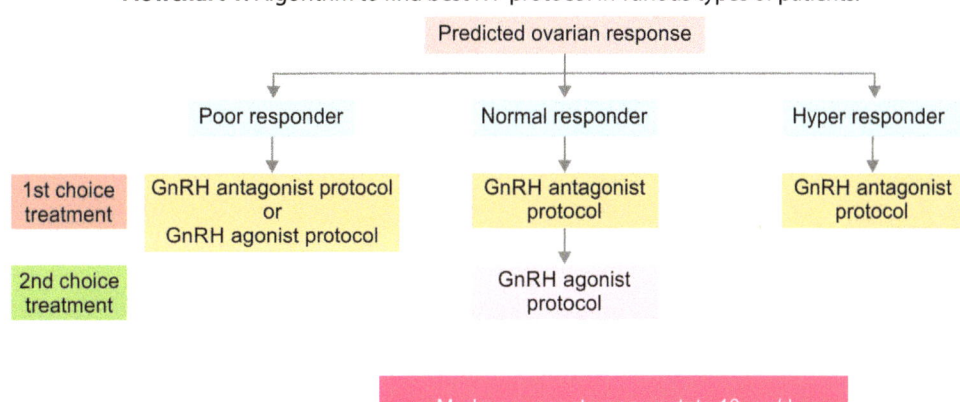

Flowchart 1: Algorithm to find best IVF protocol in various types of patients.

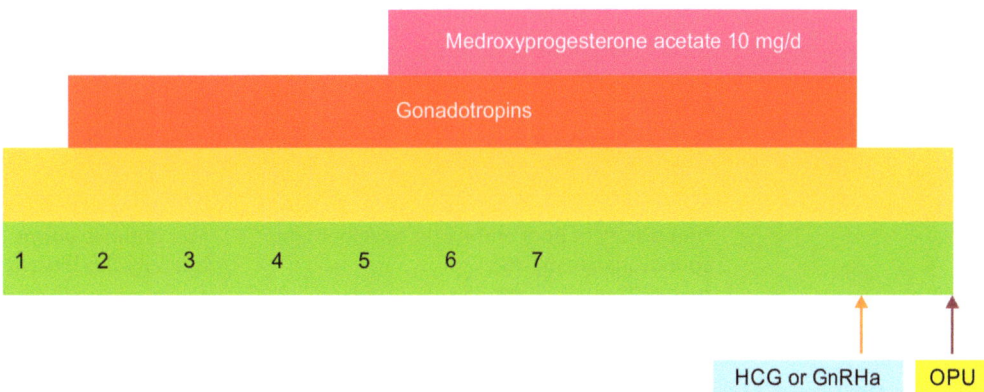

Fig. 14: Progesterone primed ovarian stimulation.

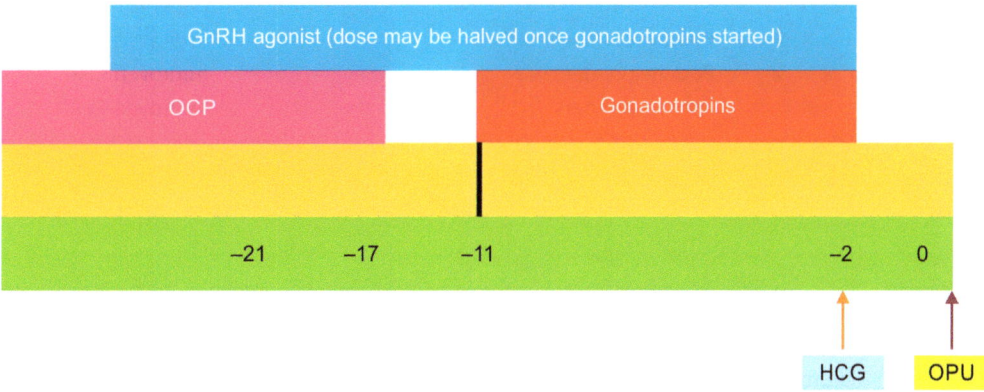

Fig. 15: Batch IVF long GnRH protocol.

RANDOM START CONTROLLED OVARIAN STIMULATION (TABLE 5; FIG. 16)[19]

For women in the reproductive years who have diagnosed with cancer, fertility preservation is important and urgent. Controlled ovarian stimulation (COS) for oocyte or embryo cryopreservation in cancer patients can be initiated within 2–3 days of initial visit, irrespective of their day in menstrual cycle; this is due to multiple waves of follicular recruitment in each menstrual cycle. Antagonist protocol is used along with additional letrozole in those with estrogen sensitive malignancy.

Adjuvants have been used in IVF cycles but there is limited evidence of their usefulness **(Table 6)**.[13]

TABLE 5: Random start IVF protocols.

Time in menstrual cycle	Random start IVF protocol
Early follicular phase	GnRH antagonist 0.25 mg is given daily for 3 days till estradiol <50 pg/mL. Standard antagonist protocol follows. **(Fig. 16)**
Late follicular phase (>day 7)	• Ovarian stimulation started without GnRH antagonist. Antagonist added when secondary follicles reached size >12 mm. • Ovulation induced with GnRH agonist or hCG followed by stimulation in 2–3 days
Luteal phase	Stimulation started and GnRH antagonist added when secondary follicles reached size >12 mm

(GnRH: gonadotropin-releasing hormone; hCG: human chorionic gonadotropin; IVF: in vitro fertilization).

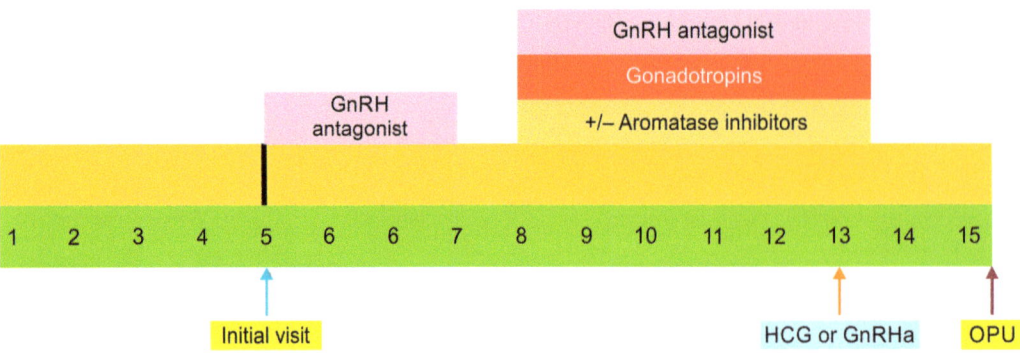

Fig. 16: Random start protocol-early follicular phase.

TABLE 6: Adjuvants used in IVF cycles.

Adjuvant	Patient	Evidence
Metformin	PCOS, hyperresponders	Reduces incidence of OHSS[14]
Aspirin	Poor responders, endometrial preparation in frozen embryo transfer cycles	Not much useful in ovarian stimulation[15]
Growth hormone	Prior history of poor embryonic development, poor ovarian responses	May improve oocyte and embryo quantity, live birth rate[16,17]
Vasodilators—sildenafil, glyceryl trinitrate (GTN), nifedipine, nimodipine, pentoxifylline and isosorbide monohydrate	Thin endometrium, RIF, poor responders	May increase the clinical pregnancy rate[18]
Antiestrogens—letrozole or tamoxifen	Oncofertility patients	Decreases estradiol levels in women with estrogen sensitive malignancy[19]
Testosterone	Poor responder	Improves success rates in POR patients[20] by increasing LBR, CPR[21]
DHEA	Poor responder	Improved CPR[21]
CoQ 10	Poor responder	Improved CPR[21]
rLH	Poor responders	Improved CPR[22]

(CoQ 10: Coenzyme Q10; CPR: clinical pregnancy rate; DHEA: dehydroepiandrosterone; LBR: livebirth rate; rLH: recombinant LH; RIF: repeated implantation failure)

TABLE 7: Common complications in in vitro fertilization cycles.

Complication	Risk factors	Prevention
OHSS	PCOS, High AMH/AFC, HCG trigger, Agonist protocols, young age, low BMI	GnRH agonist trigger, freeze all, antagonist protocol, metformin[14]
Multiple pregnancy	Multiple embryo transfer, advanced age, ovulation induction	Single embryo transfer, Fetal reduction
Ectopic pregnancy and heterotopic pregnancy	Tubal factor infertility, PID, endometriosis, previous surgery, STI, previous ectopic	Single embryo transfer, blastocyst transfer, FET cycle

(PCOS: polycystic ovary syndrome; AFC: antral follicle count; AMH: anti-Müllerian hormone; BMI: body mass index; FET: frozen embryo transfer; GnRH: gonadotropin-releasing hormone; HCG: human chorionic gonadotropin; PID: pelvic inflammatory disease; STI: sexually transmitted infections;).

COMPLICATIONS[3]

The following complications are more common in IVF cycles and thus require vigilance for their prevention **(Table 7)**.

REFERENCES

1. Macklon NS, Stouffer RL, Giudice LC, Fauser BC. The science behind 25 years of ovarian stimulation for in vitro fertilization. Endocr Rev. 2006;27(2):170-207.
2. Humaidan P, Bungum L, Bungum M, Hald F, Agerholm I, Blaabjerg J, et al. Reproductive outcome using a GnRH antagonist (cetrorelix) for luteolysis and follicular synchronization in poor responder IVF/ICSI patients treated with a flexible GnRH antagonist protocol. Reprod Biomed Online. 2005;11(6):679-84.
3. Ovarian Stimulation TEGGO, Bosch E, Broer S, Griesinger G, Grynberg M, Humaidan P, et al. ESHRE guideline: ovarian stimulation for IVF/ICSI. Hum Reprod Open. 2020;2020(2): hoaa009.

4. Van Wely M, Westergaard LG, Bossuyt PM, Van der Veen F. Human menopausal gonadotropin versus recombinant follicle stimulation hormone for ovarian stimulation in assisted reproductive cycles. Cochrane Database Syst Rev. 2003;(1):CD003973.
5. Sallam HN, Garcia-Velasco JA, Dias S, Arici A, Abou-Setta AM. Long-term pituitary down-regulation before in vitro fertilization (IVF) for women with endometriosis. Cochrane Database Syst Rev. 2006 Jan 25;2006(1):CD004635.
6. Yang R, Guan Y, Perrot V, Ma J, Li R. Comparison of the long-acting GnRH agonist follicular protocol with the GnRH antagonist protocol in women undergoing in vitro fertilization: a systematic review and meta-analysis. Adv Ther. 38(5):2027-37.
7. Badawy A, Wageah A, Gharib MEL, Osman EE. Strategies for pituitary down-regulation to optimize IVF/ICSI outcome in poor ovarian responders. J Reprod Infertil. 2012;13(3):124-30.
8. Nargund G, Datta AK, Fauser BCJM. Mild stimulation for in vitro fertilisation. Fertil Steril. 2017;108(4):558-67.
9. Cozzolino M, Vitagliano A, Cecchino GN, Ambrosini G, Garcia-Velasco JA. Corifollitropin alfa for ovarian stimulation in in vitro fertilisation: a systematic review and meta-analysis of randomised controlled trials. Fertil Steril. 2019;111(4):722-33.
10. Kuang Y, Chen Q, Hong Q, Lyu Q, Ai A, Fu Y. Double stimulations during the follicular and luteal phases in patients with poor ovarian response in IVF/ICSI programs (the shanghai protocol). Reprod Biomed Online. 2014;29(6):684-91.
11. Yildiz S, Turkgeldi E, Angun B, Eraslan A, Urman B, Ata B. Comparison of a novel flexible progestin primed ovarian stimulation protocol and the flexible gonadotropin-releasing hormone antagonist protocol for assisted reproductive technology. Fertil Steril. 2019;112(4):677-83.
12. Gutgutia R, Rao S, Garcia-Velasco J, Basu S. Scheduling cycles with gonadotropin-releasing hormone antagonist protocol in in vitro fertilisation: Is there a scope in batch in vitro fertilisation? J Hum Reprod Sci. 2014;7(4):230-5.
13. ESHRE Reproductive Endocrinology Guideline Group. (2019). Ovarian Stimulation for IVF/ICSI. [online] Available from https://www.eshre.eu/Guidelines-and-Legal/Guidelines/Ovarian-Stimulation-in-IVF-ICSI [Last accessed April, 2023].
14. Tso LO, Costello MF, Albuquerque LE, Andriolo RB, Freitas V. Metformin treatment before and during IVF or ICSI in women with polycystic ovary syndrome. Cochrane Database Syst Rev. 2009;(2):CD006105.
15. Mourad A, Antaki R, Jamal W, Albaini O. Aspirin for endometrial preparation in patients undergoing IVF: a systematic review and meta-analysis. J Obstet Gynaecol Can. 2021;43(8):984-992.e2.
16. Li J, Chen Q, Wang J, Huang G, Ye H. Does growth hormone supplementation improve oocyte competence and IVF outcomes in patients with poor embryonic development? A randomized controlled trial. BMC Pregnancy Childbirth.2020;20(1):310.
17. Duffy JMN, Ahmad G, Mohiyiddeen L, Nardo LG, Watson A. Growth hormone for in vitro fertilization. Cochrane Database Syst Rev. 2010 Jan 20;2010(1):CD000099.
18. Gutarra-Vilchez RB, Bonfill Cosp X, Glujovsky D, Viteri-García A, Runzer-Colmenares FM, Martinez-Zapata MJ. Vasodilators for women undergoing fertility treatment. Cochrane Database Syst Rev. 2018;10(10):CD010001.
19. Cakmak H, Katz A, Cedars MI, Rosen MP. Effective method for emergency fertility preservation: random-start controlled ovarian hyperstimulation. Fertil Steril. 2013;100(6):1673-80.
20. Noventa M, Vitagliano A, Andrisani A, Blaganje M, Viganò P, Papaelo E, et al. Testosterone therapy for women with poor ovarian response undergoing IVF: a meta-analysis of randomized controlled trials . J Assist Reprod Genet. 2019;36(4):673-83.
21. Zhang Y, Zhang C, Shu J, Guo J, Chang HM, Leung PCK, et al. Adjuvant treatment strategies in ovarian stimulation for poor responders undergoing IVF: a systematic review and network meta-analysis. Hum Reprod Update. 2020;26(2): 247-63.
22. Lehert P, Kolibianakis EM, Venetis CA, Schertz J, Saunders H, Arriagada P, Copt S, et al. Recombinant human follicle-stimulating hormone (r-hFSH) plus recombinant luteinizing hormone versus r-hFSH alone for ovarian stimulation during assisted reproductive technology: systematic review and meta-analysis. Reprod Biol Endocrinol. 2014;12:17.

CHAPTER 20: Management of Ovarian Hyperstimulation Syndrome

Deepika Krishna

INTRODUCTION
- Ovarian hyperstimulation syndrome (OHSS) is an iatrogenic complication of ovarian stimulation (OS) resulting in a wide spectrum of symptoms, with one end characterized by mild abdominal pain and distension due to enlarged ovaries to the other end of the spectrum manifested with signs and symptoms of massive ovarian enlargement and shift of fluid from the intravascular compartment to third space.
- This is one of the complications of OS which can be fatal and is largely preventable, if appropriate preventive measures are undertaken.

INCIDENCE
- *Incidence of OHSS:* 1–14% of all cycles[1]
- *Mild:* About 20–33% of stimulated cycles[1-3]
- *Moderate:* In about 3–8%[1-3]
- *Severe:* 0.1–0.5%[3]

TYPES OF OVARIAN HYPERSTIMULATION SYNDROME
Based on the onset, types of OHSS are presented in **Table 1**.

SPONTANEOUS OVARIAN HYPERSTIMULATION SYNDROME
- Rarely occurs spontaneously in patients not undergoing OS.
- Modified classification (De Leener et al.[5]) **(Table 2)**.

CLASSIFICATION OF OVARIAN HYPERSTIMULATION SYNDROME
Various classifications have been proposed based on the severity, laboratory parameters, and ultrasound findings. Proposed Royal College of Obstetricians and Gynaecologists (RCOG) classification of OHSS is given in **Table 3**.

TABLE 1: Types of ovarian hyperstimulation syndrome (OHSS).

Early	Late
• Occurs 3–9 days after human chorionic gonadotropin (hCG) trigger[4] • Due to excessive ovarian response to exogenous hCG	• Occurs after 10–17 days of hCG trigger[4] • Due to endogenous hCG which is produced by the implanting embryo • More likely to be severe and long-lasting[4] • Can also be seen when hCG is used for luteal phase support

TABLE 2: Modified classification of spontaneous ovarian hyperstimulation syndrome (OHSS).

Types	Cause	Associated conditions
Type I	Mutated follicle-stimulating hormone receptor (FSHR) increasing its sensitivity to trophoblastic human chorionic gonadotropin (hCG)	Cause of familial recurrent spontaneous OHSS
Type II	Elevated β-hCG	• Multiple pregnancies • Gestational trophoblastic disorders (GTD) • This type is the most frequently encountered.
Type III	• Elevated thyroid-stimulating hormone (TSH) • Similarity of the binding receptors of TSH and follicle-stimulating hormone (FSH)	Severe hypothyroidism
Type IV	Elevated FSH/luteinizing hormone (LH)	Pituitary adenomas (FSH/LH secreting), resulting in a huge rise in estradiol (E2) levels with ovarian enlargement

TABLE 3: Proposed Royal College of Obstetricians and Gynaecologists (RCOG) classification of severity of ovarian hyperstimulation syndrome (OHSS).[6]

Category	Features
Mild	• Abdominal bloating • Mild abdominal pain • Ovarian size usually <8 cm*
Moderate	• Moderate abdominal pain • Nausea ± vomiting • Ultrasound evidence of ascites • Ovarian size usually 8–12 cm*
Severe	• Clinical ascites (± hydrothorax) • Oliguria (<300 mL/day or <30 mL/hour) • Hematocrit >0.45 • Hyponatremia (sodium <135 mmol/L) • Hypo-osmolality (osmolality <282 mOsm/kg) • Hyperkalemia (potassium >5 mmol/L) • Hypoproteinemia (serum albumin <35 g/L) • Ovarian size usually >12 cm*
Critical	• Tense ascites/large hydrothorax • Hematocrit >0.55 • White cell count >25,000/mL • Oliguria/anuria • Thromboembolism • Acute respiratory distress syndrome (ARDS)

*Ovarian size may not correlate with severity in cases of assisted reproduction because of the effect of follicular aspiration. Women demonstrating any feature of severe or critical OHSS should be classified in that category.

PATHOPHYSIOLOGY

- Massive transudation of protein-rich fluid (mainly albumin) from intravascular to extravascular space **(Fig. 1)**.[3,7]
- *Triggering factor:* Human chorionic gonadotropin (hCG), either exogenous or endogenous.[8]
- Release of various vasoactive angiogenic factors, vascular endothelial growth factor (VEGF) playing a key role **(Fig. 2)**.[9-12]
- VEGF levels correlates with the severity of OHSS.[3,13]
- Activation of Intraovarian renin-angiotensin system (RAS) by hCG potentiates the development of OHSS.[14]

PREDICTING OVARIAN HYPERSTIMULATION SYNDROME

Identifying patients at risk of OHSS can be done as depicted in **Table 4.**

CLINICAL FEATURES OF OVARIAN HYPERSTIMULATION SYNDROME

Clinical features of OHSS are given in **Table 5**.

INVESTIGATIONS IN A CASE OF OVARIAN HYPERSTIMULATION SYNDROME

Investigations to be done in a case of OHSS are presented in **Table 6**.

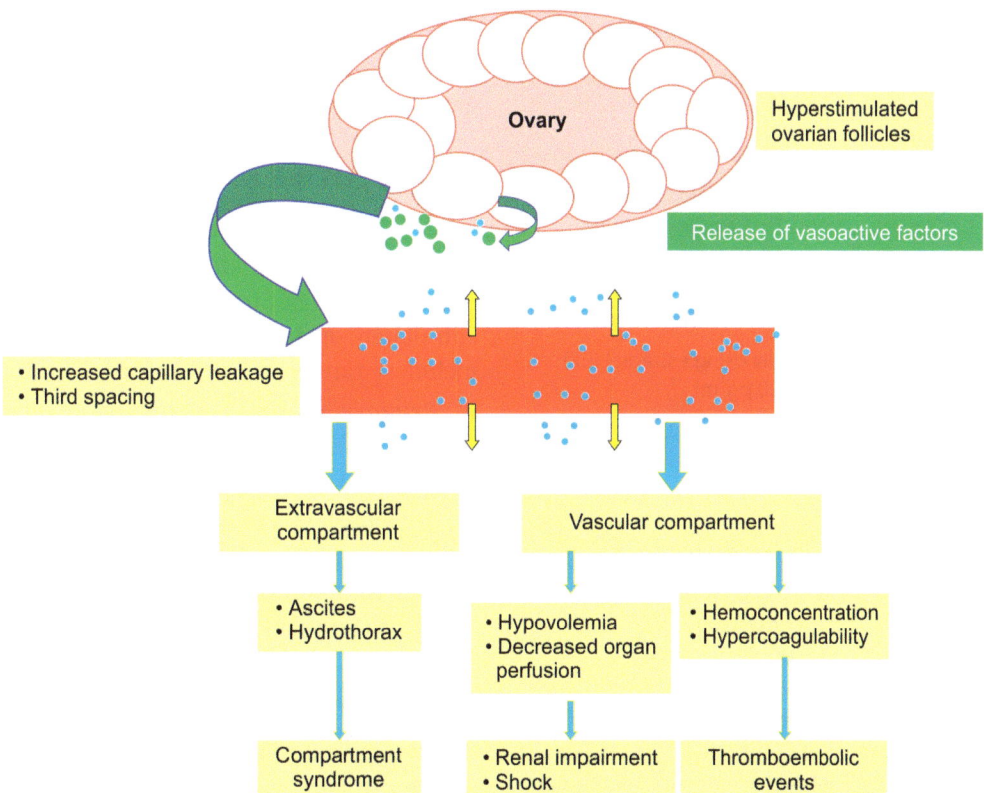

Fig. 1: Pathophysiology of ovarian hyperstimulation syndrome (OHSS).

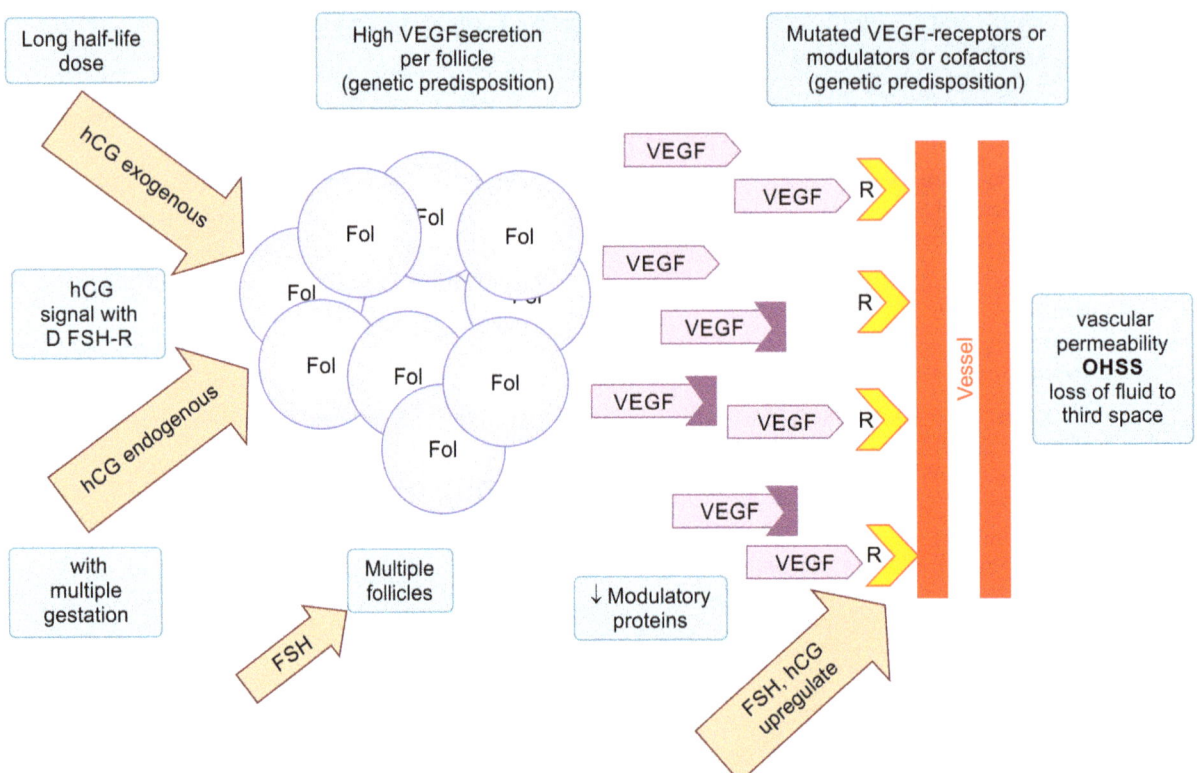

Fig. 2: Pathogenesis of OHSS.
(FSH: follicle-stimulating hormone; hCG: human chorionic gonadotropin; OHSS: ovarian hyperstimulation syndrome; VEGF: vascular endothelial growth factor)
(*Source:* Humaidan P, Quartarolo J, Papanikolaou EG. Preventing ovarian hyperstimulation syndrome: guidance for the clinician. Fertil Steril. 2010;94:389-400.)

TABLE 4: Risk factors for OHSS.[15-19]	
Primary (patient related)	**Secondary (ovarian response)**
Young age <33 years[15]	Stimulation protocol-GnRHa downregulated
Low body mass index (BMI)	High doses of gonadotropins
High basal anti-müllerian hormone (AMH) >3.36 ng/mL (sensitivity: 90.5%, specificity: 81.3%)[16]	Multiple stimulated follicles [(ART >19 large/medium-sized follicles before trigger; >25 follicles at retrieval); in ovulation induction >6][17,18]
Polycystic ovarian morphology (PCOM) [follicles of 2–9 mm ≥12) and/or increased ovarian volume ≥10 cc3) in one or both ovaries on transvaginal sonography][15]	Rapidly rising estradiol (E2) >3,500 pg/mL.[17]
Previous history of OHSS	>24 oocytes retrieved[17]
High antral follicle count (AFC) >24 follicles[19]	• Exogenous hCG—trigger • Luteal phase hCG supplementation • Endogenous hCG production—pregnancy

ART: assisted reproductive technology; GnRHa: gonadotropin-releasing hormone agonist; hCG: human chorionic gonadotropin; OHSS: ovarian hyperstimulation syndrome)

COMPLICATIONS OF OVARIAN HYPERSTIMULATION SYNDROME

Complications of ovarian hyperstimulation syndrome are given in **Box 1**.

PREVENTIVE STRATEGIES

Prevention of OHSS becomes paramount importance with an exponential increase in the number of ART cycles over the decades. Strategies can be implied to avoid OHSS completely or decrease its incidence and severity, which includes primary and secondary.

- *Primary prevention:* Begins with identification of risk factors and individualized stimulation protocols **(Table 7)**.
- *Secondary prevention:* Undertaken in patients with an exaggerated response to OS to avert further progression and worsening of OHSS and involves modifications in the components of stimulation protocol **(Table 8)**.

MANAGEMENT

It depends on the severity of presentation—mild, moderate, severe/critical, complications, and presence/absence of pregnancy **(Flowchart 1)**.

TABLE 5: Clinical features in a case of ovarian hyperstimulation syndrome (OHSS).		
History	*Symptoms*[6]	*Examination*[6,17]
• Diagnosis of polycystic ovary syndrome (PCOS) • History of ovarian stimulation for intrauterine insemination (IUI)/in vitro fertilization (IVF) cycle • Number of follicles (dominant + intermediate) on scan • Trigger agent used [human chorionic gonadotropin (hCG) or gonadotropin-releasing hormone (GnRH) agonist] • Time of onset of symptoms since hCG trigger • Number of oocytes retrieved in IVF cycle • If fresh embryo transfer was done (number of embryos transferred)	• Lower abdominal distension • Heaviness and pain in the lower abdomen • Nausea and vomiting • Diarrhea • Dizziness or syncope • Difficulty in breathing • Rapid gain in weight (>2 Lb/day) • Reduced urine output • Swelling of legs • Associated comorbidities such as thrombosis	*General:* • Assessment for dehydration – Edema (pedal, vulval, and sacral) • Monitor vitals (temperature, pulse rate, respiratory rate, and blood pressure) • Check body weight *Abdominal:* • Measure girth (at the level of umbilicus) • Assessment for ascites, palpable mass, and peritonism *Respiratory:* Assessment for: • Pleural effusion • Acute respiratory distress syndrome (ARDS) • Pulmonary edema • Pneumonia *Cardiac:* Assessment for: • Arrhythmia • Pericardial effusion

TABLE 6: Investigations.		
Blood tests	*Imaging*	*Other tests that may be required*
• Complete blood count • Hematocrit (HCT) (hemoconcentration) • C-reactive protein (severity) • Renal function tests (RFT) (urea and creatinine) • Liver function tests (LFTs) (reduced albumin and elevated enzymes) • Serum electrolytes (hyperkalemia and hyponatremia) • Serum osmolality (hypo-osmolality) • Coagulation profile (elevated fibrinogen and reduced antithrombin) • Human chorionic gonadotropin (hCG) (if conception is suspected)	• *Ultrasound:* Ovaries size, free fluid in the pelvis and abdomen • *Doppler of the ovaries:* if torsion is suspected.	• Chest X-ray • Electrocardiogram (ECG) • Echocardiogram • Arterial blood gases • D-dimers • Computerized tomography pulmonary angiogram (CTPA) or ventilation/perfusion (V/Q) scan

BOX 1: Complications of ovarian hyperstimulation syndrome (OHSS).

- Thromboembolism (both arterial and venous)
- Acute renal insufficiency
- Hepatocellular and cholestatic changes
- Pleural effusion
- Pericardial effusion
- Pulmonary dysfunction (due to intra-abdominal or pleural fluid accumulation)
- Acute respiratory distress syndrome (ARDS)
- Increased risk for infection
- Electrolyte imbalance complications (hyperkalemia and azotemia)
- Shock
- Death

OVARIAN HYPERSTIMULATION SYNDROME AND PREGNANCY OUTCOME

- In rare cases of critical OHSS, termination of pregnancy has been reported as in progressive thrombosis despite anticoagulation.[49]
- Increased rate of preclinical pregnancy loss in women with early OHSS but not late.[50]
- Higher incidence of preeclampsia (21.2% vs. 9.2%) and prematurity (36% vs. 10.7%).[51]
- In singleton pregnancies, OHSS was associated with increased risk of low birth weight and preterm delivery. In twin pregnancies, OHSS was accompanied with increased risk of second trimester loss, low birth weight and preterm delivery.[52]

TABLE 7: Primary prevention strategies.

Interventions for primary prevention	Recommendations
Regimens to be followed during ovulation induction (OI) and ovarian stimulation (OS)	• Recognition of risk factors based on age, examination, ultrasound, and antral follicle count (AFC)[3,20] • Reducing the gonadotropin dose[3] • Reducing the gonadotropin duration[3] • Chronic step-up low-dose protocol in polycystic ovary syndrome (PCOS)—yields a higher rate of monofollicular development[21] • Use of aromatase inhibitors (AIs) for OI—AI inhibit aromatase enzyme, decreases estrogen production, thereby increasing follicle-stimulating hormone (FSH) secretion and promotes folliculogenesis. With the negative feedback mechanisms remaining intact, the incidence of ovarian hyperstimulation syndrome (OHSS) is decreased.[22] However, Cochrane review failed to show any difference in OHSS rates with AI[23] • Laparoscopic ovarian drilling: To induce ovulation in anovulatory PCOS. Beneficial in lean PCOS with high-serum levels of luteinizing hormone (LH)[24]
Individualizing in vitro fertilization (IVF) treatment regimens	• Individualized controlled ovarian stimulation (iCOS)—based on algorithm of these biomarkers, age, AFC and anti-müllerian hormone (AMH), starting dose of FSH is calculated.[25] Additionally, previous response to OS to be considered • Use of gonadotropin-releasing hormone antagonist (GnRHA) protocol as an alternative to the long agonist IVF protocol[26,27] • Mild stimulation regimens—administration of FSH is delayed until the mid-to-late follicular phase[17]

Use of adjuvants:
• Insulin sensitizers (metformin)
• Low-dose aspirin
	• *Metformin:*
	  – By inducing intraovarian hyperandrogenism, reduces the number of nonperiovulatory follicles and thereby reducing estradiol (E2) secretion[17]
	  – Inhibits secretion of vasoactive molecules [vascular endothelial growth factor (VEGF)] during OI[17]
	  – Dose: 1,000–2,000 mg daily at least 2 months prior to OS
	  – Good evidence that metformin decreases OHSS risk in PCOS patients (Grade A)[17]
	• *Aspirin:*
	  – Prevents platelet activation and release of inflammatory mediators
	  – Dose: 100 mg daily, starting on the first day of OS in IVF cycle decreases the severity (fair evidence)[17]

Modifications in human chorionic gonadotropin (hCG) trigger	• Low-dose hCG (1,000–1,500 IU) or dual trigger (low-dose hCG + GnRHa) • Insufficient evidence to recommend a lower dose of hCG for OHSS risk reduction[17]

Alternatives for hCG trigger:
• Gonadotropin-releasing hormone agonist (GnRHa)
• Recombinant LH (rLH)
• Kisspeptin (KP)-54
	• GnRHa:
	  – Induces a short (24–36 hours) endogenous gonadotropin (FSH + LH) surge
	  – Due to massive luteolysis, freeze-all strategy needs to be followed
	  – *Dose:* Triptorelin (0.2 mg)/leuprolide (0.5–1 mg)/buserelin acetate (2 mg), subcutaneous
	  – In IVF cycle—use of GnRHA + GnRHa + freeze-all, virtually eliminates OHSS risk (good evidence)[17]
	• rLH:
	  – Used to mimic endogenous LH surge (T1/2 = 10 hours)
	  – However, routine use not recommended due to high cost and lower pregnancy rate[7]
	• Kisspeptin-54:
	  – Neuropeptide acts at the hypothalamus to release endogenous GnRH resulting in an LH surge (~12–14 hours)
	  – Dose: 6.4–12.8 nmol/kg as a single bolus, or 19.2 nmol/kg as a split dosing over 10 hours[28]
	  – Use of KP in high-risk patients decreases OHSS risk[28]

To avoid hCG as luteal phase support (LPS)	• hCG, similar to LH in its physiological actions, has been used as LPS drug. This increases the risk of OHSS with no effect on clinical pregnancy or live birth rate • The risk of OHSS is approximately half with use of progesterone only as LPS compared with hCG[17]
In vitro maturation (IVM)	• Retrieval of immature oocytes to prevent OHSS in PCOS, PCO-like ovaries and previous history of severe OHSS • IVM is not used widely due to low implantation, pregnancy, and live birth rates as with standard IVF treatment • However due to recent advancements in cryopreservation techniques, there has been an improvement in the clinical outcomes[29]

TABLE 8: Secondary prevention strategies.

Interventions for secondary prevention	Recommendations
Coasting	• Gonadotropins are withdrawn whilst continuing agonist until E2 levels significantly decrease or plateau • Delaying hCG trigger • Generally employed up to 4 days • Results in fewer oocytes being retrieved, decreases clinical pregnancy with no benefit on OHSS risk reduction (Cochrane review)[30]
Cryopreservation of all oocytes/embryos	Elective cryopreservation of all oocytes/embryos and their transfer in subsequent cycles to avoid endogenous hCG rise in fresh transfer cycles, which can exacerbate late-onset OHSS (fair evidence ASRM)[17]
Cycle cancellation	• Cancellation and withholding of hCG in GnRHa IVF protocol are the definitive methods to completely eliminate OHSS risk[17] • Causes financial and emotional burden

Colloid infusion-plasma expanders
• Human albumin
• Hydroxyethyl starch
• Mannitol
	• Human albumin:
	  – Acts as a carrier protein, binds and inactivates vasoactive molecules and by its oncotic function, maintains intravascular volume
	  – *Dose:* 50 g of 25% albumin in 500 mL of saline around the time of oocyte retrieval
	  – *Risks:* Allergic reactions, transmission of viruses and prions
	  – Decreases the pregnancy rate
	• Hydroxyethyl starch:
	  – Synthetic colloid alternative to albumin with similar properties
	  – *Dose:* 6% of 500–1,000 mL on the day of oocyte retrieval
	  – Cheaper and potentially safer alternative to human albumin
	• Mannitol:
	  – Osmotic diuretic
	  – *Dose:* 1–1.5 g/kg/dose, daily or twice a day
	  – Evidence suggests that plasma expanders reduce the rates of moderate and severe OHSS in high-risk women (Cochrane review)[31]

Dopamine agonist	• *Cabergoline:* Dopamine D2 receptor agonist inactivates VEGF receptor 2, thereby reduces vascular permeability • *Dose:* 0.5 mg/day × 8 days from the day of hCG trigger • Reduces the incidence of moderate or severe OHSS in high-risk women without any negative impact on the oocytes retrieved or clinical pregnancy • Recommended (good evidence)[32]
Intravenous (IV) calcium gluconate	• 10 mL of 10% calcium gluconate in 200 mL saline on the day of oocyte retrieval and for 3 days thereafter lowers the risk of OHSS risk[33,34] • *Mechanism:* Inhibits cAMP synthesis and cAMP-dependent renin secretion, which decreases angiotensin II synthesis and thus reduced VEGF levels
Vasopressin-induced VEGF secretion blockade	• Vasopressin V1a receptor antagonist, relcovaptan, inhibits VEGF in rat models[35] • Further research required
Miscellaneous: • Glucocorticoids • Luteal antagonist administration • Intramuscular progesterone • Ketoconazole	• Glucocorticoids have an inhibitory effect on VEGF gene expression in the vascular smooth muscle cells • Insufficient data to make recommendations of these to alleviate OHSS risk (ASRM 2016)[17]
Nonrecommended strategies Follicular aspiration	Aspiration of granulosa cells from one ovary so as to limit the production of OHSS mediators while allowing continued development of contralateral ovary[3]

(ASRM: American Society for Reproductive Medicine; cAMP: cyclic adenosine monophosphate; E2: estradiol; GnRHa: gonadotropin-releasing hormone agonist; hCG: human chorionic gonadotropin; IVF: in vitro fertilization; OHSS: ovarian hyperstimulation syndrome; VEGF: vascular endothelial growth factor)

Flowchart 1: Management of ovarian hyperstimulation syndrome (OHSS).

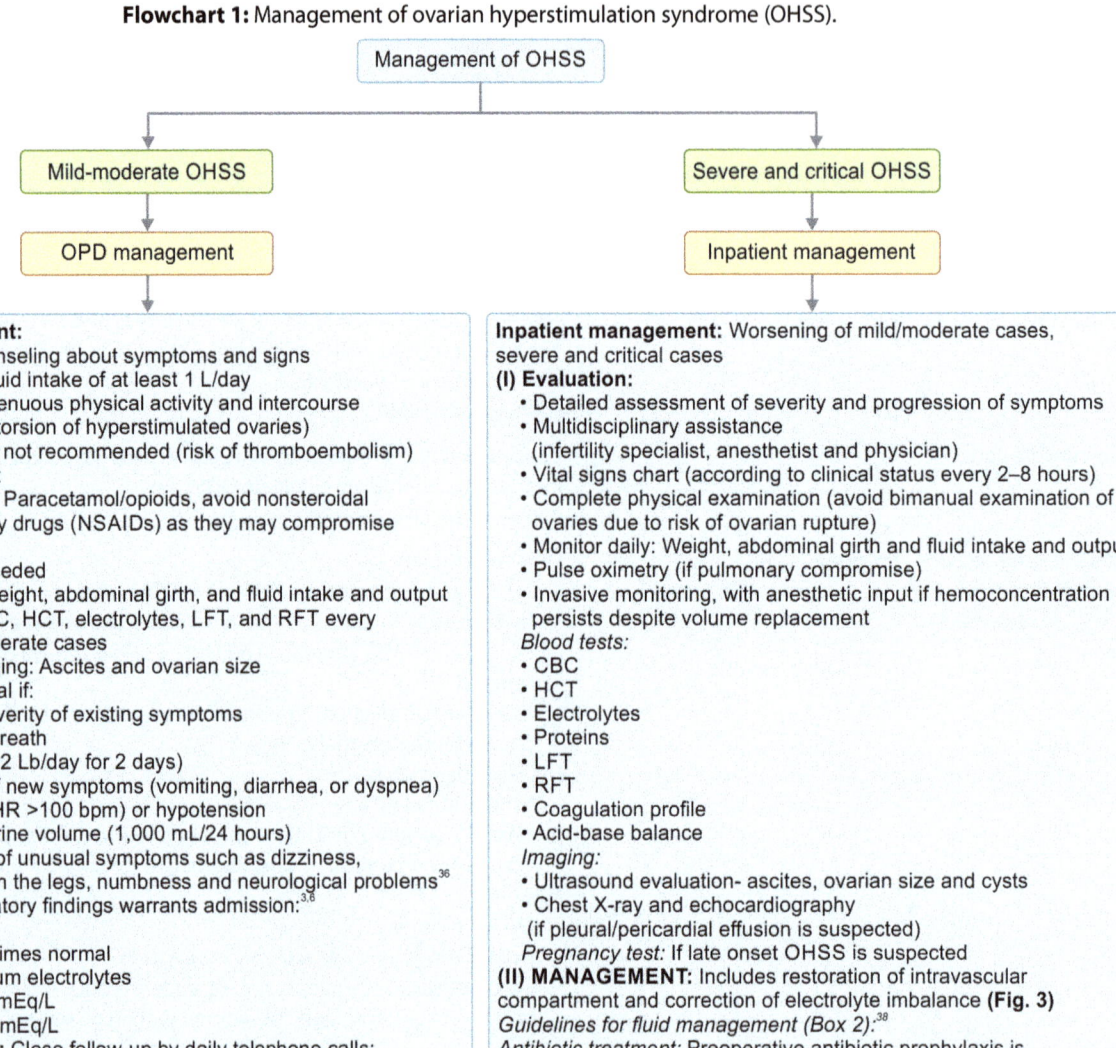

(CBC: complete blood count; HCT: hematocrit; HR: heart rate; LFT: liver function test; OHSS: ovarian hyperstimulation syndrome; OPD: outpatient department; RFT: renal function test)

OHSS-FREE CLINIC

- Segmentation strategy has been described by Dr Paul Devroey for an OHSS free clinic **(Fig. 4)**.[53]
- PCOS phenotype A (hyperandrogenism + PCOM + ovulatory dysfunction) seems to have a highest risk of OHSS and use of this strategy is beneficial.[54]

Measures to be taken by a Clinician for an OHSS-Free Clinic

The concept of "OHSS-free clinic" can soon be a reality if these preventive steps are resorted to **(Table 9)**.

SUMMARY

- OHSS is an iatrogenic complication of ovarian stimulation resulting in a spectrum of symptoms, with one end characterized by mild abdominal pain and distension due to enlarged ovaries to the other end manifested with signs and symptoms of massive ovarian enlargement and shift of fluid from the intravascular compartment to third space.
- Incidence of OHSS being 1–14% of all cycles, with mild accounting to about 20%–33% of stimulated cycles and severe to about 0.1-0.5%.
- Pathophysiology, being transudation of protein-rich fluid (mainly albumin) from intravascular to extravascular space with release of various vasoactive angiogenic factors, vascular endothelial growth factor (VEGF) playing a major role.
- Early OHSS occurs due to excessive ovarian response to exogenous hCG, whilst Late OHSS occurs due to endogenous hCG, from the implanting embryo and is more likely to be severe and long-lasting.

Fig. 3: Inpatient management of OHSS

[I] Maintain intravascular compartment
- IV fluids
- Plasma expanders

[II] Correction of electrolyte imbalance
Hyperkalemia: may lead to cardiac dysrhythmia
Treatment:[40,41]
- Use of sodium bicarbonate, insulin, and glucose, and albuterol—shifts potassium into the intracellular space
- Use of calcium gluconate to protect the cardiac tissue (if ECG shows changes) against hyperkalemia
- Kayexalate, administered orally or rectally as a retention enema

[III] Thromboprophylaxis
Incidence of thrombosis with OHSS: 0.7–10%[6]
Thromboprophylaxis is indicated in:[42-46]
- Immobilization
- Severe and critical OHSS
- Moderate OHSS (activation of intrinsic coagulation cascade) with risk factors for thrombosis
- Hypercoagulable state due to pregnancy or high estrogen
- Obesity
- Factor V Leiden mutation, antithrombin III deficiency, protein C and S deficiency
- Personal or familial history of thrombosis

Use of full-length venous support stockings

Low-molecular weight heparin: Enoxaparin (40 mg) or dalteparin (5,000 IU) daily is recommended and continued at least until discharge from hospital and possibly longer, depending on other risk factors[6,45]

[IV] Paracentesis
Paracentesis (aspiration of ascitic fluid), indications:[46,47]
- Tense painful ascites
- Respiratory compromise (tachypnea, hypoxia, hydrothorax) secondary to ascites and increased intra-abdominal pressure
- Oliguria/anuria despite adequate volume restoration, secondary to increased abdominal pressure causing reduced renal perfusion

Paracentesis is effective in resolving hydrothorax and thoracentesis, indicated for those with persistent bilateral or severe pleural effusions.[46,48]

Done under ultrasound guidance, either abdominally or vaginally, slowly and maximum of 4 L over 12 hours to be aspirated

Monitoring of plasma proteins is required and IV colloid therapy to be given when large amount of fluids has been removed.[37]

[V] Surgery
- Adnexal torsion: Laparoscopic untwisting of torted hyperstimulated ovaries
- Rupture of ovarian cyst
- Ectopic/heterotopic pregnancy

Fig. 3: Inpatient management of OHSS. (ECG: electrocardiogram; IV: intravenous; OHSS: ovarian hyperstimulation syndrome)

BOX 2: Fluid management in severe/critical OHSS.

- Oral fluid intake guided by thirst (at least 1 L/day)
- IV crystalloids: Started at a rate of 125–150 mL/hour
- Initial rapid hydration may be done with a bolus of IV fluids (500–1,000 mL)
- IV fluid administration should be carefully titrated so as to reverse hemoconcentration and to maintain an adequate urine output (20–30 mL/hour)
- 5% dextrose in normal saline is preferred to Ringer lactate (RL) solution (RL, avoided for the tendency of hyponatremia)
- Administration of IV fluids should be reduced when symptoms improve or when brisk diuresis starts and oral fluids being encouraged
- Plasma expanders: 25% albumin (50–100 g) infused over 4 hours, repeated 4- to 12-hourly, when infusion of IV fluids fails to maintain hemodynamic stability and adequate urine output.
- Diuretics: (Furosemide 20 mg IV) may be considered after restoring adequate intravascular volume (hematocrit <38%) if: (1) oliguria persists despite adequate fluid replacement, and drainage of ascites and (2) in the management of pulmonary edema

(IV: intravenous; OHSS: ovarian hyperstimulation syndrome)

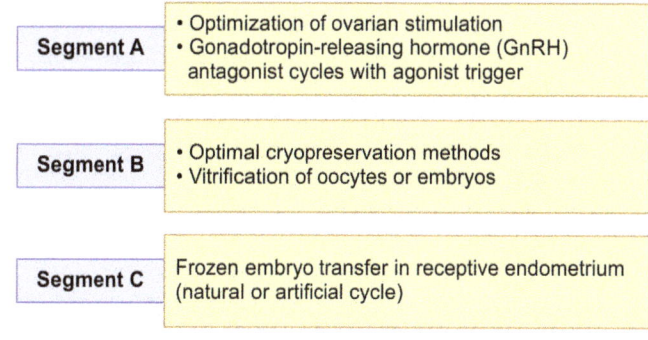

Segment A
- Optimization of ovarian stimulation
- Gonadotropin-releasing hormone (GnRH) antagonist cycles with agonist trigger

Segment B
- Optimal cryopreservation methods
- Vitrification of oocytes or embryos

Segment C
Frozen embryo transfer in receptive endometrium (natural or artificial cycle)

Fig. 4: Segmentation strategy.

- The first step to predict OHSS is to identify patients who are at risk of OHSS; younger age, Lean PCOS with high AMH>3.36ng/ml, PCOM on USG and previous history of OHSS.
- Mild and moderate OHSS cases can be managed on OPD basis by appropriate counselling about the symptoms and signs and regular follow-up.

TABLE 9: Measures to be taken for an OHSS-free clinic.

Before stimulation	• Identify patients at risk of OHSS • Antagonist protocol • Individualizing IVF treatment
During stimulation	• iCOS • Mild stimulation • Chronic low-dose step-up protocol • Insulin-sensitizing agents • Low-dose aspirin • Trigger-GnRH agonist
After OPU	• Freeze all oocytes/embryos • Intravenous albumin/hydroxyethyl starch • Calcium gluconate infusion • Dopamine agonists
Luteal phase support	Avoid hCG for LPS

(GnRH: gonadotropin-releasing hormone; hCG: human chorionic gonadotropin; LPS: luteal phase support; iCOS: individualized controlled ovarian stimulation; IVF: in vitro fertilization; OHSS: ovarian hyperstimulation syndrome)

- An OHSS free clinic can be attained by opting for an antagonist protocol, individualizing IVF Treatment, use of mild stimulation, chronic low-dose step-up protocol, Dopamine agonists and segmentation strategy.

Key Learning Points

- OHSS is an iatrogenic complication of ovarian over stimulation resulting in fatal systemic complications if severe, and is largely preventable, if appropriate preventive measures are undertaken.
- Triggering factor for OHSS, being hCG (exogenous/endogenous).
- Prevention of OHSS becomes paramount importance with an exponential increase in the number of ART cycles over the decades.
- Prevention begins with identification of risk factors and individualized stimulation protocols.
- Segmentation strategy-GnRH antagonist cycles with agonist trigger, freezing all oocytes/embryos followed by frozen embryo transfer needs to be followed for an OHSS-free clinic.
- Identification and close monitoring of patients with mild to moderate OHSS is important to prevent its progression to severe/critical stage.

■ REFERENCES

1. Papanikolaou EG, Pozzobon C, Kolibianakis EM, Camus M, Tournaye H, Fatemi HM. Incidence and prediction of ovarian hyperstimulation syndrome in women undergoing gonadotropin-releasing hormone antagonist in vitro fertilization cycles. Fertil Steril. 2006;85:112-20.
2. Golan A, Ron-El R, Herman A, Soffer Y, Weinraub Z, Caspi E. Ovarian hyperstimulation syndrome: an update review. Obstet Gynecol Surv. 1989;44:430-40.
3. Humaidan P, Quartarolo J, Papanikolaou EG. Preventing ovarian hyperstimulation syndrome: guidance for the clinician. Fertil Steril. 2010;94:389-400.
4. Mathur RS, Akande VA, Keay SD, Hunt LP, Jenkins NM. Distinction between early and late ovarian hyperstimulation syndrome. Fertil Steril. 2000;73:901-7.
5. De Leener A, Montanelli L, Van Durme J, Chae H, Smits G, Vassart G, et al. Presence and absence of follicle-stimulating hormone receptor mutations provide some insights into spontaneous ovarian hyperstimulation syndrome physiopathology. J Clin Endocrinol Metab. 2006;91(2):555-62.
6. Royal College of Obstetricians and Gynaecologists. The Management of Ovarian Hyperstimulation Syndrome. Green-top Guideline No. 5. London: RCOG; 2016.
7. Schenker JG, Polishuk WZ. The role of prostaglandins in ovarian hyperstimulation syndrome. Eur J Obstet Gynecol Reprod Biol. 1976;6:47-52.
8. Smith V, Osianlis T, Vollenhoven B. Prevention of Ovarian Hyperstimulation syndrome: A review. Obstet Gynecol Int. 2015;2015:514159.
9. Pellicer A, Albert C, Mercader A, Bonilla-Musoles F, Remohi J, Simon C. The pathogenesis of ovarian hyperstimulation syndrome: In vivo studies investigating the role of interleukin-1beta, interleukin-6, and vascular endothelial growth factor. Fertil Steril. 1999;71:482-9.
10. Aboulghar MA, Mansour RT, Serour GI, El Helw BA, Shaarawy M. Elevated levels of interleukin-2, soluble interleukin-2 receptor alpha, interleukin-6, soluble interleukin-6 receptor and vascular endothelial growth factor in serum and ascitic fluid of patients with severe ovarian hyperstimulation syndrome. Eur J Obstet Gynecol Reprod Biol. 1999;87:81-5.
11. Whelan JG, Vlahos NF. The ovarian hyperstimulation syndrome. Fertil Steril. 2000;73:883-96.
12. Levin ER, Rosen GF, Cassidenti DL, Yee B, Meldrum D, Wisot A, et al. Role of vascular endothelial growth factor in ovarian hyperstimulation syndrome. J Clin Invest. 1998;102:1978-85.
13. Neulen J, Yan Z, Raczek S, Weindel K, Keck C, Weich HA, et al. Human chorionic gonadotropin-dependent expression of vascular endothelial growth factor/vascular permeability factor in human granulosa cells: importance in ovarian hyperstimulation syndrome. J Clin Endocrinol Metab. 1995;80:1967-71.
14. Herr D, Bekes I, Wulff C. Local Renin-Angiotensin system in the reproductive system. Front Endocrinol (Lausanne). 2013;4:150.
15. Rotterdam ESHRE-ASRM Sponsored PCOS Consensus Workshop Group. Revised 2003 consensus on diagnostic criteria and long-term health risks related to polycystic ovary syndrome. Hum Reprod. 2004;81(1):19-25.
16. Lee TH, Liu CH, Huang CC, Wu YL, Shih YT, Ho HN, et al. Serum anti-müllerian hormone and estradiol levels as predictors of ovarian hyperstimulation syndrome in assisted reproduction technology cycles. Hum Reprod. 2008;23:160-7.
17. Practice Committee of the American Society for Reproductive Medicine. Prevention and treatment of moderate and severe ovarian hyperstimulation syndrome: a guideline. Fertil Steril. 2016;106:1634-47.
18. Kahnberg A, Enskog A, Brannstrom M, Lundin K, Bergh C. Prediction of ovarian hyperstimulation syndrome in women undergoing in vitro fertilization. Acta Obstet Gynecol Scand. 2009;88:1373-81.
19. Jayaprakasan K, Chan Y, Islam R, Haoula Z, Hopkisson J, Coomarasamy A, et al. Prediction of in vitro fertilization outcome at different antral follicle count thresholds in a prospective cohort of 1,012 women. Fertil Steril. 2012;98:657-63.

20. Lamazou F, Legouez A, Letouzey V, Grynberg M, Deffieux X, Trichot C, et al. Ovarian hyperstimulation syndrome: Pathophysiology, risk factors, prevention, diagnosis and treatment]. J Gynecol Obstet Biol Reprod (Paris). 2011;40:593-611.
21. Howles CM, Alam V, Tredway D, Homburg R, Warne DW. Factors related to successful ovulation induction in patients with WHO group II anovulatory infertility. Reprod Biomed Online. 2010;20:182-90.
22. Lee VC, Ledger W. Aromatase inhibitors for ovulation induction and ovarian stimulation. Clin Endocrinol (Oxf). 2011;74:537-46.
23. Franik S, Kremer JA, Nelen WL, Farquhar C. Aromatase inhibitors for subfertile women with polycystic ovary syndrome. Cochrane Database Syst Rev. 2014;(2):CD010287.
24. Homburg R. Management of infertility and prevention of ovarian hyperstimulation in women with polycystic ovary syndrome. Best Pract Res Clin Obstet Gynaecol. 2004;18:773-88.
25. Bosch E, Ezcurra D. Individualised controlled ovarian stimulation (iCOS): Maximising success rates for assisted reproductive technology patients. Reprod Biol Endocrinol. 2011;9:82.
26. Al-Inany HG, Abou-Setta AM, Aboulghar M. Gonadotrophin-releasing hormone antagonists for assisted conception. Cochrane Database Syst Rev. 2006;4:CD001750.
27. Kolibianakis EM, Collins J, Tarlatzis BC, Devroey P, Diedrich K, Griesinger G. Among patients treated for IVF with gonadotrophins and GnRH analogues, is the probability of live birth dependent on the type of analogue used? A systematic review and meta-analysis. Hum Reprod Update. 2006;12:651-71.
28. Abbara A, Islam R, Clarke SA, Jeffers L, Christopoulos G, Comninos AN, et al. Clinical parameters of ovarian hyperstimulation syndrome following different hormonal triggers of oocyte maturation in IVF treatment. Clinical Endocrinology. 2018;88:920-7.
29. Hatırnaz S, Ata B, Saynur E, Hatırnaz ES. Oocyte in vitro maturation: A systematic review. Turk J Obstet Gynecol. 2018;15:112-25.
30. D'Angelo A, Brown J, Amso NN. Coasting (withholding gonadotrophins) for preventing ovarian hyperstimulation syndrome. Cochrane Database Syst Rev. 2001;(3):CD002811.
31. Youssef MA, Mourad S. Volume expanders for the prevention of ovarian hyperstimulation syndrome. Cochrane Database Syst Rev. 2016;(8):CD001302.
32. Leitao VMS, Moroni RM, Seko LMD, Nastri CO, Martins WP. Cabergoline for the prevention of ovarian hyperstimulation syndrome: systematic review and meta-analysis of randomized controlled trials. Fertil Steril. 2014;101(3):664-75.e7.
33. Yakovenko S, Sivozhelezov V, Zorina I, Dmitrieva N, Apryshko V, Voznesenskaya J. Prevention of OHSS by intravenous calcium. Hum Reprod. 2009;24:i61.
34. Naredi N, Karunakaran S. Calcium gluconate infusion is as effective as the vascular endothelial growth factor antagonist cabergoline for the prevention of ovarian hyperstimulation syndrome. J Hum Reprod Sci. 2013;6:248-52.
35. Cenksoy C, Cenksoy PO, Erdem O, Sancak B, Gursoy R. A potential novel strategy, inhibition of vasopressin induced VEGF secretion by relcovaptan, for decreasing the incidence of ovarian hyperstimulation syndrome in the hyperstimulated rat model. Eur J Obstet Gynecol Reprod Biol. 2014;174:86-90.
36. Delvigne A, Rozenberg S. Review of clinical course and treatment of ovarian hyperstimulation syndrome (OHSS). Hum Reprod Update. 2003;9:77-96.
37. Rizk B. Ovarian Hyperstimulation Syndrome: Epidemiology, Pathophysiology, Prevention and Management, 1st edition. Cambridge: Cambridge University Press; 2006.
38. Youssef MA, Al-Inany HG, Evers JL, Aboulghar M. Intravenous fluids for the prevention of severe ovarian hyperstimulation syndrome. Cochrane Database Syst Rev. 2011;(2):CD001302.
39. Jakimiuk AJ, Fritz A, Grzybowski W, Walecka I, Lewandowski P. Diagnosing and management of iatrogenic moderate and severe ovarian hyperstimulation syndrome (OHSS) in clinical material. Folia Histochem Cytobiol. 2007;45 Suppl 1:S105-8.
40. Budev MM, Arroliga AC, Falcone T. Ovarian hyperstimulation syndrome. Crit Care Med. 2005;33:S301-6.
41. Alper MM, Smith LP, Sills ES. Ovarian hyperstimulation syndrome: Current views on pathophysiology, risk factors, prevention, and management. J Exp Clin Assist Reprod. 2009;6:3.
42. Rizk B, Meagher S, Fisher AM. Severe ovarian hyperstimulation syndrome and cerebrovascular accidents. Hum Reprod. 1990;5:697-8.
43. Fabregues F, Tassies D, Reverter JC, Carmona F, Ordinas A, Balasch J. Prevalence of thrombophilia in women with severe ovarian hyperstimulation syndrome and cost-effectiveness of screening. Fertil Steril. 2004;81:989-95.
44. Chen CD, Chen SU, Yang YS. Prevention and management of ovarian hyperstimulation syndrome. Best Pract Res Clin Obstet Gynaecol. 2012;26:817-27.
45. Nelson SM, Greer IA. The potential role of heparin in assisted conception. Hum Reprod Update. 2008;14:623-45.
46. Abramov Y, Elchalal U, Schenker JG. Pulmonary manifestations of severe ovarian hyperstimulation syndrome: A multicentre study. Fertil Steril. 1999;71:645-51.
47. ASRM Educational Bulletin. Ovarian hyperstimulation syndrome. Fertil Steril. 2008;90:S188-93.
48. Rinaldi ML, Spirtos NJ. Chest tube drainage of pleural effusion correcting abdominal ascites in a patient with severe ovarian hyperstimulation syndrome: A case report. Fertil Steril. 1995;63:1114-7.
49. Cupisti S, Emran J, Mueller A, Dittrich R, Beckmann MW, Binder H. Course of ovarian hyperstimulation syndrome in 19 intact twin pregnancies after assisted reproduction techniques, with a case report of severe thrombo embolism. Twin Res Hum Genet. 2006;9:691-6.
50. Papanikolaou EG, Tournaye H, Verpoest W, Camus M, Vernaeve V, Van Steirteghem A, et al. Early and late ovarian hyperstimulation syndrome: early pregnancy outcome and profile. Hum Reprod. 2005;20:636-41.
51. Courbiere B, Oborski V, Braunstein D, Desparoir A, Noizet A, Gamerre M. Obstetric outcome of women with in vitro fertilization pregnancies hospitalized for ovarian hyper stimulation syndrome: a case-control study. Fertil Steril. 2011;95:1629-32.
52. Schirmer DA, Kulkarni AD, Zhang Y, Kawwass JF. Ovarian hyperstimulation syndrome after assisted reproductive technologies: trends, predictors, and pregnancy outcomes. Fertil Steril. 2020;114:567-78.
53. Devroey P, Polyzos NP, Blockeel C. An OHSS-Free Clinic by segmentation of IVF treatment. Hum Reprod. 2011; 26(10):2593-7.
54. Cela V, Obino MER, Alberga Y, Pinelli S, Sergiampietri C, Casarosa E, et al. Ovarian response to controlled ovarian stimulation in women with different polycystic ovary syndrome phenotypes. Gynecol Endocrinol. 2018;34(6):518-23.

CHAPTER 21

Pregnancy of Unknown Location

Veronica Irene Yuel

■ OVERVIEW

An increasing awareness of women has led to many women attending pregnancy care units earlier and more frequent. This has led to an increase in the detection of pregnancy of unknown location—a condition marked by positive pregnancy tests but no ultrasonographic evidence of intrauterine or extrauterine pregnancy.

Diagnosis is important to avoid a catastrophic event like ectopic pregnancy, biomarkers and ultrasonography help one establish a diagnosis.

Management here is mainly conservative, with surgical intervention to be resorted to only in very few cases.

A point of concern—treatment may sometimes disturb a healthy viable intrauterine pregnancy.

Keywords: Pregnancy unknown location; viable/nonviable pregnancy/methotrexate management.

■ INTRODUCTION

Pregnancy of unknown location or origin (PUL) is a condition where the pregnancy test of women is positive but there are no demonstrable signs of either an intrauterine or extrauterine pregnancy, on a transvaginal ultrasonography (USG).[1]

This condition is different from an ectopic pregnancy (EP) also. Many times no diagnosis can be made as the location of such a pregnancy remains unidentified, and also, at times early miscarriages and ectopic may also resolve on its own.

■ INCIDENCE

An incidence between 5 and 42% has been reported in various studies. The incidence differs on availability of resources for detecting these pregnancies. A high-resolution USG performed by skilled physicians may report a higher incidence.[2,3] On an average, the overall incidence may be between 8 and 15% as the majority of the places have good USG machines and expertise.

■ CLASSIFICATION OF PREGNANCY OF UNKNOWN LOCATION

Pregnancy of unknown location is classified retrospectively, mainly on the basis of the outcome on follow-up.[1] Thus they can be classified into:

- *Intrauterine pregnancy (IUP):* Based on early ultrasonographic assessment, comprising of nearly 30–47% of women with a positive test, these are classified into:[4,5]
  - Viable IUP—where the ultrasonographic findings are compatible with the gestation
  - IUP of uncertain viability—where the ultrasound shows definite features of IUP but is uncertain about viability
  - *Nonviable IUP:* Where the ultrasound features show nonviable pregnancy
- *Failed PUL (PULF):* In this scenario, there is a positive pregnancy test with ultrasound findings suggestive of an early pregnancy but eventually early in the pregnancy the beta-human chorionic gonadotropin (β-hCG) falls and the end result is a spontaneous resolution of pregnancy.
- *EP:* Those EPs which are resolved spontaneously before actually getting detected as a demonstrable EP.
- *Persistent PUL (PPUL):* It consists in around 2% of patients of PUL.[6] These cases are marked by a plateauing or abnormal rise of the hCG levels (<15% rise in hCG levels over three consecutive 48-hour interval) or if at all a fall occurs it is very slow.

Transvaginal sonography does not reveal any intrauterine/EP. These pregnancies may also be either small ectopic pregnancies that have not been visualized on ultrasound or they may be small retained products of conception where a small portion of the trophoblast may be active. Based on the outcome PPUL may be grouped into:[1]

- EP not visualized—here hCG levels continue to rise despite an evacuation.
- Treated PUL—treatment is administered without any localization of the pregnancy.
- Resolved PUL—as the name suggests, PUL that resolves without any management.

- Histopathological IUP—pregnancy identified by presence of chorionic tissue in histopathology specimen obtained after evacuation.

CLINICAL FEATURES

No definite clinical features are found to be present. Some of the commonly associated features are:

- *Positive pregnancy test:* A women who has either missed her periods or has had very scanty menses compared to the last cycle with a positive pregnancy test either a card test or hCG levels in blood; and no demonstrable ultrasound parameters of a pregnancy anywhere. This may be associated with or without other features mentioned here.
- *Pelvic pain:* It is also a feature in many women during early pregnancy.
- *Vaginal bleeding:* In the presence of other features, this symptom may or may not be there.
- PUL constitutes a good number of patients attending antenatal clinics with this early pregnancy complication.

DIAGNOSIS

Diagnosis is based on the measurements of biomarkers (enumerated here) in the absence of ultrasound or laparoscopic visualization[6] of a pregnancy anywhere in the abdomen. These biomarkers are:

- *Serum hCG:* Measurements of serum hCG levels and correlating it with ultrasound findings is an important feature in diagnosing PULs. hCG levels >1,500–2000[7,8] have been able to document a gestation sac on transvaginal sonography. A value above 6,500 and above will demonstrate a gestation sac on transabdominal ultrasound.[9] A diagnosis of PUL can be made only once no ultrasonographic evidence of a pregnancy is there even after the hCG levels have gone up beyond the discriminatory level findings on ultrasound. Along with this, the studies have advocated single as well as serial measurements of hCG levels are good enough in the diagnosis of PULs though single levels have limited value.[10]
- *Serum hCG and USG:* Women where the hCG levels have gone beyond the above expected values but there is no evidence of a gestational sac in the uterus should raise the suspicion of EP. A careful high-resolution sonography in the hands of an expert should be done to exclude an EP. There may also be presence of fluid in the uterine cavity suggesting a pseudo sac. Along with this, serial measurements of hCG levels coupled with ultrasound findings can fairly distinguish between an EP, viable early IUP, or a failing pregnancy.[11-13]

Measurement of endometrial thickness on ultrasound is another parameter that can be taken into consideration. Endometrial thickness has been reported to be thinner in women with ectopic compared with intrauterine gestations[14,15] although there may be a significant overlap of endometrial thickness, hence, it cannot be used as a single marker in the diagnosis of EP. Transvaginal color Doppler when used may not increase the detection rates of EP when compared to 2D ultrasound but may be useful in showing presence of trophoblastic flow.[16]

In nonviable pregnancies ending up as miscarriages or spontaneous abortions, the serial measurements of hCG will give a good clinch to the diagnosis. The levels will eventually fall serially and come down to zero. The fall in hCG levels in a women undergoing dilation and curettage (D&C) for a miscarriage has been reported to be around 12–16 days.[12]

- *Serum progesterone:* Measurement of serum progesterone levels helps us to establish the viability of a pregnancy, but, they are not good indicators for establishing the location of a pregnancy.[10] Progesterone level <20 nmol/L indicates a failing pregnancy, while level >60 nmol/L is strongly associated with a viable pregnancy. Serum progesterone is the best single marker for viability while progesterone and hCG levels when used together are the best predictors of a spontaneously resolving PUL.[17]
- *Serum CA-125:* Another biomarker that has been suggested in the measurement of PULs, though CA-125 ratio at 48 and 0 hours have been found to be more discriminatory in differentiating a failing PUL from a viable one.[18]
- *Inhibin A levels:* Another useful marker in identifying spontaneously resolving PUL where its levels are significantly lower when compared to the levels seen in IUP or ectopic pregnancies. All pregnancies for which the inhibin A level is <11 pmol/L are considered spontaneously resolving PULs.[17]
- *Other biomarkers:* Insulin-like growth factor-binding protein-1 (IGFBP-1) levels for spontaneously resolving PULs, inhibin pro-aC-RI levels, IGFBPs, and creatine kinase (CK) are nonspecific markers, CK and CK-MB levels are some of the other markers that have been mentioned; however, their role in determining PUL is yet to be established.[19]
- *Magnetic resonance imaging:* A good tool in diagnosing EP thus helps in differentiating a PUL from an ectopic gestation.[20]

DIFFERENTIAL DIAGNOSIS

Pregnancy of unknown location may have four possibilities:
1. Very early pregnancy, not yet detected with ultrasound
2. Nonviable IUP not detected with ultrasound
3. Complete miscarriage
4. Unidentified EP.

MANAGEMENT OF PREGNANCY OF UNKNOWN LOCATION

Management of women with PUL is based on correct identification of the case with the risk associated and its categorization into the various class of PUL. Management of these cases is therefore based on the fact that a timely identification of an EP versus a viable or nonviable gestation should be done so that timely intervention may save a patient from a catastrophic event. An algorithm for management of these patients may be defined on these norms.

According to the Association of Early Pregnancy Units guidelines,[21] advocate conservation management of these pregnancies so long as a definite sign of ectopic, viable, or nonviable pregnancy is documented. Conservative management is based on:

- *Serum hCG pattern at 48 hours:* Rise or fall in hCG levels has been very helpful in differentiating between an ectopic, viable IUP, and a failing PUL. A healthy viable pregnancy is marked by a doubling of hCG levels in 48 hours reported in many studies.[13,22] When the rise is there but it does not double in 48 hours or the rise is suboptimal, it points more toward an EP.[22,23] Falling hCG levels are indicative of a failing PUL.[23]
- *hCG ratio:* Formed by taking hCG levels at 48 hours: hCG levels at 0 hours. Studies have mentioned a cutoff level <0.87 is helpful in predicting failing PULs, ectopic, and nonviable pregnancies.[24,25]
- *Serum hCG and progesterone:*
- Serum progesterone <20 ng/mL and serum β-hCG >25 IU/L indicates a resolving pregnancy, repeat urine pregnancy test in 7 days.
- Serum progesterone 20–60 ng/mL and serum β-hCG >25 IU/L (<1,000 IU/L), most likely an EP, repeat serum hCG at 48 hours.
- Serum progesterone >60 ng/mL and serum β-hCG <1,000 IU/L, likely to be a normal pregnancy, transvaginal USG should be performed at hCG levels above 1,000 IU/L.
- Serum progesterone >20 ng/mL and serum β-hCG >1,000 IU/L, then the possible diagnosis is EP, transvaginal USG should be repeated as soon as possible or laparoscopy may be performed.[17]

Treatment

Expectant management is the mainstay in these pregnancies as majority of them resolve spontaneously to a diagnosis. Therefore, strict monitoring both with biochemical markers and USG should be done and treated accordingly.

Based on the various markers and tests, high risk patients are identified, and categorized into medical management versus those requiring surgical management.

TABLE 1: Methotrexate regimen for PUL—based on diagnosis and hCG level monitoring.

Day	Investigations and methotrexate
0	Blood group, complete blood count, renal function tests, and liver function tests
1	Serum β-hCG, injection methotrexate 50 mg/m^2
4	Serum hCG
7	Serum hCG

If hCG decrease >15% repeat hCG weekly until 10 IU/L

Second dose of methotrexate if hCG decrease <15% on days 4–7

Methotrexate may be repeated weekly till the decrease >15% is consistently achieved

(hCG: human chorionic gonadotropin; PUL: pregnancy of unknown location)

Medical Management

Medical management of PUL has a limited role. Methotrexate has been advocated only in certain cases of ectopic pregnancies with careful monitoring. Methotrexate 50 mg/m^2 has been found to be 90% effective[21] without resorting to surgical management. Monitoring that needs to be done and protocol to be followed has been tabulated in **Table 1**.

Single dose regimen is usually the most tolerated and accepted, however, some may need a multidose regime with a folinic acid rescue.

After methotrexate has been used, the patient should be advised to defer pregnancy for 3 months post therapy.

Surgical Management

Uterine curettage and laparoscopy have been two methods used in the treatment of PUL.[10] Uterine curettage has been advocated by some in cases of nonviable pregnancies. It helps one to establish those PULs which are to be categorized as miscarriages and need further evaluation. Presence of chorionic villi in the curettage material helps one to establish this diagnosis. Another favorable point for uterine evacuation is that the unnecessary use of methotrexate would be avoided in up to 50% of cases.[26] However, presence of chorionic villi may not be there in every case of nonviable pregnancy. So, in such cases, an EP should be ruled out by doing an hCG titer. A fall in the hCG titer by ≥15% is suggestive of a nonviable pregnancy. If the titer is plateaued or the fall is less than a suspicion of EP then methotrexate is indicated in such cases. Uterine curettage is advocated only after a viable IUP has been carefully ruled out, as this procedure carries a risk of disturbing a viable IUP.[27]

Laparoscopy/laparotomy is performed in cases of ectopic pregnancies after a failed medical management or if the patient is hemodynamically unstable.

Both the surgical methods are not used routinely in the management of PUL.[10]

Flowchart 1: Algorithm for management of pregnancy of unknown location (PUL).

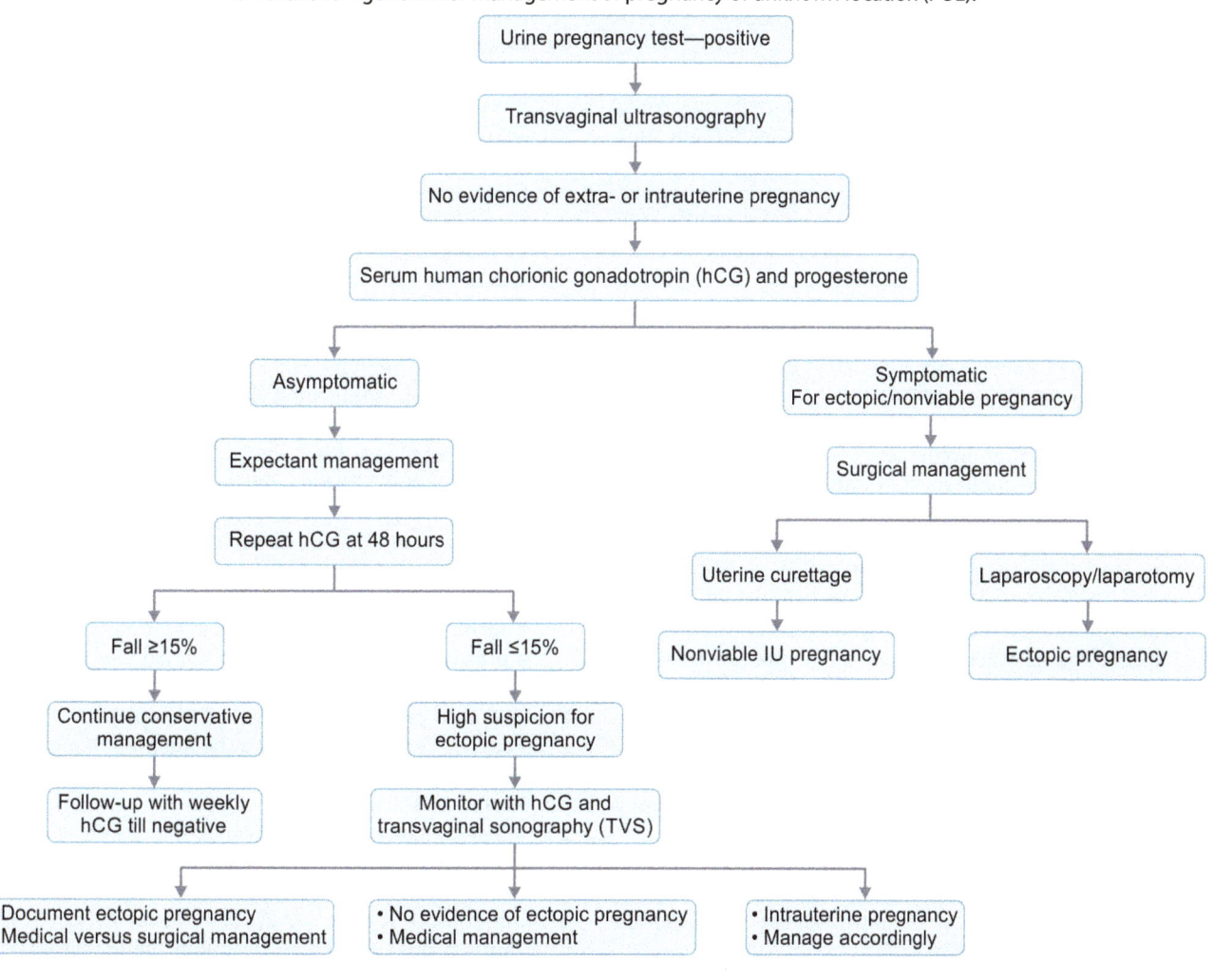

Algorithm for the management of PUL is presented in **Flowchart 1**.

CONCLUSION

Incidence of women with PUL has increased due to an increase in the detection rate, occurring due to the advances in technology and expertise.

Serum hCG, progesterone, CA-125, and inhibin are some of the prime markers that help in prediction of these pregnancies.

Regular follow-up and frequent visits help one to carefully establish the diagnosis.

No specific algorithm is there to manage these patients. Expectant management is advocated in majority, medical management with methotrexate for some and surgical management in select cases. Laparoscopy/laparotomy is performed in hemodynamically unstable patients.

REFERENCES

1. Barnhart K, van Mello NM, Bourne T, Kirk E, Van Calster B, Bottomley C, et al. Pregnancy of unknown location: a consensus statement of nomenclature, definitions, and outcome. Fertil Steril. 2011;95:857-66.
2. Cordina M, Schramm-Gajraj K, Ross JA, Lautman K, Jurkovic D. Introduction of a single visit protocol in the management of selected patients with pregnancy of unknown location: a prospective study. BJOG. 2011;118:693-7.
3. Banerjee S, Aslam N, Woelfer B, Lawrence A, Elson J, Jurkovic D. Expectant management of early pregnancies of unknown location: a prospective evaluation of methods to predict spontaneous resolution of pregnancy. BJOG. 2001;108:158-63.
4. Kirk E, Bottomley C, Bourne T. Diagnosing ectopic pregnancy and current concepts in the management of pregnancy of unknown location. Hum Reprod Update. 2014;20(2):250-61.
5. Reid S, Condous G. Is there a need to definitively diagnose the location of a pregnancy of unknown location? The case for "no". Fertil Steril. 2012;98(5):1085-90.
6. Condous G, Lu C, Van Huffel S, Timmerman D, Bourne T. Human chorionic gonadotrophin and progesterone levels for the investigation of pregnancies of unknown location. Int J Gynecol Obstet. 2004;86:351-7.
7. Barnhart KT, Simhan H, Kamelle SA. Diagnostic accuracy of ultrasound above and below the β-hCG discriminatory zone. Obstet Gynecol. 1999;94:583-7.
8. Condous G, Kirk E, Lu C, Van Huffel S, Gevaert O, De Moor B, et al. Diagnostic accuracy of varying discriminatory zones

for the prediction of ectopic pregnancy in women with a pregnancy of unknown location. Ultrasound Obstet Gynaecol. 2005;26:770-5.
9. Romero R, Kadar N, Jeanty P, Copel JA, Chervenak FA, DeCherney A, et al. Diagnosis of ectopic pregnancy: value of the discriminatory human chorionic gonadotropin zone. Obstet Gynecol. 1985;66:357-60.
10. Kirk E, Condous G, Bourne T. Pregnancies of unknown location. Best Pract Res Clin Obstet Gynaecol. 2009;23:493-9.
11. Barnhart KT. Clinical practice. Ectopic pregnancy. N Engl J Med. 2009;361:379-87.
12. Barnhart K, Sammel MD, Chung K, Zhou L, Hummel AC, Guo W. Decline of serum human chorionic gonadotropin and spontaneous complete abortion: defining the normal curve. Obstet Gynecol. 2004;104:975-81.
13. Barnhart KT, Sammel MD, Rinaudo PF, Zhou L, Hummel AC, Guo W. Symptomatic patients with an early viable intrauterine pregnancy: HCG curves redefined. Obstet Gynecol. 2004;104:50-5.
14. Hammoud AO, Hammoud I, Bujold E, Gonik B, Diamond MP, Johnson SC. The role of sonographic endometrial patterns and endometrial thickness in the differential diagnosis of ectopic pregnancy. Am J Obstet Gynecol. 2005;192:1370-5.
15. Dart RG, Dart L, Mitchell P, Berty C. The predictive value of endometrial stripe thickness in patients with suspected ectopic pregnancy who have an empty uterus at ultrasonography. Acad Emerg Med. 1999;6:602-8.
16. Ardaens Y, Guérin B, Perrot N, Legoeff F. Contribution of ultrasonography in the diagnosis of ectopic pregnancy. J Gynecol Obstet Biol Reprod. 2003;32 Suppl 7:S28-38.
17. Chetty M, Sawyer E, Dew T, Chapman AJ, Elson J. The use of novel biochemical markers in predicting spontaneously resolving 'pregnancies of unknown location'. Hum Reprod. 2011;26:1318-23.
18. Condous G, Kirk E, Syed A, Van Calster B, Van Huffel S, Timmerman D, et al. Do levels of serum cancer antigen 125 and creatine kinase predict the outcome in pregnancies of unknown location? Hum Reprod. 2005;20:3348-54.
19. Kruchkovich J, Orvieto R, Fytlovich S, Lavie O, Anteby EY, Gemer O. The role of CPK isoenzymes in predicting extrauterine early pregnancy. Arch Gynecol Obstet. 2012;286:135-7.
20. Yoshigi J, Yashiro N, Kinoshita T, O'uchi T, Kitagaki H. Diagnosis of ectopic pregnancy with MRI: efficacy of T2-weighted imaging. Magn Reson Med Sci. 2006;5:25-32.
21. Earlypregnancy.org. Association of Early Pregnancy Units. Guidelines 2007. [online] available from www.earlypregnancy.org.uk/documents/AEPUGuidelines2007.pdf. [Last accessed November, 2022].
22. Seeber BE, Sammel MD, Guo W, Zhou L, Hummel A, Barnhart KT. Application of redefined human chorionic gonadotropin curves for the diagnosis of women at risk for ectopic pregnancy. Fertil Steril. 2006;86:454-9.
23. Ling FW, Stovall TG. Update on the diagnosis and management of ectopic pregnancy. In: Rock JA (Ed). Advances in Obstetrics and Gynaecology, 1st edition. Chicago: Mosby Inc.; 1994. pp. 55-83.
24. Condous G, Kirk E, Van Calster B, Van Huffel S, Timmerman D, Bourne T. Failing pregnancies of unknown location: a prospective evaluation of the human chorionic gonadotrophin ratio. BJOG. 2006;113:521-7.
25. Condous G, Van Calster B, Kirk E, Timmerman D, Van Huffel S, Bourne T. Prospective cross-validation of three methods of predicting failing pregnancies of unknown location. Hum Reprod. 2007;22:1156-60.
26. Rubal L, Chung K. Do you need to definitively diagnose the location of a pregnancy of unknown location? The case for "yes". Fertil Steril. 2012;98(5):1078-84.
27. Condous G, Kirk E, Lu C, Van Calster B, Van Huffel S, Timmerman D, et al. There is no role for uterine curettage in the contemporary diagnostic workup of women with a pregnancy of unknown location. Hum Reprod. 2006;21(10):2706-10.

CHAPTER 22: Diagnosis and Management of Ovarian Torsion

Divya Sardana, Aashna Arora

INTRODUCTION

Definition

Adnexal torsion refers to the partial or complete rotation of adnexa (ovary, fallopian tube, or both) on its own vascular pedicle. It is one of the common gynecological surgical emergencies, with a prevalence of 2.7%.[1]

It is most often seen in women of reproductive age. It can occur during pregnancy also. However, it can also be seen in infants, children, adolescents, and postmenopausal women.

ANATOMICAL CONSIDERATION

The infundibulopelvic (IP) ligaments suspend the ovary (suspensory ligament), allowing the ovary to remain in its anatomical position, lateral or posterior to the uterus. The ovarian vessels traverse along the IP ligaments which attach to the pelvic sidewall.[2]

The other side of the ovary is attached to the uterus by the utero-ovarian (UO) ligament. The UO ligament is made up of muscular and fibrous tissues. Besides providing support to the ovary, it also carries blood from the uterine artery to the ovary **(Fig. 1)**.

PATHOPHYSIOLOGY

Ovarian torsion happens when both IP and UO ligaments are rotated due to an ovarian cyst or mass or an enlarged ovary due to stimulation. However, this can happen even with normal ovaries.

In the early process, there is impairment of the venous blood flow and later on, there is impairment of arterial blood flow also. The underlying pathophysiology involves torsion of the ovarian tissue on its pedicle leading to reduced venous return, stromal edema, internal hemorrhage, and infarction with the subsequent sequelae and ultimately necrosis.[3]

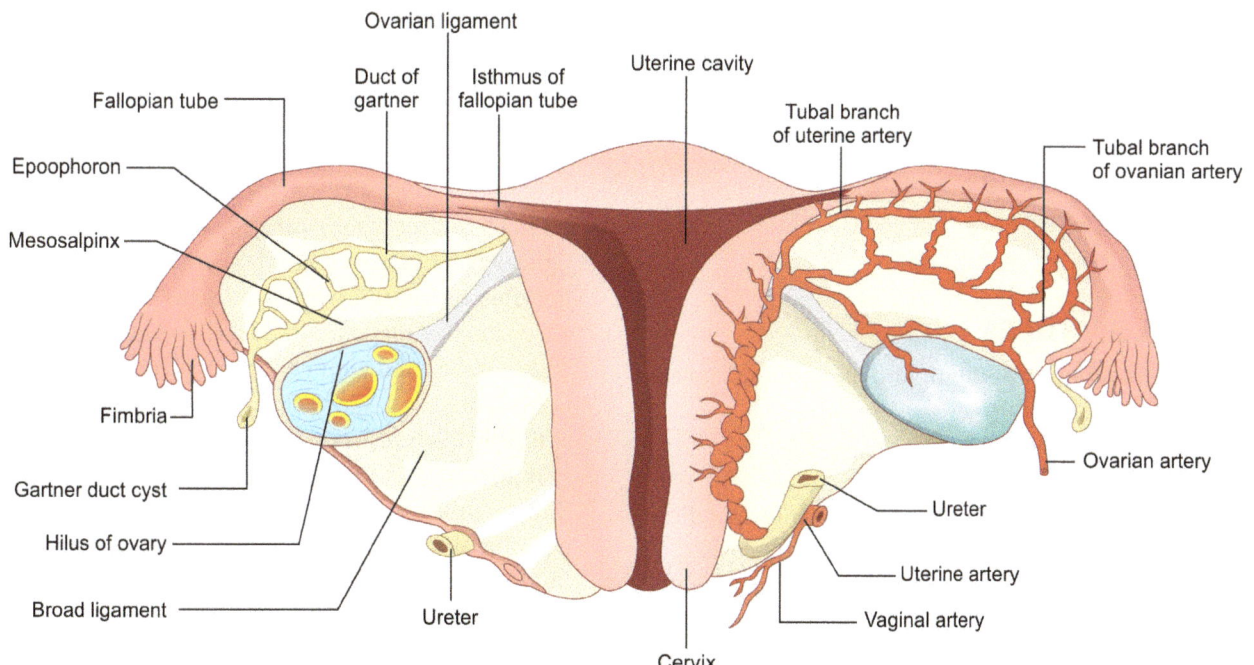

Fig. 1: Support system of ovary.
(*Source:* Adapted from Berek JS. Berek & Novak's Gynecology, 16th edition. India, Gurugram: Wolters Kluwer India Pvt. Ltd.; 2019)

Involvement of right adnexa is slightly more often (66%) than the left adnexa which suggests that sigmoid colon on left side may be helpful in preventing torsion.

RISK FACTORS FOR OVARIAN TORSION

- Ovarian cysts (particularly ≥5 cm)
- Ovarian tumors (more with benign than malignant tumors, particularly mature cystic teratoma)
- Stimulated ovaries [e.g., in vitro fertilization (IVF)]
- Congenitally malformed and elongated fallopian tubes
- Increased length of IP ligament (particularly in premenarcheal girls)
- Pregnancy (around 10–20% torsion cases), (particularly in the early second trimester and with ovarian cysts)
- Patient with a history of adnexal surgery (mainly tubal ligation).

STEP BY STEP APPROACH IN DIAGNOSIS

- Detailed history—onset, nature, site, and duration of pain
- Associated symptoms—anorexia, nausea, vomiting, and bowel/urinary symptoms

↓

Urine pregnancy test (UPT) to rule out ectopic and abnormal early pregnancy

↓

- General examination: General condition, temperature, pulse, respiratory rate, blood pressure (BP), pallor, and icterus
- Per abdomen: Location and severity of pain, tenderness, guarding and rigidity, rebound tenderness, organomegaly, and presence of free fluid
- Gynecological examination: Local examination, per speculum and per vaginum examination

↓

- Stabilize—ABCs (airway, breathing, and circulations)
- Rule out non gynecological cause

↓

- Ultrasonography (USG) with color Doppler is the mainstay for diagnosis
- Definitive diagnosis is surgical

↓

Management involves detorsion with or without cystectomy in most of the cases

CLINICAL FEATURES

- Acute onset of lower abdominal pain (sudden, severe, and worsens with time)[4]
- Nausea and vomiting
- Peritonitis features in some cases
- Associated bladder and bowel symptoms (nonspecific)
- Fever is a late feature suggestive of ovarian necrosis
- On examination: Unilateral tender adnexal mass which may become palpable over time with increasing venous congestion
- Per vaginum examination—cervical motion tenderness, adnexal mass (size, tenderness, and mobility).

INVESTIGATIONS

- *Complete blood count (CBC):* This may show leukocytosis or anemia if hemorrhage is present[5]
- *Beta-human chorionic gonadotropin (hCG):* It can reveal pregnancy or ovarian germ cell tumors[6]
- *Raised C-reactive protein (CRP) levels:* If necrosis present, nonspecific marker
- No specific serum marker for ovarian torsion but serum markers can hint at other pathologies
- *CA-125:* It indicates malignant ovarian tumors or endometriomas
- Some studies have found association between increased levels of inflammatory marker interleukin-6 (IL-6) and ovarian torsion; IL-6 level >10 pg/dL is considered significant.[7]

EVALUATION

Ultrasonography with color Doppler is the mainstay for diagnosis;[8] however, definitive diagnosis is surgical.[1]

Ultrasonography and Doppler Findings

- Abnormal position of the ovaries (ovaries are usually suspended high after torsion)
- Small cystic structures scattered around the periphery of the ovary (up to 25 mm) (most likely displaced ovarian follicles due to edema and venous congestion)
- Unilateral ovarian enlargement due to edema and congestion of ovary (most consistent finding)
- Central stroma shows ground glass appearance
- Associated ovarian cyst or tumor can be seen
- Free fluid in pouch of Douglas[9]
- *Doppler:* Twisted ovarian vascular pedicle is pathognomonic. Normally the vascular pedicle of the ovary, which connects the ovary with the uterus, when seen on ultrasound, has either a straight or a tortuous course. In case of a twisted vascular pedicle, where the vascular pedicle rotates itself, on gray-scale ultrasound it is typically seen as an echogenic round or beaked mass with multiple concentric, hypoechoic, and target-like stripes.
- *Early-stage of torsion:* Firstly the venous and lymphatic flows are blocked with continued arterial perfusion. On color Doppler, arterial flow around the ovarian mass will show high resistance, some amount of venous flow may remain but will soon disappear.[10] There may be diffuse enlargement of ovarian parenchyma and often peripheral follicular distension due to transudation of fluid into cysts.
- *Later stages of torsion:* Even the arterial flow will disappear (due to thrombosis) and thus the torsed ovary will show no arterial or venous flow.[11] Free fluid may be seen in most of the patients.

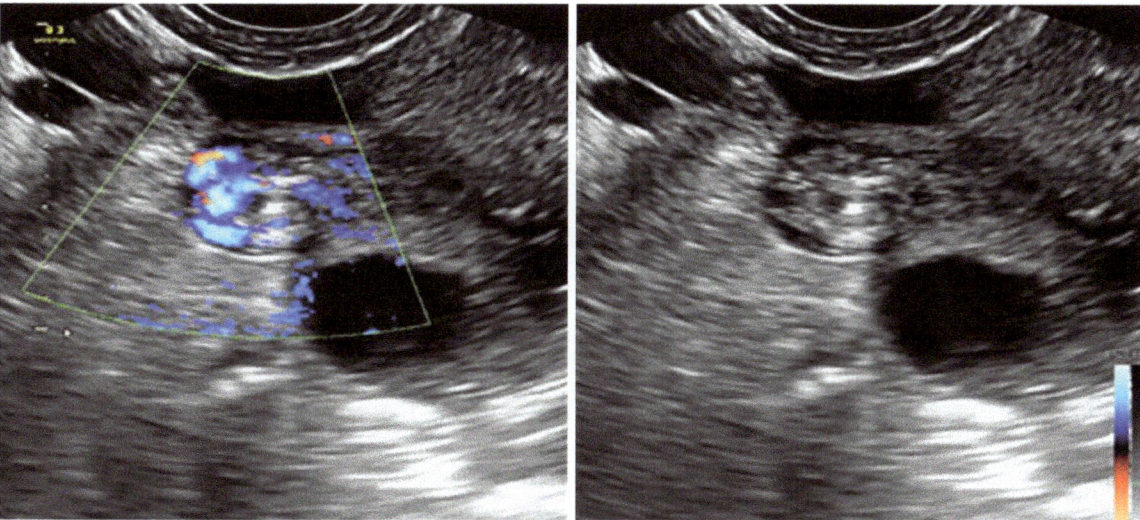

Fig. 2: Ultrasound image of twisted adnexa showing whirlpool sign.[13]
(*Source:* Adapted from Moro F, Bolomini G, Sibal M, Vijayaraghavan SB, Venkatesh P, Nardelli F, et al. Imaging in gynecological disease (20): clinical and ultrasound characteristics of adnexal torsion. Ultrasound Obstet Gynecol. 2020;56(6):934-43.)

- *Ovary viability in torsion:* Viability of the ovary is possible when both arterial and venous flow can be seen within the pedicle.
- *Chronic torsion:* In chronic torsion, collaterals may develop and thus flow in the arteries may remain or mild flow (arterial type) may be seen around periphery due to inflammation. Thus, such a condition may be difficult to separate from normal ovaries. With partial torsion low vascularity may be seen within the mass.
- Normal flow may be seen in some cases of ovarian torsion if:
  - Ovary has transient detorsion
  - Partial torsion
  - In the early process of torsion, when only venous and lymphatic drainage is obstructed and arterial perfusion is still preserved
- *Whirlpool sign:* It is the most definitive sign. It refers to band in the twisted pedicle representing clockwise and anticlockwise wrapping of vessels around central axis (coiling of vascular pedicle) **(Fig. 2)**.[12]

However, Doppler is not a sensitive modality to diagnose ovarian torsion, and even if the flow is normal, it does not rule out torsion. In one of the studies done earlier, as many as 60% of patients who had surgically confirmed ovarian torsion had normal flow within the ovary on Doppler examination prior to surgery.[1]

CT and MRI Findings

These are expensive but may be done particularly when ultrasound findings are equivocal.
- Fallopian tube thickening[14]
- Smooth wall thickening of adnexal cystic mass
- Ascites
- Uterine deviation toward the affected side.

DIFFERENTIAL DIAGNOSIS

A diagram to represent before explaining these will be better. There are many differentials for female with acute abdominal pain.
- *Ectopic pregnancy:* If the female is of childbearing age, ectopic pregnancy must be ruled out with a beta-hCG. Negative beta-hCG rules out ectopic pregnancy. If beta-hCG is positive, ultrasound needs to be done to diagnose whether it is intrauterine pregnancy, ectopic pregnancy, or heterotopic pregnancy.[15]
- *Ruptured ovarian cyst:* Patient with ruptured ovarian cyst may present with a similar picture. In both the cases, ultrasound may show free fluid in pelvis. Pain due to cyst rupture is usually sharp pain, sudden in onset and it gradually decreases with time.[15]
- *Tubo-ovarian abscess:* Patient may present with pelvic pain, gradual in onset and it is associated with fever.[16]
- *Appendicitis:* Patient usually presents with right-sided pelvic pain, associated with nausea, vomiting, and fever. Ultrasound and CT can differentiate it from ovarian pathology.[16]
- *Other differential diagnosis:* Pyelonephritis, diverticulitis, and pelvic inflammatory disease.

MANAGEMENT

- Try to minimize the time from diagnosis to treatment to improve the likelihood of ovarian salvage.[17,18]
- Laparoscopy/laparotomy is the mainstay for confirmation of diagnosis and treatment.[19,20]
- Detorsion with or without cystectomy even in case of blue-black ovary (black-blue appearance of adnexa is due to vascular stasis and not due to gangrene.[21]
- In case of an ovary with true cyst, cystectomy at the time of detorsion is often risky because tissues are friable at

that time. Early elective cystectomy after an interval of 2–3 weeks is a better approach as it allows time for the edema and congestion to resolve.[8]

- *Salpingo-oophorectomy:* In postmenopausal female, or population where there is increased risk of malignancy.
- One must consider a torsed ovary to be potentially viable as it is rare to find ovary to be necrosed. In most of the cases, torsed ovaries can be salvaged (unless some malignancy is suspected).
- According to a recent study conducted by Avantika et al. in a 5-year review of ovarian torsion cases, ovarian salvage rate was 43.2%. Ovarian salvage rate in previous studies was ranging from Hibbard et al. 7%, Houry et al. 9.5%, Huang et al. 35.8%, Nair et al. 54.3%, Balci et al. 60%, and Resapu et al. 82%.[22]
- In cases of torsion, there is no intraoperative approach which is highly effective in determining the viability of ovary.
- Dark and enlarged ovary with or without hemorrhagic lesion is usually viable in most of the cases. So in most of the cases, tube and ovary should be preserved with acknowledgment that in some patients tube and ovary will not survive and it will either result in involution or it may need removal at a later date.
- In rare cases where the ovary is necrotic, it appears as gelatinous or poorly defined structure and it tends to fall apart on being manipulated.
- In cases where adnexa is not salvageable, unilateral salpingo-oophorectomy is the treatment of choice.
- There are several methods to decrease the risk of recurrence: Suppression of ovarian cysts by oral contraceptives; another method is oophoropexy.
- *Oophoropexy:* To correct anatomical hypermobility of the tube and ovary.[23,24] It can be done by suturing the ovary to the lateral pelvic wall, plication of ovarian ligament or fixing the ovary to the posterior surface of uterus.[24]

  It is done in certain cases:
  - Congenitally long ovarian ligament
  - Repeated torsion
  - In cases where there is no obvious cause for torsion found
  - Childhood torsion of normal ovaries.

Key Learning Points

- Ovarian torsion refers to the complete or partial rotation of the ovary on its supporting ligaments causing ischemia.
- It is one of the most common gynecological emergencies.
- It occurs in females of all age groups, most commonly in reproductive age group.
- Presenting symptom is acute onset of abdominal pain associated with nausea and vomiting.
- Ultrasound is the common modality used to make the diagnosis. However, definitive diagnosis can be made only after direct visualization at the time of surgery.
- Surgery involves detorsion with or without cystectomy.

REFERENCES

1. Peña JE, Ufberg D, Cooney N, Denis AL. Usefulness of Doppler sonography in the diagnosis of ovarian torsion. Fertil Steril. 2000;73(5):1047-50.
2. Huang C, Hong MK, Ding DC. A review of ovary torsion. Tzu Chi Med J. 2017;29(3):143-7.
3. Asfour V, Varma R, Menon P. Clinical risk factors for ovarian torsion. J Obstet Gynaecol. 2015;35(7):721-5.
4. Sintim-Damoa A, Majmudar AS, Cohen HL, Parvey LS. Pediatric Ovarian Torsion: Spectrum of Imaging Findings. Radiographics. 2017;37(6):1892-908.
5. Tasset J, Rosen MW, Bell S, Smith YR, Quint EH. Ovarian Torsion in Premenarchal Girls. J Pediatr Adolesc Gynecol. 2019;32(3):254-8.
6. Kroger-Jarvis MA, Pavlik-Maus T, Mullins K. Ovarian Torsion: ED Recognition and Management. J Emerg Nurs. 2018;44(6):647-9.
7. Cohen SB, Wattiez A, Stockheim D, Seidman DS, Lidor AL, Mashiach S, et al. The accuracy of serum interleukin-6 and tumour necrosis factor as markers for ovarian torsion. Hum Reprod. 2001;16(10):2195-7.
8. Bottomley C, Bourne T. Diagnosis and management of ovarian cyst accidents. Best Pract Res Clin Obstet Gynaecol. 2009;23(5):711-24.
9. Gounder S, Strudwick M. Multimodality imaging review for suspected ovarian torsion cases in children. Radiography (Lond). 2021;27(1):236-42.
10. Sugi MD, Patel AG, Yi J, Patel MD. The Flipped Ovary Sign in Ovarian Torsion. J Ultrasound Med. 2021;40(4):839-43.
11. Duigenan S, Oliva E, Lee SI. Ovarian torsion: diagnostic features on CT and MRI with pathologic correlation. AJR Am J Roentgenol. 2012;198(2):W122-31.
12. Vijayaraghavan SB, Senthil S. Isolated torsion of the fallopian tube: the sonographic whirlpool sign. J Ultrasound Med. 2009;28(5):657-62.
13. Moro F, Bolomini G, Sibal M, Vijayaraghavan SB, Venkatesh P, Nardelli F, et al. Imaging in gynecological disease (20): clinical and ultrasound characteristics of adnexal torsion. Ultrasound Obstet Gynecol. 2020;56(6):934-43.
14. Lourenco AP, Swenson D, Tubbs RJ, Lazarus E. Ovarian and tubal torsion: imaging findings on US, CT, and MRI. Emerg Radiol. 2014;21(2):179-87.
15. Rey-Bellet Gasser C, Gehri M, Joseph JM, Pauchard JY. Is It Ovarian Torsion? A Systematic Literature Review and Evaluation of Prediction Signs. Pediatr Emerg Care. 2016;32(4):256-61.
16. Guile SL, Mathai JK. Ovarian Torsion. Treasure Island (FL): StatPearls Publishing; 2022.
17. Robertson JJ, Long B, Koyfman A. Myths in the evaluation and management of ovarian torsion. J Emerg Med. 2017;52(4):449-56.
18. Dasgupta R, Renaud E, Goldin AB, Baird R, Cameron DB, Arnold MA, et al. Ovarian torsion in pediatric and adolescent patients: A systematic review. J Pediatr Surg. 2018;53(7):1387-91.
19. Winton C, Yamoah K. Ovarian torsion and laparoscopy in the paediatric and adolescent population. BMJ Case Rep. 2020;13(5):e232610.

20. Nur Azurah AG, Zainol ZW, Zainuddin AA, Lim PS, Sulaiman AS, Ng BK. Update on the management of ovarian torsion in children and adolescents. World J Pediatr. 2015;11(1):35-40.
21. Novoa M, Friedman J, Mayrink M. Ovarian torsion: can we save the ovary? Arch Gynecol Obstet. 2021;304(1):191-5.
22. Gupta A, Gadipudi A, Nayak D. A Five-Year Review of Ovarian Torsion Cases: Lessons Learnt. J Obstet Gynaecol India. 2020;70(3):220-4.
23. Fuchs N, Smorgick N, Tovbin Y, Ben Ami I, Maymon R, Halperin R, et al. Oophoropexy to Prevent Adnexal Torsion: How, When, and for Whom? J Minim Invasive Gynecol. 2010;17(2):205-8.
24. Obut M, Değer U. A New Technique of Oophoropexy: Folding and Fixating of Utero-Ovarian Ligament to Round Ligament in a Patient with Reccurrent Ovarian Torsion. Case Rep Obstet Gynecol. 2019;2019:7647091.

CHAPTER 23

Work-up and Management of Thin Endometrium

Runa Acharya

■ INTRODUCTION

Endometrium plays one of the critical factors involved in the process of implantation. Thin endometrial lining is an important limiting factor determining the success of in vitro fertilization and embryo transfer (IVF-ET) cycles and managing these patients still remains one of the most challenging arena for IVF clinicians.

■ DEFINITION

Endometrial thickness below 7 mm is the most frequently reported cutoff to define a thin endometrium.[1,2] Though many studies prefer >8 mm in case of fresh embryo transfers, anything <7 mm should be considered as thin endometrium.

The latest systematic review and meta-analysis revealed that the probability of clinical pregnancy for a patient with endometrial thickness 7 mm or less was significantly lower than that for a patient with ET over 7 mm.[3]

Live birth rates have been observed to be 33.7, 25.5, 24.6, and 18.1% for endometrial thickness ≥8, 7–7.9, 6–6.9, and 5–5.9 mm, respectively. In frozen-thaw embryo transfer cycles, clinical pregnancy, and live birth rates reduced with every millimeter decline in endometrial thickness below 7 mm, without any significant difference in pregnancy loss rates. The likelihood of achieving an endometrial thickness ≥8 mm decreased with age (89.7, 87.8, and 83.9%) in women <35, 35–39, and ≥40, respectively.[4]

Cause of thin endometrium is very important factor determining response to treatment and from management perspective. The postulated hypotheses behind thin endometrium are as follows:
- Permanent damage to the basal endometrium
- Endometrial resistance to estrogen
- Reduced blood flow
- Overexposure to testosterone.[5]

■ CAUSES

They can be classified as given in **Flowchart 1**.

■ EVALUATION/WORK-UP

The etiology behind thin endometrium needs to be understood for proper management to improve pregnancy outcomes **(Flowchart 2)**.

Flowchart 1: Causes of thin endometrium.

Causes
- Reversible
  - Central/Genetic (Hypoestrogenic state)
    - Kallmann syndrome
    - Tumor
    - Idiopathic hypogonadotropic Hypogonadism[6]
    - Prolactin disorders
  - Hormonal and structural
    - POF
    - Fibroids[7]
    - Müllerian anomalies[8]
- Irreversible
  - Inflammatory
    - TB
    - Nontuberculous endometritis
    - Change in normal microbiome
  - Iatrogenic
    - OI (inadvertent usage of CC)[9]
    - Asherman's
    - Trauma
    - Previous surgery/D and C[9,10]
    - Pelvic radiation[11,12]
    - Postpartum endometritis[7]
    - Septic abortion[7]
    - In utero diethylstilbestrol[7]
  - Idiopathic

(CC: clomiphene citrate; D&C: dilation and curettage; OI: ovulation induction; POF: premature ovarian failure; TB: tuberculosis)

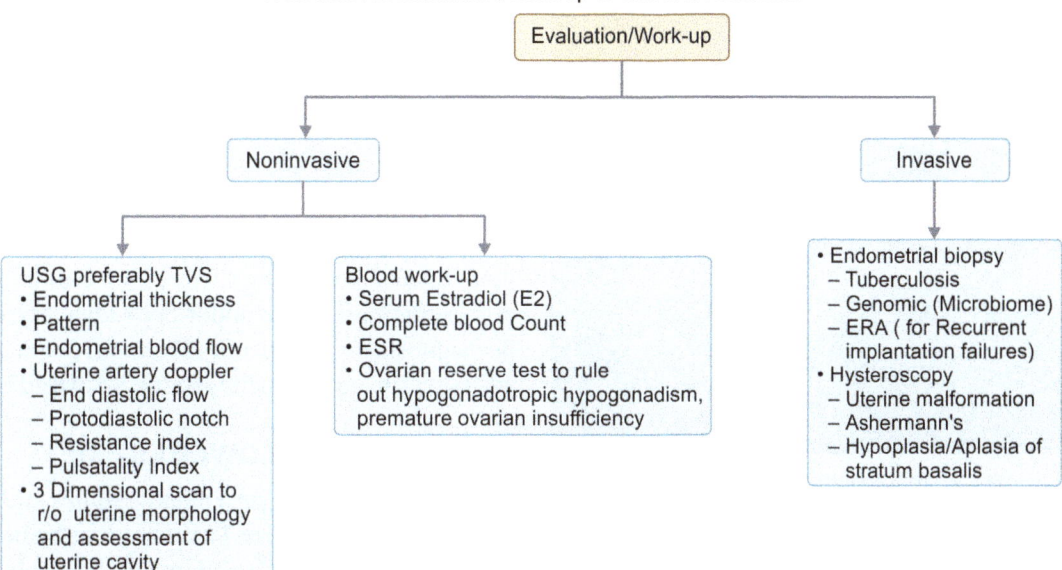

Flowchart 2: Evaluation/Work-up of thin endometrium.

(ERA: endometrial receptivity array; ESR: erythrocyte sedimentation rate; TVS: transvaginal sonography; USG: ultrasonography)

Essential work-up includes blood investigations, ultrasonography (USG), hysteroscopy, and magnetic resonance imaging (MRI).

Noninvasive Tests

Ultrasonography is the most important tool to study the endometrium. However there appears to be a lot of interobserver or intraobserver variation in the measurement of endometrial thickness. To reduce the bias and improve reproducibility of the test following methodology needs to followed:

- *Endometrial thickness:* The endometrium has to be measured using a transvaginal probe on an empty bladder.[13] The transvaginal probe of frequency ≥5–8 MHz needs to be kept closer to the endometrial lining in a longitudinal axis of uterus. The measurement has to be begin from the thickest echogenic part of the lining (endomyometrial junction) from one side across to the other interface. The thickness is calculated in sagittal or longitudinal axis **(Figs. 1 and 2)**.
- *The endometrial pattern:* (1) Homogenous-characterized by homogeneous isoechoic endometrium and (2) Trilaminar-characterized by an outer hyperechoic layer surrounding a central hypoechoic area and inner hyperechogenic layer.

The uterine artery pulsatility index (PI) is measured at the level of uterine isthmus in a transverse plane. The uterine artery PI is the maximum on the day 1 of menstrual cycle and reduces over the follicular phase to improve the blood flow to the endometrium. Color Doppler signals are obtained from the right and left ascending branches of the uterine arteries at the time of trigger. PI <3 is considered normal and ≥3 is abnormal.[14]

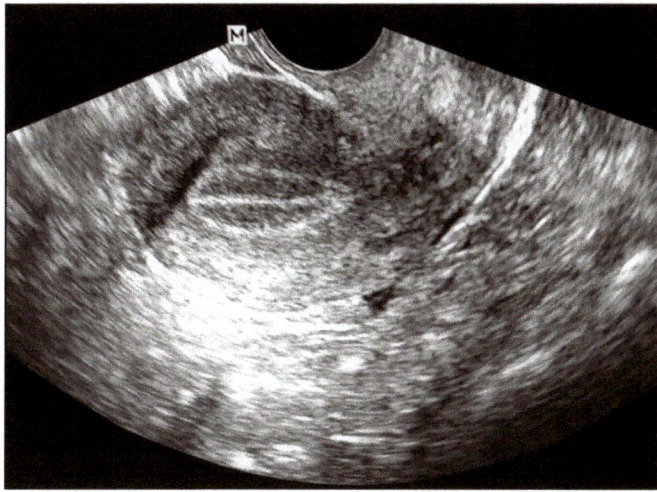

Fig. 1: Normal endometrium.

- *Radial artery-resistance index (RA-RI):* Endometrial thickness is found to be significantly and negatively correlated with RA-RI (single regression analysis). The cutoff value of 0.81 provides the best combination, with 89.3% sensitivity and 87.6% specificity to discriminate between normal and thin endometrium.[14]

Endometrial vascularization is assessed on a longitudinal axis of the uterus. The color gate is placed over the thickest part of the endometrium. According to Applebaum classification, zone 1-vessels penetrating the outer hypoechogenic area surrounding the endometrium but not entering the hyperechogenic outer margin; zone 2-vessels penetrating the hyperechogenic outer margin of the endometrium but not entering the hypoechogenic inner area; zone 3-vessels entering the hypoechogenic inner area; and zone 4-vascularity noted in central

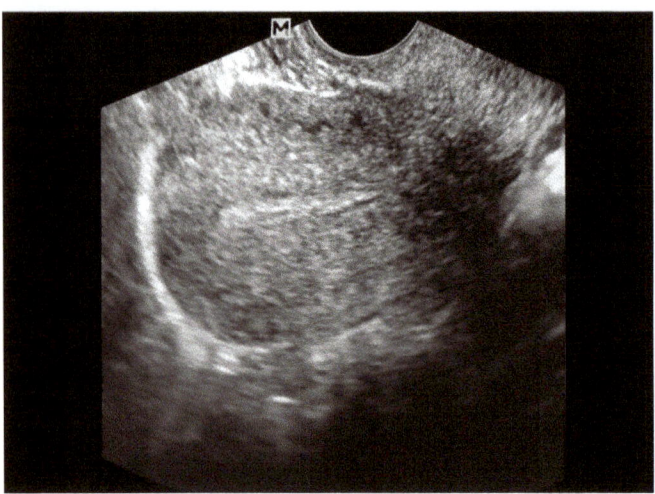

Fig. 2: Thin endometrium.

echogenic line (Applebaum, 1995). The vascularization was considered positive if vessels entered the hypoechogenic inner area. The other Doppler positive findings are presence of protodiastolic notch and end-diastolic flow (EDF).

- *Serum estradiol (E2):* During natural cycles, E2 progressively rises, triggering a luteinizing hormone (LH) surge at levels >200–250 pg/mL for at least 50 hours,[15] and peaks at approximately 300–400 pg/mL around the time of ovulation followed by an abrupt and a steep decline.[16]

  Studies have also shown that ongoing pregnancy and live birth rates decrease from 54% for peak serum E2 levels below 234 pg/mL to 9% for peak serum E2 levels above 692 pg/mL.[17]

  Ovarian reserve tests to rule out ovarian insufficiency and hypogonadotropic hypogonadism wherein low E2 could be the cause of thin endometrium.

- *Uterine microbiota:* Lot of research lately has been attributing to altered physiological microbiota in uterine cavity to be a cause for chronic endometritis (CE) and thin endometrium leading to implantation failures. CE, characterized by an inflammation of endometrium caused by infiltration and overgrowth of different bacteria, e.g., *Escherichia coli*, *Streptococcus* spp., *Staphylococcus* spp., *Chlamydia*, *Mycoplasma*, and *Ureaplasma*. Pathologic species such as *Gardnerella*, *Acinetobacterium*, *Bacteroidetes*, etc., along with decreased abundance of *Lactobacillus* spp. has been postulated as one of the causes for thin endometrium and implantation failures.

Invasive Tests

Endometrial biopsy helps to diagnose the phase of endometrium whether it is proliferative, secretory, out of phase, disordered proliferation, and if any findings suggestive of endometritis. The diagnosis of CE is currently diagnosed based on the histological demonstration of plasma cells within endometrial stromal tissue; however, immunohistochemical staining with CD138 allows simple and reliable identification of plasma cells in the endometrial tissue.[18]

Hysteroscopy

Hysteroscopy is one of the most reliable and common modality for diagnosing CE in expert hands, but its overall accuracy is markedly operator-dependent. Hysteroscopy can be diagnostic or therapeutic in terms of treating Asherman's, adhesiolysis, and evaluating the cause of thin endometrium.

■ TREATMENT (FLOWCHART 3)

- *E2 progressive step up:* Different routes and preparations of estrogen are in use. E2 valerate has been the main stay of treatment for thin endometrium. Significant increase in endometrial thickness from 6.7 mm to 8.6 mm has been noted after an extended estrogen therapy for 14–82 days.[19] Change in administration route to transdermal or vaginal pellets may increase E2 serum concentration through bypassing of first-pass hepatic metabolism.[20] The doses and routes of administration have been discussed in the final algorithm.

- *Ecosprin:* Low-dose aspirin (75 mg/day) is known to improve uterine blood flow. Currently available evidence does not support the use of aspirin in IVF or intracytoplasmic sperm injection (ICSI) treatment. However, there is a noted trend of improvement in clinical pregnancy. The lack of power even when the studies were pooled highlights the need for a definitive trial.[21] A randomized control trial (RCT) explored the effect of aspirin in oocyte recipients with refractory endometrium receiving Hormone replacement therapy (HRT).[22] Patients treated with aspirin showed significantly higher implantation rate (24% vs. 9%, $p < 0.05$). However, this was not associated with a demonstrable increase in endometrial thickness.

- *Sildenafil citrate:* Sildenafil citrate is a potent and selective inhibitor of cyclic guanosine monophosphate (cGMP)-specific phosphodiesterase type 5 (PDE5) that prevents the breakdown of cGMP and potentiates the effect of nitric oxide (NO) on vascular smooth muscles. Sildenafil citrate could lead to an improvement in uterine blood flow and in conjunction with estrogen, led to the estrogen-induced proliferation of the endometrial lining.[5,7,14,20] However there is no conclusive evidence about its role in improving endometrial thickness.

- *Nitric oxide:* Estrogen-induced endometrial proliferation is in large part dependent upon blood flow to the basal endometrium. NO leads to relaxation of vascular smooth muscles through a cGMP mediated pathway. L-arginine

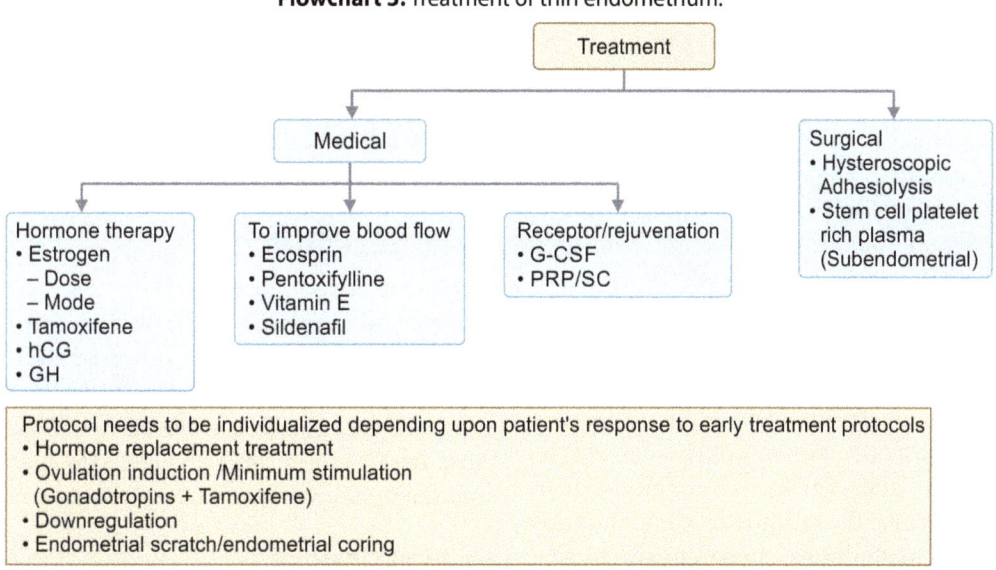

Flowchart 3: Treatment of thin endometrium.

(G-CSF: granulocyte colony-stimulating factor; GH: growth hormone; hCG: human chorionic gonadotropin; PRP: platelet-rich plasma; SC: stem cell)

improves RA-RI and may be useful for the patients with a thin endometrium.[5,14]

- *Pentoxifylline and vitamin E:* Pentoxifylline is a non-specific phosphodiesterase inhibitor with vasodilating effect that improves the blood flow by decreasing its viscosity. Alpha-tocopherol (vitamin E) is an antioxidant reinforcing pentoxifylline action when administered together and acting as well as a vasodilator itself. Two observational studies with a small number of patients explored the impact of the association of pentoxifylline and tocopherol during 3–6 months and have reported improved endometrial thickness and pregnancies.[6,11,12]
- *Human chorionic gonadotropin (hCG):* hCG is a glycopeptide secreted by syncytiotrophoblasts which helps in implantation of the embryo and at the same time supports progesterone production by the corpus luteum. A significant increase in endometrial thickness after hCG priming has been observed in few prospective studies. However, this needs to be interpreted with caution as hCG during follicular phase at higher doses has also been shown to adversely affect endometrial thickness.
- *Granulocyte colony-stimulating factor (G-CSF):* G-CSF, a member of the colony-stimulating factor family of cytokines, has been widely studied in assisted reproduction techniques. It contributes to oocyte and embryo development; therefore, it can be used as a biomarker to assess oocyte and embryo implantation potential.[23] Furthermore, it enhances cyclic adenosine monophosphate-mediated decidualization of human endometrial stromal cells and trophoblast invasion into the maternal tissue,[24] and is predictive of IVF outcome. 300 µg of G-CSF (100 µg/0.6 mL) is introduced into the uterine cavity through an IUI catheter. Higher embryo implantation rate (31.5%) and clinical pregnancy rate (48.1%), as well as a trend toward higher live birth rate (33.3%) has been demonstrated,[25-28] though there are lot of conflicting evidence on its routine use. Low-quality evidence suggests that G-CSF administration may improve clinical pregnancy rate in women with two or more IVF failures (Cochrane 2015).
- *Stem cell platelet-rich plasma (SCPRP):* Stem cells are undifferentiated cells with a potential to differentiate and regenerate into specific cell lines and evolve to multiple mature cell types. These mechanisms involve paracrine effects such as the secretion of certain cytokines, including vascular endothelial growth factor (VEGF), insulin-like growth factor, and hepatocyte growth factor, which are helpful for angiogenesis, anti-inflammation, immunoregulation, antiapoptosis, and antifibrosis to help endometrial regeneration. Also the regenerative properties of transplanted mesenchymal stem cells (MSCs) promote tissue repair, thereby inhibiting scarring, modulating inflammatory and immune reactions, and activating tissue specific progenitor cells. Improvement in endometrial thickness, blood flow to zone 3 of endometrium, blood flow in ovarian Doppler, and FSH levels were noted in 1–3 months.[29,30] Chang et al. reported the efficacy of intrauterine infusion of PRP for endometrial growth in women with thin endometrium for the first time in 2015.[31]

Platelet-rich plasma has multiple growth factors which stimulate cellular processes and activate multipotent stem cells to generate newer younger tissue. Platelets play an important role in local tissue repair and secrete significant amount of autologous growth factors that stimulate proliferation and growth like VEGF, epidermal growth factor (EGF), platelet-derived growth factor (PDGF), transforming growth factor (TGF), and other cytokines. Studies have shown significantly high implantation rate and per-cycle clinical pregnancy rate in PRP-treated group.[31-34]

- *Luteal phase agonist:* The results of a prospective randomized controlled trial showed that the implantation and pregnancy rates improved significantly in the group of patients who received GnRH-a for luteal phase, possibly through a direct effect on the endometrium and corpus luteum, and activation of an endocrine paracrine mechanism.[35,36]
- *Endometrial coring or scratch:* Scratching or coring is a process of stimulating the endometrium so as to create a proinflammatory state apt for implantation. It has been shown to enhance the receptivity of endometrium, though numbers of pathologies have been postulated for implantation failure. The present studies observe that scratching may not be helpful in unselected and subfertile women. In contrast, it appears to be a successful measure for enhancing the chances of implantation in women with recurrent implantation failure (**Fig. 3**). The results of the Cochrane meta-analyses are consistent with an increased chance, no effect, and a small reduction in these outcomes concluding that current evidence does not support the routine use of endometrial injury for women undergoing IVF.[37,38]
- Hysteroscopic adhesiolysis could be helpful in case of Asherman's syndrome. This can be followed by few cycles of estrogen plus progesterone therapy to cyclically regrow and shed the endometrium. Hysteroscopic coring is a procedure wherein the thickness of the endometrial layer can also be assessed along with scratching (**Fig. 3**).
- *Role of antibiotics in case of endometritis:* In cases positive for gram-negative bacteria, ciprofloxacin 500 mg twice a day for 10 days whereas in the case of gram-positive bacteria, amoxicillin and clavulanate 1 g twice a day for 8 days can be prescribed. In women with negative cultures, a treatment based on ceftriaxone 250 mg intramuscular injection in a single dose plus doxycycline 100 mg orally twice a day for 14 days with metronidazole 500 mg orally twice a day for 14 days is recommended, according to the Centre for Disease Control guidelines.[18]

CONCLUSION

Endometrial receptivity is one of the key factors determining successful implantation and hence pregnancy. Well-designed and adequately powered RCT are required to understand better modalities to evaluate endometrium and suggest appropriate measures to improve endometrial thickness. More insights are needed to upgrade and optimize endometrial investigation for better outcomes.

REFERENCES

1. El-Toukhy T, Coomarasamy A, Khairy M, Sunkara K, Seed P, Khalaf Y, et al. The relationship between endometrial thickness and outcome of medicated frozen embryo replacement cycles. Fertil Steril. 2008;89:832-9.
2. Kumbak B, Erden HF, Tosun S, Akbas H, Ulug U, Bahçeci M. Outcome of assisted reproduction treatment in patients with endometrial thickness less than 7 mm. Reprod Biomed Online. 2009;18:79-84.
3. Kasius A, Smit JG, Torrance HL, Eijkemans MJC, Mol BW, Opmeer BC, et al. Endometrial thickness and pregnancy rates after IVF: a systematic review and meta-analysis. Hum. Reprod. Update. 2014;20;530-41.
4. Liu KE, Hartman M, Hartman A, Luo Z-C, Mahutte N. The impact of a thin endometrial lining on fresh and frozen–thaw IVF outcomes: an analysis of over 40000 embryo transfers. Hum Reprod. 2018;33(10):1883-8.
5. Firouzabadi RD, Davar R, Hojjat F, Mahdavi M. Effect of sildenafil citrate on endometrial preparation and outcome of frozen-thawed embryo transfer cycles: a randomized clinical trial. Iran J Reprod Med. 2013;11(2):151-8.
6. Acharya S, Yasmin E, Balen AH. The use of a combination of pentoxifylline and tocopherol in women with a thin endometrium undergoing assisted conception therapies–a report of 20 cases. Hum Fertil (Camb). 2009;12:198-203.
7. Sher G, Fisch JD. Effect of vaginal sildenafil on the outcome of in vitro fertilization (IVF) after multiple IVF failures attributed to poor endometrial development. Fertil Steril. 2002;78:1073-6.
8. Check JH, Cohen R, Choe JK. Failure to improve a thin endometrium in the late proliferative phase with uterine infusion of granulocyte-colony stimulating factor. Clin Exp Obstet Gynecol. 2014;41:473-5.
9. Santamaria X, Cabanillas S, Cervello I, Arbona C, Raga F, Ferro J, et al. Autologous cell therapy with CD133+ bone marrow-derived stem cells for refractory Asherman's syndrome and endometrial atrophy: a pilot cohort study. Hum. Reprod. 2016;31:1087-96.
10. Shufaro Y, Simon A, Laufer N, Fatum M. Thin unresponsive endometrium–a possible complication of surgical curettage

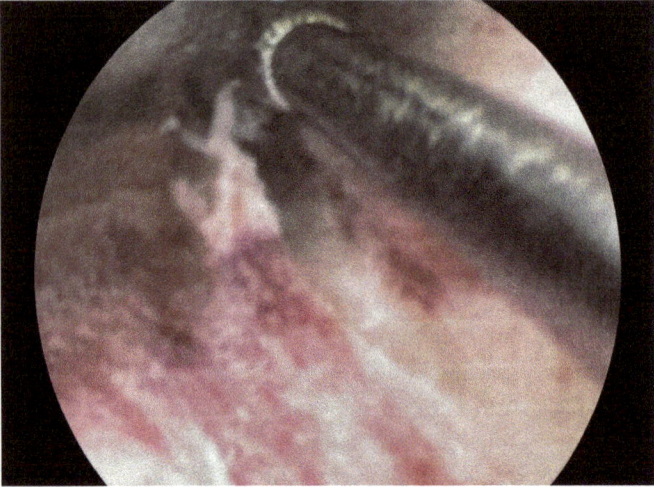

Fig. 3: Endometrial coring.

compromising ART outcome. J Assist Reprod Genet. 2008;25:421-5.
11. Ledee-Bataille N, Olivennes F, Lefaix JL, Chaouat G, Frydman R, Delanian S. Combined treatment by pentoxifylline and tocopherol for recipient women with a thin endometrium enrolled in an oocyte donation programme. Hum Reprod. 2002;17:1249-53.
12. .Letur-Konirsch H, Guis F, Delanian S. Uterine restoration by radiation sequelae regression with combined pentoxifylline-tocopherol: a phase II study. Fertil Steril. 2002;77:1219-26.
13. Persadie RJ. Ultrasonographic assessment of endometrial thickness: a review. J Obstet Gynaecol Can. 2002;24:131-6.
14. Takasaki A, Tamura H, Miwa I, Taketani T, Shimamura K, Sugino N. Endometrial growth and uterine blood flow: a pilot study for improving endometrial thickness in the patients with a thin endometrium. Fertil Steril. 2010;93(6):1851-8.
15. Reed BG, Carr BR. The normal menstrual cycle and the control of ovulation. In: De Groot LJ, Chrousos G, Dungan K (Eds). Endotext. South Dartmouth: MDText.com, Inc.; 2000.
16. Hoff JD, Quigley ME, Yen SS. Hormonal dynamics at midcycle: a reevaluation. J Clin Endocrinol Metab. 1983;57(4):792-6.
17. Fritz R, Jindal S, Feil H, Buyuk E. Elevated serum estradiol levels in artificial autologous frozen embryo transfer cycles negatively impact ongoing pregnancy and live birth rates. J Assist Reprod Genet.2017;34:1633-8.
18. Cicinelli E, Resta L, Loizzi V, Pinto V, Santarsiero C, Cicinelli R, et al. Antibiotic therapy versus no treatment for chronic endometritis: a case-control study. Fertil Steril. 2021;115(6):1541-8.
19. Chen MJ, Yang JH, Peng FH, Chen SU, Ho HN, Yang YS. Extended estrogen administration for women with thin endometrium in frozen-thawed in-vitro fertilization programs. J Assist Reprod Genet. 2006;23(7-8):337-42.
20. Ranisavljevic N, Raad J, Anahory T, Grynberg M. Embryo transfer strategy and therapeutic options in infertile patients with thin endometrium: a systematic review. J Assist Reprod Genet. 2019;36(11):2217-31.
21. Khairy M, Banerjee K, El-Toukhy T, Coomarasamy A, Khalaf Y. Aspirin in women undergoing in vitro fertilization treatment: a systematic review and meta-analysis. Fertil Steril. 2007;88:822-31.
22. Weckstein LN, Jacobson A, Galen D, Hampton K, Hammel J. Lowdose aspirin for oocyte donation recipients with a thin endometrium: prospective, randomized study. Fertil Steril. 1997;68:927-30.
23. Ledee N, Lombroso R, Lombardelli L, Selva J, Dubanchet S, Chaouat G, et al. Cytokines and chemokines in follicular fluids and potential of the corresponding embryo: the role of granulocyte colony-stimulating factor. Hum Reprod. 2008;23:2001-9.
24. Litwin S, Lagadari M, Barrientos G, et al. Comparative immunohistochemical study of M-CSF and G-CSF in feto-maternal interface in a multiparity mouse model. Am J Reprod Immunol. 2005;54:311-20.
25. Gleicher N, Vidali A, Barad DH. Successful treatment of unresponsive thin endometrium. Fertil Steril. 2011;95:e13-7.
26. Gleicher N, Kim A, Michaeli T, Lee H-J, Shohat-Tal A, Lazzaroni E, et al. A pilot cohort study of granulocyte colony-stimulating factor in the treatment of unresponsive thin endometrium resistant to standard therapies. Hum Reprod. 2013;28:172-7.
27. Li Y, Pan P, Chen X, Li L, Li Y, Yang D. Granulocyte colony-stimulating factor administration for infertile women with thin endometrium in frozen embryo transfer program. Reprod Sci. 2014;21:381-5.
28. Bin Xu, Zhang Q, Hao J, Xu D, Li Y. Two protocols to treat thin endometrium with granulocyte colony-stimulating factor during frozen embryo transfer cycles. Reprod Biomed Online. 2015;30:349-58.
29. Anagani M, Agrawal P, Reddy BV, Mishra PC. Role of autologous bone marrow derived stem cells and platelet rich plasma for endometrial regeneration and repair and ovarian rejuvenation. Int J Reprod Contracept Obstet Gynecol. 2021; 10(2):597-604.
30. Yun-xia Zhao, Shao-rong Chen, Ping-ping Su, et al. Using mesenchymal stem cells to treat female infertility: an update on female reproductive diseases. Stem Cells Int. 2019: 9071720.
31. Chang Y, Li J, Chen Y, Wei L, Yang X, Shi Y, et al. Autologous platelet-rich plasma promotes endometrial growth and improves pregnancy outcome during in vitro fertilization. Int J Clin Exp Med. 2015;8:1286-90.
32. Anagani M, Agrawal P, Radhika B, et al. Preliminary Study of Role of Autologous Platelet Rich Plasma for Endometrial Regeneration, Repair and Ovarian Rejuvenation. AAF JRAFM. 10.25096/aafjrafm.00103.112017.
33. Eftekhar M, Neghab N, Naghshineh E, Khani P. Can autologous platelet rich plasma expand endometrial thickness and improve pregnancy rate during frozen-thawed embryo transfer cycle? A randomized clinical trial. Taiwan J Obstet Gynecol. 2018;57(6):810-3.
34. Tandulwadkar SR, Naralkar MV, Surana AD, Selvakarthick M, Kharat AH. Autologous intrauterine platelet-rich plasma instillation for suboptimal endometrium in frozen embryo transfer cycles: a pilot study. J Hum Reprod Sci. 2017;10(3):208-12.
35. Qublah H, Amarin Z, Al-Quda M, Diab F, Nawasreh M, et al. Luteal phase support with GnRH-a improves implantation and pregnancy rates in IVF cycles with endometrium of <7 mm on day of egg retrieval. Hum Fertil (Camb). 2008; 11(1):43-7.
36. Pirard C, Donnez J, Loumaye E. GnRH agonist as luteal phase support in assisted reproduction technique cycles: Results of a pilot study. Hum Reprod. 2006;21:1894-900.
37. Günther V, von Otte S, Maass N, Alkatout I. Endometrial "Scratching" An update and overview of current research. J Turk Ger Gynecol Assoc. 2020;21:124-9.
38. Lensen SF, Armstrong S, Gibreel A, Nastri CO, Raine-Fenning N, Martins WP. Endometrial injury in women undergoing IVF. Cochrane Database Syst Rev. 2021;6(6):CD009517.

CHAPTER 24

Endometrial Preparation for Frozen Embryo Transfer

Manishi Mittal, Umesh Nandani Jindal

■ INTRODUCTION

Assisted reproductive technology (ART) practices have undergone a sea change in recent years owing to progressively improving techniques in the embryology laboratory. Foremost among these is refinement in the technique of vitrification which has provided increasing flexibility in the stimulation protocols, while maintaining an excellent pregnancy rate. In particular, the use of "freeze all" cycles has been expanding to include indications such as prevention of ovarian hyperstimulation syndrome, preimplantation genetic testing, and fertility preservation. Moreover, few studies have shown that frozen embryo transfer (FET) cycles have higher pregnancy rates, when compared to fresh cycles.[1]

The proportion of FET cycles has been consistently increasing globally (from 20.8% in 2010 to 26.9% in 2016 in Europe; 16.8% in 2010 to 28.6% in 2016 in USA).[2] In fact, the number of FET cycles crossed fresh cycles in USA in 2015. The proportion of FET cycles was reported as 77% of all embryo transfers in the latest United States nationwide database report.[3] Moreover, the number of freeze-all cycles is also rising rapidly (fraction of all ART cycles in 2016 being 26.5% in Australia and New Zealand, 19.2% in USA).[2] In addition, the pregnancy rates per cycle in FET cycles have also been increasing, being 23.1% in 2015 from 21.3% in 2011.[4]

■ INDICATIONS FOR FROZEN EMBRYO TRANSFER

The standard indication for freezing of embryos is when surplus embryos are obtained in an ART cycle. In such a case, after fresh transfer, extra embryos are kept for future use as and when required. The other increasingly common scenario is when all embryos are frozen (**Box 1**).

■ PREPARATION PRIOR TO FROZEN EMBRYO TRANSFER

The patient needs to be thoroughly investigated before starting therapy for FET:

BOX 1: Indications for "freeze all" cycles.

- High risk for OHSS
- Poor endometrium:
  – Fluid in endometrial cavity
  – Endometrial thickness <7 mm or >14 mm
  – Applebaum score <14
- Previous failed fresh embryo transfers
- Spotting on day of ET
- High serum progesterone (>1.5 ng/mL) prior to ET
- Difficult ET
- Preimplantation genetic testing
- For fertility preservation
- Use of random start ovarian stimulation protocol
- Use of medroxyprogesterone acetate or other progesterone during stimulation
- Embryo pooling in poor responders
- Batch IVF
- Patient convenience
- Ovum donation and surrogacy cycles
- Personalized ET after ERA test

(ERA: endometrial receptivity analysis; ET: embryo transfer; IVF: in vitro fertilization; OHSS: ovarian hyperstimulation syndrome)

- Detailed history and complete physical examination of female along with correction of any abnormalities/optimization of any comorbid condition, if present.
- Investigations of female—ultrasonography [transvaginal sonography (TVS)], complete blood count, liver and kidney function (when indicated), blood sugar levels, viral markers, coronavirus disease-2019 (COVID-19) testing (according to local guideline), and thyroid function
- *Counseling of couple:*
  • Availability of number and quality of embryos
  • Pros and cons of different days of embryo (day-2, day-3, or day-5) transfer
  • Number of embryos to be transferred
  • Any doubts regarding procedure
  • Quality of embryos to be expected after thawing and risk of cancellation if no embryos available

- Chances of implantation and miscarriage after transfer
- Written consent for embryo transfer procedure.

FROZEN EMBRYO TRANSFER PLANNING AFTER EMBRYO FREEZING

Frozen embryo transfer can be done in the cycle immediately following the stimulation cycle, or after a gap of few months. The arguments in favor of a gap are that the effect of high estrogen levels on the endometrium will be normalized in addition to the psychological and physical recovery after ovarian stimulation and ovum pickup (OPU). However, the actual time required for the genetic and immunological environment in the uterus to restore to normal, is not known. Moreover, delaying FET leads to an increase of stress and anxiety, along with the time to pregnancy. In a meta-analysis, no advantage was seen of either waiting one cycle for FET, or performing it immediately.[5] Hence, the decision should be individualized.

WINDOW OF IMPLANTATION

The objective of endometrial preparation for FET is to prepare receptive endometrium for embryo transfer. The endometrium becomes receptive under the influence of progesterone (P) after estrogen (E) priming during proliferative phase of menstrual cycle. Similar to ovulation, endometrial preparation is also a highly programmed event. Within secretory phase, there is a very short period on day 21–24 of an idealized 28 day menstrual cycle during which the window of implantation (WOI) opens. This WOI involves morphological and functional change from proliferative endometrium to secretory endometrium and then decidualization. There is growth of glands and microvasculature without an increase in thickness making the endometrium more compact. In addition, there are multiple molecular changes. While receptors for estrogen and progesterone are downregulated, several others protein and biochemical markers have been described. Endometrial receptivity tests which can assess these markers at molecular level and on day-to-day basis have been described. The detailed description of assessment of receptivity tests is beyond the scope of this chapter.

Success of FET depends mainly upon three factors:
1. Availability and selection of good embryo
2. Appropriate preparation of endometrium and synchronization
3. Adequate luteal support.

SYNCHRONIZATION OF EMBRYO AND ENDOMETRIUM

The day of embryo transfer needs to be synchronized with the age of embryos. Embryos are thawed and transferred depending on the stage at which they were frozen. In protocols integrating ovulation, the day of ovulation is taken as corresponding to day of OPU in fresh cycle. Age of the embryos is then coordinated with day post ovulation. In artificial cycles (ACs), the day P starts is called P0 and subsequent days labeled P1 to P5; age of embryos is synchronized accordingly. The endometrium can be prepared using many different protocols.

FROZEN EMBRYO TRANSFER PROTOCOLS (FLOWCHART 1)

These can be broadly classified as natural cycle along with its various modifications or artificial cycles. The development of corpus luteum provides the benefits of endogenous hormones for support of implantation. The Artificial cycles on the other hand are exclusively dependent upon exogenous hormones to support implantation and early pregnancy.

True Natural Cycle (Fig. 1)

Description

The embryos are transferred in natural cycle (NC) without any exogenous medications.

Best Suited For

It can only be used in women with regular cycles. The protocol is most suitable for young women with male factor infertility and in the absence of any female factor.

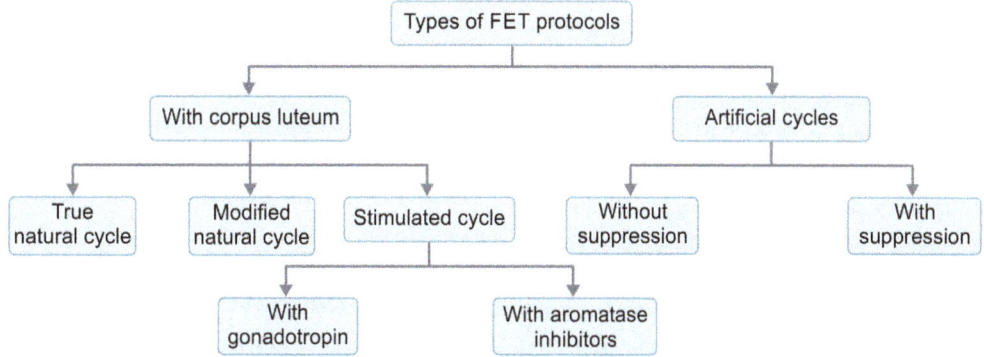

Flowchart 1: Types of frozen embryo transfer (FET) modified natural cycle.

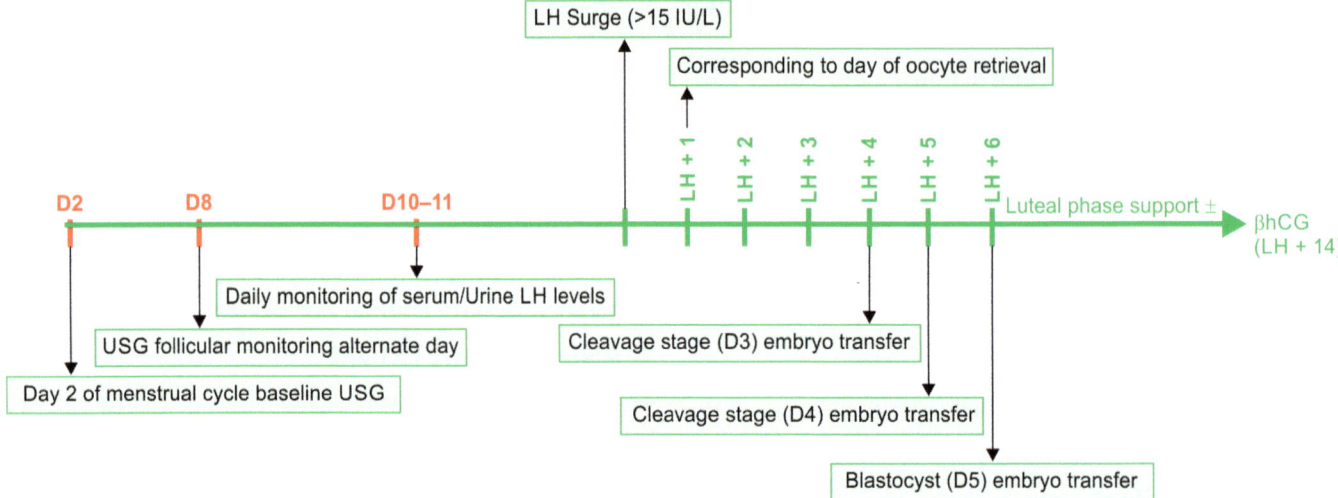

Fig. 1: True natural cycle. (βhCG: β-human chorionic gonadotropin; LH: luteinizing hormone; USG: ultrasonography)

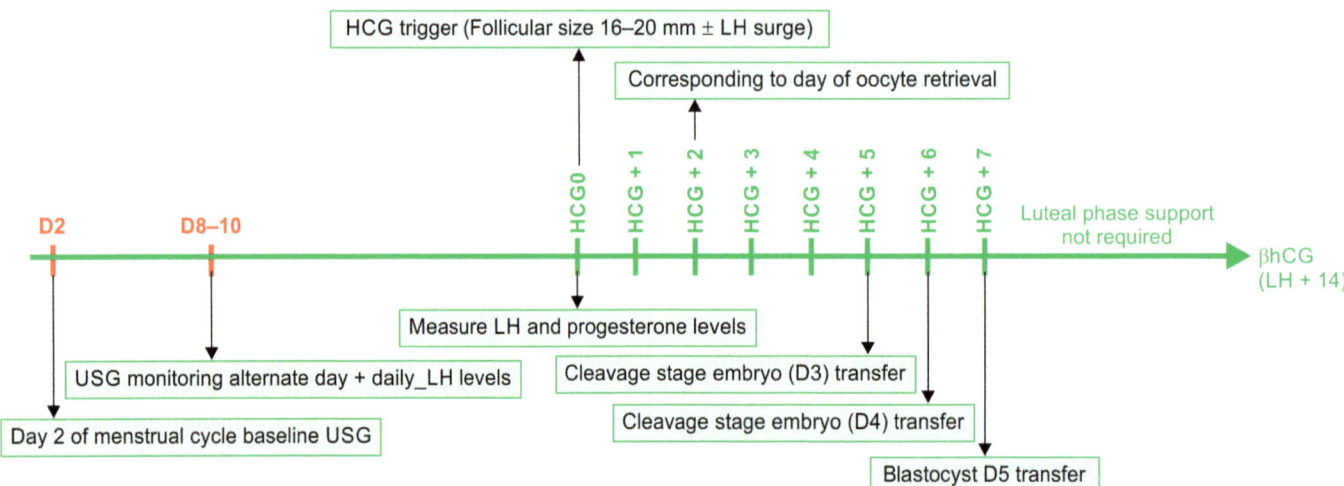

Fig. 2: Modified natural cycle. (βhCG: β-human chorionic gonadotropin; LH: luteinizing hormone; USG: ultrasonography)

Monitoring

Serial follicular study is the main monitoring modality. A baseline scan is done on day one/two of the menstrual cycle to ensure complete shedding of endometrium, resolution of corpus luteum and absence of any other abnormality. From day 8/9, serial scans are conducted for follicular and endometrial development. The objective is to assess day of ovulation with synchronous endometrial development. Additionally, daily urinary or serum LH may be done to detect LH surge. Regarding the diagnosis of LH surge, opinions are divided. Most commonly, a rise of LH >180% of the mean level in prior 24 hours is defined as LH surge. A rise of 180% more than latest serum levels available, with rising titers, and concentration of 10 IU/L or more is also considered.[6,7] Measurement of other hormone levels is controversial. Estimation of progesterone levels can be done one day prior to FET in true natural cycles. Level lesser than 10 ng/mL were seen to have a lower live birth rate and clinical pregnancy rate.[8] This may be because of suboptimal corpus luteum function in an infertile patient. Therefore, Progesterone measurement may be used to customize the luteal phase support according to patient's requirement.

Medications

In true natural cycles, no medications are required. However, there is a controversy regarding use of P in luteal phase. The incidence of luteal phase defect in ovulating patients has been seen to be 8%.[9] In a NC, midluteal serum P levels lower than 10 ng/mL have been ascribed to luteal phase defect.[10] Hence, luteal phase support (LPS) may be given in NC FET cycle. However, evidence both for and against LPS in NC is present.[11]

Modified Natural Cycle

Modified natural cycle is depicted in **Figure 2**.

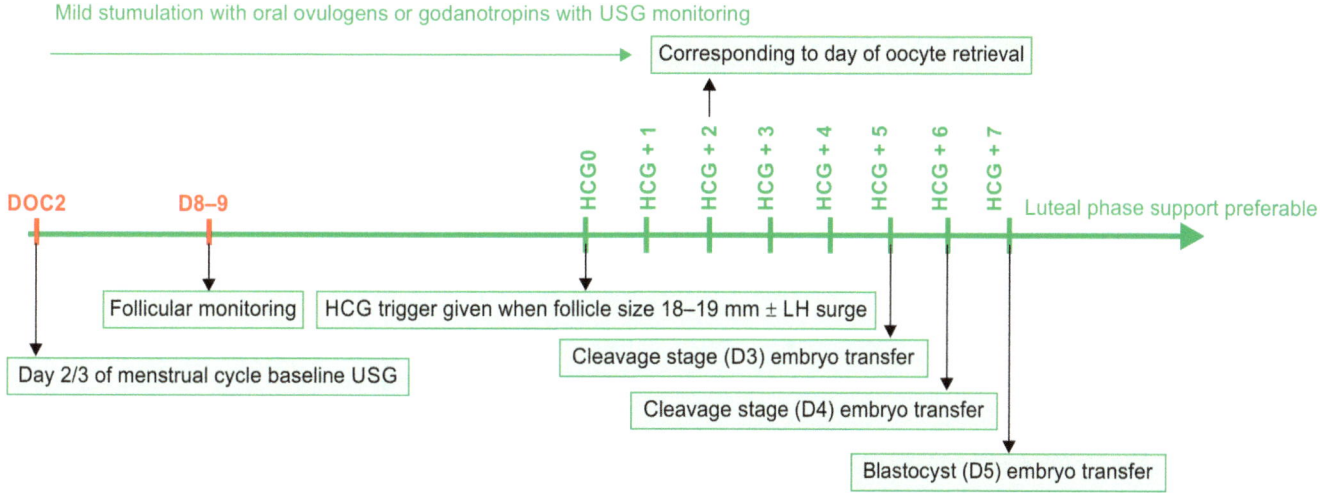

Fig. 3: Stimulated cycle. (hCG: human chorionic gonadotropin; USG: ultrasonography)

Description

Instead of relying on natural LH surge, human chorionic gonadotropin (hCG) is given to trigger ovulation.

Best Suited For

It is best suited for ovulatory women willing for slight hormonal modification in the cycle.

Monitoring

Monitoring is similar to the NC. The ovulation is timed when the follicular size reaches >18–20 mm, endometrium is ready and there is no detectable LH surge or premature P rise.

Medications

Luteal phase support is not required due to long half-life of hCG.[12] However, it can be added.

Stimulated Cycle (Fig. 3)

Description

Mild ovarian stimulation mimicking a natural menstrual cycle is used.

Best Suited For

The protocol can be used in ovulatory or anovulatory women presenting with male factor or anovulatory infertility. It is not preferred for women with endometriosis or unexplained infertility as the intrinsic inflammation may reduce implantation rate.[13]

Monitoring

Monitoring is like modified NC with similar criteria for giving hCG trigger.

Medications

One may use Letrozole (2.5 to 5 mg daily for 5 days starting from day 2/3 of cycle) with or without gonadotrophins, for stimulation, depending upon patient profile. Many PCOS women respond best to Letrozole while gonadotrophins are required for some to achieve a follicle and good endometrium. Dose and frequency of gonadotrophins is individualized according to response seen on follicular monitoring. Clomiphene citrate is usually not used because of its adverse impact on endometrium. Tamoxifen is a selective estrogen receptor modulator used commonly in breast cancer management. It is also occasionally used for ovulation induction, due to action similar to clomiphene. However, unlike clomiphene, it has a positive effect on endometrium through both estrogenic and non estrogenic pathways. Tamoxifen, when used in women undergoing FET with persistent thin endometrium, was seen to improve endometrial thickness as compared to other regimens.[14] Nonetheless, evidence regarding improvement in clinical pregnancy rate and miscarriage rate is insufficient. HCG is given to synchronize the endometrium regardless of stimulation agent used. LPS with Progesterone is usually required in these women.

Artificial Cycle without Suppression (Fig. 4)

Description

The endometrial preparation is achieved with exogenous E and P administration. No follicular development occurs because of suppression of follicle-stimulating hormone (FSH) secretion at the start of follicular phase. Consequently, no corpus luteum develops. The hormonal support is totally exogenous. Since there is no corpus luteum, E and P support is required during early pregnancy also, until placenta takes over, that is around 8-10 weeks.[15]

Best Suited For

Artificial cycles are suitable for all women undergoing FET. In anovulatory women (amenorrhea, ovum donation cycles,

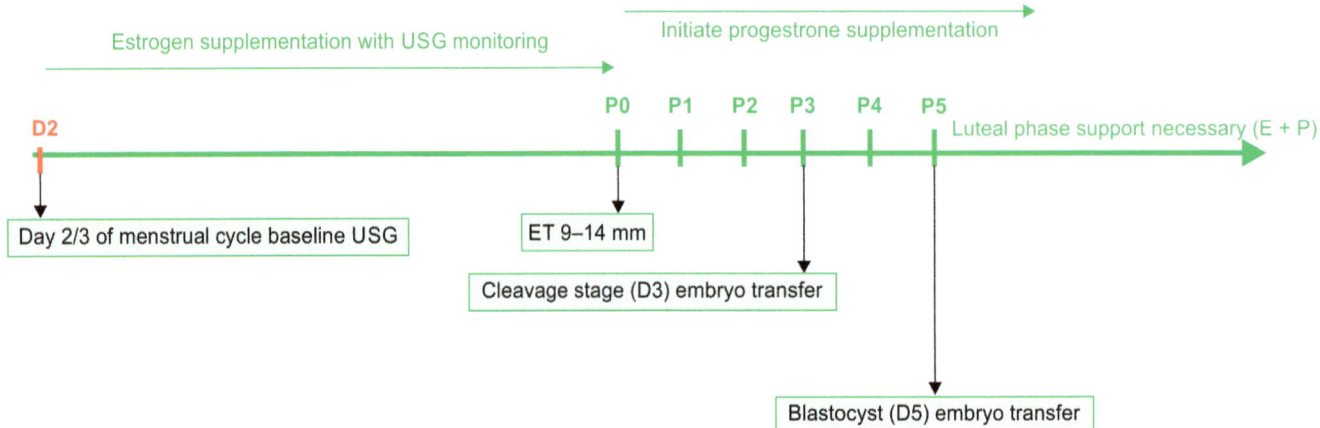

Fig. 4: Protocol for artificial cycle without suppression. (P0 – corresponding to day of oocyte retrieval).

and perimenopausal women), NC is not an option, hence AC is used.

Evidence regarding preference of route and preparation is limited. However, no advantage of any particular type of E or route of administration has been found in FET cycles.[16] Transdermal route may be preferred where oral route is contraindicated.

- Risk of thromboembolism [here NC/modified NC (mNC) are preferred over hormone replacement therapy (HRT)]
- Liver disorders
- Intolerance to oral preparations.

Different dosing techniques are as follows:

- *Fixed:* Oral estradiol valerate 4–6 mg per days in divided doses.[17]
- *Incremental:* Most frequently used starting dose is 4–6 mg per day in divided doses, which can be increased depending on sonographic appearance of endometrium.[18]

Comparison of both methods has not shown any significant difference in live birth rates.[19] Cancellation of cycle may occur due to escape ovulation, which may result from late start of replacement or inadequate dose. Starting with 6 mg estradiol per day, from day 1 to 3 of the cycle, is useful to prevent cancellation.

Different estrogen preparations used are discussed in **Table 1**.

Duration of Estrogen Replacement

The duration of E replacement before starting P does not affect FET outcome. Once appropriate endometrial thickness and pattern is achieved, P can be started according to patient and physician convenience. Estrogen supplementation has been given varying from minimum 10 to maximum 36 days without affecting pregnancy outcome.[20] Still, the aim is to mimic a natural cycle in which the follicular phase usually lasts 14 days.

Monitoring of FET Cycles

Frozen embryo transfer cycle is monitored sonographically, during which endometrial thickness and pattern is noted. A baseline ultrasound on second day of menstrual cycle helps to rule out occurrence of a pre-ovulatory follicle, corpus luteum or luteinized endometrium before preparing for FET. Traditionally, embryo transfer is planned when endometrial thickness is 9–14 mm with a trilaminar pattern.[21] However, when euploid blastocyst transfers were analyzed, endometrial pattern and thickness were not seen to have any impact on subsequent pregnancy rates.[22] Still, they found an association with endometrial pattern, specifically that, type 3 endometrium (mid-late secretory and homogeneous hyperechoic endometrium) prior to FET, demonstrated poor implantation rate.[19] A lower limit of 7 mm endometrial thickness has been established in fresh in vitro fertilization (IVF) cycles, and the same is being followed for FET cycles too, though further research to specify thickness in FET cycles should be done.

Role of serum P levels at time of FET has been investigated in AC. A lower pregnancy rate and live birth rate, and a higher pregnancy loss rate was seen when P levels were higher than 20 ng/dL.[23] However, these levels do not necessarily represent endometrial concentration or WOI. Few studies have propounded midluteal P levels between 22 and 31 ng/mL as being ideal for implantation.[24] Progesterone supplements being taken by the patient also should be considered while monitoring hormonal levels. In addition, intercourse in women using vaginal progesterone gel has been seen to reduce serum P levels.[25] Assessment of serum estradiol, LH or P levels has not been seen to provide benefit in terms of improvement of FET results.

Frozen Embryo Transfer Timing

The WOI is the time period during which the secretory transformation of the endometrium is optimal for blastocyst implantation. Therefore, timing of FET needs to be matched to the WOI. It is especially important to identify the time

TABLE 1: Estrogen preparations used in FET.		
Estrogen	**Route of administration**	**Dose**
Estradiol valerate	Tablets – can be used orally or vaginally	2 mg
Estradiol hemihydrate	Oral tablets	2 mg
17-β-Estradiol	Transdermal gel	One pump actuation delivers 1.25 g of gel which contains 0.75 mg estradiol

Approximate conversion values[41] –0.75 mg of micronised estradiol (oral administration) = 1.25 g of estradiol gel (transdermal administration) = 1 mg of estradiol valerate (oral or vaginal administration).

limit. Even though trials to identify biomarkers assessing WOI are being done, no fully validated test is available yet.

In cases where further in vitro culture is done for cryopreserved embryos after thawing, embryo transfer should be timed according to the expected developmental stage of embryo after culture.[26] The type of freezing procedure followed (slow freezing versus vitrification) affects post thaw development of embryos.

Exogenous Progesterone Initiation

Progesterone supplementation is started once appropriate endometrium is seen on ultrasound. It helps in final preparation of endometrium for embryo transfer. Additional hCG supplementation was not seen to improve pregnancy rates.[27] The timing of initiating P is controversial. Usually, P in AC is started 3 days before transfer of a cleavage stage embryo, giving a pregnancy rate of up to 40.5%.[28] Longer P supplementation was seen to have a higher early pregnancy loss rate.[29] Therefore, starting P on the day equivalent to oocyte retrieval results in better pregnancy rates.[11] Shorter duration of supplementation also led to more pregnancy loss, giving credence to the concept of WOI.[30]

There is no consensus about the type of P to be used **(Table 2)**. Vaginal P is considered more patient friendly as compared to injectable. However, injectable P has been more commonly used, with few retrospective studies showing beneficial results with this route.[31]

Artificial Cycle with Suppression (Fig. 5)

Description

In this protocol, downregulation is done with the help of gonadotropin-releasing hormone (GnRH) agonist (depot or daily low dose) given in luteal phase of previous cycle. Ultralong downregulation for 2-3 months can also be done in cases of endometriosis and adenomyosis. After appearance of menstrual bleeding, same protocol as that of AC without suppression is followed.

Best Suited For

It is used in women with endometriosis and adenomyosis, recurrent luteinized unruptured follicle (LUF), ovarian cysts, and very high basal LH in PCOS. The strategy may be used in cases of batch IVF for convenient scheduling of FET.

LUTEAL PHASE SUPPORT

Different preparations are available which are as follows:
- Progesterone—micronized progesterone capsules, dydrogesterone tablets, injections, and vaginal gel
- GnRH agonist
- hCG.

Regarding route of administration of P, few studies show better pregnancy rates with vaginal and intramuscular routes, while majority studies show no difference **(Table 2)**.[29,32] A recent three-armed, randomized controlled noninferiority trial comparing different progesterone regimens has shown lower early pregnancy loss rates with use of P injections.[33] Vaginal absorption of P is variable and peak levels in serum are achieved after 6–8 hours. The progestational activity provided by hCG in stimulated cycles, with the corpus luteum, is thought to be more consistent.[34]

WHICH PROTOCOL IS BETTER? (TABLE 3)

The choice of ideal protocol is based on multiple factors. The protocol selected should give the best implantation, clinical pregnancy and live birth rates. Simultaneously, it should be safe for the mother as well as the baby. Currently available evidence does not support or condemn any particular method of endometrial preparation.[35,36] Few studies have demonstrated a higher early pregnancy loss rate with AC.[37] On the other hand, AC are often preferred because of both patient and clinician's convenience. Few studies demonstrate the advantage of stimulated cycles and natural cycles, due to presence of natural LPS from the corpus luteum.[38] Presence of corpus luteum is now increasingly recognized to improve perinatal outcome.[39] There is clear evidence that FET reduces the risk of low birth infants, placenta previa and placental abruption when compared to fresh transfers. However, there are reports of a twofold increased risk of hypertensive disorders of pregnancy, 1.5 fold increase in postpartum haemorrhage and twofold increase in large for gestational age newborns, with artificial cycles.[40] The reasons proposed for such differences are presence or absence of corpus luteum and various other vasoactive substances secreted by it which help in placentation. All these aspects should be considered before starting FET protocol.

Endometrial Preparation for Frozen Embryo Transfer

TABLE 2: Types of progesterone supplements used in FET.[42,43]

Type of progesterone	Preparation	Dose in AC cycles	Advantages	Disadvantages
Progesterone in oil	50 mg, 100 mg Intramuscular	100 mg/day once daily	• High and sustained plasma concentration • Better results reported	• Painful injections • Self administration not possible
Aqueous progesterone	25 mg, 50 mg subcutaneous, Intramuscular	50–100 mg/day once daily	• Comparable pregnancy and live birth rates to intramuscular injections[44] • Less painful than intramuscular injections	• Less acceptable and more painful as compared to vaginal or oral • Less experience with its use
Oral micronized sustained released tablets	Oral tablets 200 mg, 300 mg, 400 mg	200–400 mg once or twice/day	Convenient, high acceptability	Absorption erratic side effects - constipation
Dydrogesterone	Oral tablets 10 mg	10 mg twice or thrice per day	• Convenient, high acceptability • Comparable results with vaginal Progesterone. Can be used in combination with vaginal progesterone • Preferred LPS in fresh ET	Experience limited in FET when compared to intramuscular injections
Micronized Progesterone vaginal/ oral capsules	Vaginal capsules 100, 200, 300, 400 mg	300 to 400 mg twice daily	• Some women have better acceptability • Comparable pregnancy rates • Progesterone is transported directly from the vagina to the uterus leading to adequate uterine tissue levels	• Injections may reduce uterine contractility and endometrial wave activity better than vaginal progesterone • Vaginal irritation, less acceptable • Oral use – high first pass metabolism, more side effects like dizziness and constipation • Higher miscarriage rate after FET as compared to injectable[45]
Micronized Progesterone vaginal gel	Bioadhesive gel 90 mg/ application	90 mg twice daily	• Some women have better acceptability • Comparable pregnancy rates • Progesterone is transported directly from the vagina to the uterus leading to adequate uterine tissue levels	Injections may reduce uterine contractility and endometrial wave activity better than vaginal progesterone Vaginal irritation, less acceptable

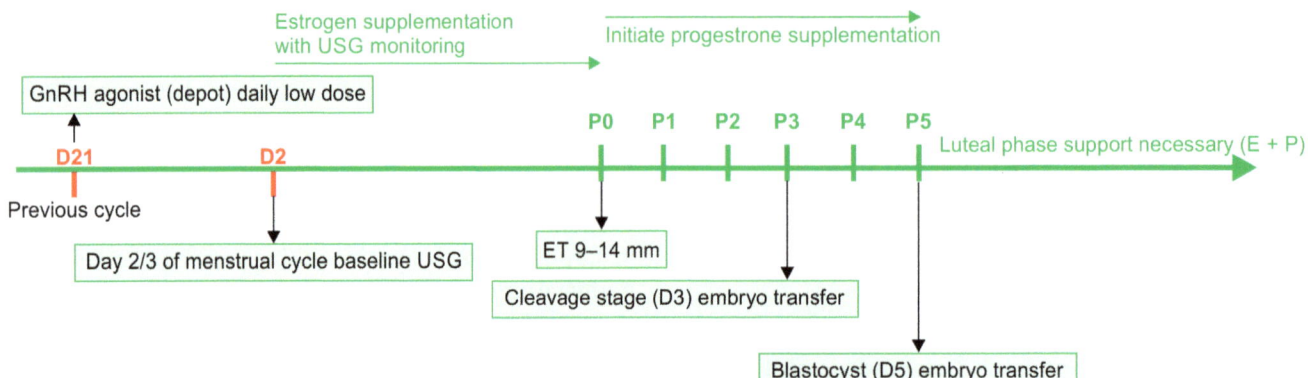

Fig. 5: Protocol for artificial cycle with suppression.

Choice of protocol should be based on various factors:
- Previous cycle cancellations
- Number of hospital visits expected
- Possible adverse effects of medicines
- Hospital & IVF Lab logistics
- Convenience & cost efficiency
- Patient & doctor preference.

Troubleshooting

Troubleshooting is explained in **Table 4** and **Flowchart 2**.

Endometrial Preparation for Frozen Embryo Transfer

TABLE 3: Comparison of different protocols for frozen embryo transfer (FET).

Protocol	Advantages	Disadvantages
Natural cycle	• Patient friendly—less requirement of medication, less cost • Better perinatal outcome • Comparable pregnancy rates with other methods	• More frequent and careful monitoring required (both sonographic and hormonal) • No flexibility • Cannot be used in women with anovulatory cycles
Modified natural cycle	• Patient friendly—less requirement of medication, less cost • Better perinatal outcome • Comparable pregnancy rates with other methods • More flexibility than true natural cycle—continuous hormonal monitoring not required • Luteal phase support not required	Cannot be used in women with anovulatory cycles
Artificial cycle without suppression	• Patient friendly—no injections, less frequent visits • More flexibility • Can be used in women with both ovulatory and nonovulatory cycles • Time tested method	• Side effects of high dose estrogen • Avoided in patients at risk for thromboembolic disorders • More chances of escape ovulation • High cost • High risk of hypertensive disorders of pregnancy
Artificial cycle with suppression	• Less risk of escape ovulation • More flexibility	• More injections—less patient friendly • High cost • High risk of hypertensive disorders of pregnancy
Stimulated cycle	• Overcomes minor endometrial defects • Better pregnancy rates according to few reports	• High cost • Less flexibility

TABLE 4: Comparison of different protocols for FET.

Protocol	Advantages	Disadvantages
Natural cycle	• Patient friendly—less requirement of medication, less cost • Better perinatal outcome, pregnancy grows in a completely natural environment without any exogenous medicines • Comparable pregnancy rates with other methods	• More frequent and careful monitoring required (both sonographic and hormonal) • No flexibility • Applicable in minority of women - cannot be used in women with anovulatory cycles • Cancellation of cycle due to various reasons like nonresolution of previous corpus luteum, premature Progesterone rise, Luteinized unruptured follicle, missed LH surge etc may occur in a significant number of cases
Modified natural cycle	• Patient friendly—less requirement of medication, less cost • Better perinatal outcome • Comparable pregnancy rates with other methods • More flexibility than true natural cycle—continuous hormonal monitoring not required • Luteal phase support not required	Cannot be used in women with anovulatory cycles
Artificial cycle without suppression	• Patient friendly—no injections, less frequent visits, convenient scheduling • More flexibility. Supplementation may be extended without affecting pregnancy rates • Can be used in women with both ovulatory and nonovulatory cycles • Time tested method with high success rates • Applicable to all • Acceptable cost	• Side effects of high dose estrogen eg thrombosis • Avoided in patients at risk for thromboembolic disorders • More chances of escape ovulation. Seen in 1.9–7.4% cycles[19] • High risk of hypertensive disorders of pregnancy[46] • Total dependence on exogenous E and P during peri-implantation phase and early pregnancy raises questions regarding safety of these medicines for the baby
Artificial cycle with suppression	• Less risk of escape ovulation • More flexibility, convenient scheduling • Downregulation helps to reduce inflammation associated with endometriosis and adenomyosis–improved implantation	• More injections—less patient friendly • High cost • Treatment duration spread over 2 or even 3 menstrual cycles • High risk of hypertensive disorders of pregnancy
Stimulated cycle	• Overcomes minor endometrial defects • Better pregnancy rates according to few reports	• High cost • Less flexibility • Some evidence claiming detrimental effects[47]

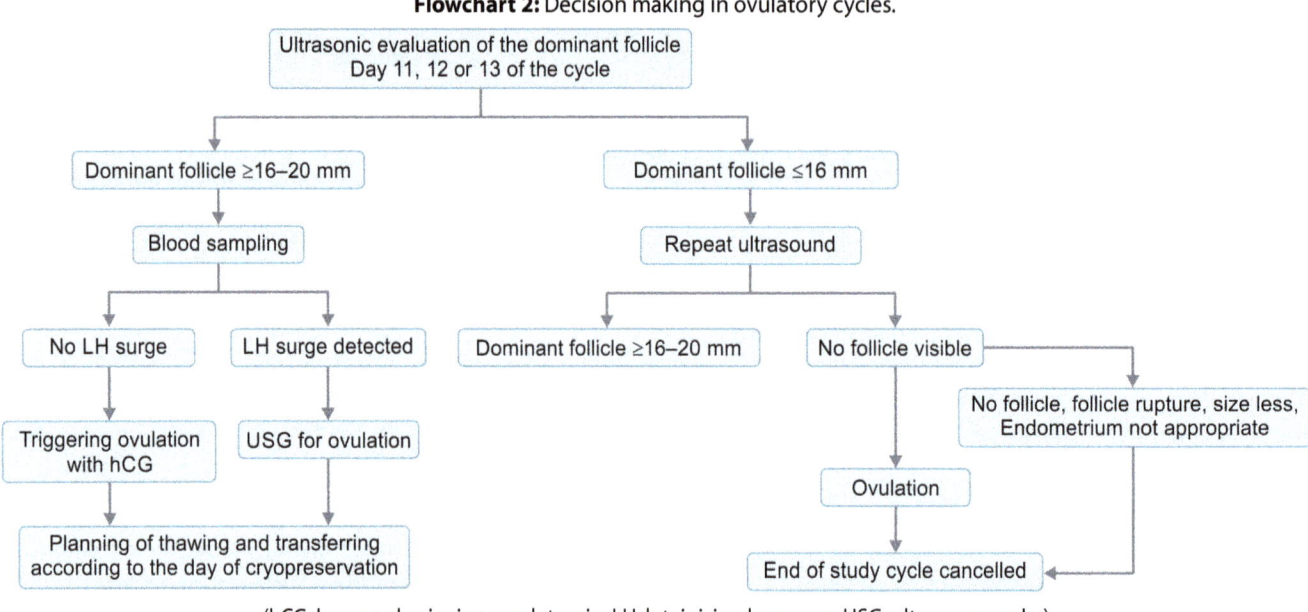

Flowchart 2: Decision making in ovulatory cycles.

(hCG: human chorionic gonadotropin; LH: luteinizing hormone; USG: ultrasonography)

TABLE 5: Adjuvants used in IVF.		
Adjuvant	*Usage*	*Evidence*
Filgrastim (G-CSF analog)	Subcutaneous injection (on day of ET) or intrauterine infusion (2 days prior to ET)	Conflicting reports regarding benefit (add reference)
Low molecular weight heparin	Daily subcutaneous injections along with LPS	No proven benefit in FET, but should be carefully considered in women with thrombophilia (reference)
Intralipid infusion	Prior to FET cycle	No proven benefit in RIF. No specific studies for FET (reference)
Antibiotics	Prior to FET	• No proven benefit in IVF • No specific studies for FET
Aspirin	80–100 mg orally daily	Conflicting reports
Steroids	Oral glucocorticoids daily	Limited evidence showing improved live birth rates in conventional IVF
Vasodilators—nitroglycerine (NTG), sildenafil, and L-arginine	Vaginal tablet of sildenafil 100 mg daily from day 8 of cycle	Improved live birth rates in few studies with FET, though no robust evidence available for routine use in FET
Autologous platelet rich plasma	Intrauterine infusion 2 days prior to FET	No proven benefit
Uterine relaxants—β2 adrenergic antagonists, piroxicam, and atosiban	Single dose 1–2 hours prior to FET	No proven benefit
Endometrial scratching/endometrial injury (EI)		Conflicting body of evidence. No robust evidence available for routine use in FET
Intrauterine hCG administration		No robust evidence available for routine use in FET
Anti-tumor necrosis factor-α (TNF-α) agents		No robust evidence available for routine use in FET
Autologous peripheral blood mononuclear cells (PBMC)		No robust evidence available for routine use in FET
PRP		

(ET: embryo transfer; FET: frozen embryo transfer; G-CSF: granulocyte colony-stimulating factor; hCG: human chorionic gonadotropin; IVF: in vitro fertilization; LPS: luteal phase support; RIF: repeated implantation failure)

ADJUVANTS (TABLE 5)

Various adjuvants have been tried for improving endometrial receptivity in ART, which could be extrapolated to FET. However, none of these is standard practice.

CONCLUSION

The choice of endometrial preparation needs to be individualized taking into account age of the patient and etiology of infertility (e.g., endometriosis). In patients with anovulation, only AC can be used. For women with regular cycles, true or modified NC may be used. Nevertheless, women with advanced age tend to exhibit abnormal ovulatory patterns such as premature ovulation and anovulatory cycles. Therefore, for these women, AC, with or without suppression are preferred. Adequately powered randomized control trials need to be performed for optimization of the FET and improvement of results along with better patient compliance and satisfaction. Also, identification of different groups of women, who benefit from different protocols need to be identified.

Key Learning Points

- Frozen Embryo Transfer has become the preferred choice over fresh embryo transfer.
- The objective of endometrial preparation for FET is to prepare receptive endometrium for embryo transfer. Similar to ovulation, endometrial preparation is also a highly programmed event.
- The success of FET depends upon embryo quality, appropriate decidualized endometrium, endometrial embryonic age synchronization, adequate luteal support.
- Endometrial preparation protocols can be broadly divided into two groups. First in which the endogenous production of hormones, with or without exogenous hormone supplementation, through ovulation and presence of corpus luteum are used. The others are completely artificial cycles.
- The protocols need to be individualized according to the patient profile.

REFERENCES

1. Casper RF, Yanushpolsky EH. Optimal endometrial preparation for frozen embryo transfer cycles: window of implantation and progesterone support. Fertil Steril. 2016;105(4):867-72.
2. Geyter CH DE, Wyns C, Calhaz-Jorge C, de Mouzon J, Ferraretti AP, Kupka M, et al. 20 years of the European IVF-monitoring Consortium registry: what have we learned? A comparison with registries from two other regions. Hum Reprod. 2020;35(12):2832-49.
3. Centers for Disease Control and Prevention. Assisted Reproductive Technology Fertility Clinic Success Rates Report. Atlanta, GA: US Department of Health and Human Services; 2020.
4. Calhaz-Jorge C, de Geyter C, Kupka MS, de Mouzon J, Erb K, Mocanu E, et al. Assisted reproductive technology in Europe, 2012: results generated from European registers by ESHRE. European IVF-Monitoring Consortium (EIM) for the European Society of Human Reproduction and Embryology (ESHRE). Hum Reprod. 2016;31:1638-52.
5. Matorras R, Pijoan JI, Perez-Ruiz I, Lainz L, Malaina I, Borjaba S. Meta-analysis of the embryo freezing transfer interval. Reprod Medi Biol. 2021;20(2):144-58.
6. Testart J, Frydman R, Feinstein MC, Thebault A, Roger M, Scholler R. Interpretation of plasma luteinizing hormone assay for the collection of mature oocytes from women: definition of a luteinizing hormone surge-initiating rise. Fertil Steril. 1981;36(1):50-4.
7. Groenewoud ER, Macklon NS, Cohlen BJ, Al-Oraiby A, Brinkhuis EA, Broekmans FJ, et al. The effect of elevated progesterone levels before HCG triggering in modified natural cycle frozen-thawed embryo transfer cycles. Reprod Biomed Online. 2017;34(5):546-54.
8. Gaggiotti-Marre S, Álvarez M, González-Foruria I, Parriego M, Garcia S, Martínez F, Barri PN, Polyzos NP, Coroleu B. Low progesterone levels on the day before natural cycle frozen embryo transfer are negatively associated with live birth rates. Human Reproduction. 2020;35(7):1623-9.
9. Rosenberg SM, Luciano AA, Riddick DH. The luteal phase defect: the relative frequency of, and encouraging response to, treatment with vaginal progesterone. Fertil Steril. 1980;34(1):17-20.
10. Jordan J, Craig K, Clifton DK, Soules MR. Luteal phase defect: the sensitivity and specificity of diagnostic methods in common clinical use. Fertil Steril. 1994;62(1):54-62.
11. Bjuresten K, Landgren BM, Hovatta O, Stavreus-Evers A. Luteal phase progesterone increases live birth rate after frozen embryo transfer. Fertil Steril. 2011;95(2):534-7.
12. Eftekhar M, Rahsepar M, Rahmani E. Effect of progesterone supplementation on natural frozen-thawed embryo transfer cycles: a randomized controlled trial. Int J Fertil Steril. 2013;7(1):13-20.
13. Qi Q, Luo J, Wang Y, Xie Q. Effects of artificial cycles with and without gonadotropin-releasing hormone agonist pretreatment on frozen embryo transfer outcomes. Journal of International Medical Research. 2020;48(6): 0300060520918474.
14. Zhongying Huang, Zhun Xiao, Qianhong Ma, Yu Bai, Feilang Li. Efficacy of tamoxifen for infertile women with thin endometrium undergoing frozen embryo transfer: a meta-analysis. Clin. Exp. Obstet. Gynecol. 2021;48(4):806-11.
15. Weissman A. IVF worldwide survey results: frozen-thawed embryo transfer.
16. Glujovsky D, Pesce R, Fiszbajn G, Sueldo C, Hart RJ, Ciapponi A. Endometrial preparation for women undergoing embryo transfer with frozen embryos or embryos derived from donor oocytes. Cochrane Database Syst Rev. 2010;(1):CD006359.
17. Cobo A, de los Santos MJ, Castelló D, Gámiz P, Campos P, Remohí J. Outcomes of vitrified early cleavage-stage and blastocyst-stage embryos in a cryopreservation program: evaluation of 3,150 warming cycles. Fertil Steril. 2012;98(5):1138-46.
18. Van De Vijver A, Polyzos NP, Van Landuyt L, De Vos M, Camus M, Stoop D, et al. Cryopreserved embryo transfer in an artificial cycle: is GnRH agonist down-regulation necessary? Reprod Biomed Online. 2014;29(5):588-94.
19. Madero S, Rodriguez A, Vassena R, Vernaeve V. Endometrial preparation: effect of estrogen dose and administration route on reproductive outcomes in oocyte donation cycles with fresh embryo transfer. Hum Reprod. 2016;31(8):1755-64.
20. Sekhon L, Feuerstein J, Pan S, Overbey J, Lee JA, Briton-Jones C, et al. Endometrial preparation before the transfer of single, vitrified-warmed, euploid blastocysts: does the duration of estradiol treatment influence clinical outcome? Fertil Steril. 2019;111(6):1177-85.
21. El-Toukhy T, Coomarasamy A, Khairy M, Sunkara K, Seed P, Khalaf Y, et al. The relationship between endometrial thickness

and outcome of medicated frozen embryo replacement cycles. Fertil Steril. 2008;89(4):832-9.
22. Gingold JA, Lee JA, Rodriguez-Purata J, Whitehouse MC, Sandler B, Grunfeld L, et al. Endometrial pattern, but not endometrial thickness, affects implantation rates in euploid embryo transfers. Fertil Steril. 2015;104(3):620-8.
23. Kofinas JD, Blakemore J, McCulloh DH, Grifo J. Serum progesterone levels greater than 20 ng/dl on day of embryo transfer are associated with lower live birth and higher pregnancy loss rates. J Assist Reprod Genet. 2015;32:1395-9.
24. Yovich JL, Conceicao JL, Stanger JD, Hinchliffe PM, Keane KN. Mid-luteal serum progesterone concentrations govern implantation rates for cryopreserved embryo transfers conducted under hormone replacement. Reprod Biomed Online. 2015;31(2):180-91.
25. Merriam KS, Leake KA, Elliot M, Matthews ML, Usadi RS, Hurst BS. Sexual absorption of vaginal progesterone: a randomized control trial. Int J Endocrinol. 2015;2015:685281.
26. Cercas R, Villas C, Pons I, Brana C, Fernandez-Shaw S. Vitrification can modify embryo cleavage stage after warming. Should we change endometrial preparation? J Assist Reprod Genet. 2012;29(12):1363-8.
27. Ben-Meir A, Aboo-Dia M, Revel A, Eizenman E, Laufer N, Simon A. The benefit of human chorionic gonadotropin supplementation throughout the secretory phase of frozen-thawed embryo transfer cycles. Fertil Steril. 2010;93(2):351-4.
28. Givens CR, Markun LC, Ryan IP, Chenette PE, Herbert CM, Schriock ED. Outcomes of natural cycles versus programmed cycles for 1677 frozen–thawed embryo transfers. Reprod Biomed Online. 2009;19(3):380-4.
29. Escribá MJ, Bellver J, Bosch E, Sánchez M, Pellicer A, Remohí J. Delaying the initiation of progesterone supplementation until the day of fertilization does not compromise cycle outcome in patients receiving donated oocytes: a randomized study. Fertil Steril. 2006;86(1):92-7.
30. van de Vijver A, Polyzos NP, Van Landuyt L, Mackens S, Stoop D, Camus M, et al. What is the optimal duration of progesterone administration before transferring a vitrified-warmed cleavage stage embryo? A randomized controlled trial. Hum Reprod. 2016;31(5):1097-104.
31. Haddad G, Saguan DA, Maxwell R, Thomas MA. Intramuscular route of progesterone administration increases pregnancy rates during non-downregulated frozen embryo transfer cycles. J Assist Reprod Genet. 2007;24(10):467-70.
32. Shapiro DB, Pappadakis JA, Ellsworth NM, Hait HI, Nagy ZP. Progesterone replacement with vaginal gel versus IM injection: cycle and pregnancy outcomes in IVF patients receiving vitrified blastocysts. Hum Reprod. 2014;29(8):1706-11.
33. Devine K, Richter KS, Jahandideh S, Widra EA, McKeeby JL. Intramuscular progesterone optimizes live birth from programmed frozen embryo transfer: a randomized clinical trial. Fertil Steril. 2021;116:633-43.
34. El-Toukhy T, Taylor A, Khalaf Y, Al-Darazi K, Rowell P, Seed P, et al. Pituitary suppression in ultrasound-monitored frozen embryo replacement cycles. A randomised study. Human Reprod. 2004;19(4):874-9.
35. Yarali H, Polat M, Mumusoglu S, Yarali I, Bozdag G. Preparation of endometrium for frozen embryo replacement cycles: a systematic review and meta-analysis. J Assist Reprod Genet. 2016;33(10):1287-304.
36. Groenewoud ER, Cantineau AE, Kollen BJ, Macklon NS, Cohlen BJ. What is the optimal means of preparing the endometrium in frozen–thawed embryo transfer cycles? A systematic review and meta-analysis. Hum Reprod Update. 2013;19(5):458-70.
37. Tomás C, Alsbjerg B, Martikainen H, Humaidan P. Pregnancy loss after frozen-embryo transfer a comparison of three protocols. Fertil Steril. 2012;98:1165-9.
38. Hatoum I, Bellon L, Swierkowski N, Ouazana M, Bouba S, Fathallah K, et al. Disparities in reproductive outcomes according to the endometrial preparation protocol in frozen embryo transfer. J Assist Reprod Genet. 2018;35(3):425-9.
39. Gan J, Rozen G, Polyakov A. Treatment outcomes of blastocysts thaw cycles, comparing the presence and absence of a corpus luteum: a systematic review and meta-analysis. BMJ open. 2022;12(4):e051489.
40. Sha T, Yin X, Cheng W, Massey IY. Pregnancy-related complications and perinatal outcomes resulting from transfer of cryopreserved versus fresh embryos in vitro fertilization: a meta-analysis. Fertility and sterility. 2018; 109(2):330-42.
41. Mackens S, Santos-Ribeiro S, Van De Vijver A, Racca A, Van Landuyt L, Tournaye H, Blockeel C. Frozen embryo transfer: a review on the optimal endometrial preparation and timing. Human Reproduction. 2017;32(11):2234-42.
42. Mumusoglu S, Polat M, Ozbek IY, Bozdag G, Papanikolaou EG, Esteves SC, Humaidan P, Yarali H. Preparation of the endometrium for frozen embryo transfer: a systematic review. Frontiers in Endocrinology. 2021;12:831.
43. Dashti S, Eftekhar M. Luteal-phase support in assisted reproductive technology: An ongoing challenge. International Journal of Reproductive BioMedicine. 2021;19(9):761.
44. Conforti A, Carbone L, Iorio GG, Cariati F, Bagnulo F, Marrone V, et al. Luteal phase support using subcutaneous progesterone: a systematic review. Frontiers in Reproductive Health. 2021;3:634813.
45. de Ziegler D, Pirtea P, Ayoubi JM. Implantation Failures and Miscarriages in Frozen Embryo Transfers Timed in Hormone Replacement Cycles (HRT): A Narrative Review. Life. 2021; 11(12):1357.
46. Dall'Agnol H, Velasco JA. Frozen embryo transfer and preeclampsia: where is the link? Current Opinion in Obstetrics and Gynecology. 2020;32(3):213-8.
47. Horcajadas JA, Minguez P, Dopazo J, Esteban FJ, Dominguez F, Giudice LC, et al. Controlled ovarian stimulation induces a func- tional genomic delay of the endometrium with potential clinical implications. J Clin Endocrinol Metab. 2008;93(11):4500-10.

CHAPTER 25

Work-up of Azoospermia

Divyashree PS

◼ DEFINITION

- *Azoospermia* is defined as absence of sperm, even after centrifugation in two separate ejaculates. The centrifugation is done at 3,000 g for 15 minutes and then thorough examination by phase contrast optics at 200X magnification.[1]
- *Cryptozoospermia*—Sperms found in the pellet post-centrifugation in 20% cases.[2]
- The incidence of azoospermia is 1% in all men and 10–15% in all infertile men.[3]
  Classification and etiology of azoospermia are given in **Box 1**.
  Classification system of azoospermia employed in clinical practice is depicted in **Figure 1**.

BOX 1: Classification and etiology of azoospermia.[4]

Pretesticular (secondary testicular failure/secondary hypogonadism)
- *Hypogonadotropic hypogonadism (HH)*
  – Congenital-Kallmann syndrome, normosmic HH, and Prader–Willi syndrome
  – Acquired pituitary tumor, trauma, radiation, hyperprolactinemia, chronic opioid use, and steroid abuse
  – Idiopathic

Testicular (primary testicular failure/primary hypogonadism)
- Genetic abnormalities—Klinefelter's syndrome and Y chromosome microdeletion
- Acquired—Torsion, trauma, postinflammatory, chemoradiation, cancer, systemic illnesses [chronic kidney disease/chronic liverdisease (CKD/CLD)], and varicocele
- Idiopathic

Post-testicular
- Ejaculatory dysfunction—retrograde ejaculation
- Obstructive
  – Congenital—congenital bilateral absence of the vas deferens (CBAVD)
  – Accquired
    - Prostatectomy, vasectomy, scrotal surgery, epididymal cyst removal, and hernia repair
    - Postinfectious
- Idiopathic

◼ DIAGNOSIS (FIG. 2)

The work-up of azoospermia follows the standard principles of thorough history (**Fig. 3**), detailed physical examination (**Table 1**), and aided by investigations (**Table 2**).[5]

◼ OBSTRUCTIVE AZOOSPERMIA (FLOWCHART 1)

- Accounts for approximately 40% of all cases of azoospermia.[6]
- Semen volume, testicular volume, and serum follicle-stimulating hormone (FSH) are the key factors in determining the etiology of azoospermia in the absence of vasal agenesis and testicular atrophy.
- In men with low ejaculate volume (<1.5 mL) and normal FSH and testis volume:
  - Determine collection error—loss of sample and abstinence of 2–3 days
  - Check postejaculate urinalysis (PEU) to evaluate possible retrograde ejaculation

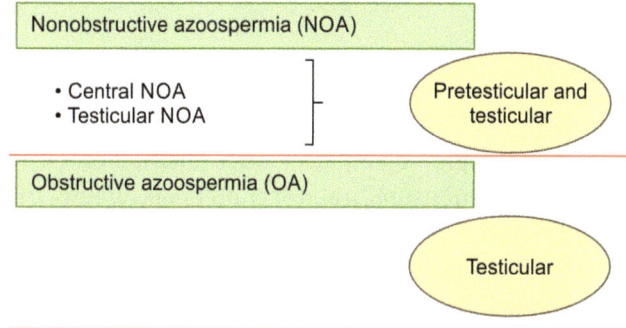

Fig. 1: Classification system employed in clinical practice.

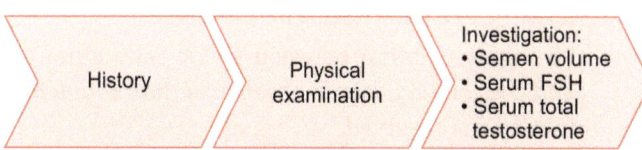

Fig. 2: Diagnostic work-up of a case defined as azoospermia.[5]
(FSH: follicle-stimulating hormone)

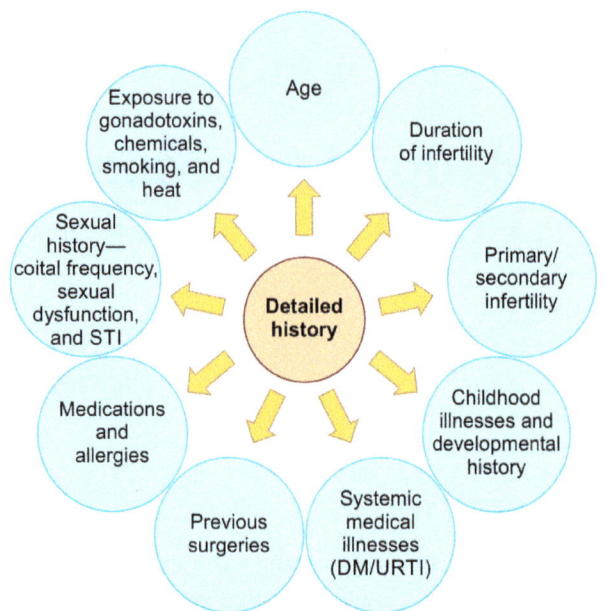

Fig. 3: Detailed history in a case of azoospermia.[3]
(DM: diabetes mellitus; STI: sexually transmitted infection; URTI: upper respiratory tract infection)

TABLE 1: Physical examination in a case of azoospermia.[3]

General examination	Genitourinary examination	Digital rectal examination
• Body habitus/gait • *Secondary sexual characteristics:* Facial and body hair distribution/voice • Height/weight/BP • Thyroid examination • *CVS and respiratory system:* Dextrocardia, bronchiectasis, and TB • *Abdominal examination:* Hepatomegaly, scars of previous surgery	• *Scrotum:* Hypoplasia/hydrocele • *Testis:* Size/volume/consistency • *Epididymis:* If palpable then size/texture • *Spermatic cord:* Vas deferens–palpable or not, beaded vas • Presence of varicocele	Indicated in case of suspicion of prostate adenoma or seminal vesicle cysts

(BP: blood pressure; CVS: cardiovascular system; TB: tuberculosis)

TABLE 2: Basic laboratory investigations in azoospermia.[3]

Etiology	Semen volume	Total testosterone	FSH
Pretesticular • Hypogonadotropic hypogonadism • Exogenous androgens	• Normal/decreased • Normal/decreased	• Decreased • Increased/normal/decreased	• Decreased • Decreased
Testicular • Primary testicular failure • Genetic etiology varicocele	Normal	Decreased	Increased
Post-testicular • Vasectomy • Epididymal obstruction	Normal	Normal	Normal
• Ejaculatory dysfunction, ejaculatory duct obstruction	Decreased	Normal	Normal

Semen volume <1.5 mL—decreased; serum FSH >7.6 mIU/mL—increased; serum FSH <1.4 mIU/mL—decreased; serum testosterone <300 ng/dL—decreased
(FSH: follicle-stimulating hormone)

- If vas palpable—ejaculatory duct obstruction (EDO) suspected—transurethral resection of ejaculatory duct (TRUS) performed:
  - To identify causes of EDO such as midline cysts, dilated ejaculatory ducts, and/or dilated seminal vesicles (>1.5 cm in diameter)
- If vas not palpable—unilateral or bilateral vasal agenesis—CFTR gene testing performed:
  - Strong association between CFTR gene mutation and congenital bilateral absence of the vas deferens (CBAVD) is observed
  - Most of the men with clinical cystic fibrosis have CBAVD to exclude the possibility of carrier state in female partner (4%) genetic testing should be offered before using sperm from a man with CBVAD or congenital unilateral absence of the vas deferens (CUAVD).[7]
- Almost all men with clinical cystic fibrosis have CBAVD.
- At least three quarters of men with CBAVD have mutations of the CFTR gene.[8]
- Before any treatment using sperm from a man with CBAVD or CUAVD, testing should be offered to his female partner to exclude the possibility (4%) that she too may be a carrier. Genetic counseling should be offered both before and after genetic testing of both partners.[3]

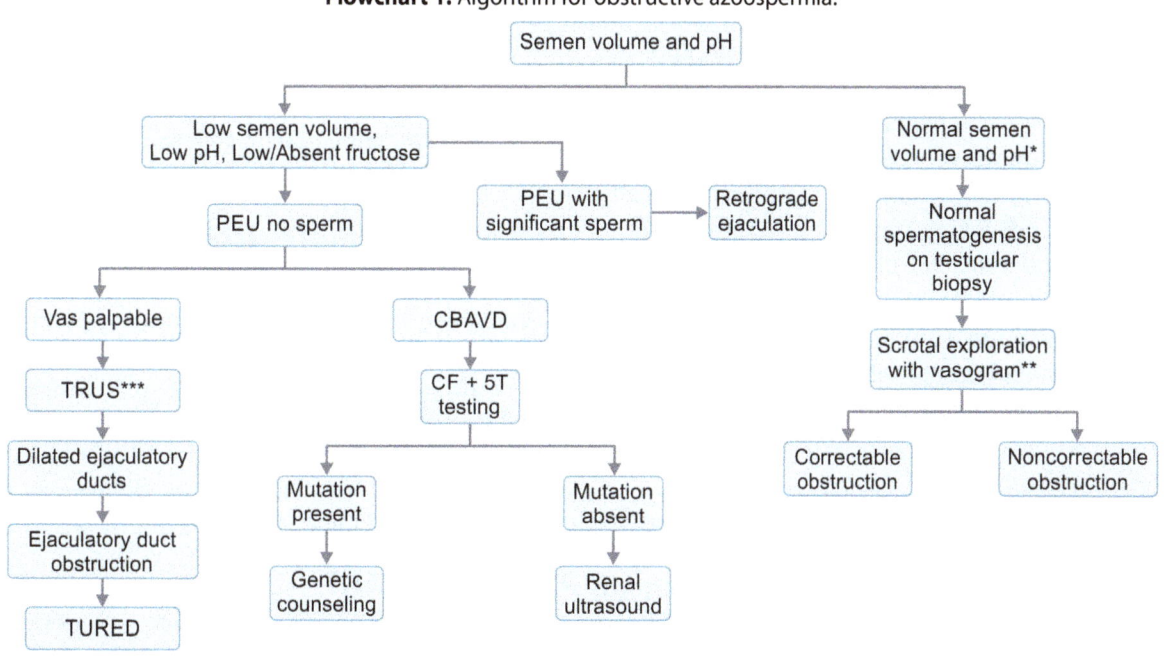

Flowchart 1: Algorithm for obstructive azoospermia.[3]

*Normal testis volume and normal FSH
**Vasogram: includes saline, methylene blue, and contrast
***If negative TRUS, genetic testing is recommended

(CBAVD: congenital bilateral absence of the vas deferens; FSH: follicle-stimulating hormone; PEU: postejaculate urinalysis; TRUS: transurethral resection of ejaculatory duct)

- Unilateral renal agenesis is found in 25% of men with unilateral vasal agenesis and 10-15% of men with CBAVD.[9]
- Due to the embryologic association between the vasa and seminal vesicles, most men with vasal agenesis also have seminal vesicle hypoplasia or agenesis leading to low volume ejaculate.
- In men with normal ejaculate volume and normal FSH and testis volume:
  - A diagnostic testicular biopsy may be helpful to assess spermatogenesis.
  - A normal testicular biopsy or aspirate implies obstruction at some level in the reproductive system, and the location can be determined using *vasography*.
  - Vasography should not be performed at the time of diagnostic testicular biopsy unless reconstructive surgery is planned simultaneously as it can result in vasal scarring and obstruction.
  - In case assisted reproductive technology (ART) becomes necessary in future, reconstruction should be coupled with sperm retrieval and cryopreservation in the setting of likely epididymal obstruction.

NONOBSTRUCTIVE AZOOSPERMIA

- Accounts for approximately 40% of all cases of azoospermia.
- Pretesticular causes account for around 2-3% and testicular causes account for 55-60%.[10]
- Patients typically demonstrate small, soft, and atrophic testes unlike normal volume testes in obstructive azoospermia (OA).

Genetic Analysis

- Karyotype and Y chromosome microdeletion (YCMD) tests are warranted in men with nonobstructive azoospermia (NOA) without history of prior fertility, obstruction of male reproductive tract, or toxic exposures.[11]
- Karyotype found abnormal in up to 19% of men with NOA.
- The most common abnormality is Klinefelter syndrome (47,XXY; found in 1/600 men) and Robertsonian translocations (fusion of long arms of two acrocentric chromosomes 13, 14, 15, 21, or 22).[10]
- Men with Klinefelter syndrome have successful sperm retrieval rate of 30-70% which is better than all men with NOA.[12]
- YCMD of three azoospermic factor (AZF) regions located in Yq11 which encode proteins influencing spermatogenesis.
- The abnormalities in the AZF regions (AZFa, AZFb, and AZFc) are present in 10-20% NOA cases.
  - AZFa and AZFb—no successful sperm retrieval
  - AZFc—50-60% of chances of successful sperm retrieval by microsurgical testicular sperm extraction (microTESE); however, male offspring will also manifest AZFc microdeletion and have the same fertility problem as their fathers.[13,14]

Hypogonadotropic Hypogonadism

- Hypogonadotropic hypogonadism (HH) affects approximately 1–2% of infertile men.
- HH is characterized by hypothalamic or pituitary dysfunction, low/suppressed serum gonadotropins, and decreased testicular function that manifests clinically as testosterone deficiency, oligospermia/azoospermia, and/or decreased testicular volume.
- Among congenital HH, the most common form is Kallmann syndrome in which due to absence of hypothalamic gonadotropin-releasing hormone (GnRH) the pituitary is not stimulated to produce luteinizing hormone (LH) and FSH, although pituitary gonadotrophs are present and normal.
- Both spermatogenesis and testosterone production by the testes are not stimulated.
- X-linked or autosomal for KAL1 (Xp22.32), FGFR1 (8p11.2-11.1), and other genes testing is warranted and varies depending on the inheritance pattern.[15]
- *Genetic testing in HH:*
  - Gives the opportunity to counsel patients about the risks of HH in their offspring
  - Gives an option to screen for unaffected embryos using preimplantation genetic testing for aneuploidy (PGT-A).[3]

Role of Diagnostic Testicular Biopsy (Flowchart 2)[3]

- Indicated in case of doubt regarding obstructive and NOA
- *For example:* For patients with normal testicular size, at least one palpable vas deferens and a normal serum FSH level, to determine presence of focal spermatogenesis
- Cryopreservation of sperm to be done along with it, to avoid the need for a second procedure.

■ MANAGEMENT

Algorithm for the management of obstructive azoospermia is presented in **Flowchart 3**.

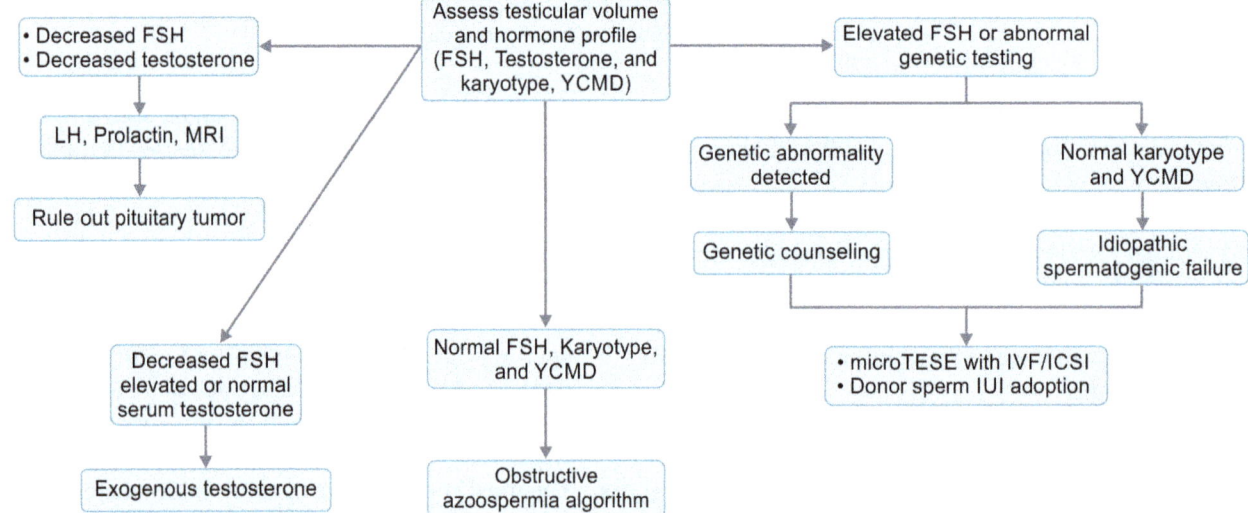

Flowchart 2: Evaluation of nonobstructive azoospermia (normal semen volume).[3]

(CF: cystic fibrosis; FSH: follicle-stimulating hormone; LH: luteinizing hormone; IUI: intrauterine insemination; IVF/ICSI: in vitro fertilization with intracytoplasmic sperm injection; microTESE: microsurgical testicular sperm extraction; YCMD: Y-chromosome microdeletion)

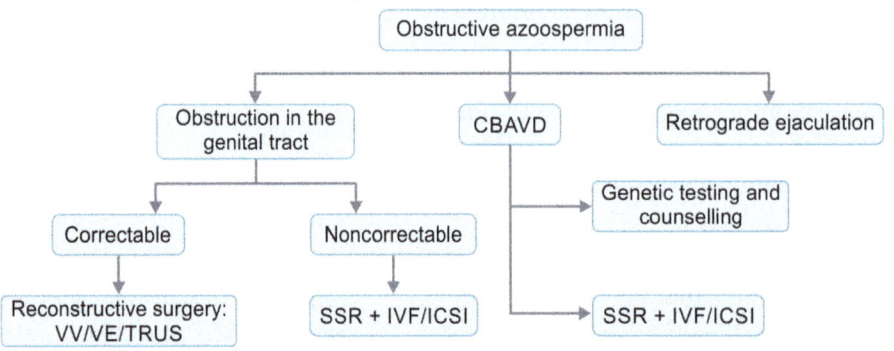

Flowchart 3: Management of obstructive azoospermia.[13]

(CBAVD: congenital bilateral absence of the vas deferens; IVF/ICSI: in vitro fertilization with intracytoplasmic sperm injection; SSR: surgical sperm retrieval; TRUS: transurethral resection of ejaculatory duct; VE: vasoepididymostomy; VV: vasovasostomy)

Reconstructive Surgery

- *Decision for reconstruction surgery* is multifactorial, based upon female partner characteristics, prior fertility, past surgical history, number of offspring desired, as well as religious and financial background.[16]
- *Predictors of microsurgical reconstruction outcomes* include intraoperative vasal fluid quality and sperm granuloma presence, vasal obstructive interval, and microsurgeon experience.[17]
- *Success rate:* Outcomes of microsurgical reconstruction have improved over the past four decades **(Table 3)**.

TABLE 3: Outcome post reconstructive surgery in obstructive azoospermia (OA).[10,18]

Type of reconstruction surgery	Patency rates	Pregnancy rates	Postoperative reobstruction
Vasovasostomy (VV)	70–99.5%	36–92%	12%
Vasoepididymostomy (VE)	30–90%	20–50%	21%

- *Monitoring postsurgery:* Sperm may return to the ejaculate as early as 1 month after surgery, especially in the case of vasovasostomy. Semen analyses done every 8–12 weeks in the postoperative period until sperm concentration and motility return to normal or until a pregnancy occurs.
- Surgery is considered to have failed if sperm do not return to the ejaculate by 6 months after vasovasostomy or by 18 months after vasoepididymostomy.[19]

Advantages of reconstructive surgery over surgical sperm retrieval (SSR) + intracytoplasmic sperm injection (ICSI):

- Surgery will allow the couple to achieve many pregnancies, whereas a new ICSI cycle is needed for each attempt.
- Surgery avoids the high chance of multiple pregnancy associated with ICSI and multiple embryo transfer.
- Performing corrective surgery may be more cost-effective than sperm retrieval and ICSI.[19] Therefore, SSR/ICSI should only be offered where the obstruction is not amenable to surgical correction or after failed surgery.

Management of nonobstructive azoospermia is depicted in **Figure 4**.

Surgical Sperm Retrieval Techniques

Indications *(Table 4)*

- For OA cases not amenable to surgical intervention or failure of surgery—SSR + IVF/ICSI is the treatment of choice.
- For testicular causes of NOA cases—SSR + ICSI but only postgenetic testing and counseling.

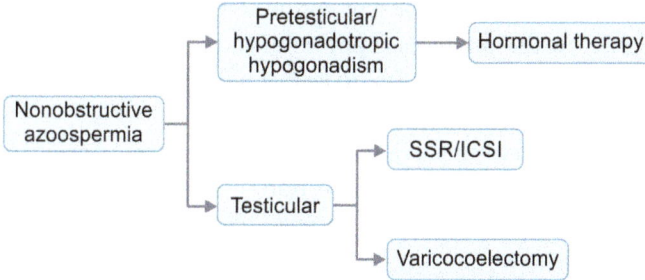

Fig. 4: Management of nonobstructive azoospermia.[20]

TABLE 4: Indications and procedure of sperm retrieval techniques.

Technique	Indications	Procedure
PESA	OA: Postepididymal obstruction	Epididymis is first stabilized between thumb and the index finger and epididymal sperm aspiration is done using a fine needle percutaneously
MESA	OA: Postepididymal obstruction	A fine incision is made on the epididymis and using operating microscope single tubule of the epididymis is identified, contents aspirated
TESA	• OA: Pre-epididymal obstruction • Failed epididymal retrievals • NOA	A wide bore needle (20–22 G scalp vein needle) attached to a 10 or 20 mL syringe is inserted through the scrotal skin into the testis, along the anteromedial or anterolateral side of the testis at an oblique angle to avoid any injury to the blood vessels under tunica albuginea. The fluid is aspirated after creating negative pressure
cTESE	• OA: Pre-epididymal obstruction • Failed epididymal retrievals • Failed TESA attempts • NOA	It is an open surgical method where in the testicular tissue is excised without the help of operating microscope. Biopsy sample, approximately around 450–500 g, is put in the petri dish with culture media and sent to the laboratory
microTESE	NOA	In it, the scrotum is incised and the testis is exteriorized. A transverse incision is taken and testicular parenchyma is exposed. With the help of operative stereo microscope of up to 14–25X magnification, seminiferous tubules are examined and more turgid tubules which look healthier with increased diameter are selected and microsurgical multiple biopsies taken. Hemostasis is better achieved as vessels can be easily identified under the microscope and injury avoided. The tunica is then closed with 5-0 or 6-0 polypropylene sutures

(cTESE: conventional testicular sperm extraction; MESA: microscopic ependymal sperm aspiration; microTESE: microsurgical testicular sperm extraction; NOA: nonobstructive azoospermia; OA: obstructive azoospermia; PESA: percutaneous ependymal sperm aspiration; TESA: testicular sperm aspiration)

TABLE 5: Advantages and disadvantages of sperm retrieval techniques.

Technique	Advantages	Disadvantages
PESA	Fast and low cost, no microsurgical expertise required, local anesthesia, fast and repeatable, and minimal morbidity	Few sperm retrieved, risk of hematoma, and damage to adjacent tissue
MESA	Minimal postoperative discomfort, large number of sperm retrieved, and reduced risk of hematoma	Requires microsurgical expertise, increased cost, general or local anesthesia, and incision required
TESA	Fast and low cost, no microsurgical expertise required, repeatable, and minimal to mild morbidity	Few sperm retrieved in NOA, risk of hematoma, and risk of testicular atrophy
cTESE	No microsurgical expertise required, local or general anesthesia, few instruments, and fast and repeatable	Few sperm retrieved in NOA, risk of testicular atrophy, and postoperative discomfort
microTESE	Higher success rates in NOA and larger number of sperm retrieved	Increased cost and time-demanding, require microsurgical expertise, postoperative discomfort, and limited risk of testicular atrophy (with multiple biopsies)

(cTESE: conventional testicular sperm extraction; MESA: microscopic ependymal sperm aspiration; microTESE: microsurgical testicular sperm extraction; NOA: nonobstructive azoospermia; PESA: percutaneous ependymal sperm aspiration; TESA: testicular sperm aspiration)

Objectives[21]

- To retrieve adequate number of sperms to be used for ICSI
- To retrieve adequate number of sperms to be used for cryopreservation as well
- To try to find morphologically better sperms
- To minimize complications and limit testicular damage
  Advantages and disadvantages of sperm retrieval techniques are given in **Table 5**.
- *In testicular azoospermia:*
  - Studies have suggested that microTESE is 1.5-fold more effective than cTESE, which is twofold more effective than TESA.[22]
  - More recent reports have found similar retrieval rates (46%) in both microTESE and cTESE.[23]
  - Pre-SSR patient hormonal optimization:[20,24]
    - In testicular azoospermia no role of clomiphene citrate, aromatase inhibitors, and human chorionic gonadotropin (hCG) to improve the sperm retrieval rate.
  - In hypogonadal men with NOA, there is no relationship between preoperative testicular volume, FSH levels, or testosterone response to hormonal therapy and TESE sperm retrieval outcomes.[25]
- Cryopreserved testicular sperm are as good as fresh testicular sperm in their fertilizing ability and pregnancy rates.[26]
- The transient changes in the testis, due to hematoma formation and inflammation can negatively affect spermatogenesis therefore a repeat procedure is less likely to yield sperm if performed <3-6 months after the initial SSR.[27,28]

Varicocele Treatment in Men with Nonobstructive Azoospermia

- Varicocele is found in 4.3-13.3% of men with severely impaired spermatogenesis or azoospermia.[29]
- The causal link between varicocele and NOA, however, is weakly established.[30]
- A clinical benefit is observed when correcting a clinical varicocele in NOA men before IVF/ICSI.[31]
- This benefit is most pronounced in patients with histological evidence of hypospermatogenesis.
- Varicocele therapy may be less effective in NOA patients with maturation arrest or Sertoli cell-only syndrome.
- Given the prognostic potential of testicular histology, biopsy at the time of varicocele repair may provide useful information for patient counseling.
- Semen cryopreservation should be performed as azoospermia relapse has been noted in several studies at varying intervals in this population.[32,33]

Hormonal Therapy

- Indicated in in pretesticular azoospermia—HH
- Irrespective of etiology, HH is one of the most medically treatable causes of NOA.[20]

Gonadotropin-releasing Hormone Therapy[20]

- It is as effective as gonadotropin therapy in achieving spermatogenesis and pregnancy in patients with hypothalamic disorders who have intact pituitary function.
- Pulsatile administration of 5-20 mg every 2 hours via an infusion pump is used.
- It is less likely to be used than gonadotropin therapy due to its cumbersome nature and its ineffectiveness in men with panhypopituitarism.

Gonadotropin

- hCG monotherapy (1,000-1,500 IU, two to three times/week)—advised for individuals with testicular volume >4 mL and/or no history of cryptorchidism. If the patient remains azoospermic after 3-6 months of treatment, FSH supplementation is added.[34]
- *Combined therapy:* hCG (1,000-1,500 IU, two to three times/week) and FSH (75-150 IU, two to three times/week)

is the "gold standard" for patients with prepubertal testicular volume, i.e., <4 mL.
- *FSH priming followed by hCG:* A 2-4 months FSH-priming stimulates Sertoli and spermatogonial cell proliferation leading to increase in testicular volume, and then hCG can be added when testicular volume reaches around 8 mL.
- The first sign of response can be observed after 3-6 months, but fertility induction may take up to 24 months to reach the maximal effect.[35]
- *For men with anabolic steroid-induced hypogonadism:*[36-39]
  - Discontinuation of exogenous androgens/steroids and prevention of further use is recommended
  - Time to recovery in suppressed individuals is variable[36]

REFERENCES

1. WHO. (2010). WHO laboratory manual for the examination and processing of human semen, 5th ed. [online] Available from https://apps.who.int/iris/handle/10665/44261. [Last accessed April, 2023].
2. Jaffe TM, Kim ED, Hoekstra TH, Lipshultz LI. Sperm pellet analysis: a technique to detect the presence of sperm in men considered to have azoospermia by routine semen analysis. J Urol. 1998;159(5):1548-50.
3. Practice Committee of the American Society for Reproductive Medicine in collaboration with the Society for Male Reproduction and Urology. Evaluation of the azoospermic male: a committee opinion. Fertil Steril. 2018;109(5):777-82.
4. Cocuzza M, Alvarenga C, Pagani R. The epidemiology and etiology of azoospermia. Clinics (Sao Paulo). 2013;68 Suppl 1(Suppl 1):15-26.
5. Schlegel PN, Sigman M, Collura B, De Jonge CJ, Eisenberg ML, Lamb DJ, et al. Diagnosis and Treatment of Infertility in Men: AUA/ASRM Guideline Part I. J Urol. 2021;205(1):36-43.
6. Jarow JP, Espeland MA, Lipshultz LI. Evaluation of the azoospermic patient. J Urol. 1989;142:62-5.
7. Chillon M, Casals T, Mercier B, Bassas L, Lissens W, Silber S, et al. Mutations in the cystic fibrosis gene in patients with congenital absence of the vas deferens. N Engl J Med. 1995;332(22):1475-80.
8. Yu J, Chen Z, Ni Y, Li Z. CFTR mutations in men with congenital bilateral absence of the vas deferens (CBAVD): a systemic review and meta-analysis. Hum Reprod. 2012;27(1):25-35.
9. Schlegel PN, Shin D, Goldstein M. Urogenital anomalies in men with congenital absence of the vas deferens. J Urol. 1996;155(5):1644-8.
10. Wosnitzer M, Goldstein M, Hardy MP. Review of Azoospermia. Spermatogenesis. 2014;4:e28218.
11. Male Infertility Best Practice Policy Committee of the American Urological Association; Practice Committee of the American Society for Reproductive Medicine. Report on evaluation of the azoospermic male. Fertil Steril. 2006; 86(5 Suppl 1):S210-5.
12. Plotton I, Brosse A, Cuzin B, Lejeune H. Klinefelter syndrome and TESE-ICSI. Ann Endocrinol (Paris). 2014;75:118-25.
13. Hopps CV, Mielnik A, Goldstein M, Palermo GD, Rosenwaks Z, Schlegel PN. Detection of sperm in men with Y chromosome microdeletions of the AZFa, AZFb and AZFc regions. Hum Reprod. 2003;18:1660-5.
14. Choi JM, Chung P, Veeck L, Mielnik A, Palermo GD, Schlegel PN. AZF microdeletions of the Y chromosome and in vitro fertilization outcome. Fertil Steril. 2004;81:337-41.
15. Silveira LF, Trarbach EB, Latronico AC. Genetics basis for GnRH-dependent pubertal disorders in humans. Mol Cell Endocrinol. 2010;324(1-2):30-8.
16. Practice Committee of the American Society for Reproductive Medicine in collaboration with the Society for Male Reproduction and Urology. The management of obstructive azoospermia: a committee opinion. Fertil Steril. 2019;111(5):873-80.
17. Hsiao W, Goldstein M, Rosoff JS, Piccorelli A, Kattan MW, Greenwood EA, et al. Nomograms to predict patency after microsurgical vasectomy reversal. J Urol. 2012;187:607-12.
18. Matthews GJ, Schlegel PN, Goldstein M. Patency following microsurgical vasoepididymostomy and vasovasostomy: temporal considerations. J Urol. 1995;154:2070-3.
19. Wolter S, Neubauer S, Heidenreich A. Vasovasostomy versus MESA/TESE combined with ICSI. A cost benefit analysis. J Urol. 1999;161:312.
20. Practice Committee of the American Society for Reproductive Medicine. Management of nonobstructive azoospermia: a committee opinion. Fertil Steril. 2018;110(7):1239-45.
21. Esteves SC, Miyaoka R, Orosz JE, Agarwal A. An update on sperm retrieval techniques for azoospermic males. Clinics. 2013;68(S1):99-110.
22. Bernie AM, Mata DA, Ramasamy R, Schlegel PN. Comparison of microdissection testicular sperm extraction, conventional testicular sperm extraction, and testicular sperm aspiration for nonobstructive azoospermia: A systematic review and meta-analysis. Fertil Steril. 2015;104(5):1099-103.e3.
23. Corona G, Minhas S, Giwercman A, Bettocchi C, Dinkelman-Smit M, Dohle G, et al. Sperm recovery and ICSI outcomes in men with non-obstructive azoospermia: a systematic review and meta-analysis. Hum Reprod Update. 2019;25(6):733-57.
24. Flannigan RK, Schlegel PN. Microdissection testicular sperm extraction: preoperative patient optimization, surgical technique, and tissue processing. Fertil Steril. 2019;111(3):420-6.
25. Reifsnyder JE, Ramasamy R, Husseini J, Schlegel PN. Role of optimizing testosterone before microdissection testicular sperm extraction in men with nonobstructive azoospermia. J Urol. 2012;188(2):532-6.
26. Friedler S, Raziel A, Strassburger D, Komarovsky D, Ron-El R. Intracytoplasmic injection of fresh and cryopreserved testicular spermatozoa in patients with nonobstructive azoospermia—a comparative study. Fertil Steril. 1997;68:892-7.
27. Schlegel PN, Su LM. Physiological consequences of testicular sperm extraction. Hum Reprod. 1997;12(8):1688-92.
28. Amer M, El Haggar S, Moustafa T, El-Naser TA, Zohdy W. Testicular sperm extraction: Impact of testicular histology on outcome, number of biopsies to be performed and optimal time for repetition. Hum Reprod. 1999;14(12):3030-4.
29. Ishikawa T, Kondo Y, Yamaguchi K, Sakamoto Y, Fujisawa M. Effect of varicocelectomy on patients with unobstructive

azoospermia and severe oligospermia. BJU Int. 2008;101: 216-8.
30. Persad E, O'Loughlin CAA, Kaur S, Wagner G, Matyas N, Hassler-Di Fratta MR, et al. Surgical or radiological treatment for varicoceles in subfertile men. Cochrane Database Syst Rev. 2021;4: CD000479.
31. Kohn TP, Kohn JR, Pastuszak AW. Varicocelectomy before assisted reproductive technology: are outcomes improved? Fertil Steril. 2017;108(3):385-91.
32. Lee JS, Park HJ, Seo JT. What is the indication of varicocelectomy in men with nonobstructive azoospermia? Urology. 2007;69:352-5.
33. Pasqualotto FF, Sobreiro BP, Hallak J, Pasqualotto EB, Lucon AM. Induction of spermatogenesis in azoospermic men after varicocelectomy repair: an up-date. Fertil Steril. 2006;85:635-9.
34. Bhasin S. Approach to the infertile man. J Clin Endocrinol Metab. 2007;92:1995-2004.
35. Burgues S, Calderon MD. Subcutaneous self-administration of highly purified follicle stimulating hormone and human chorionic gonadotrophin for the treatment of male hypogonadotrophic hypogonadism. Spanish Collaborative Group on Male Hypogonadotropic Hypogonadism. Hum Reprod. 1997;12:980-6.
36. Liu PY, Swerdloff RS, Christenson PD, Handelsman DJ, Wang C, Hormonal Male Contraception Summit Group. Rate, extent, and modifiers of spermatogenic recovery after hormonal male contraception: an integrated analysis. Lancet. 2006;367:1412-20.
37. Menon DK. Successful treatment of anabolic steroid-induced azoospermia with human chorionic gonadotropin and human menopausal gonadotropin. Fertil Steril. 2003;79(Suppl 3):1659-61.
38. Turek PJ, Williams RH, Gilbaugh JH 3rd, Lipshultz LI. The reversibility of anabolic steroid-induced azoospermia. J Urol. 1995;153:1628-30.
39. Coward RM, Rajanahally S, Kovac JR, Smith RP, Pastuszak AW, Lipshultz LI. Anabolic steroid induced hypogonadism in young men. J Urol. 2013;190:2200-5.

Ejaculatory/Erectile Dysfunction—Work-up and Management

Vivek Kakkad, Harsh Nihlani

■ INTRODUCTION

Sexual dysfunctions have been reported very frequently among a large proportion of men and it has profound impact on the quality of life and male infertility might be a consequence of these sexual dysfunctions. There is a vicious cycle here because the majority of men with infertility are anxious, depressed, and emotionally labile and this, in turn, affects the overall sexual health of the couple. Data from population-based studies suggest that 50% of men report at least one or the other form of sexual development during their lifetime. The prevalence of sexual dysfunctions among Indian males is grossly underreported due to paucity of good quality data and the social stigma and taboo associated with this issue.[1]

Sexual dysfunctions may affect any of the five stages of male sexual function—sexual desire, erection, sexual intercourse, ejaculation, and orgasm. Psychological factors tend to play a greater role in the pathogenesis of these dysfunctions than organic factors. This makes it even more difficult to elucidate the cause and obscures the management options. These disorders can be either lifelong, always present, or situational, limited to a certain time frame of life. Ejaculatory dysfunction is the most common form of sexual dysfunction experienced by men and may directly or indirectly lead to infertility among 2–4% of couples by affecting the frequency of vaginal intercourse.[2]

This chapter will shed some light into the common causes of sexual dysfunction, evaluation pathways, and management options targeting the fertility concerns and sexual health of men.

■ ERECTILE DYSFUNCTION

A normal erection is a result of an articulated interplay between the nervous system (peripheral and autonomic) and hemodynamic alterations in the penis on the background of unique anatomical features of the penis. Erectile dysfunction (ED) is defined as a man's continuous inability (≥3 months) to attain and/or maintain a penile erection sufficient for satisfactory sexual intercourse. Prevalence of ED increases with the advancing age and the presence of ED is a hallmark of cardiovascular dysfunction and it should be received as an opportunity to improve men's health.[3]

Erectile dysfunction is most commonly due to psychogenic causes—generalized (generalized inhibition or unresponsiveness) or situational (partner or performance related) and less commonly due to organic causes vascular, neurogenic, endocrine, anatomical factors, and exogenous drug intake (thiazides and antipsychotics). Proper history taking remains the hallmark in differentiating organic from psychogenic ED and there are patient questionnaires such as Sexual Health Inventory for Men (SHIM) and International Index of Erectile Function (IIEF) to facilitate dialogue and diagnosis.[4,5] General physical examination should evaluate the anthropometric variables [height, weight, and body mass index (BMI)], signs of androgenization, detailed urogenital examination, rectal examination, and nervous system examination to confirm the integrity to reflex arcs (cremasteric and anal wink reflex).

Men with ED should undergo a psychological evaluation to find out immediate and deeper causes of sexual dysfunction. General blood investigations should be performed to check the well-being (hemogram, lipid profile, and blood sugars) and specific hormonal tests [testosterone, prolactin, and follicle-stimulating hormone (FSH)/luteinizing hormone (LH)/thyroid-stimulating hormone (TSH)] in men with reduced libido and signs of hypogonadism **(Flowchart 1)**. Penile Doppler clubbed with intracavernous injection and stimulation may help in evaluating the vascular factors leading to ED and may serve both diagnostic and therapeutic purposes.[6] Psychophysiological evaluation [nocturnal penile tumescence (NPT), RigiScan, and NPT electrobioimpedance] can be done in patients with sleep disorders, legally sensitive cases and when the cause of ED is obscure and there is no response to medical therapy.[7]

Lifestyle modifications and psychosexual therapy are the first line of supportive therapies for ED aiming to eliminate the modifiable risk factors. Phosphodiesterase-5 (PDE-5) inhibitors (sildenafil and tadalafil) form the first line of pharmacotherapy and require careful monitoring

Flowchart 1: Evaluation and management of erectile dysfunction.

Suspicion of erectile dysfunction

First-line evaluation

- **Proper history taking** (organic vs. psychogenic)
- **Patient questionnaires** (SHIM and IIEF)
- **Clinical examination**
  - Anthropometry, androgenization
  - Genitourinary examination
  - Rectal examination
  - Nervous system examination (cremasteric reflex, anal wink reflex, bulbocavernosus reflex)

Second-line evaluation

- **Psychological evaluation**
- **General blood screening tests**
  - Hemogram, lipid profile, blood sugars
  - **Hormonal tests** (decreased libido, signs of hypogonadism)
    - Testosterone, FSH, LH TSH, prolactin, estradiol
- **Imaging**
  - Combined Intravenous injection and stimulation
  - Penile duplex ultrasonography
  - Cavernous arterial occlusion pressure
- **Psychophysiological tests**
  - Nocturnal penile tumescence (NPT)
  - RigiScan
  - NPT electrobioimpedance
- **Neurophysiological tests**
  - EMG, NCV, SSEPs

Management options

- **Lifestyle modifications** (exercise, weight loss, dietary changes)
- **Psychosexual therapy** (behavioral techniques, couples' therapy)
- **Medical therapy**
  - PDE-5 inhibitors (**first-line therapy**; sildenafil, tadalafil)
  - Intracavernosal agents (**second line**; PGE1 analogs—alprostadil)
  - Intraurethral agents (MUSE) (**second line**)
  - Testosterone therapy
  - Treatment for hyperprolactinemia
- **Surgical therapy**
  - Vacuum device (**second line**)
  - Penile prosthesis (**third line**)
  - Penile revascularization procedures (**third line**)
- **Experimental therapies**
  - Platelet rich plasma
  - Shock wave therapy
  - Stem cell therapy

(EMG: electromyography; FSH: follicle-stimulating hormone; IIEF: International Index of Erectile Function; LH: luteinizing hormone; MUSE: Medicated Urethral System for Erection; NCV: nerve conduction velocity; SHIM: Sexual Health Inventory for Men; SSEPs: somatosensory evoked potentials; TSH: thyroid-stimulating hormone)

of side effects (priapism, worsening of heart disease, and drug interactions) and some men with hypogonadism not desiring fertility can receive testosterone replacement therapy as well. Agents like alprostadil (prostaglandin E1 analog) can be used via intracavernous or intraurethral routes [Medicated Urethral System for Erection (MUSE)]. Patients with ED refractory to medical management may opt for vacuum constriction devices, penile implants, and revascularization procedures.[8]

EJACULATORY DYSFUNCTION

Ejaculation is predominantly controlled by the nervous system—both peripheral and central nervous system. Ejaculatory reflex has three phases—emission (deposition of semen in posterior urethra and bladder neck closure, mediated by sympathetic nervous system), expulsion (regulated by pudendal nerve and perineal muscles), and orgasm (pleasurable sensation due to increasing pressure of posterior urethra). Ejaculatory dysfunction can be either due to the inability to ejaculate [retrograde ejaculation (RE), anejaculation] or due to abnormal time taken for ejaculation [premature ejaculation (PE), delayed ejaculation (DE)] or sometimes, painful ejaculation **(Flowchart 2)**. There is a growing concern to label intravaginal ejaculatory dysfunction (ejaculation during masturbation but not during sexual intercourse) as a separate diagnostic entity.[9]

Premature Ejaculation

Premature ejaculation is the most common ejaculatory disorder and it affects almost 40–50% of sexually active men. PE is the inability to control ejaculation for a sufficient length of time during intravaginal containment to satisfy the female in at least 50% of coital events. There are multiple definitions on the basis of intravaginal ejaculation latency time (IELT) and generally a time interval of <1 minute is suggestive of PE in the absence of other disorders.[10,11]

Premature ejaculation can be either lifelong or acquired, generalized or situational, mild (30 seconds to 1 minute), moderate (15–30 seconds), or severe (<15 seconds) depending on the latency time. PE can be due to psychological causes (fear, guilt, and anxiety), neurobiological causes, infections, hormonal alterations (hypogonadism), or due to exogenous drug intake. Evaluation should focus on medical and a detailed sexual history to ascertain the latency time, control of ejaculation and the impact on quality of life. IELT is defined as the time interval between penetration and ejaculation and it can be assessed by stopwatch method or sexual assessment monitor.[11] Hormonal tests are

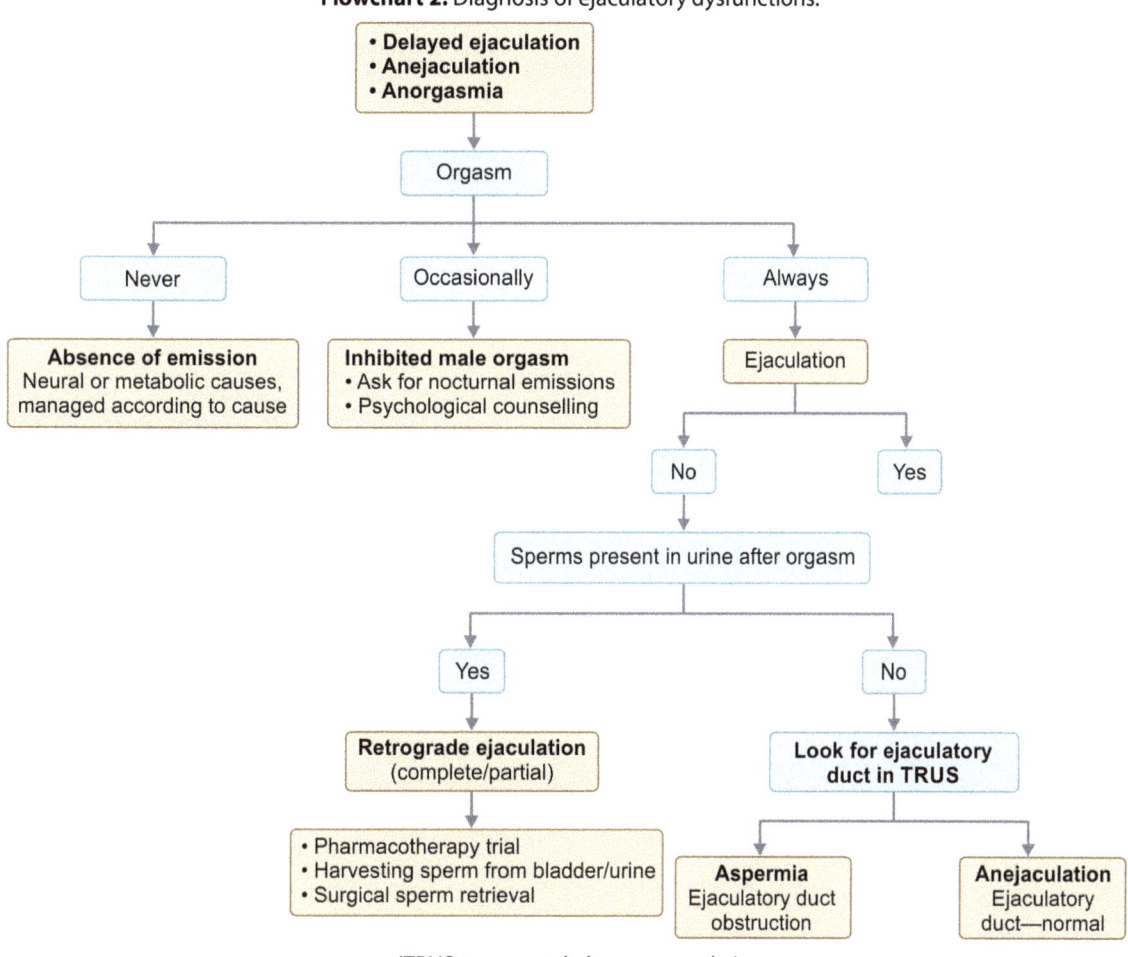

Flowchart 2: Diagnosis of ejaculatory dysfunctions.

(TRUS: transrectal ultrasonography)

indicated only if PE is associated with decreased libido and neurophysiological tests can be done but they have limited diagnostic potential.[12]

Psychosexual therapy is the first step of management and the strategies are designed to re-instill confidence in the male partner, reduce performance anxiety, and modify maladaptive sexual notions. The "start-stop" technique and "squeeze" technique are frequently combined with other distraction therapies **(Flowchart 3)**. Pharmacotherapy **(Table 1)** includes selective serotonin reuptake inhibitors (SSRIs) (paroxetine—most efficacious), topical local anaesthetics (to be applied before intercourse), alpha-blockers, and intracavernosal injection of vasoactive agents (for coexistent ED). Surgical therapies such as selective dorsal nerve neurotomy, glans penis augmentation, and circumcision do not have much acceptance and have conflicting evidence regarding their efficacy.[13]

Delayed Ejaculation/Anejaculation

Delayed ejaculation (DE) includes a spectrum of disorders ranging from increased latency to ejaculation to absent ejaculation. There is no firm consensus on latency time but latencies beyond 25–30 minutes are assumed to suffer from DE. Anejaculation is the complete failure to achieve ejaculation despite adequate stimulation whereas anorgasmia is the perceived absence of orgasm experience irrespective of the physiological concomitants of ejaculation.[14]

These disorders occur when any psychogenic cause (inadequate stimulation), medical disease (diabetes mellitus, hypogonadism, hypothyroidism, and multiple sclerosis) or surgical procedure (prostate surgeries, retroperitoneal surgeries, and spinal cord injuries) affects the central control of ejaculation, sympathetic nerve supply to the bladder neck or vas deferens, and nerve supply to the pelvic floor or penis. Obstructive pathologies secondary to infections, posterior urethral valves, pelvic trauma, or pelvic radiotherapy can also lead to similar consequences.[15]

History taking should include details about the age of first masturbation, frequency, the strength of erection, time interval for ejaculation, volume of ejaculate, and whether orgasm is attained or not. All patients should undergo general physical and detailed systemic examination to identify organic causes. Screening and specific blood tests (testosterone) should be done depending on the probable cause of concern. The patients should undergo routine urine

Flowchart 3: Evaluation and management of premature ejaculation.

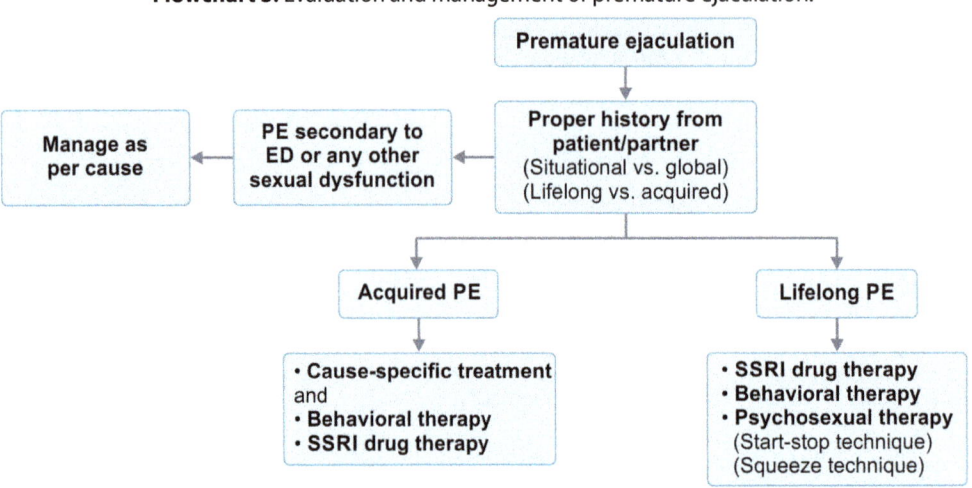

(ED: erectile dysfunction; PE: premature ejaculation; SSRI: selective serotonin reuptake inhibitor)

TABLE 1: Pharmacotherapy for premature ejaculation.					
Drug	**Dose**	**Dosing instructions**	**Route**	**Side effects**	**Remarks**
Dapoxetine	30–60 mg	On demand, 1–3 hours before intercourse	Oral	• Nausea • Headache • Diarrhea • Dizziness	
Paroxetine	10–40 mg	Once daily	Oral	• Fatigue • Decreased libido	
Sertraline	50–200 mg	Once daily	Oral	Nausea	
Clomipramine	12.5–50 mg	Once daily or on demand, 3–4 hours before intercourse	Oral	Yawning	
Fluoxetine	20–40 mg	Once daily	Oral	Diarrhea	
Citalopram	20–40 mg	Once daily	Oral	Perspiration	
Tramadol	25–50 mg	On demand, 3–4 hours before intercourse	Oral	• Headache • Dry mouth • Sleepiness	Risk for opiate addiction
Topical lignocaine/prilocaine	Patient titrated	On demand, 20–30 minutes before intercourse	Topical	Allergic reactions	
Alprostadil	5–20 µg	Patient administered intracavernous injection 5 minutes before intercourse	Intracavernous	• Priapism • Corporal fibrosis	Very low evidence
PDE-5 inhibitors	• Sildenafil 25–100 mg • Tadalafil 10–20 mg • Vardenafil 10–20 mg	On demand, 30–50 minutes before intercourse	Oral	• Headache • Flushing • Dizziness	Only with coexistent ED

(ED: erectile dysfunction; PDE-5: phosphodiesterase-5)

analysis and postejaculatory urine analysis to rule out RE. Perineal and transrectal ultrasound are useful noninvasive adjuncts in uncovering the reasons for absent/low volume antegrade seminal emission.[16]

The first step of management is to differentiate RE form failure of emission by doing a postejaculatory urine analysis. Further management depends on whether the man desires fertility or not and all the patients should undergo psychological counseling aiming at masturbatory retraining and adjustment of sexual fantasies. Pharmacotherapy, although less effective, can be tried in certain situations such as dopamine agonists for hyperprolactinemia and testosterone therapy in hypogonadal cases. The next step is targeted at collecting spermatozoa by collection of nocturnal sperm emissions in spermicide free condoms, stimulation of ejaculation by prostatic massage, penile vibratory stimulation (PVS), or electroejaculation. Spermatozoa retrieved by these methods can be used for assisted reproductive technology (ART) and surgical sperm retrieval methods (percutaneous sperm aspiration or testicular extraction) should be preferred in couples committed to ART.[17]

Retrograde Ejaculation

Antegrade ejaculation is possible due to the closure of the bladder neck and proximal urethra and the contraction of urethral smooth muscle at the verumontanum is essential to prevent RE. RE accounts for 0.3–2% of male infertility and it can be due to anatomical causes (prostatic surgeries and posterior urethral valves), drugs (alpha-blockers and antipsychotics), and neurogenic factors (spinal cord injuries, retroperitoneal surgeries, and neuropathies).

Postejaculatory urine analysis showing 5–10 sperms/hpf confirms the presence of RE and more sperms in urine than antegrade ejaculate suggests a significant component of RE.[18] Medical therapy includes sympathomimetic agents (pseudoephedrine) and tricyclic antidepressants (TCAs; imipramine 25 mg BD) but these agents only help in some form of antegrade ejaculation and do not ensure complete recovery. The other forms of therapy include sperm harvesting from the urinary bladder (first step), bladder neck reconstruction/collagen injection and surgical sperm retrieval (most effective).[19] Sperm harvesting from urinary bladder is done after obtaining a postejaculatory urine specimen either by voiding or catheterization usually after alkalinization of urine using oral sodium bicarbonate or increasing intake of oral fluids to dilute urine. The urine specimen is then suspended in medium, centrifuged, and resuspended to be used for either intravaginal insemination, intrauterine insemination (IUI), in vitro fertilization (IVF), or intracytoplasmic sperm injection (ICSI). The ongoing pregnancy rate per cycle was around 17% and live birth rate was 15% per cycle in couples in which urinary sperm retrieval was done.[19]

Painful Ejaculation

It is defined as penile, perineal, scrotal, or testicular pain during or shortly after ejaculation and is mostly due to infectious causes followed by obstructive etiologies. Evaluation should be targeted to detect chronic infections—routine urine analysis, culture, screening for sexually transmitted infections (STIs) and imaging (transrectal ultrasound), and cystoscopy for specific causes. Treatment includes anti-inflammatory agents, antibiotics, and promotion of perineal hygiene measures.[20]

REFERENCES

1. McCabe MP, Sharlip ID, Lewis R, Atalla E, Balon R, Fisher AD, et al. Incidence and prevalence of sexual dysfunction in women and men: a consensus statement from the fourth international consultation on sexual medicine 2015. J Sex Med. 2016;13(2):144-52.
2. Perlis N, Lo KC, Grober ED, Spencer L, Jarvi K. Coital frequency and infertility: which male factors predict less frequent coitus among infertile couples? Fertil Steril. 2013;100(2):511-5.
3. Yannas D, Frizza F, Vignozzi L, Corona G, Maggi M, Rastrelli G. Erectile Dysfunction Is a Hallmark of Cardiovascular Disease: Unavoidable Matter of Fact or Opportunity to Improve Men's Health? J Clin Med. 2021;10(10):2221.
4. Cappelleri JC, Rosen RC. The Sexual Health Inventory for Men (SHIM): a 5-year review of research and clinical experience. Int J Impot Res. 2005;17(4):307-19.
5. Rosen RC, Riley A, Wagner G, Osterloh IH, Kirkpatrick J, Mishra A. The international index of erectile function (IIEF): a multidimensional scale for assessment of erectile dysfunction. Urology. 1997;49(6):822-30.
6. Jung DC, Park SY, Lee JY. Penile Doppler ultrasonography revisited. Ultrason Seoul Korea. 2018;37(1):16-24.
7. Liu T, Xu Z, Guan Y, Yuan M. Comparison of RigiScan and penile color duplex ultrasound in evaluation of erectile dysfunction. Ann Palliat Med. 2020;9(5):2988-92.
8. Yafi FA, Jenkins L, Albersen M, Corona G, Isidori AM, Goldfarb S, et al. Erectile dysfunction. Nat Rev Dis Primer. 2016;2:16003.
9. Otani T. Clinical review of ejaculatory dysfunction. Reprod Med Biol. 2019;18(4):331-43.
10. Parnham A, Serefoglu EC. Classification and definition of premature ejaculation. Transl Androl Urol. 2016;5(4):416-23.
11. Althof SE, McMahon CG, Waldinger MD, Serefoglu EC, Shindel AW, Adaikan PG, et al. An Update of the International Society of Sexual Medicine's Guidelines for the Diagnosis and Treatment of Premature Ejaculation (PE). Sex Med. 2014;2(2):60-90.
12. Rowland DL, Althof SE, McMahon CG. The Unfinished Business of Defining Premature Ejaculation: The Need for Targeted Research. Sex Med Rev. 2022;10(2):323-40.
13. Mitsogiannis I, Dellis A, Papatsoris A, Moussa M. An up-to-date overview of the pharmacotherapeutic options for premature ejaculation. Expert Opin Pharmacother. 2022;23(9):1043-50.
14. Abdel-Hamid IA, Ali OI. Delayed Ejaculation: Pathophysiology, Diagnosis, and Treatment. World J Mens Health. 2018;36(1):22-40.
15. Shindel AW. Anejaculation: relevance to sexual enjoyment in men and women. J Sex Med. 2019;16(9):1324-7.
16. Forbes CM, Flannigan R, Paduch DA. Perineal Ultrasound: a Review in the Context of Ejaculatory Dysfunction. Sex Med Rev. 2018;6(3):419-28.
17. Capogrosso P, Jensen C, Rastrelli G, Torremade Barreda J, Russo G, Raheem A, et al. Male Sexual Dysfunctions in the Infertile Couple–Recommendations From the European Society of Sexual Medicine (ESSM). Sex Med. 2021;9:100377.
18. Mehta A, Jarow JP, Maples P, Sigman M. Defining the "normal" postejaculate urinalysis. J Androl. 2012;33(5):917-20.
19. Jefferys A, Siassakos D, Wardle P. The management of retrograde ejaculation: a systematic review and update. Fertil Steril. 2012;97(2):306-12.
20. Fan D, Mao W, Wang G, Shi H, Wu Z, Xie J, et al. Study on the relationship between sex hormone changes and erectile dysfunction in patients with chronic prostatitis/chronic pelvic pain syndrome. Ann Palliat Med. 2021;10(2):1739-47.

CHAPTER 27: Dyspareunia—Work-up and Management

Sudha Prasad, Saumya Prasad, Shrinkhla Khandelwal, Priyanka Kar

■ INTRODUCTION

Expression of sexuality is one of the most complex aspects of the human behavior, and sexual function is its key aspect. Sexual dysfunction is more common in women than men, yet it is less investigated. If left untreated, sexual problems are associated with decreased quality of life, depression, and interpersonal conflicts.

The Diagnostic and Statistical Manual of Mental Disorders (DSM) defines female sexual dysfunction (FSD)[1] as "any sexual complaint or problem resulting from disorders of desire, arousal, orgasm, or sexual pain that causes marked distress or interpersonal difficulty" **(Table 1)**. To qualify as a dysfunction, the problem must be present >75% of the time, for >6 months, affecting the quality of life of the patient.

Dyspareunia is one of the most challenging complaints that a healthcare provider can come across. Ensuring adequate time and a comfortable setting to address a woman's concern is of utmost importance. It can significantly affect a woman's well-being and quality of life.

The medical term for painful intercourse is dyspareunia, defined as, persistent or recurrent genital pain that occurs just before, during or after sexual intercourse. It is a common condition in both young and elderly women with somatic and psychological elements.[3] Hence the providers should feel empowered to treat this condition with adequate information.

TABLE 1: Categories of FSD.

DSM-4[2]	DSM-5
Desire disorders	Desire/arousal disorders
Arousal disorders	
Orgasm disorder	Female orgasm disorders
Sexual pain disorder: • Dyspareunia: Pelvic pain with intercourse • Vaginismus: Pelvic floor muscle spasm leading to pain and obstruction to penetration	Genitopelvic pain/penetration disorder: Vaginismus + dyspareunia

(DSM: Diagnostic and Statistical Manual of Mental Disorders; FSD: female sexual dysfunction)

■ ETIOLOGY AND CLASSIFICATION

Dyspareunia can be classified on the basis of the following:[4]

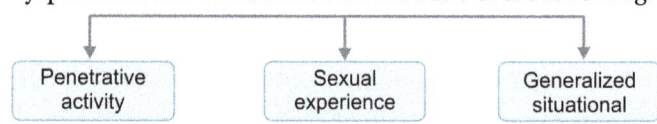

Dyspareunia is classified on the basis of a penetrative activity as **(Table 2)**:
- Superficial—insertional dyspareunia
- Deep—seen with deep penetration
- Both.

Some of the common causes observed are as follows:
- *Vaginismus:*
  - It is caused by the involuntary contraction of pelvic floor muscles, leading to dyspareunia.
  - It can also be experienced during tampon insertion and any gynecological examination.
  - There are different forms of vaginismus. Symptoms vary within individuals and range from mild to severe pain.
  - It can be due to medical or emotional factors, or both.
  - Dyspareunia with vaginismus is now termed as *genitopelvic pain or penetration disorder.*
- *Vaginal dryness and age-related factors:*
  - During sexual arousal, glands at the vaginal opening secrete lubricants to aid in intercourse. A lesser quantity of fluid secretion can lead to painful intercourse.[6]
  - Inadequate lubrication can be due to many factors such as hypoestrogenism, old age factors such as lichen sclerosis or lichen planus, medications, and lack of foreplay.
- *Vaginitis:*[5,6]
  - Differences in pH from normal vaginal pH can lead to excessive discharge and pain during intercourse.
- *Vulvodynia:*[7]
  - It is a type of chronic pain which affects a woman's external sexual organs, collectively known as vulva, which includes, labia, clitoris, and vaginal orifice.

TABLE 2: Classification of dyspareunia on the basis of a penetrative activity.

Superficial	Deep	Both
Anatomical: • Imperforate hymen • Vaginal septum	Endometriosis	Anxiety
Accessory gland involvement: • Bartholin cyst/abscess • Skene's cyst	Adenomyosis	Iatrogenic pain after instrumentation
Vaginitis: • Candidal vulvovaginitis • Chlamydial vaginitis • Bacterial vaginosis • Group A Streptococcus • Trichomonas vaginitis	Leiomyoma	Insufficient lubrication: • Urogenital atrophy • Vaginitis • Infective causes
Vestibulitis	Pelvic inflammatory diseases	Perineal ulcers
Atopic dermatitis	Pelvic organ prolapse	Surgery
Genital mutilation	Cervical pathology • Polyps • Cervicitis	Sexual abuse
Age-related changes: • Lichen sclerosis • Lichen planus • Atrophic vaginitis[5] • Vaginal stenosis	Urological: • Cystitis • Urethral stone • Urethral diverticulum	Vaginal or pelvic trauma
UTI	• Pelvic congestion syndrome • Dysmenorrhea	Sjögren's syndrome
Vaginismus[5]	Pelvic adhesions	
Herpetic neuralgia	Female genital TB	
Vulvodynia[5]	Gastrointestinal: • Ulcerative colitis • Crohn's disease • Diverticular diseases • Chronic constipation	
Pudendal neuropathy	Psychological diagnosis: • Depression • Anxiety • Psychosomatic disorders	
Hemorrhoids	Iatrogenic: • Chemotherapy • Radiation • Surgical scars	
Autoimmune causes: • Lichen planus • Desquamative • Inflammatory vaginitis • Pemphigus vulgaris	Pelvic malignancies	
	Musculoskeletal conditions: • Myofascial pain syndrome • Levator ani spasm • Osteitis pubis • Pelvic fractures	
	Clitoral pathology	
	Malfunction of IUD	

(IUD: intrauterine device; TB: tuberculosis; UTI: urinary tract infection)

- It may occur in just a single spot or affect different areas from one time to the next.
- Its cause is still unknown, but self-care with medical and psychosexual treatment can bring relief.
- *Endometriosis-associated dyspareunia:*
  - Endometriotic spots release excessive amounts of inflammatory cytokines such as tumor necrosis factor-α (TNF-α) and interleukins which trigger the pain.[8]
  - Sexual intercourse can stretch, pull, and mechanically cause pain.
- *Pelvic inflammatory disease (PID) and female genital tuberculosis (TB):*
  - PID and TB cause the formation of hydrosalpinx and an increase in inflammatory markers along with the accumulation of exudates in the system which triggers pain.[9]
- *Malfunction of intrauterine device (IUD):*
  - No direct causal relationship has been identified between IUD and dyspareunia. However, the presence of IUD causing PID or IUD migration to the bladder/peritoneum can also cause dyspareunia.
  - IUD causing endometrial rupture is a rare entity.
- *Anatomical causes:*
  - Müllerian anomalies such as septum in the vagina or imperforate hymen can cause mechanical obstruction and hence greater force during penetration leading to dyspareunia.
  - Any previous surgical scars (e.g., episiotomy) or history of any perineal trauma sustained due to accidents or as a result of female genital mutilation causes fibrosis of tissue at the vulval opening and increased sensitivity of the nerve endings at the perineum.

It can be classified on basis of sexual experience **(Table 3)**:
- Primary—coincides with coitarche
- Secondary—follows an early period of pain-free sexual activity.

TABLE 3: Classification of dyspareunia on the basis of sexual experience.

Primary	Secondary
Sexual abuse	Endometriosis
Female genital mutilation	Pelvic inflammatory disease (PID)
Congenital anomalies • Imperforate hymen • Vaginal septum • Mayer–Rokitansky–Küuster–Hauser syndrome	Fibroids
	Pelvic infections
	Vaginal atrophy

It can also be:
- Generalized—present during all the acts of intercourse
- Situational—seen during intercourse with specific partners or positions.

SIGNS AND SYMPTOMS

Symptoms
- Pain (burning or aching) occurs at entry or with deep penetration.
- Thin sparse pubic hair. This is usually seen in cases with menopause associated genital atrophy or associated with other autoimmune causes of atrophy and vaginitis.
- Pain with every penetration including tampons.
- Pain that lasts for hours after intercourse.

Signs
- *Clitoral atrophy:* It is seen in postmenopausal patients mostly due to a lack of adequate hormone environment. Treatment with vaginal estrogen, low-dose testosterone or dehydroepiandrosterone sulfate (DHEA-S), and oxytocin have shown promising results.
- Bacterial or fungal growth in case of an infective etiology.
- Vaginal pH >5.0. Normal vaginal pH is between 3.8 and 5. A slightly acidic pH protects the vaginal mucosa from harmful pathogens. Any increase in alkalinity of the vaginal environment acts as an incubator of microbial growth.
- The unnatural appearance of the epithelium as seen in lichen sclerosis or lichen planus, pemphigoid, and atrophic vulva.

MANAGEMENT (TABLE 4)

Diagnosis
- History of vaginal discharge, vulvar pain, dysmenorrhea, or any chronic pelvic pain.
- Past history of pelvic surgery, surgery for an abscess, or an obstetric delivery.
- On local examination—the presence of any generalized erythema, episiotomy scar, vulval or vaginal wall atrophy, prolapse, or any infection.
- Very rarely it may be after lactation caused hypoestrogenism which will indirectly cause vaginal atrophy.
- Decreased lubrication.

Physical Examination
- *On inspection:*
  - Look for any vulvar rashes, redness or pustules and warts, any scratch marks due to repeated itching, which may indicate venereal diseases or genital infections.

TABLE 4: Common causes of dyspareunia and its management.

S. no.	Etiological cause	History at presentation	Examination and diagnosis	Treatment
1.	Imperforate hymen (anatomical cause)	• Amenorrhea • Cryptomenorrhea	• On examination: Bluish bulging membrane • Investigations: On USG, hematometra and hematocolpos	Cruciate incision and drainage
2.	• MRKH • Vaginal septum	• Amenorrhea • Inability to consummate marriage	• On examination: Vaginal dimple and septum present • Investigations: On USG, absent uterus, uterine, and/or cervical septum	• Vaginoplasty • Septal resection
3.	Bartholin cyst/abscess	Pain and tenderness at introitus, if large	On examination: Tender cystic swelling in lower third of the vestibule	• Antibiotics • Marsupialization • Sclerotherapy • Incision and drainage
4.	Vaginismus	Inability to consummate marriage	On examination: Resistance to digital examination	• Self-manual dilatation • Psychosexual counseling
5.	Age related	Elderly woman with complaints of recurrent vaginal infections, UTI, dysuria, dribbling of urine	On examination: Loss of vaginal rugosities, pale and thin vaginal epithelium, and ±discharge	Lubrication local estradiol cream
6.	Vaginitis	Complaints of itching, rashes over vulva, and foul smelling discharge	• On examination: Bright red vagina and vaginal discharge • Investigations: Vaginal and cervical culture will rule out the cause of vaginitis. • Vaginal pH >4.5	Antibiotics
7.	Endometriosis	Deep dyspareunia, ±dysmenorrhea, ±dyschezia	• On examination: Nonmobile uterus with forniceal fullness and tenderness in cases with endometrioma, uterosacral nodularity in rectovaginal endometriosis • Investigations: On USG-ground glass appearance of an endometrioma	• Endometrioma excision • Cautery of endometriotic spots • GnRH agonists • Hormonal therapy • Androgens • LUNA/ablation of endometriotic spots
8.	PID and hydrosalpinx	Abdominal pain, fever, and vaginal discharge	• On examination: Uterine and forniceal tenderness • Investigations: USG clearly delineates hydrosalpinges, leukocytosis and increased C-reactive protein. Laparoscopy is gold standard	• Antibiotics • Delinking of tubes • Salpingectomy
9.	Adhesions	Lower abdominal dull pain, past history of surgery, chronic PID, or history of genital TB	• On examination: Fixed uterus, ±tenderness • Investigations: Laparoscopy and hysteroscopy will show dense wedge-like projections from one wall of the uterus to the other, Fitz-Hugh-Curtis syndrome seen.	Adhesiolysis
10.	Female genital tuberculosis	History of primary infection, recurrent pregnancy loss or recurrent implantation failures	• On examination: Fixed uterus • Investigations: Asherman's syndrome seen on hysteroscopy • HSG findings: Lead pipe abnormality • Tobacco pouch appearance • Golf club appearance • Diverticula • Peritubal adhesions • Beaded tubal abnormalities	• AKT • Adhesiolysis
11.	Vulvodynia	Past history of trauma or surgery at perineum or vulval area, history of chronic pain at a single spot or affecting various areas	On history (diagnosis of exclusion), pain during digital examination	Psychotherapy

(GnRH: gonadotropin-releasing hormone; HSG: Hysterosalpingography; LUNA: laparoscopic uterosacral nerve ablation; MRKH: Mayer–Rokitansky–Küster–Hauser; PID: pelvic inflammatory disease; TB: tuberculosis; USG: ultrasonography; UTI urinary tract infection)

- On per speculum examination, note any offensive and discolored discharge from the cervix. Note the vaginal walls color and rugae.
- Note for any excoriation marks on the vulva. Look for shiny silvery scaly lesions on vulva as seen in age-related atrophy or autoimmune causes of vaginitis such as lichen planus and pemphigoid.
- *On palpation:*
  - Bartholin and paraurethral gland palpation
  - Single digit insertion into distal vagina to diagnose vaginismus
  - Anterior vaginal palpation to rule out interstitial cystitis
  - Deeper digital palpation to rule out mid-vaginal pain
  - Palpation of insertion points of uterosacral ligaments to rule out endometriosis
  - Palpation of pelvic floor muscles
  - Cervical motion tenderness
  - Bimanual palpation of uterus to rule out leiomyoma, PID-like features
- *On per-rectal examination* and palpation of rectovaginal septum is done to look for any:
  - Hemorrhoids
  - Endometriotic nodularity
  - Myofascial tenderness
- Stool to be checked for occult blood.

Diagnostic Testing

- Saline slide preparation for diagnosis of different pathogens which can cause vaginitis.
- Vaginal pH test. A patient with bacterial vaginosis presents with an alkaline pH test. Vaginal pH is maintained in an acidic environment and any infection can swing the pH in the opposite direction.
- Vaginal and urine culture and sensitivity
- Fungal culture, if applicable. KOH slides and culture and sensitivity help in diagnosis of vulvovaginal candidiasis. Fungal hyphae can be seen on KOH slides.
- Radiological examination to rule out any structural abnormality such as Müllerian anomalies such as vaginal septum and imperforate hymen.

Treatment

- *Home care:*[10]
  - Water-soluble lubricants
  - Emptying bladder prior to intercourse
  - Intercourse to happen in a relaxed and inter-communication between both partners' minds.
  - Pain relievers may be taken before sex.
  - An ice pack may be applied over the vulva after having sex.
  - Water-based vaginal lubricants (KY jelly, Astroglide). It is applied before intercourse.
  - Polycarbophil-based gel can hold water to add moistness to vagina. However, its acidity lowers the vaginal pH. It is used up to three times weekly.
- *Drugs:*
  - Pharmacotherapy of dyspareunia is based on the etiology of the symptom.
  - Antibiotics
  - Antifungals
  - Topical or injectable corticosteroids
  - Hormone therapy
  - Estrogen cream—17-beta-estradiol
  - Vaginal estradiol tablet—10 µg daily for 2 weeks, followed by twice weekly
  - Vaginal ring—17-beta-estradiol or estradiol acetate. Replaced every 3 months
  - Selective estrogen receptor modulator (SERM)—ospemifene 60 mg is used to treat vulvar and vaginal atrophy
- *Surgery:*
  - For correction of any structural abnormality such as adhesiolysis, endometrial ablation[11]
  - Uterine suspension in a retroverted uterus
  - Fenton procedure
- Botox injections in the pelvic floor muscle. Refractory vaginismus may respond to the Botox injections into the puborectalis and pubococcygeus. Patient selection is of utmost importance due to limited evidence.[12]
- *Psychotherapies:*[13]
  - Cognitive behavioral therapies or sex therapies
  - Psychosexual counseling—for patients of abuse or any trauma or any associated emotional source. It is also important for maintenance of sexual and reproductive health.[14]
  - Relaxation techniques—Kegels exercise.

CONCLUSION

- Dyspareunia is the medical term for painful intercourse and its etiology encompasses both organic and psychosomatic causes.
- The diagnosis of dyspareunia should be made after addressing all of the woman's concern and after finding the cause for the same.
- The clinician should be able to outline the history and review the psychosocial considerations before embarking on the management of the condition.
- Patients with dyspareunia should be counseled regarding the cause of their condition, and the follow-up treatment of the enticing cause, be executed accordingly.
- Even in patients with a known anatomic cause, we should always ask a psychologist for a psychosexual analysis of the patient and hence improve, self-confidence of the patient and interpersonal relationships of the couple intending.

REFERENCES

1. Kershaw V, Jha S. Female sexual dysfunction. Obstet Gynaecol. 2022;24:12-23.
2. Binik YM. Should dyspareunia be retained as a sexual dysfunction in DSM-V? A painful classification decision. Arch Sex Behav. 2005;34(1):11-21.
3. Alizadeh A, Farnam F. Coping with dyspareunia, the importance of inter and intrapersonal context on women's sexual distress: a population-based study. Reprod Health. 2021;18:161.
4. Hoffman BL. Pelvic pain. In: Hoffman BL, Schorge J, Bradshaw K, Halvorson L, Schaffer J, Corton M (Eds). William's Gynecology, 3rd edition. USA: McGraw-Hill Education; 2016. pp. 253-63.
5. Tayyeb M, Gupta V. Dyspareunia. Treasure Island (FL): StatPearls Publishing; 2022.
6. Hoffman BL. Menopausal transition. In: Hoffman BL, Schorge J, Bradshaw K, Halvorson L, Schaffer J, Corton M (Eds). William's Gynecology, 3rd edition. USA: McGraw-Hill Education; 2016. pp. 486-87.
7. Bornstein J, Goldstein AT, Stockdale CK, Bergeron S, Pukall C, Zolnoun D, et al. 2015 ISSVD, ISSWSH and IPPS Consensus Terminology and Classification of Persistent Vulvar Pain and Vulvodynia. Obstet Gynecol. 2016;127(4):745-51.
8. Hoffman BL. Endometriosis. In: Hoffman BL, Schorge J, Bradshaw K, Halvorson L, Schaffer J, Corton M (Eds). William's Gynecology, 3rd edition. USA: McGraw-Hill Education; 2016. pp. 234.
9. Nikki MW Li, Adam D Jakes, Jillian Loyd, Leila CG Frodsham. Dypareunia. BMJ. 2018;19;361.
10. Sorensen J, Bautista KE, Lamvu G, Feranec J. Evaluation and Treatment of Female Sexual Pain: A Clinical Review. Cureus. 2018;10(3):e2379.
11. Hoffman BL. Surgeries for benign gynecological disorders. In: Hoffman BL, Schorge J, Bradshaw K, Halvorson L, Schaffer J, Corton M (Eds). William's Gynecology, 3rd edition. USA: McGraw-Hill Education; 2016. p. 962.
12. Moga MA, Dimienescu OG, Bălan A, Scârneciu I, Barabaș B, Pleș L. Therapeutic Approaches of Botulinum Toxin in Gynecology. Toxins (Basel). 2018;10(4):169.
13. Morin M, Carroll MS, Bergeron S. Systematic review of the effectiveness of physical therapy modalities in women with provoked vestibulodynia. Sex Med Rev. 2017;5:295-322.
14. Weijmar Schultz W, Basson R, Binik Y, Eschenbach D, Wesselmann U, Van Lankveld J. Women's sexual pain and its management. J Sex Med. 2005;2(3):301-16.

Work-up and Management of Premature Ovarian Insufficiency

Nivedita Shetty, Prakash B Savanur

■ INTRODUCTION

More cases of POI are being identified, most likely secondary to improved recognition and awareness. It is even more important in the era of assisted reproduction since there are solutions for fertility preservation. However, the important goal in recognising this condition is to improve the overall health of the woman by identifying and preventing the development of secondary complications.

■ TERMINOLOGY

It was previously called as premature ovarian failure. The term premature ovarian insufficiency (POI) was first used by the American endocrinologist, Fuller Albright in 1942[1] and accepted by the American consensus meeting and The European Society of Human Reproduction and Embryology ESHRE guideline committee.[2,3]

■ DEFINITION

Premature ovarian insufficiency is a clinical condition where there is a loss of ovarian activity before the age of 40 years resulting in menstrual disturbances like oligomenorrhea or amenorrhea with raised gonadotropins and low estradiol.[3]

■ PREVALENCE[4,11,12]

- Ranges from 1 to 4% of the overall population
- Prevalence is higher in low and medium human development index countries.

■ RISK FACTORS[9,10]

- Family history—mother and sister having similar problem
- Early menarche and nulliparity
- Child of a multiple pregnancy
- Smoking and low body mass index (BMI).

■ CAUSES[6,7]

Autoimmune

- Polyglandular autoimmune syndrome types I and II
- Primary adrenal insufficiency
- Autoimmune thyroiditis
- Nonendocrine conditions (systemic lupus erythematosus, pernicious anemia, and myasthenia gravis).

Enzyme Deficiencies

- Galactosemia [galactose-1-phosphate uridylyltransferase (GALT)]
- 17 alpha-hydroxylase
- Aromatase.

Infections

- Viral [mumps, cytomegalovirus (CMV), and varicella]
- Bacterial (tuberculosis and *Shigella*)
- Parasite (malaria).

Genetic Syndromes

- Ataxia telangiectasia
- Fanconi anemia
- Premature aging syndromes (Bloom and Werner)
- Blepharophimosis, ptosis, and epicanthus inversus syndrome (BPES).

Toxins and Injury

- Chemotherapy (e.g., alkylating agent)
- Radiation
- Pelvic surgery (oophorectomy)
- Smoking.

X Chromosome Disorders

- Turner syndrome (TS) (XO and mosaics)
- Triple X syndrome (XXX)
- Fragile X [*fragile X mental retardation gene 1 (FMR1)* gene premutation carrier]
- Diaphanous-related formin 2 (DIAPH2) translocation
- Bone morphogenetic protein 15 (BMP15) variants
- Progesterone receptor membrane component 1 (PGRMC1) variants
- X chromosome deletions, inversions, duplications, and balanced translocations.

Other Single Gene Variants

- Ovarian function genes: *BMP15, GDF9, FIGLA, FSHR*, etc.
- DNA repair genes: *MCM8/9, FANCA/M/C/G, RAD51*, etc.

Idiopathic

- Majority still idiopathic
- *More genetic cases being identified:* Account up to 25% cases.

■ RECOMMENDED DIAGNOSTIC CRITERIA[8]

Oligomenorrhea/amenorrhea for 4 months in a woman <40 years supported by the laboratory tests.

The diagnostic algorithm for a woman suspected of POI is presented in **Flowcharts 1 and 2**.

Points to Remember

- *Good clinical history* including history of surgery, medical treatment, radiotherapy, and family history.
- *Physical examination*: Turner's signs, scars from previous surgery, BMI, and any other phenotypically abnormal features.
- *Hormonal assay:* Follicle-stimulating hormone (FSH) should have been done for diagnosis. Following hormone assay is necessary after diagnosis: Baseline serum estradiol, thyroid function tests (TFTs), prolactin, serum testosterone, sex hormone binding globulin (SHBG), and vitamin D.
- *Genetic testing:*
  - Karyotype for aneuploidy, mosaicism, deletion, and duplications
  - Fragile X premutation carrier screening
- *Autoimmune screening:*
  - *Thyroid autoantibodies:* Thyroid peroxidase antibody and thyroglobulin antibody
  - 21-hydroxylase antibodies
- *Imaging studies:* Dual X-ray absorptiometry for bone mineral density (BMD) at the time of diagnosis.

Further referral depending on the test results:[3] Referral to a *menopause specialist* could be considered if there is any doubt about the diagnosis **(Table 1)**.

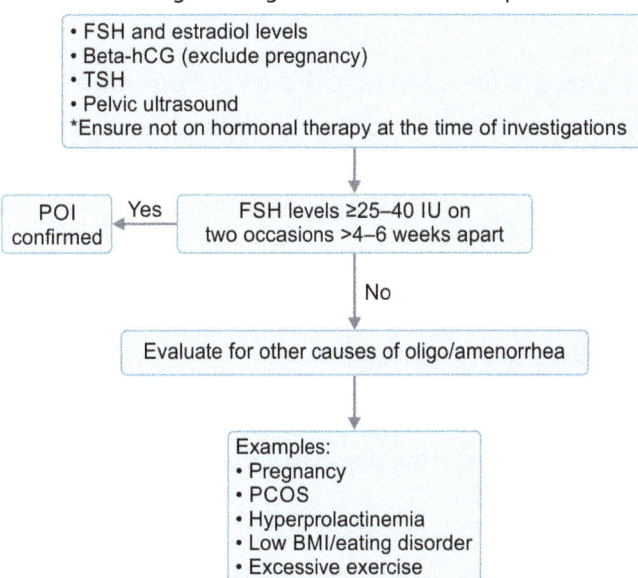

Flowchart 1: Diagnostic algorithm for a woman suspected of POI.

(BMI: body mass index; FSH: follicle-stimulating hormone; hCG: human chorionic gonadotropin; PCOS: polycystic ovary syndrome; POI: premature ovarian insufficiency; TSH: thyroid-stimulating hormone)

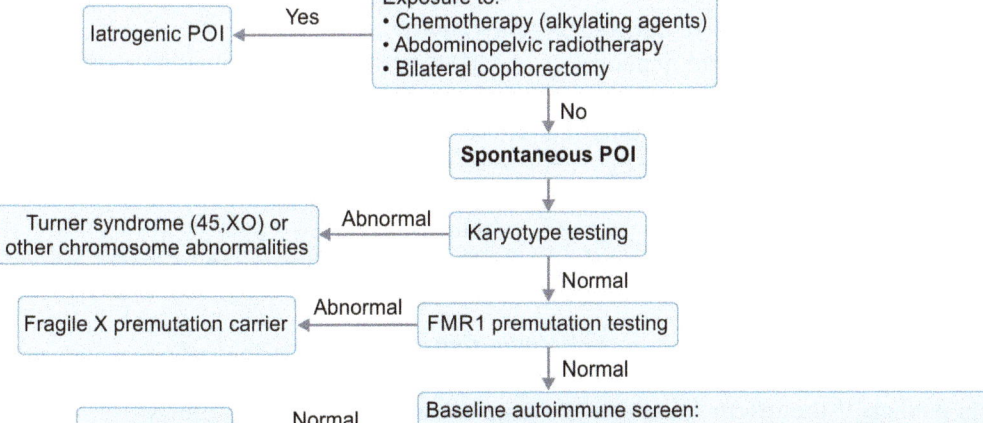

Flowchart 2: Work-up when POI is diagnosed.[8]

(FMR1: fragile X mental retardation gene 1; POI: premature ovarian insufficiency; TSH: thyroid-stimulating hormone)

TABLE 1: Considerations after test results.

Test	Positive	Negative
Karyotyping (Turner syndrome)	Refer to endocrinologist, cardiologist, and geneticist	If there is high clinical suspicion repeat test in epithelial cells
Y chromosome	Discuss gonadectomy	
FRA-X	Refer to geneticist	
ACA/21OH antibodies	Refer to endocrinologist	Retest if clinical signs or symptoms
Anti-TPO	Check thyroid-stimulating hormone (TSH) every year	

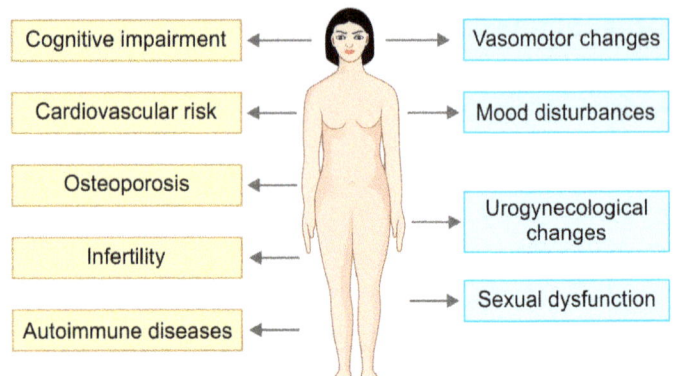

Fig. 1: Premature ovarian insufficiency sequelae.

Premature Ovarian Insufficiency Sequelae[8]

Premature ovarian insufficiency sequelae is depicted in **Figure 1**.

■ TREATMENT

Lifestyle Modifications[5]

- Balanced diet including vitamin D3 800–1,000 IU/day with calcium supplementation
- *Maintain healthy weight:* BMI <25
- *Regular exercise:* Weight-bearing exercises such as walking and strength training exercises for upper body
- Avoid smoking
- *Limit alcohol:* No alcohol is better.

Hormone Replacement Treatment[5,13]

- Hormone replacement treatment (HRT) is the cornerstone in the management of POI unless contraindicated. It is indicated till the age of natural menopause to avoid adverse effects of early cessation of ovarian function on cardiovascular and bone health.
- Estrogen is essential for bone, cardiovascular, neurological, sexual and genitourinary health, and general well-being.
- Either HRT or combined hormonal contraceptive pills (COCPs) should be offered unless contraindicated (e.g., in women with hormone-sensitive cancer).
- It is recommended to use HRT until at least the age of natural menopause (around 50 years) unless contraindicated. HRT is preferable to COCPs.
- HRT as either tablets or patches is acceptable.
- Combined HRT is required if uterus is present and estrogen-only HRT is enough if the uterus has been removed for other reasons.
- 17β-estradiol is preferred to ethinylestradiol or conjugated equine estrogens for estrogen replacement. Estradiol can be started with 2 mg and increased up to 4 mg as required.
- Suggested HRT preparations and doses are given in **Table 2**.[8]

TABLE 2: Hormone replacement treatment preparations and doses.

Estrogen component	Dose recommended
Estradiol valerate	2 mg/day
Ethinylestradiol	10 μg/day
Conjugated equine estrogen	1.25 mg/day
Transdermal estradiol	75–100 μg/24 hours patch, twice weekly application
Progesterone component-in intact uterus	
Long-acting intrauterine system (Mirena)	52 mg in the device. 20 μg delivery per day
Medroxyprogesterone acetate	• Cyclical regime: 10 mg/day, for 12 days/month • Continuous regime: 2.5–5 mg/day
Micronized progesterone	• Cyclical regime: 200 mg/day for 12 days/month • Continuous regime: 100 mg/day

Route and method of administration of HRT:[5]
- Patient preference and availability
- *First choice:*
  • Transdermal estrogen and progestogen
  • Transdermal estrogen as patch or gel with progestogen as IUS or tablets
- *Second choice:*
  • Oral estradiol/norethisterone as 2 mg/500 μg tablets daily.
  • The dose of estrogen can be increased up to 4 mg as necessary.

Monitoring HRT:
- Review at 3 months after initiating treatment and then annual review.
- Check compliance and blood pressure (BP).
- No need to check for blood levels of estradiol if asymptomatic.

Options for Fertility[6]

- Chance of spontaneous pregnancy is very low. About 5% within 2 years of diagnosis and very unlikely after that.

- However, if pregnancy is not desired, contraception is necessary.
- *Donor oocyte* is the main option for the fertility.
- With early diagnosis and timely intervention, might be able to *salvage reproductive potential* by elective *freezing of oocytes and ovarian tissue*. Particularly useful in those at risk for POI, such as young girls and women with genetic predispositions, pediatric and reproductive age cancer survivors, or women with autoimmune diseases.
- Breakthrough therapies still in experimental stages:
  - In vitro activation (IVA)
  - Mitochondrial activation
  - Stem cell and exosomes therapy
  - Intraovarian infusion of platelet-rich plasma (PRP).

Pregnancy in Premature Ovarian Insufficiency Patient[3]

- *High-risk pregnancy* depending on the cause of POI and the type of fertility treatment and comorbidity like cardiovascular problems.
- *Multidisciplinary approach* in pregnancy management is required: Obstetric medicine and other specialists depending on the cause of POI such as cardiologist, endocrinologist, and fetal medicine.

Pregnancy in Turner Mosaic/Turner Syndrome[14]

- Full preconception evaluation and counseling
- Counseled about increased cardiovascular risk in pregnancy
- Cardiac assessment with Holter BP monitoring, echocardiography ± thoracic MRI
- Management of pregnant women with TS should be undertaken by a *multidisciplinary team* including maternal-fetal medicine specialists and cardiologists with expertise in managing women with TS.
- ART or spontaneous conception should be avoided in case of an ascending aortic size index (ASI) of >2.5 cm/m^2 or an ascending ASI 2.0–2.5 cm/m^2 with associated risk factors for aortic dissection (AoD), which include bicuspid aortic valve, elongation of the transverse aorta, coarctation of the aorta, and hypertension.
- Vaginal delivery is reasonable in women with TS with an ascending ASI below 2.0 cm/m^2
- In women with TS with an ascending ASI of 2.0–2.5 cm/m^2, a vaginal delivery with epidural anesthesia and expedited second stage is preferred or a caesarean section may be considered.

Bone Health Management[3,5]

- Lifestyle modifications with emphasis on balanced diet with recommended calcium and vitamin D intake.
- HRT as described earlier
- Bisphosphonates if BMD in osteoporotic range should only be considered with advice from rheumatologists or related specialists.
- If BMD is normal at diagnosis and HRT commenced appropriately, no need to repeat dual-energy X-ray absorptiometry (DEXA).
- If BMD in the osteoporotic range at diagnosis, DEXA every 5 years and managed in association with rheumatologists.
- If HRT is contraindicated discuss with rheumatologists or other related specialists for bone health.

Cardiovascular Health Management[3,5]

- Lifestyle modifications as mentioned earlier
- HRT until the average of menopause
- Regular BP check
- *Important in TS:* Annual CV checkup with BP, lipid profile, fasting glucose, hemoglobin A1C (HbA1C), and echocardiogram (ECHO) when necessary.

Sexual and Genitourinary Function[3,5]

- HRT as described earlier and if required the following:
  - Vaginal lubricants
  - Vaginal estrogen
- Testosterone supplementation in the form of gel.

POI and BRCA 1/2 Gene Mutation/Breast Cancer Patient[3]

- Conventional HRT is contraindicated in breast cancer survivors.
- HRT can be prescribed in those without prior cancer after prophylactic bilateral salpingo-oophorectomy (BSO).
- Bisphosphonates might be considered for bone protection.
- Nonhormonal alternatives can be considered for symptom control.

POI and Hypertension[3]

- HRT not an absolute contraindication in women with hypertension.
- Transdermal estradiol is the preferred method.

POI and Venous Thromboembolism[3]

- Small increased risk of stroke and venous thromboembolism (VTE)
- Managed in association with hematologists/cardiologists
- Transdermal estradiol is preferred
- HRT with oral anticoagulants is an option in rare situations.

POI and Migraine[3]

- Migraine is not a contraindication for HRT
- Transdermal delivery carries lowest risk

- Consider changing dose, regimen, and route of administration when migraine worsens during HRT.

POI and Genetics[3]

- Genetic factors might be identified in 20–25% cases of POI.
- Among the genetic causes, X chromosome numerical and structural alterations are the most common—TS (45X), turner mosaic (45X/46XX), and trisomy X (47XXX)
- Genetic diagnosis is valuable in early intervention, possible fertility preservation, detection of associated problems, and counseling family members.

POI and Implications of Close Relatives[3]

Genetic counseling and testing should be offered for women with Fragile X premutation.

Counseling regarding their risk of developing POI:
- Except a known mutation, there is not reliable test to predict POI
- No established preventive measures
- Fertility preservation is an option as required
- Risk of early menopause should be taken into consideration if planning family.

Key Learning Points

- Women with POI are at risk of cardiovascular, bone, cognitive, and other chronic conditions.
- Management of women with POI should be a multidisciplinary approach.
- HRT should be given until the age of natural menopause unless contraindicated.
- Infertility is a significant condition in women with POI. Fertility treatment needs to be individualized and women counseled in detail about available options.
- Lifestyle, weight management, diet, and exercise should be optimized.

REFERENCES

1. Albright F, Smith PH, Fraser R. A syndrome characterized by primary ovarian insufficiency and decreased stature: report of 11 cases with a digression on hormonal control of axillary and pubic hair. Am J Med Sci. 1942;204:625-48.
2. Welt CK. Primary ovarian insufficiency: a more accurate term for premature ovarian failure. Clin Endocrinol (Oxf). 2008;68(4):499-509.
3. European Society for Human Reproduction and Embryology (ESHRE) Guideline Group on POI; Webber L, Davies M, Anderson R, Bartlett J, Braat D, et al. ESHRE Guideline: Management of women with premature ovarian insufficiency. Hum Reprod. 2016;31(5):926-37.
4. Huang QY, Chen SR, Chen JM, Shi QY, Lin S. Therapeutic options for premature ovarian insufficiency: an updated review. Reprod Biol Endocrinol. 2022;20:28.
5. Panay N, Anderson RA, Nappi RE, Vincent AJ, Vujovic S, Webber L, et al. Premature ovarian insufficiency: an International Menopause Society White Paper. Climacteric. 2020;23(5):426-46.
6. Wesevich V, Kellen AN, Pal L. Recent advances in understanding primary ovarian insufficiency. F1000Res. 2020;9:F1000 Faculty Rev-1101.
7. Chon SJ, Umair Z, Yoon MS. Premature Ovarian Insufficiency: Past, Present, and Future. Front Cell Dev Biol. 2021;9:672890.
8. Nguyen HH, Milat F, Vincent A. Premature ovarian insufficiency in general practice: Meeting the needs of women. Aust Fam Physician. 2017;46(6):360-6.
9. Di-Battista A, Moysés-Oliveira M, Melaragno MI. Genetics of premature ovarian insufficiency and the association with X-autosome translocations. Reproduction. 2020;160:R55-R64.
10. Silvén H, Savukoski SM, Pesonen P, Pukkala E, Gissler M, Suvanto E, et al. Incidence and familial risk of premature ovarian insufficiency in the Finnish female population. Hum Reprod. 2022;37(5):1030-6.
11. Gruber N, Kugler S, de Vries L, Brener A, Zung A, Eyal O, et al. Primary Ovarian Insufficiency Nationwide Incidence Rate and Etiology Among Israeli Adolescents. J Adolesc Health. 2020;66(5):603-9.
12. Gosden RG, Treloar SA, Martin NG, Cherkas LF, Spector TD, Faddy MJ, et al. Prevalence of premature ovarian failure in monozygotic and dizygotic twins. Hum Reprod. 2007;22(2):610-5.
13. Tao XY, Zuo AZ, Wang JQ, Tao FB. Effect of primary ovarian insufficiency and early natural menopause on mortality: a meta-analysis. Climacteric. 2016;19(1):27-36.
14. Gravholt CH, Andersen NH, Conway GS, Dekkers OM, Geffner ME, Klein KO, et al. Clinical practice guidelines for the care of girls and women with Turner syndrome: proceedings from the 2016 Cincinnati International Turner Syndrome Meeting. Eur J Endocrinol. 2017;177(3):G1-G70.

CHAPTER 29

Recurrent Pregnancy Loss: Work-up and Management

Shalini Gainder, Plabani Sarkar

INTRODUCTION

Diagnosis of recurrent pregnancy loss (RPL) could be considered after the loss of two or more pregnancies.[1] RPL affects 1–5% of all pregnancies. The true incidence of RPL escapes accurate estimation as most of the losses occur either before clinical recognition or sometimes even before the first missed period. Of the total pregnancies, 70% of female fails to report a pregnancy loss as 50% of these pregnancies tend to undergo spontaneous miscarriage before the first cycle and 20% are clinically unrecognized.[1,2]

Any pregnancy loss has a significant negative impact on a women's life and the repetitive nature of RPL could be the source of overwhelming grief experienced by these couples. Clinicians and clinics should take the psychosocial needs of couples faced with RPL into account when offering and organizing care for these couples.

Recurrent pregnancy loss is a broader terminology and encompasses the pregnancy losses due to:
- Recurrent miscarriages (first or second trimester)
- Recurrent preterm pregnancy losses
- Recurrent abruptio placentae
- Recurrent intrauterine fetal deaths
- RPLs due to hypertensive disorders of pregnancy.

In this chapter, we would discuss recurrent miscarriage and pregnancy losses due to preterm labor which are dependent on management in first and second trimester of pregnancy.

DEFINITION

Recurrent pregnancy loss has been the most ambiguous with the American Society of Reproductive Medicine defining RPL as "distinct disorder defined by two or more failed clinical pregnancies". The Royal College of Obstetricians and Gynaecologists (RCOG) guidelines for RPL[3] define recurrent miscarriage as "loss of three or more consecutive pregnancies". The most recent is the guidelines by the European Society of Human Reproduction and Embryology[1] where the diagnosis of RPL can be considered after the loss of two or more pregnancy loses.

A pregnancy loss (miscarriage) is defined as the spontaneous demise of a pregnancy before the fetus reaches viability including all pregnancy losses from the time of conception until 24 weeks of gestation. Primary RPL is described as RPL without a previous ongoing pregnancy (viable pregnancy) beyond 24 weeks of gestation, while secondary RPL is defined as an episode of RPL after one or more previous pregnancies progressing beyond 24 weeks of gestation.

RISK FACTORS FOR RECURRENT MISCARRIAGE

- A woman's risk of a pregnancy loss is directly related to the outcome of her previous pregnancies
- The risk of recurrence increases with each added pregnancy loss **(Table 1)**

TABLE 1: Etiological factors implicated in RPL.

Genetic (2–5%)	Aneuploidies, balanced, and other structural translocations
Endocrinological 5–8%	Thyroid disorders, uncontrolled diabetes, and hyperprolactinemia
Anatomical abnormality of uterus (1.8–37.6%)	• Congenital—septate, bicornuate, unicornuate, and didelphic uterus • Acquired—submucosal fibroids, polyps, and adhesions
Thrombophilia mainly APLS (8–42%)	• APLA syndrome—lupus, anticardiolipin, and anti-β2 glycoprotein 1 • Inherited—prothrombin gene *(PTG20210A)* mutation, factor V Leiden, and protein C and S deficiencies
Environmental and lifestyle related	Obesity, extreme underweight, smoking, excess alcohol, heavy metals, drug addiction-cocaine, and heroine
Immunological	HLA and ANA
Miscellaneous	Chronic endometritis
Unexplained (50%)	

(ANA: antinuclear antibody; APLA: antiphospholipid antibody; HLA: human leukocyte antigen; RPL: recurrent pregnancy loss)

TABLE 2: Age-related risk of miscarriage.

Age of the woman in years	Probability to have abortion[4]
<19	13%
20–24	11%
25–29	12%
30–34	15%
35–39	25%
40–44	51%
45–49	93%

TABLE 3: Risk factors for recurrent miscarriage.

	Other risk factors for recurrent miscarriage	Evidence level
I	Black ethnic groups	2+
II	Excess alcohol consumption	2+
III	Smoking	2+
IV	Excess caffeine intake	2++
V	Women with body mass index (BMI) < 19	2++
VI	Women with BMI > 25	2++
VII	Paternal age > 40 years	2++

- The recurrence may occur even if there is no genetic abnormality
- The age of the woman is the greatest determinant of recurrent miscarriage. With advancing age the risk of abortion rises remarkably probably related to increased incidence of aneuploidy in the conceptus.

RISK FACTORS AND SUGGESTED BEHAVIORAL MODIFICATIONS

- *Age:* Age-related risk of miscarriage **(Table 2)** in recognized pregnancies has been found to be 12% in 25–29 years, 15% in 30–34 years, 25% in 35–39 years, 51% in 40–44 years, and 93% in ≥ 45 years.[4] Advancing maternal age results in decline in number and quality of residual oocytes thereby increasing losses due to aneuploidy of the resulting embryos leading to recurrent implantation failure and recurrent miscarriages.
- *Healthy normal range body mass index (BMI):* Higher prevalence of RPL in obese women (30 kg/m^2) compared to women with normal BMI (19–24.9 kg/m^2) (0.45% vs. 0.1%). Another study by Metwally et al. concluded obese and underweight patients had a small but significant increased risk of miscarriage in subsequent pregnancy.[5,6]
- *Smoking:* Impact of smoking or its cessation on pregnancy loss in women of RPL needs further evaluation. Smoking has been strongly associated with adverse obstetric and neonatal outcomes. Impact of male smoking was more in heavy smokers compared to moderate smokers (<20 cigarettes/day).[7]
- *Alcohol:* It has clear negative impact on pregnancy and neonatal outcomes. Increased risk of pregnancy loss has been observed with more than two to four drinks per week.[8,9]
- *Stress:* Higher stress levels have been found to be a risk factor for RPL in smaller studies.[10,11]

Table 3 details other risk factors which can contribute to the woman's poor pregnancy outcome.

EVALUATION

Referral to a Dedicated Recurrent Pregnancy Loss Clinic

Dedicated RPL clinic requisites include qualified clinicians and specialists, trained staff, psychological counselor and social worker, necessary testing equipment, and most importantly well-organized set up to address the needs of these "distressed couples" can dramatically uplift the care experienced by these patients.

Provision of adequate information is one of the core principles in management of RPL couples. They should be aptly sensitized that definite cause may not be always elucidated and investigations may not lead to treatment options always.

Evaluation should be individualized as appropriate to each woman or couple, based on age, fertility, pregnancy history, family history, previous investigations, and treatments. When diagnosed with a problem for which treatment is uncertain, couples need more information about possible benefits and disadvantages. It is important to show good listening skills, awareness of the patient's obstetric history, and respect toward her previous pregnancy losses. Providing sensitive ear to the couple and assessing their emotional needs enables improvement in overall treatment of the patients. **Flowchart 1** gives a protocol of evaluation of recurrent pregnancy loss in a woman who visits her physician.

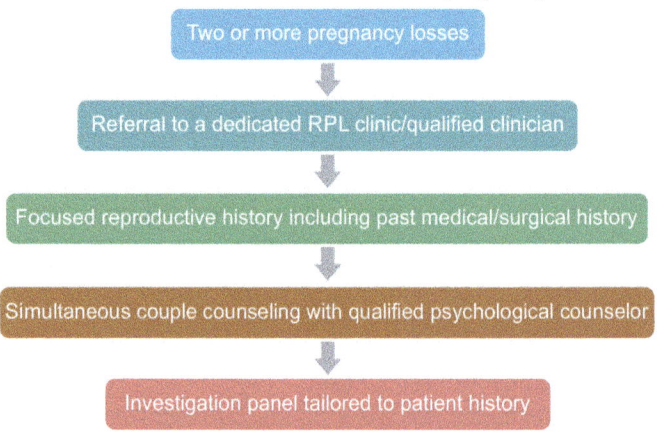

Flowchart 1: Evaluation of a woman with pregnancy losses.

PROGNOSTICATION AND MANAGEMENT

Prognostication should be guided by patients' exact history and maternal age. A complete pregnancy history (i.e.,

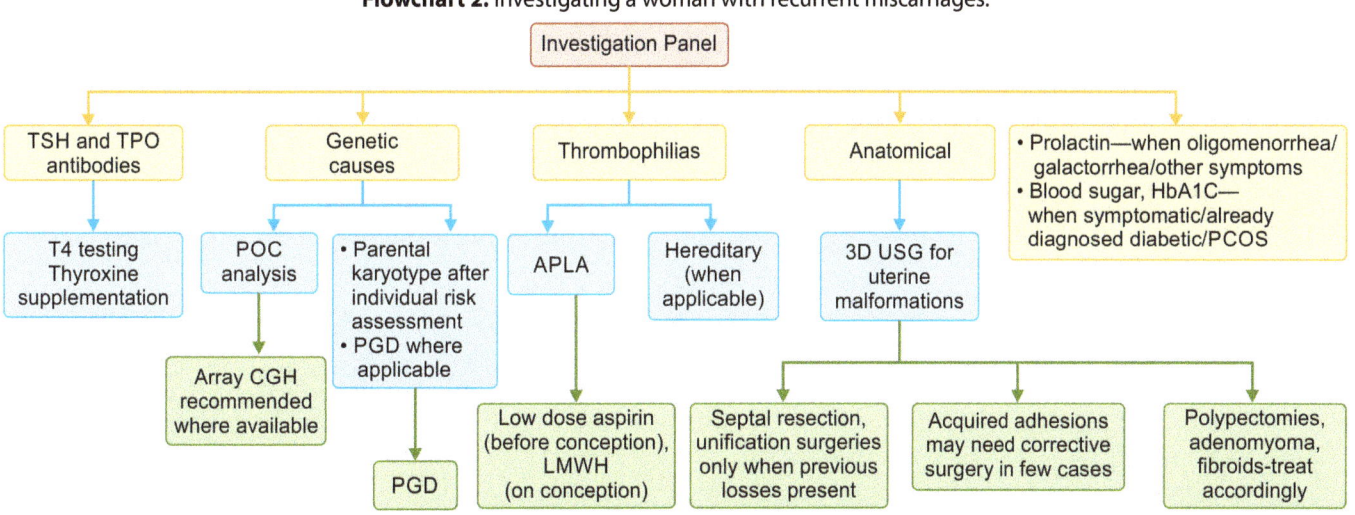

Flowchart 2: Investigating a woman with recurrent miscarriages.

(APLA: antiphospholipid antibody; CGH: comparative genomic hybridization; HbA1C: hemoglobin A1C; LMWH: Low-molecular-weight heparin; PCOS: polycystic ovary syndrome; PGD: preimplantation genetic diagnosis; POC: products of conception; USG: ultrasonography)

number of previous pregnancy losses, live births, and their sequence) is important in estimating chance of live birth in next pregnancy.

Use of several prediction models such as Brigham model and the Lund model, Kolte and Westergaard[12-14] yet to be validated, can be used to gauge estimates of subsequent live births in unexplained RPL. RPL couples have a good prognosis for the next live birth, especially if female age and the number of previous miscarriages are low.

EVALUATION OF RECURRENT PREGNANCY LOSSES

- *Thrombophilia:*
  - *Acquired*: Any woman reporting with RPL needs to undergo testing for acquired thrombophilia. To diagnose antiphospholipid syndrome (APS), it is recommended that the woman should have two positive tests at least 12 weeks apart.
  - *Inherited*
- Genetic factors
- *Anatomical factors:*
  - Congenital
  - Acquired uterine anomalies
- Cervical integrity
- Endocrine
- Infective
- Male factors

Flowchart 2 gives the algorithm for investigating a woman with recurrent pregnancy losses.

INVESTIGATIONS FOR EXPLANATORY PURPOSES

- The radiological evaluation of the uterus to rule out uterine anomalies/abnormality: In a woman with recurrent pregnancy losses who do not have APLA and have recurrent abortions in second trimester or at increasing gestations in subsequent pregnancies or with associated painless cervical dilatation, ultrasound helps to find out the cause of any abnormality in uterus and if indicated an MRI can be considered to define the anomaly necessitating further intervention for corrective surgery. The Abnormalities can be both congenital or acquired in the form of intrauterine adhesions or fibroids **(Flowchart 3)**.

- *Products of conception (POC) karyotyping:* A systematic review found prevalence of chromosomal abnormalities in a single sporadic miscarriage to be 45% and prevalence in subsequent miscarriages to be similar. Variety of genetic techniques [conventional karyotyping and fluorescence in situ hybridization (FISH)], array-based comparative genomic hybridization (A-CGH), can be used for finding the defect which may be the cause of abortion **(Flowchart 4)**, A-CGH preferred (avoids maternal contamination) technique, avoids limitation of FISH, and karyotyping. Newer techniques such as single-nucleotide polymorphism (SNP), next-generation sequencing (NGS), and whole-genome sequencing (WGS) yet to be extensively investigated.[15] No clear effect of genetic testing on prognosis (subsequent live birth) has been described.

- *Parental genetic analysis:* Abnormal parental karyotype has been found in 1.9% of couples in large retrospective studies.[16] Other study reported chromosomal abnormalities in 3.5% of couples with two or more pregnancy losses.[17] Couples with abnormal fetal or parental karyotype reports should receive genetic counseling. Possible treatment options in form of preimplantation

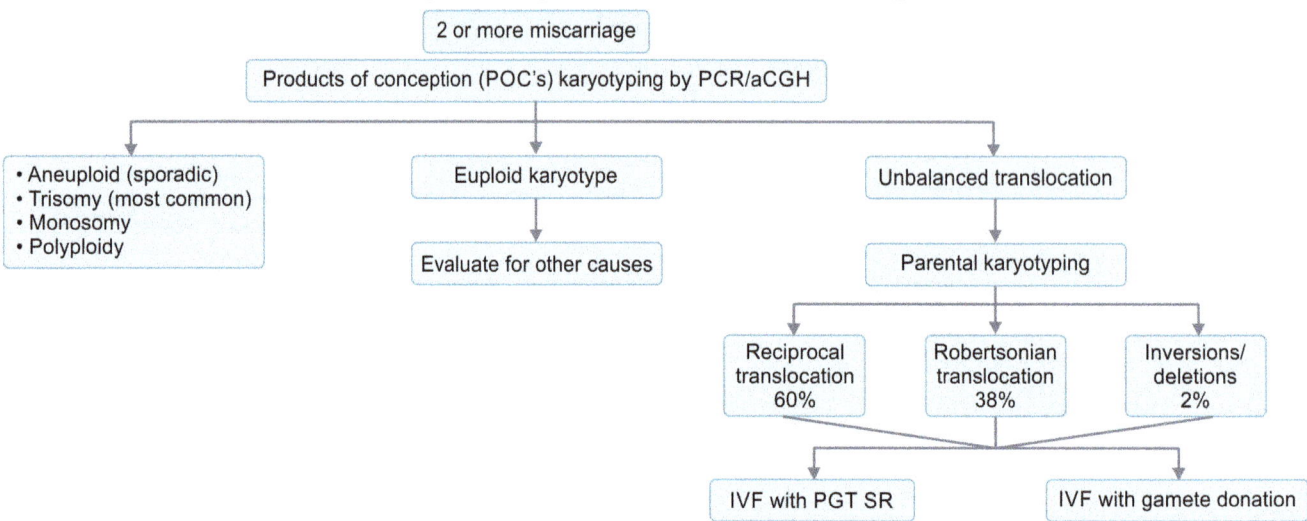

Flowchart 3: Algorithm for genetic evaluation and further management of RPL.

(aCGH: array comparative genomic hybridization; IVF: in vitro fertilization; PCR: polymerase chain reaction; PGT-SR: preimplantation genetic testing for structural chromosomal rearrangement; RPL: recurrent pregnancy loss)

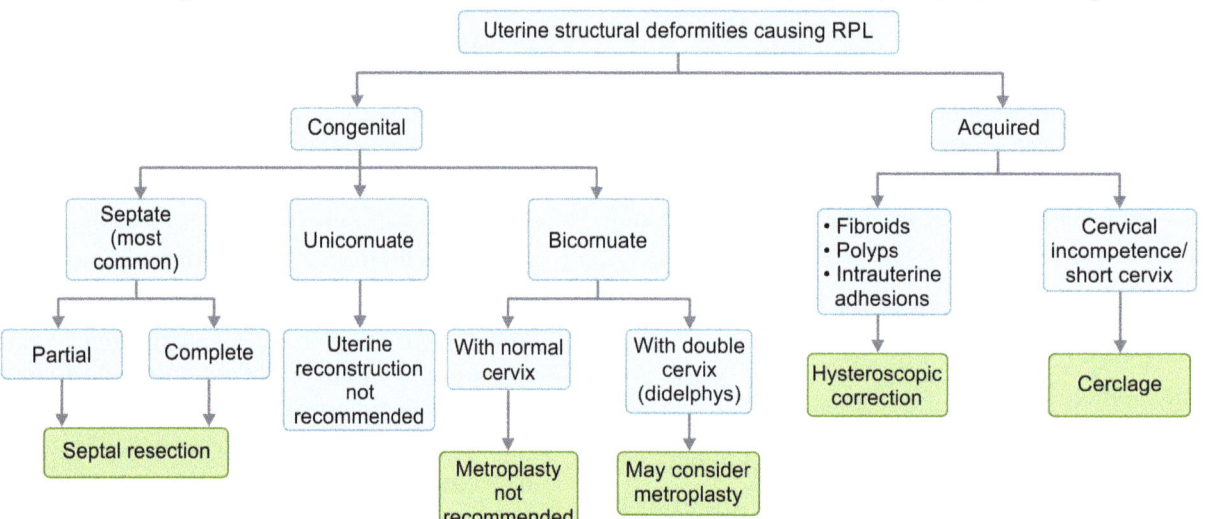

Flowchart 4: Algorithm for uterine structural malformations causing recurrent pregnancy loss (RPL) and management.

genetic diagnosis (PGD) with in vitro fertilization (IVF) with advantages and disadvantages should be explained.

- *Antinuclear antibody (ANA) testing:* Studies reported ANA positivity was more prevalent in women with RPL compared to those who gave live birth.[18] Direct pathophysiological link yet to be documented. HLA DRB1*03 allele is the only known genetic predisposing factor associated with production of various autoantibodies including ANA and risk of RPL.
- *Sperm DNA fragmentation:* Major causes of DNA damage are smoking, obesity, and excessive exercise. Male partners of couples with RPL with the mentioned risk factors may be considered for DNA fragmentation index (DFI) testing **(Figure 1)**. Most recent WHO manual for semen analysis recommends extended testing using sperm DNA fragmentation where indicated.
- RCOG 2021 draft[19] gives a systematic protocol to proceed in the work-up of woman with repeated pregnancy loss **(Flowchart 5)** and helps the treating doctor in reaching a diagnosis of the cause and its management. The evaluation and investigations in a woman with previous pregnancy losses in the form of recurrent abortions should be evidence based and not begun after a single pregnancy loss. Unnecessary evaluation and investigations can only add to anxiety as well as financial burden for the couple and can lead to confusion rather than diagnosis. **Box 1** incorporates investigations not required for evaluation as the evidence is not supportive for them and **Box 2** enumerates a list of investigations which can be done in an individualized manner to improve future pregnancy outcome.

Recurrent Pregnancy Loss: Work-up and Management

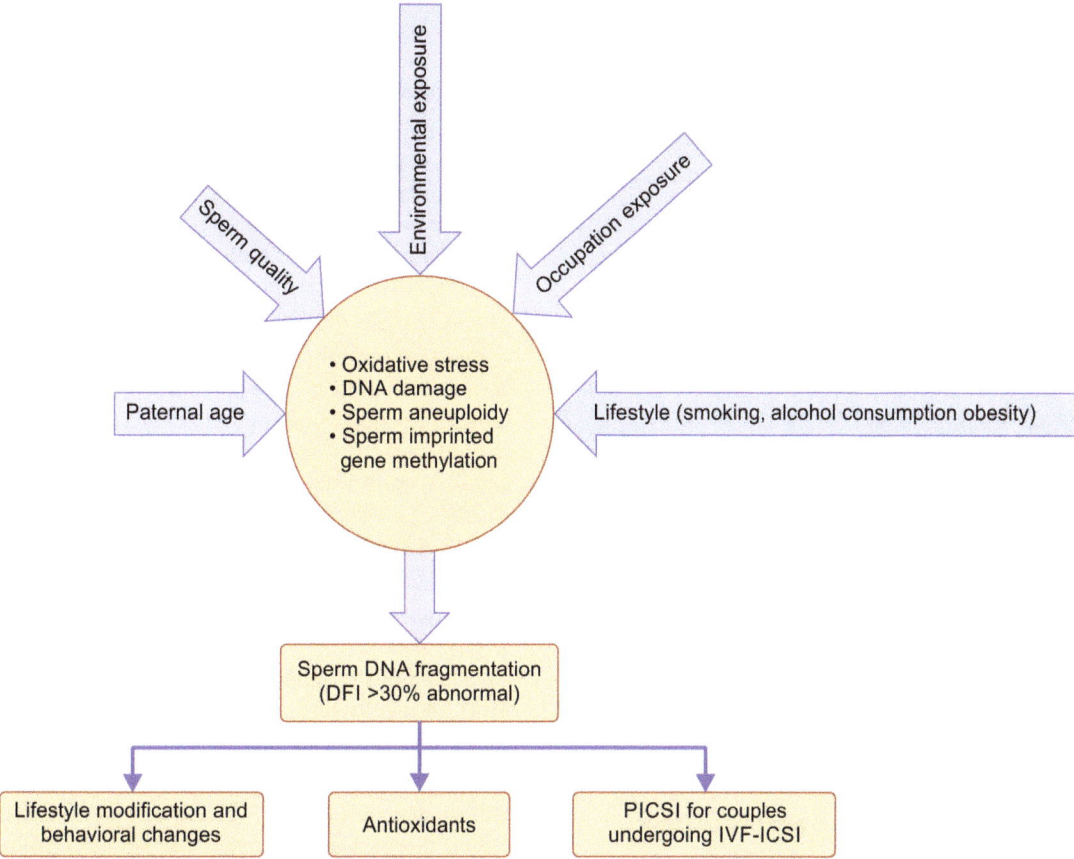

Fig. 1: Male factor contribution to RPL and management.
(DFI: DNA fragmentation index; DNA: deoxyribonucleic acid; IVF: in vitro fertilization; PICSI: physiological intracytoplasmic sperm injection; RPL: recurrent pregnancy loss)

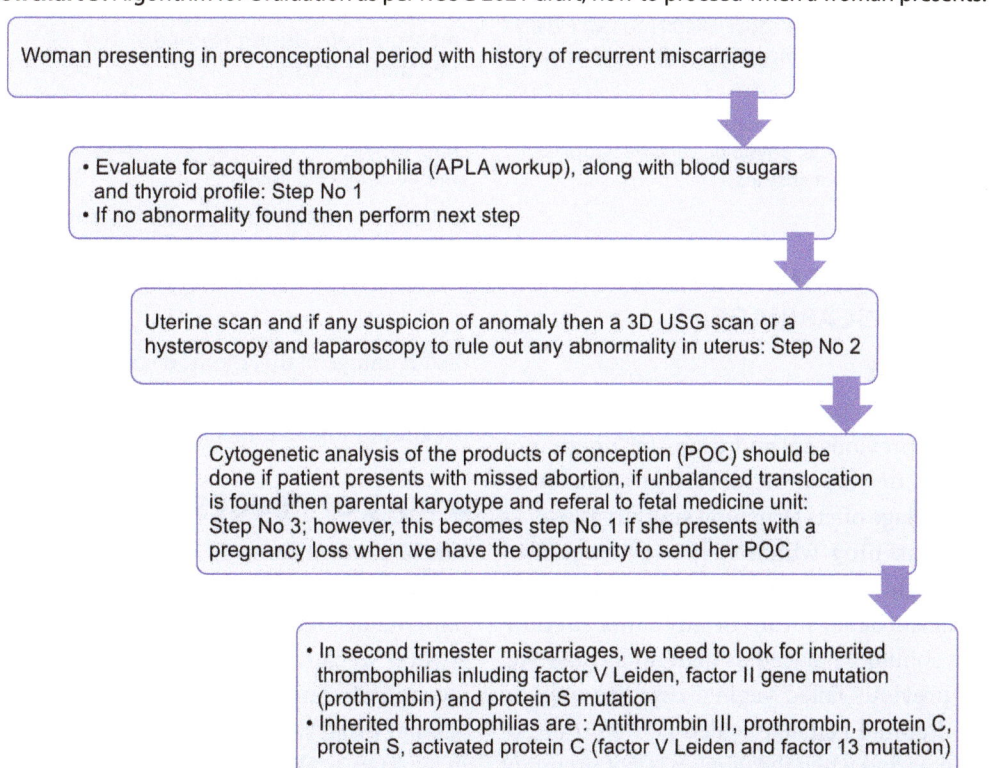

Flowchart 5: Algorithm for evaluation as per RCOG 2021 draft, how to proceed when a woman presents.

(APLA: antiphospholipid antibody; RCOG; Royal College of Obstetricians and Gynaecologists; USG: ultrasonography)

BOX 1: Investigations not recommended (lack of good quality evidence).

- Natural killer (NK) cell (peripheral/endometrial tissue)
- Anti-HY antibodies
- Cytokine polymorphism
- Anti-human leukocyte antigen (HLA) antibodies
- Luteinizing hormone (LH) testing
- Ovarian reserve testing
- Androgen testing
- Homocysteine levels

BOX 2: Suggested recommendations to increase chance of live birth in couples with RPL (ESHRE 2017 RPL guidelines).[1]

- Genetic counseling for couples with abnormal fetal/parental karyotype report
- Anticoagulant treatment for two or more pregnancy loss with APS
- Treatment of overt hypothyroidism
- Subclinical hypothyroidism (treatment after risk vs. benefit assessment)
- Bromocriptine treatment for hyperprolactinemia
- Prophylactic vitamin D supplementation
- Septal resection (low quality evidence)
- Unification surgeries not recommended (for bicorporeal uterus with normal cervix)
- Uterine reconstruction for hemiuterus with RPL no longer recommended
- Removal of fibroids distorting cavity (insufficient evidence in favor)
- Second trimester pregnancy losses, suspected cervical weakness—sonographic cervical length surveillance and cerclage
- Women >35 years (unexplained RPL)—sperm selection by PICSI
- Vaginal progesterone in women with unexplained RPL with vaginal bleeding in early pregnancy (dose of 400 mg twice daily from presentation to 16 weeks to improve live birth rate in a subsequent pregnancy)[20]

(APS: antiphospholipid syndrome; ESHRE: European Society of Human Reproduction and Embryology; PICSI: physiological intracytoplasmic sperm injection; RPL: recurrent pregnancy loss)

TABLE 4: Cervical cerclage: When to perform as per RCOG 2022 and ACOG guideline.

Indications	Not indicated
History-based cerclage Women with previous two or higher order second trimester losses or preterm birth. The RCOG states three losses then only perform cerclage between 11 and 14 weeks of pregnancy	Women with multiple pregnancy should not be offered
USG-based cerclage Women with previous one preterm loss or mid trimester loss should undergo USG-based cervical monitoring between 16 and 24 weeks of gestation, if cervical length <25 mm then cerclage should be considered	In any singleton pregnancy, where chance detection of short cervix would benefit from progesterone therapy alone where there is no previous pregnancy loss
Rescue cerclage Women detected to have cervical dilated or shortened cervix after 24 weeks but <27 + 6 weeks may be considered for emergency cerclage	Once membranes are absent and leakage is already there
Women with previous cervical trauma due to conization may be considered	If any fetal anomaly is detected or amniotic fluid is less then anomaly scan should be performed and no cerclage should be done
Women with previous cesarean section at full dilation may be offered cervical length measurement during routine mid-trimester USG	Pregnancy following IVF should not be offered cerclage
Women with anomalous uterus may be offered cervical length monitoring/ cerclage	Any sign of infection in the mother

(ACOG: American College of Obstetricians and Gynecologists; IVF: in vitro fertilization; RCOG: Royal College of Obstetricians and Gynaecologists; USG: ultrasonography)

CERVICAL CERCLAGE AND ITS ROLE IN RECURRENT MISCARRIAGE

Cervical Insufficiency

Cervical cerclage has been used in the prevention of preterm birth in women with previous second trimester pregnancy loss or risk factors such as short cervix at ultrasound examination. The cerclage offers structural support as well as maintains the mucus plug which helps in pregnancy continuation. McDonald's is a preferred method worldwide with usage of nonabsorbable suture or any other method may be used but it should be placed as high up as possible. The woman with previous failed vaginal cerclage may be considered for abdominal cerclage which can be done in the interconception period when the woman is not pregnant as it does not affect the pregnancy **(Table 4)**. However, the disadvantage of this method should be clearly discussed with the woman that it may need an added surgery for removal if pregnancy loss occurs which may need hysterotomy **(Box 3)**.

ROLE OF PROGESTERONE

While progesterone is essential for the maintenance of pregnancy, its role in prevention of pregnancy loss for patients at high risk of miscarriage is still debatable after several decades. A multicenter, double blind, placebo-controlled, randomized trial (PROMISE trial) investigating vaginal progesterone as a treatment to improve live births in women with unexplained RPL found no difference in the rate of live births in the progesterone group compared

BOX 3: Treatment modalities not recommended (lack of evidence), (ESHRE 2017 RPL guidelines).[1]

- Intralipids
- IVIG
- G-CSF
- Endometrial scratching
- Glucocorticoids in unexplained/immunological RPL
- Lymphocyte immunization therapy

(ESHRE: European Society of Human Reproduction and Embryology; G-CSF: granulocyte colony-stimulating factor; IVIG: intravenous immunoglobulin; RPL: recurrent pregnancy loss)

to the placebo group. In a meta-analysis combined of 10 trials, the intervention group receiving progesterone had a lower risk of subsequent pregnancy loss and higher live birth rate compared with those who did not.[21] Combining the PROMISE trial of 836 women with RPL and from the PRISM study of 4,153 women with bleeding in early pregnancy the risk ratio of subsequent live birth in progesterone-treated women with a minimum of three previous pregnancy losses and current bleeding significantly increased.[22] Vaginal progesterone in early pregnancy (started <12 weeks) may have a beneficial effect in women with unexplained RPL with vaginal bleeding and therefore may be recommended to use vaginal progesterone (twice daily 400 mg progesterone from presentation to 16 weeks of gestation) to improve live birth rate in subsequent pregnancy.[23]

EVIDENCE FOR OTHER TREATMENT MODALITIES

Nonconventional treatment modalities such as Chinese herbal medicine, acupuncture, dietary antioxidants, homeopathy bioresonance therapy and NaProTechnology have been suggested as treatment options for pregnancy loss, but data supporting their use in clinical practice is lacking.

CONCLUSION

Thorough reproductive history combined with guided physical examination and individualized investigations such as thyroid-stimulating hormone, prolactin (in presence of symptoms), transvaginal ultrasonography (USG-TVS), (3D) preferably or sonohysterography, and antiphospholipid antibody test [lupus anticoagulant (LAC), anticardiolipin lipid (ACL), and anti-beta-2 glycoprotein antibody 12 weeks apart. A systematic approach with appropriate counseling by qualified personnel should be provided to all couples of RPL. Specific cause-related treatment such as surgical treatment for uterine septum, submucous fibroid, cervical cerclage for cervical incompetence, thyroxin supplementation for subclinical or over hypothyroidism, low dose aspirin and heparin for APS and dopamine agonist for hyperprolactinemia should be given. More than 50% of the women with RPL, definite etiology cannot be found that could become source of grave distress for these couples. Empathetic dealing and information of a better prognosis should be provided to such couples. Patient-tailored approach is the way to go and forms the basis for practice of modern medicine.

REFERENCES

1. Christiansen OB, Elson J, Kolte AM, Lewis S, Middeldorp S, Nelen W, et al. ESHRE guideline: recurrent pregnancy loss. Hum Reprod Open. 2018;2018(2):hoy004.
2. Practice Committee of the American Society for Reproductive Medicine. Evaluation and treatment of recurrent pregnancy loss: committee opinion. Fertil Steril. 2012:98(5)1103-11.
3. Sharma R, Agarwal A, Rohra VK, Assidi M, Abu-Elmagd M, Turki RF. Effects of increased paternal age on sperm quality, reproductive outcome and associated epigenetic risks to offspring. Reprod Biol Endocrinol. 2015;13:35.
4. Nybo Anderson AM, Wohlfahrt J, Christens P, Olsen J, Melbye M. Maternal age and fetal loss: population based register linkage study. BMJ. 2000;320(7251):1708-12.
5. Lashen H, Fear K, Sturdee DW. Obesity is associated with increased risk of first trimester and recurrent miscarriage: matched case-control study. Hum Reprod. 2004;19:1644-6.
6. Metwally M, Ong KJ, Ledger WL, Li TC. Does high body mass index increase the risk of miscarriage after spontaneous and assisted conception? A meta-analysis of the evidence. Fertil Steril. 2008;90:714-26.
7. Venners SA, Wang X, Chen C, Wang L, Chen D, Guang W, et al. Paternal smoking and pregnancy loss: a prospective study using a biomarker of pregnancy. Am J Epidemiol. 2004;159:993-1001.
8. Avalos LA, Roberts SC, Kaskutas LA, Block G, Li DK. Volume and type of alcohol during early pregnancy and the risk of miscarriage. Subst Use Misuse. 2014;49:1437-45.
9. Andersen AM, Andersen PK, Olsen J, Gronbaek M, Strandberg-Larsen K. Moderate alcohol intake during pregnancy and risk of fetal death. Int J Epidemiol. 2012;41:405-13.
10. Li W, Newell-Price J, Jones GL, Ledger WL, Li TC. Relationship between psychological stress and recurrent miscarriage. Reprod Biomed Online. 2012;25:180-9.
11. Kolte AM, Olsen LR, Mikkelsen EM, Christiansen OB, Nielsen HS. Depression and emotional stress is highly prevalent among women with recurrent pregnancy loss. Hum Reprod. 2015;30:777-82.
12. Lund M, Kamper-Jorgensen M, Nielsen HS, Lidegaard O, Andersen AM, Christiansen OB. Prognosis for live birth in women with recurrent miscarriage: what is the best measure of success? Obstet Gynecol. 2012;119:37-43.
13. Brigham SA, Conlon C, Farquharson RG. A longitudinal study of pregnancy outcome following idiopathic recurrent miscarriage. Hum Reprod. 1999;14:2868-71.
14. Kolte AM, Westergaard D, Lidegaard Ø, Brunak S, Nielsen HS. Chance of live birth: a nationwide, registry-based cohort study. Hum Reprod. 2021;36:1065-73.
15. van den Berg MM, van Maarle MC, van Wely M, Goddijn M. Genetics of early miscarriage. Biochim Biophys Acta. 2012;1822:1951-9.

16. Barber JC, Cockwell AE, Grant E, Williams S, Dunn R, Ogilvie CM. Is karyotyping couples experiencing recurrent miscarriage worth the cost? BJOG. 2010;117:885-8.
17. Flynn H, Yan J, Saravelos SH, Li TC. Comparison of reproductive outcome, including the pattern of loss, between couples with chromosomal abnormalities and those with unexplained repeated miscarriages. J Obstet Gynaecol Res. 2014;40:109-16.
18. Cavalcante MB, Costa FD, Araujo Junior E, Barini R. Risk factors associated with a new pregnancy loss and perinatal outcomes in cases of recurrent miscarriage treated with lymphocyte immunotherapy. J Matern Fetal Neonatal Med. 2015;28(9):1082-6.
19. Regan L, Rai R, Saravelos S. Royal College of Obstetricians & Gynaecologists. RCOG Consultation Document. 2021;4:1-48.
20. Coomarasamy A, Devall AJ, Cheed V, Harb H, Middleton LJ, Gallos ID, et al. A Randomized Trial of Progesterone in Women with Bleeding in Early Pregnancy. N Engl J Med. 2019;380:1815-24.
21. Saccone G, Schoen C, Franasiak JM, Scott RT Jr, Berghella V. Supplementation with progestogens in the first trimester of pregnancy to prevent miscarriage in women with unexplained recurrent miscarriage: a systematic review and meta-analysis of randomized, controlled trials. Fertil Steril. 2017;107:430-8.e3.
22. Coomarasamy A, Devall AJ, Brosens JJ, Rai R, Regan L, Gallos ID, et al. Micronized vaginal progesterone to prevent miscarriage: a critical evaluation of randomized evidence. Am J Obstet Gynecol. 2020;223(2):167-76.
23. Haas DM, Hathaway TJ, Ramsey PS. Progestogen for preventing miscarriage in women with recurrent miscarriage of unclear etiology. Cochrane Database Syst Rev. 2018;10:CD003511.

CHAPTER 30

Recurrent Implantation Failure—Work-up and Management

Mandeep Kaur, Ajitabh Shukla

INTRODUCTION

The emergence of assisted reproductive technology (ART) has ushered in a new era of hope for infertile couples, and as the procedures get more refined, the success rates too have consequently risen. However, there still exist case scenarios resulting in multiple unsuccessful in vitro fertilization (IVF) attempts, leading to frustration and disappointment, for both the infertile couple, as well as the treating physicians.

Implantation of the human embryo is now believed to be a complex procedure, involving an intricate interplay/crosstalk between the embryo and the endometrium. The traditional concept of adhesion, apposition, and invasion of the embryo[1] is rendered too simplistic, in the wake of modern day information. Implantation is said to be complete, once the embryo has fully lodged itself into the endometrium, followed by the production of human chorionic gonadotropin (hCG) in the body.

Recurrent implantation failure (RIF) is an enigmatic condition, distinct from recurrent pregnancy loss (RPL), which is generally defined as the loss of two consecutive pregnancies till the gestation of 20 weeks.[2] Implantation failure, on the other hand, means a pregnancy which failed to take off from the stage of implantation of the embryo, i.e., either there was no discernible rise in the hCG production, or the hCG rose, but did not culminate in any ultrasonographic evidence of clinical pregnancy (biochemical pregnancy).[3] Implantation failure is not exclusive to IVF, and maybe applicable to regular, natural pregnancies as well. However, RIF falls specifically in the domain of IVF, as it is very arduous to prove implantation failure in a regular and spontaneous pregnancy.

There is no universally accepted definition of RIF. Generally, RIF is traditionally considered in the event of the failure of three successive embryo transfers (ETs) with good quality embryos.[4] The European Society of Human Reproduction and Embryology (ESHRE) defines RIF as "more than three failed ETs with high quality embryos, or the failed transfer of ≥10 embryos in multiple transfers".[5] Others have variously mentioned the endometrial factor,[6] maternal age and the stage of the embryo development (cleavage/blastocyst)[7] in the definition. Coughlan et al., in the backdrop of the aforementioned variations in the definitions, have holistically defined RIF as "the failure of clinical pregnancy after four good quality ETs, with at least three fresh or frozen IVF cycles, and in women under the age of 40".[3] A "good quality" embryo is again subject to variable interpretations. The British Fertility Society (BFS)[8] considers a good quality embryo in accordance with the Association of Clinical Embryologists (ACE) guidelines: A day-3 embryo which is graded 5 cell/c/c or above and a blastocyst graded 3/4/2 or above.[9]

RISK FACTORS FOR RECURRENT IMPLANTATION FAILURE

Risk factors for recurrent implantation failure are tabulated in **Table 1**.

- *Maternal age:* A study has found an increased incidence of biochemical pregnancy in frozen ETs, over the maternal age of 39 years.[10] Another detailed investigation reported lower implantation and live birth rates in these women, apart from increased chances of endometrial asynchrony with the transferred embryos.[11]
- *Body mass index (BMI):* Studies have also showed increased gonadotropin usage with fewer egg retrieval in obese patients, as compared to their healthier counterparts, suggesting intrinsic oocyte defects as well.[14]
- *Smoking:* Studies reveal especially increased abortion rates.[15]

TABLE 1: Risk factors for recurrent implantation failure.

Age	Especially maternal-poor reproductive outcomes and aneuploidies
Body mass index (BMI)	Reduced implantation and increased abortion and biochemical pregnancy rates[12,13]
Smoking	Consistently poor reproductive outcomes reported

PATHOLOGY OF RECURRENT IMPLANTATION FAILURE

Immunological

A study evaluated the serum natural killer (NK) cell levels in women perceived at a high risk for abortions and found elevated levels in those who ended up in abortions or biochemical pregnancies, as compared to the ones who had successful term pregnancies.[16] Other studies have also found increased levels of serum/peripheral NK (pNK) cells in patients of RPL as compared to the regular women.[17]

However, it is been suggested that immunological factors are one of the many responsible for RPL, and their presence in elevated levels does not necessarily indicate an increased risk of RPL. It should be tested for only in an established setting of RPL.[17]

Uterine NK cells are CD 56+ cells, found in the exclusively in the endometrial tissue, and are believed to be responsible for the variations in the local endometrial milieu, especially in the setting of trophoblast invasion. They have long been suspected of playing a role in the pathology of RIF, however, their levels are difficult to monitor, as the levels are inherently variable, depending upon the day of the menstrual cycle. A study did show higher levels of uterine NK (uNK) cells in women with RPL, but critics remain skeptical of the levels demarcated as *significant* in this study (histopathological assessment was done).[18] Moreover, other studies have failed to show any significant association of uNK cells and RPL.[19] Therefore, though promising, more data is needed to understand the role of uNK cells in conception and miscarriages. Moreover, no specific study has so far been done to evaluate the role of uNK cells in RIF.

Other immunological factors, like the relative ratios of Th1 and Th2 cells, and the cytokines produced by them, have also been evaluated, but without any conclusive results.[20] No significant differences have been found in the endometrial integrin expression in RIF patients either.[21]

Antiphospholipid antibody (APLA) syndrome, and its association with RPL, is well known. And though studies have failed to consistently demonstrate an association of RIF with the typical APLA criteria, there are some studies which prove the beneficial effects of getting an APLA screen in patients of RIF, as a prevalence of up to 9% has been reported in RIF patients.[22] Some studies have suggested an association, especially anti-beta-2 glycoprotein-1, with RIF.[23,24] These reports have influenced some voices to advocate standard APLA therapy in patients of recurrent IVF failures.[25] The role of heparin in RIF was attempted to be evaluated by Cochrane in 2018, but given up due difficulty in recruitment of patients. Similarly, hereditary thrombophilias, especially methylenetetrahydrofolate deficiency, too have been shown to be associated with RIF in a few studies,[26] though, again, an unequivocal association has not been proven. In fact, an analysis, incorporating only high quality studies, advised against testing for hereditary thrombophilias in RIF.[27]

Infections

There are studies suggesting the association of chronic endometritis with infertility, and even RIF, per se. However, the diagnosis of endometritis is often fraught with a lack of uniform acceptance, with various researchers employing methods such as histopathology, immunohistochemistry, and hysteroscopy for the diagnosis of the same. Another confounding factor is the usual lack of clinical symptoms in chronic endometritis.[28-30] Reverse transcription-polymerase chain reaction (RT-PCR) has been evaluated in the diagnosis of chronic endometritis with encouraging results. A study showed 100% specificity of this test when compared to the conventional bacterial culture methods.[31] Encouraging results, in terms of increased live birth rates, have been reported, post antibiotic treatment of diagnosed endometrial infections, in the setting of RIF.[28] The role of probiotics too, has recently emerged, after some studies showed that the presence of lactobacilli in the endometria is associated with better IVF outcomes, in terms of implantation rates.[32] Leukemia inhibitory factor (LIF), a type of interleukin, has long been accepted as an important marker of the endometrial receptivity, and so, not surprisingly, there is evidence of its association with RIF. Low levels of LIF have been showed to be associated with RIF in some studies.[33]

Tuberculosis is one of the important factors to be considered in developing countries, and should always be sought out in the setting of unexplained IVF failures. Endometrial TB treatment does improve the implantation rates, but some sequelae, like intrauterine adhesions, persist even after a successful treatment[34] and may continue to impede good fertility outcomes.

Müllerian and Acquired Uterine Anomalies

Uterine pathologies, such as endometrial polyps, myomas, intrauterine adhesions, iatrogenic endometrial injuries, and even adenomyosis, are all important factors affecting the implantation of the embryo.[35]

Role of Myomas in Recurrent Implantation Failure

Submucous myomas, in particular, have been seen to decrease the implantation and pregnancy rates even in women trying to conceive naturally.[36] A meta-analysis proved reduced implantation rates with submucous myomas, even within infertility subgroups,[37] i.e., in infertile women, with or without the submucous myomas. Multiple studies have shown the beneficial effects on fertility following the removal of submucous myomas.[37,38] The role of intramural myoma on implantation is more difficult to understand. Traditionally large (>4 cm) and cavity distorting myomas were removed prior to IVF, but now there is evidence that even though these myomas reduce the implantation and pregnancy rates, myomectomy does not always improve the clinical pregnancy rates.[37,39]

Endometrial polyps have been shown to impact the implantation[40] and their removal has been shown to increase the pregnancy rates.[38] Among müllerian anomalies, uterine septum is the most common associated with RIF,[41] and septal resection has been shown to improve the IVF success rates.[3] Other müllerian anomalies are not typically associated with RIF. Adenomyosis affects fertility and may lead to adverse pregnancy outcomes, but, is not always picked up on a vaginal ultrasound. A MRI is the most sensitive modality for its diagnosis[42] and maybe considered in suspect cases.

Hydrosalpinx

This has been definitively shown to reduce the fertility. The pregnancy rates in IVF reduce by half in the presence of hydrosalpinges.[43] Implantation too is affected by the following mechanisms:[44]
- Toxicity of the hydrosalpingeal fluid on the embryo
- Mechanical expulsion of the embryo by the fluid
- Negative effect on the endometrial receptivity.

Endometrial Thickness

Endometrial thickness plays a central role in the success of IVF. Though, no exact cut off has been universally established, but best pregnancy rates are seen between endometrial thickness of 8–16 mm.[45]

Hysteroscopy should be done to rule out any intrauterine adhesions, in cases of thin endometrium. Other modalities such as sildenafil and granulocyte colony-stimulating factor (G-CSF) too have been shown to be beneficial in some studies.[46-49]

Parental Aneuploidies

Chromosomal aneuploidies, especially translocations, have been shown to be more prevalent in the RIF patients.[50] Raziel, in his study, clearly showed the presence of increased chromosomal abnormalities in patients of high order implantation failure[51] and it is recommended to get karyotyping done in RIF, at least in the background of the additional factors such as RPL, absence of live births, or RIF with high number of embryos transferred (>15).[50]

Egg Quality

Factors such as low anti-müllerian hormone (AMH), prolonged stimulation, and unsatisfactory fertilization rate, all are potential risk factors for implantation failure.[52]

Endocrine Abnormalities

Thyroid abnormalities are recommended to be treated in all subfertile patients, even subclinical hypothyroidism is to be managed, ideally with the aim of keeping thyroid-stimulating hormone (TSH) below 2.5 mIU/L.[53] Presence of thyroid autoantibodies too has been reported in RIF patients in various studies up to the tune of 23%.[54] Lower pregnancy rates have been reported following IVF in patients with thyroid autoantibodies.[55] No studies correlating the association between hyperprolactinemia and RIF could be found, though the same for RPL exist.[56]

BASIC INVESTIGATION SUGGESTIONS FOR RECURRENT IMPLANTATION FAILURE

- Complete hemogram
- Thyroid functions and thyroid antibodies
- 3D ultrasound is one of the most important investigations for the diagnosis of intrauterine pathologies with high accuracy
- Pelvic tuberculosis needs to be ruled out
- Diagnostic hysteroscopy is the gold standard for intra uterine pathologies
- APLA
- Karyotype, especially in the setting of RPL
- AMH
- Sperm DNA fragmentation and uterine NK cells (maybe considered in unexplained cases).

MANAGEMENT OF RECURRENT IMPLANTATION FAILURE (FIG. 1)

- *Blastocyst transfer:* Some studies have shown a definite advantage of opting for blastocyst transfer over cleavage stage, in patients of RIF.[57,58] However, the methodology of these studies has come into question, especially related to the patient selection. Thus, as of now, the consensus is that blastocyst transfer cannot be unequivocally be recommended in all the RIF patients, over cleavage stage embryos.[59] However, the authors suggest that blastocyst transfer is worth a trial, especially in cases where there has not been any blast attempt in the past.
- *Assisted hatching:* There has been a belief that unusually thick zona pellucida might be a factor for the nonsuccessful "hatching" of the embryo, leading to RIF. A deliberate breach of the zona, either mechanically (laser) or chemically (acid Tyrode) might help solve this. Assisted hatching has been shown to improve the clinical pregnancy rates,[60] but the data with respect to improved live birth rates is divisive.[61,62] The American Society for Reproductive Medicine (ASRM) accepts the improved clinical pregnancy rates in RIF following assisted hatching, but does not recommend it for all cases of RIF, in the absence of further evidence on the live birth and reports of increased monozygotic twinning. The National Institute for Health and Care Excellence (NICE) too holds a similar view.[63,64]

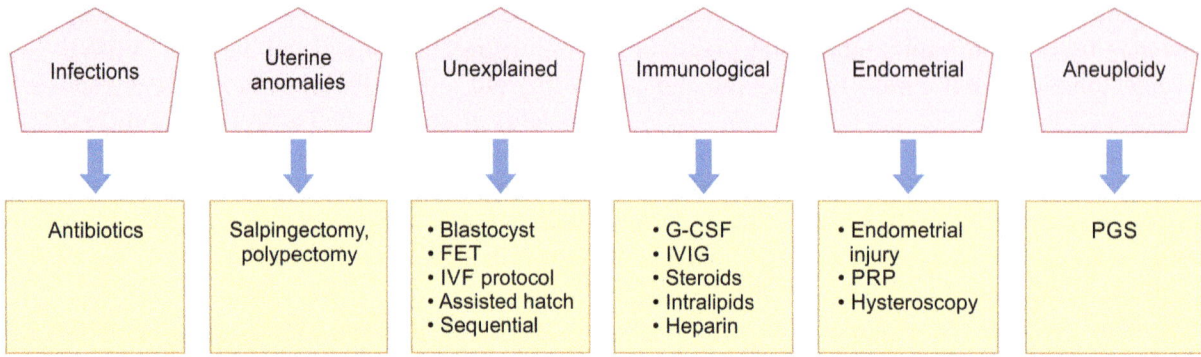

Fig. 1: Management of recurrent implantation failure.
(FET: frozen embryo transfer; G-CSF: granulocyte colony-stimulating factor; IVF: in vitro fertilization; IVIG: intravenous immunoglobulin; PGS: preimplantation genetic screening; PRP: platelet-rich plasma)

- *Frozen Embryo Transfer:* A famous study in 2011 showed that implantation rates and clinical pregnancy rates were significantly higher in frozen embryo transfer (FET) than fresh transfers, leading to a major shift in protocols favoring FETs.[65] However, latter studies could not find this association consistently, and a large randomized controlled trial (RCT) published in the New England Journal of Medicine (NEJM) too failed to establish this association.[66] There has been some evidence of the benefits of a FET in a natural cycle in RIF, though this needs further evaluation.[67]
- *IVF protocol:* Pregnancy rates in agonist versus antagonist protocols too has been a matter of debate, with studies ranging from better pregnancy rates in agonist protocol[68] to no significant difference.[69] Addition of luteinizing hormone (LH) may be beneficial in downregulated cycles, in poor responders and in women aged over 35 years.[70] Aggressive and high dose protocols may yield poor quality oocytes.[71]
- *Progesterone support:* Progesterone supplementation has an established role in RPL, with some studies claiming progesterone supplementation to be the only intervention with any proven benefit in unexplained RPL cases.[72] A meta-analysis has even shown oral dydrogesterone to be superior over other forms of progesterone.[73] However, the same association between progesterone and improved results, has not been proven in cases of RIF.
- *Heparin:* Though often employed, studies have not yet proven any significant benefit in unexplained RIF.[74] However, significantly increased live birth rates are reported in cases of RIF with known thrombophilia.[75]
- *Immunotherapy:* Multiple random protocols are in vogue for the immunological therapy for RIF, especially in a patient with established factors such as presence of autoantibodies, deranged Th1:Th2 ratio, and elevated NK cells. The modalities range from G-CSF, intravenous immunoglobulins (IVIGs), and peripheral blood mononuclear cells (PBMC) to steroids.

Tacrolimus is an immune suppressant. It suppresses inflammatory response by inhibiting the release of mainly interferon (IFN) gamma and interleukin-2 (IL-2). Increased clinical pregnancy and live birth rates have been reported in RIF patients with altered Th1:Th2 ratio.[76,77] *Sirolimus* too has shown promise in RIF cases by improving implantation and live birth rates, with no increase in the background fetal anomaly rate.[78]

- *Intravenous immunoglobulin:* This is a collection of pooled immunoglobulins of the subtype g (IgG). IVIG modulate the immune response by altering the activation of the complement system, modulating suppressor T and NK cell activity, and altering the Th1:Th2 ratio, etc.[79] It has been shown to be useful in immune-mediated cases of RIF.[80] A meta-analysis[81] showed significantly improved rates of implantation, pregnancy, and live birth following IVIG therapy. The Royal College of Obstetricians and Gynaecologists (RCOG) does not however recommend the use of IVIG in IVF, due to the lack of concrete evidence of any benefit and the possibility of serious side effects.[82] Similar success rates with increased implantation, clinical pregnancy and live birth rates have been reported with the employment of PBMCs prior to ET in RIF patients.[83] PBMC are a collection of T and B lymphocytes, apart from monocytes. These stimulate the production of growth factors and cytokines. One study showed significant improvement only in cases with a history of multiple previous implantation failures.[83,84] These mononuclear cells are thought to act by releasing pregnancy favoring cytokines. Intrauterine PBMCs have been shown to help in the invasion of the blastocyst into the endometrium.[85] They alter the maternal immune response and also favorably harmonize proimplantation molecules like metalloproteinase-2 and -9 to make the endometrial environment more favorable to implantation.[86] Most studies isolate PBMC from the blood of the patient and transfuse either fresh or after co-culture with hCG it intrauterine about 3–5 days before the ET. A meta-analysis of six studies showed significant improvement in clinical pregnancy and live birth rates following the deployment of intrauterine PBMC in RIF patients.[87] *Lymphocyte immunotherapy (LIT)* involves injecting activated leukocytes, collected generally from the husband. These act as immune modulatory agents by releasing various antibodies and influencing the regulatory T cell function. LIT transfusion before ET has been suggested to have a potential to work in cases of RPL with immune basis. It is shown to improve maternal tolerance of the fetus.[88,89] Oral *prednisolone* use has been associated with encouraging results in patients of RPL with elevated pNK cells, but implications in similar cases of RIF are unknown.[90] The use of prednisolone has been shown to reduce Th1:Th2 ratio and decrease the proinflammatory cytokines such as IL-8 and tumor necrosis factor (TNF).[91] It is also shown to reduce the cytolytic activity of uNK cells;[92] however, this has not translated into improved clinical pregnancy rates in RIF patients with increased uNK cells.[93] Steroids are thus not recommended in RIF.[94] *G-CSF* is a glycoprotein produced by macrophages and monocytes. It has multiple roles in the immunological system, the major being proliferation of neutrophils.[95] G-CSF is also expressed in decidual cells[96] and Gleicher has championed the usage of G-CSF in the world of IVF, but his work was mainly in the subset of patients with thin endometrium.[49] G-CSF has been shown to play a role in implantation by modulating the intra uterine immunal and vascular environment.[97] This principle has since been broadened to encompass RIF patients too, with some studies suggesting encouraging results[98] while others disproving any beneficial effects.[99,100] The beneficial effects of G-CSF in RIF has been shown mainly with parenteral (300 µg subcutaneous prior to ET) than intrauterine administration.[101] More high-quality studies with reporting of live birth rates are still needed to help us form an opinion.

- *Platelet-rich plasma (PRP)* is derived autologously by centrifuging the patient's blood. It contains concentrated platelets and is abundant in growth factors such as transforming growth factor-beta and platelet-derived growth factor apart from cytokines. These growth factors are delivered at the tissue of interest where these help in angiogenesis, cell proliferation, and tissue regeneration. This modality too has been used recently empirically in cases of RIF. One RCT has shown increased clinical pregnancy rates following intrauterine perfusion of autologous PRP in patients of RIF.[102] A double-blind RCT too has shown increased clinical pregnancy rates in the PRP subgroup.[103]
- *Intralipids:* These are fat emulsions containing egg phospholipids, soyabean oil and glycerin. They contain poly unsaturated fatty acids which act mainly by modulating the activity of lymphocytes and NK cells. These also reduce the inflammatory molecules by altering the activity of macrophages, TNF-α and IL-1.[104,105] Intralipids have been found to reduce the NK cell activity in cases of RPL/RIF with elevated/overactivated NK cells and there is evidence of increased live birth rates following deployment in RIF patients.[106] Another group reported 63% live births in patients with previous infertility, 70% in women with recurrent miscarriages and 55% with RIFs.[107] But more studies are necessary to advocate this intervention as a routine in RIF.
- A study has shown the efficacy of *antibiotic therapy* in patients with chronic endometritis, based on bacterial sensitivity patterns. It is important to remember; however, that the antibiotic should be carefully chosen according to the bacteria isolated, and be long term. Even repeat therapies maybe needed to clear the infection. Clinical pregnancy rates of up to 65% and live birth rates over 60% have been reported in cases where the chronic endometritis was completely obliterated.[28]
- *Müllerian and intrauterine anomalies:* It is recommended to plan a hysteroscopy in all patients of RIF. This is so because even with a normal ultrasound examination, the possibility of picking up some intrauterine pathology, with a hysteroscopy, remains high. The prevalence of such pathologies have been reported between 11%[108] and nearly 45%.[109] The best results have been reported for the removal of endometrial polyps and worst for intrauterine adhesions.[110] Myomectomy is advocated in submucous myomas and should also be considered in large myomas and in patients with failed IVF with no other discernible factors.[111]
- *Hydrosalpinges:* The deleterious effects of hydrosalpinx on endometrial receptivity have already been expounded. Salpingectomy should be seriously considered in patients with IVF failures, in the presence of hydrosalpinx. Double clinical pregnancy rates, as compared to the controls, and live birth rates of up to 40–49% has been reported post salpingectomy.[112,113]
- *Endometrial injury:* This intervention was first reported in 2003, and was shown to improve the implantation rates, clinical pregnancy rates as well as the live birth rates.[114] This concept picked up, especially when some further studies collaborated these findings.[115] This procedure is widely used, as its simple, but there multiple caveats to it. The actual extent of injury, nature of injury, and timing of injury—none has been standardized. The possibility of introducing endometrial infection always remains. Further studies have suggested that this procedure needs more evaluation to be considered as a standard intervention.[116,117] A meta-analysis reported increased clinical pregnancy rates following scratching only

after previous two failed ETs and only if conducted in a fresh cycle.[118]

- *Preimplantation genetic screening:* This is a relatively new concept, developed primarily for RPL cases, where the prevalence of chromosomal anomalies has been seen to be high. It was then transposed to RIF cases, with the same background concept. However, the studies show mixed results, with some showing no benefit in terms of clinical pregnancy or live birth rates.[119,120] However, a few studies have shown its benefit, especially in women over the age of 40.[121] The relative absence of any significant improvement in RIF with preimplantation genetic screening (PGS) may be explained by the presence of mosaicism or the fact that the cause of the implantation failure maybe something other than the embryos. Preimplantation genetic diagnosis (PGD) has been recommended in patients with RIF in the background of an abnormal karyotype.[6]
- *Endometrial receptivity assay (ERA):* ERA is a transcriptome-based assay, leaning onto the notion of the perceived aberrations in the endometrial receptivity of some women. The implantation window is thought to start from 6 days after ovulation and last for 4–5 days.[122] This window was thought to remain consistent in every woman. But, recent studies have shown that the window of implantation varies, and the adjustment of the day of the ET accordingly has been suggested to improve the implantation rates to negate this displaced window of implantation. This basically means *individualized* ET in patients of RIF. The alteration in window of implantation was reported to the tune of an astonishing 25% in patients of RIF in one study.[123] However, this study was criticized for its construction, especially with respect to the randomization of the two groups. Further studies have been rather inconclusive.[124] An RCT involving 506 cycles reported improved implantation rates following the ERA intervention.[125]
- *Male factor:* This is generally neglected, but there is some evidence that sperm abnormalities too maybe responsible for the RIF. Intracytoplasmic morphologically selected sperm injection (IMSI) involves selection of only morphologically normal sperms under high magnification, instead of random sperm selection, as in routine intracytoplasmic sperm injection (ICSI). This involves the identification of organelles like the acrosome, mitochondria and the tail, etc., under high magnification, but study reports have been mixed.[126] A study has implicated an association between sperm aneuploidy with normal male karyotype and RIF. However, this does change the management, as in there is no active intervention available.[127] While a positive relation has been shown between sperm DNA fragmentation and RPL, the same has not been proven for RIF.[128] Similarly, the concept of surgical sperm retrieval in cases of high sperm DNA fragmentation, though has some role in regular IVF success rates, it has not been shown to be of any benefit in RIF patients.[129]

Magnetic activated sperm selection, using annexin V to reject an abnormal sperm was shown to have some promise initially, but it has recently been not shown to contribute much tom the success in RIF cases.[130] Hyaluronic acid-based sperm selection for ICSI was shown to be beneficial in reducing the abortion rates in a large RCT.[131] The implications of this on RIF though needs to be sought out.

- *Time lapse imaging (TLI)* for the selection of embryos is another topic open to much debate. While a Cochrane review showed that this does not lead to an improvement in live birth rates, there has been consequent criticism regarding its study design.[132] So, for now, the place of TLI remains dubious.
- A careful review of the *previous ET* records, with special attention to any inordinate manipulation done, should be done. Full bladder, prior dilation of a stenosed cervix, change of ET catheter, should all be attempted. Assiduous ET techniques, involving a good ultrasound guidance and release of the embryo about 1.5 cm from the fundus have been shown to be useful. ET in a hyaluronic acid supplemented medium has been shown to improve the clinical pregnancy and live birth rates,[133] but its role in RIF is equivocal.[134,135]
- *Sequential embryo transfer:* This involves the transfer of cleavage stage (day 2/3) followed by blastocyst stage of the embryos in the same cycle. Not too many studies have evaluated its role in RIF, and the few studies that have been blighted by the high rates of multiple pregnancies.[136] Sequential transfers on day 2 and day 3 have been shown give good results in a study.[137]
- There is evidence that *gonadotropin-releasing hormone agonist (GnRHa)-induced downregulation* followed by frozen ET improves success rates in adenomyosis associated with RIF.[138,139]

As can be understood, there are still many "unknowns" in the field of RIF treatment, as the pathology itself is shrouded in mists of nebulousness. Many random interventions are in vogue, in the absence of appropriate, well controlled studies, providing good quality evidence. Many of these therapies are expensive, cumbersome, and even accompanied by risks, especially when it comes to the employment of blood components such as PBMC, IVIG, and LIT. Research and well-designed good quality studies are the need of the hour to address these loose ends and assist physicians into making informed and sagacious decisions.

Key Learning Points

Approach to Recurrent Implantation Failure
- Rule out infections (endometrial and vaginal), müllerian anomalies, hydrosalpinx, endocrine factors, and chromosomal anomalies
- Evaluate endometrial factor

Interventions
- Blastocyst transfer
- Hysteroscopy
- Salpingectomy, if hydrosalpinx
- Change IVF protocol, if repeat attempt
- Assisted hatching

} Good evidence

- FET
- Progesterone support
- Heparin
- Immune therapy
- Endometrial injury
- PGS
- ERA
- Sequential ET
- GnRha (adenomyosis)

} Moderate evidence

REFERENCES

1. Genbacev OD, Prakobphol A, Foulk RA, Krtolica AR, Ilic D, Singer MS, et al. Trophoblast L-selectin-mediated adhesion at the maternal-fetal interface. Science. 2003;299(5605):405-8.
2. Practice Committee of the American Society for Reproductive Medicine. Evaluation and treatment of recurrent pregnancy loss: a committee opinion. Fertil Steril. 2012;98(5):1103-11.
3. Coughlan C, Ledger W, Wang Q, Liu F, Demirol A, Gurgan T, et al. Recurrent implantation failure: definition and management. Reprod Biomed Online. 2014;28(1):14-38.
4. Orvieto R, Brengauz M, Feldman B. A novel approach to normal responder patient with repeated implantation failures: a case report. Gynecol Endocrinol. 201531(6):435-7.
5. Thornhill AR, deDie-Smulders CE, Geraedts JP, Harper JC, Harton GL, Lavery SA, et al. ESHRE PGD Consortium 'best practice guidelines for clinical preimplantation genetic diagnosis (PGD) and preimplantation genetic screening (PGS)'. Hum Reprod. 2005;20(1):35-48.
6. Simon A, Laufer N. Assessment and treatment of repeated implantation failure (RIF). J Assist Reprod Genet. 2012;29(11):1227-39.
7. Rinehart J. Recurrent implantation failure: definition. J Assist Reprod Genet. 2007;24(7):284-7.
8. Mascarenhas M, Jeve Y, Polanski L, Sharpe A, Yasmin E, Bhandari HM. Management of recurrent implantation failure: British Fertility Society policy and practice guideline. Hum Fertil (Camb). 2021;1-25.
9. Hughes, C, Association of Clinical Embryologists. Association of clinical embryologists–guidelines on good practice in clinical embryology laboratories 2012. Hum Fertil (Camb). 2012;15(4):174-89.
10. Salumets A, Suikkari AM, Mäkinen S, Karro H, Roos A, Tuuri T. Frozen embryo transfers: implications of clinical and embryological factors on the pregnancy outcome. Hum Reprod. 2006;21(9):2368-74.
11. Shapiro BS, Daneshmand ST, Desai J, Garner FC, Aguirre M, Hudson C. The risk of embryo-endometrium asynchrony increases with maternal age after ovarian stimulation and IVF. Reprod Biomed Online. 2016;33(1):50-5.
12. Orvieto R, Meltcer S, Nahum R, Rabinson J, Anteby EY, Ashkenazi J. The influence of body mass index on in vitro fertilization outcome. Int J Gynaecol Obstet. 2009;104(1):53-5.
13. Moragianni VA, Jones SM, Ryley DA. The effect of body mass index on the outcomes of first assisted reproductive technology cycles. Fertil Steril. 2012;98(1):102-8.
14. Fedorcsák P, Storeng R, Dale PO, Tanbo T, Abyholm T. Obesity is a risk factor for early pregnancy loss after IVF or ICSI. Acta Obstet Gynecol Scand. 2000;79(1):43-8.
15. Waylen AL, Metwally M, Jones GL, Wilkinson AJ, Ledger WL. Effects of cigarette smoking upon clinical outcomes of assisted reproduction: a meta-analysis. Hum Reprod Update. 2009;15(1):31-44.
16. Yamada H, Morikawa M, Kato EH, Shimada S, Kobashi G, Minakami H. Pre-conceptional natural killer cell activity and percentage as predictors of biochemical pregnancy and spontaneous abortion with normal chromosome karyotype. Am J Reprod Immunol. 2003;50(4):351-4.
17. Sacks G, Yang Y, Gowen E, Smith S, Fay L, Chapman M. Detailed analysis of peripheral blood natural killer cells in women with repeated IVF failure. Am J Reprod Immunol. 2012;67(5):434-42.
18. Santillán I, Lozano I, Illán J, Verdú V, Coca S, Bajo-Arenas JM, et al. Where and when should natural killer cells be tested in women with repeated implantation failure? J Reprod Immunol. 2015;108:142-8.
19. Seshadri S, Sunkara SK. Natural killer cells in female infertility and recurrent miscarriage: a systematic review and meta-analysis. Hum Reprod Update. 2014;20(3):429-38.
20. Kwak-Kim JY, Chung-Bang HS, Ng SC, Ntrivalas EI, Mangubat CP, Beaman KD, et al. Increased T helper 1 cytokine responses by circulating T cells are present in women with recurrent pregnancy losses and in infertile women with multiple implantation failures after IVF. Hum Reprod. 2003;18(4):767-73.
21. Coughlan C, Sinagra M, Ledger W, Li TC, Laird S. Endometrial integrin expression in women with recurrent implantation failure after in vitro fertilization and its relationship to pregnancy outcome. Fertil Steril. 2013;100(3):825-30.
22. Paulmyer-Lacroix O, Despierres L, Courbiere B, Bardin N. (2014). Antiphospholipid antibodies in women undergoing in vitro fertilization treatment: clinical value of IgA anti-b2glycoprotein I antibodies determination. Biomed Res Int. 2014;2014:1-5.
23. Geva E, Amit A, Lerner-Geva L, Yaron Y, Daniel Y, Schwartz T, et al. Prednisone and aspirin improve pregnancy rate in patients with reproductive failure and autoimmune antibodies: a prospective study. Am J Reprod Immunol. 2000;43(1):36-40.
24. Stern C, Chamley L, Hale L, Kloss M, Speirs A, Baker HW. Antibodies to β2 glycoprotein I are associated with in vitro fertilization implantation failure as well as recurrent miscarriage: results of a prevalence study. Fertil Steril. 1998;70(5):938-44.
25. Arachchillage DR, Machin SJ, Mackie IJ, Cohen H. Diagnosis and management of non-criteria obstetric antiphospholipid syndrome. Thromb Haemost. 2015;113(1):13-9.

26. Azem F, Many A, Ben Ami I, Yovel I, Amit A, Lessing JB, et al. Increased rates of thrombophilia in women with repeated IVF failures. Hum Reprod. 2004;19(2):368-70.
27. Ata B, Urman B. Thrombophilia and assisted reproduction technology-any detrimental impact or unnecessary overuse? J Assist Reprod Genet. 2016;33(10):1305-10.
28. Cicinelli E, Matteo M, Tinelli R, Lepera A, Alfonso R, Indraccolo U, et al. Prevalence of chronic endometritis in repeated unexplained implantation failure and the IVF success rate after antibiotic therapy. Hum Reprod. 2015; 30(2):323-30.
29. Kushnir VA, Solouki S, Sarig-Meth T, Vega MG, Albertini DF, Darmon SK, et al. Systemic inflammation and autoimmunity in women with chronic endometritis. Am J Reprod Immunol. 2016;75(6):672-7.
30. Bouet PE, El Hachem H, Monceau E, Gariépy G, Kadoch IJ, Sylvestre C. Chronic endometritis in women with recurrent pregnancy loss and recurrent implantation failure: prevalence and role of office hysteroscopy and immunohistochemistry in diagnosis. Fertil Steril. 2016;105(1):106-10.
31. Moreno I, Cicinelli E, Garcia-Grau I, Gonzalez-Monfort M, Bau D, Vilella F, et al. The diagnosis of chronic endometritis in infertile asymptomatic women: a comparative study of histology, microbial cultures, hysteroscopy, and molecular microbiology. Am J Obstet Gynecol. 2018;218(6):602.e1-602.e16.
32. Moreno I, Codoñer FM, Vilella F, Valbuena D, Martinez-Blanch JF, Jimenez-Almazán J, et al. Evidence that the endometrial microbiota has an effect on implantation success or failure. Am J Obstet Gynecol. 2016;215(6):684-703.
33. Hambartsoumian E. Endometrial leukemia inhibitory factor (LIF) as a possible cause of unexplained infertility and multiple failures of implantation. Am J Reprod Immunol. 1998;39(2):137-43.
34. Grace GA, Devaleenal DB, Natrajan M. Genital tuberculosis in females. Indian J Med Res. 2017;145(4):425-36.
35. Stanekova V, Woodman RJ, Tremellen K. The rate of euploid miscarriage is increased in the setting of adenomyosis. Hum Reprod Open. 2019 Jan 29;2019(1):hoy026. doi: 10.1093/hropen/hoy026. Erratum for: Hum Reprod Open. 2018;2018(3):hoy011.
36. Bernard G, Darai E, Poncelet C, Benifla JL, Madelenat P. Fertility after hysteroscopic myomectomy: effect of intramural myomas associated. Eur J Obstet Gynecol Reprod Biol. 2000;88(1):85-90.
37. Pritts EA, Parker WH, Olive DL. Fibroids and infertility: an updated systematic review of the evidence. Fertil Steril. 2009;91(4):1215-23.
38. Shokeir T, El-Shafei M, Yousef H, Allam AF, Sadek E. Submucous myomas and their implications in the pregnancy rates of patients with otherwise unexplained primary infertility undergoing hysteroscopic myomectomy: a randomized matched control study. Fertil Steril. 2010;94(2):724-9.
39. Metwally M, Farquhar CM, Li TC. Is another meta-analysis on the effects of intramural fibroids on reproductive outcomes needed? Reprod Biomed Online. 2011;23(1):2-14.
40. Richlin SS, Ramachandran S, Shanti A, Murphy AA, Parthasarathy S. Glycodelin levels in uterine flushings and in plasma of patients with leiomyomas and polyps: implications for implantation. Hum Reprod. 2002;17(10):2742-7.
41. Ban-Frangez H, Tomazevic T, Virant-Klun I, Verdenik I, Ribic-Pucelj M, -Bokal EV. The outcome of singleton pregnancies after IVF/ICSI in women before and after hysteroscopic resection of a uterine septum compared to normal controls. Eur J Obstet Gynecol Reprod Biol. 2009; 146(2):184-7.
42. Bazot M, Daraï E, Rouger J, Detchev R, Cortez A, Uzan S. Limitations of transvaginal sonography for the diagnosis of adenomyosis, with histopathological correlation. Ultrasound Obstet Gynecol. 2002:20(6):605-11.
43. Camus E, Poncelet C, Goffinet F, Wainer B, Merlet F, Nisand I, et al. Pregnancy rates after in vitro fertilization in cases of tubal infertility with and without hydrosalpinx: a meta-analysis of published comparative studies. Hum Reprod. 1999;14(5):1243-9.
44. Practice Committee of American Society for Reproductive Medicine in collaboration with Society of Reproductive Surgeons. Salpingectomy for hydrosalpinx prior to in vitro fertilization. Fertil Steril. 2008;90(5 Suppl):S66-8.
45. Richter KS, Bugge KR, Bromer JG, Levy MJ. Relationship between endometrial thickness and embryo implantation, based on 1,294 cycles of in vitro fertilization with transfer of two blastocyst-stage embryos. Fertil Steril. 2007;87(1):53-9.
46. Zinger M, Liu JH, Thomas MA. Successful use of vaginal sildenafil citrate in two infertility patients with Asherman's syndrome. J Womens Health (Larchmt). 2006;15(4):442-4.
47. Dehghani Firouzabadi R, Davar R, Hojjat F, Mahdavi M. Effect of sildenafil citrate on endometrial preparation and outcome of frozen-thawed embryo transfer cycles: a randomized clinical trial. Iran J Reprod Med. 2013;11(2):151-8.
48. Gleicher N, Vidali A, Barad DH. Successful treatment of unresponsive thin endometrium. Fertil. Steril. 2011;95(6):2123.e13-7.
49. Gleicher N, Kim A, Michaeli T, Lee HJ, Shohat-Tal A, Lazzaroni E, et al. A pilot cohort study of granulocyte colony-stimulating factor in the treatment of unresponsive thin endometrium resistant to standard therapies. Hum. Reprod. 2013;28(1):172-7.
50. De Sutter P, Stadhouders R, Dutré M, Gerris J, Dhont M. Prevalence of chromosomal abnormalities and timing of karyotype analysis in patients with recurrent implantation failure (RIF) following assisted reproduction. Facts Views Vis Obgyn. 2012;4(1):59-65.
51. Raziel A, Friedler S, Schachter M, Kasterstein E, Strassburger D, Ron-El R. Increased frequency of female partner chromosomal abnormalities in patients with high-order implantation failure after in vitro fertilization. Fertil. Steril. 2002;78(3):515-9.
52. Ferraretti AP, La Marca A, Fauser BC, Tarlatzis B, Nargund G, Gianaroli L, et al. ESHRE consensus on the definition of 'poor response' to ovarian stimulation for in vitro fertilization: the Bologna criteria. Hum. Reprod. 2011;26(7):1616-24.
53. Practice Committee of the American Society for Reproductive Medicine. Subclinical hypothyroidism in the infertile female population: a guideline. Fertil Steril. 2015;104(3):545-53.
54. Kim NY, Cho HJ, Kim HY, Yang KM, Ahn HK, Thornton S, et al. Thyroid autoimmunity and its association with cellular and humoral immunity in women with reproductive failures. Am J Reprod Immunol. 2011;65(1):78-87.
55. Geva E, Vardinon N, Lessing JB, Lerner-Geva L, Azem F, Yovel I, et al. Organ-specific autoantibodies are possible markers

56. Kaur R, Gupta K. Endocrine dysfunction and recurrent spontaneous abortion: an overview. Int J Appl Basic Med Res. 2016;6(2):79-83.
57. Guerif F, Bidault R, Gasnier O, Couet ML, Gervereau O, Lansac J, et al. Efficacy of blastocyst transfer after implantation failure. Reprod Biomed Online. 2004;9(6):630-6.
58. Levitas E, Lunenfeld E, Har-Vardi I, Albotiano S, Sonin Y, Hackmon-Ram R, et al. Blastocyst-stage embryo transfer in patients who failed to conceive in three or more day 2-3 embryo transfer cycles: a prospective, randomized study. Fertil Steril. 2004;81(3):567-71.
59. Glujovsky D, Farquhar C, Quinteiro Retamar A, Alvarez Sedo C, Blake D. Cleavage stage versus blastocyst stage embryo transfer in assisted reproductive technology. Cochrane Database Syst Rev. 2016;(6):CD002118.
60. Carney SK, Das S, Blake D, Farquhar C, Seif MM, Nelson L. Assisted hatching on assisted conception (in vitro fertilisation (IVF) and intracytoplasmic sperm injection (ICSI). Cochrane Database Syst Rev. 2012;12:CD001894.
61. Lu X, Liu Y, Cao X, Liu SY, Dong X. Laser assisted hatching and clinical outcomes in frozen-thawed cleavage-embryo transfers of patients with previous repeated failure. Lasers Med Sci. 2019;34(6):1137-45.
62. Safari S, Khalili MA, Barekati Z, Halvaei I, Anvari M, Nottola SA. Cosmetic micromanipulation of vitrified-warmed cleavage stage embryos does not improve ART outcomes: An ultrastructural study of fragments. Reprod Biol. 2017; 17(3):210-17.
63. Practice Committees of the American Society for Reproductive Medicine; Practice Committee of the Society for Assisted Reproductive Technology. Role of assisted hatching in in vitro fertilization: a guideline. Fertil Steril. 2014;102(2):348-51.
64. National Institute for Health and Care Excellence (NICE). (2017). Fertility problems: assessment and treatment ((NICE Clinical Guidelines, No. 156.). [online] Available from https://www.ncbi.nlm.nih.gov/books/NBK554709/ [Last accessed November, 2022].
65. Shapiro BS, Daneshmand ST, Garner FC, Aguirre M, Hudson C, Thomas S. Evidence of impaired endometrial receptivity after ovarian stimulation for in vitro fertilization: a prospective randomized trial comparing fresh and frozen-thawed embryo transfers in high responders. Fertil Steril. 2011;96(2):516-8.
66. Shi Y, Sun Y, Hao C, Zhang H, Wei D, Zhang Y, et al. Transfer of fresh versus frozen embryos in ovulatory women. N Engl J Med. 2018;378(2):126-36,
67. Altmäe S, Tamm-Rosenstein K, Esteban FJ, Simm J, Kolberg L, Peterson H, et al. Endometrial transcriptome analysis indicates superiority of natural over artificial cycles in recurrent implantation failure patients undergoing frozen embryo transfer. Reprod Biomed Online. 2016;32(6):597-613.
68. Lambalk CB, Banga FR, Huirne JA, Toftager M, Pinborg A, Homburg R, et al. GnRH antagonist versus long agonist protocols in IVF: a systematic review and meta-analysis accounting for patient type. Hum Reprod Update. 2017;23(5):560-79.
69. Barmat LI, Chantilis SJ, Hurst BS, Dickey RP. A randomized prospective trial comparing gonadotropinreleasing hormone (GnRH) antagonist/recombinant follicle-stimulating hormone (rFSH) versus GnRH-agonist/rFSH in women pretreated with oral contraceptives before in vitro fertilization. Fertil Steril. 2005;83(2):321-30.
70. Phelps JY, Figueira-Armada L, Levine AS, Vlahos NP, Roshanfekr D, Zacur HA, et al. Exogenous luteinizing hormone (LH) increases estradiol response patterns in poor responders with low serum LH concentrations. J Assist Reprod Genet. 1999;16(7):363-8.
71. Collins J, 2009. Mild stimulation for in vitro fertilization: making progress downward. Hum Reprod. 2009;15(1),1-3.
72. Rasmark Roepke E, Hellgren M, Hjertberg R, Blomqvist L, Matthiesen L, Henic E, et al. Treatment efficacy for idiopathic recurrent pregnancy loss: a systematic review and meta-analyses. Acta Obstet Gynecol Scand. 2018;97(8):921-41.
73. Saccone G, Schoen C, Franasiak JM, Scott RT Jr, Berghella V. Supplementation with progestogens in the first trimester of pregnancy to prevent miscarriage in women with unexplained recurrent miscarriage: a systematic review and meta-analysis of randomized, controlled trials. Fertil Steril. 2017;107(2):430-38.e3.
74. Berker B, Taşkin S, Kahraman K, Taşkin EA, Atabekoğlu C, Sönmezer M. The role of low-molecular-weight heparin in recurrent implantation failure: a prospective, quasi-randomized, controlled study. Fertil Steril. 2011;95(8):2499-502.
75. Potdar N, Gelbaya TA, Konje JC, Nardo LG. Adjunct low-molecular-weight heparin to improve live birth rate after recurrent implantation failure: a systematic review and meta-analysis. Hum Reprod Update. 2013;19(6):674-84.
76. Nakagawa K, Kwak-Kim J, Ota K, Kuroda K, Hisano M, Sugiyama R, et al. Immunosuppression with tacrolimus improved reproductive outcome of women with repeated implantation failure and elevated peripheral blood TH1/TH2 cell ratios. Am J Reprod Immunol. 2015;73(4):353-61.
77. Bahrami-Asl Z, Farzadi L, Fattahi A, Yousefi M, Quinonero A, Hakimi P, et al. Tacrolimus improves the implantation rate in patients with elevated Th1/2 helper cell ratio and repeated implantation failure (RIF). Geburtshilfe Frauenheilkd. 2020;80(8):851-62.
78. Ahmadi M, Abdolmohamadi-Vahid S, Ghaebi M, Dolati S, Abbaspour-Aghdam S, Danaii S, et al. Sirolimus as a new drug to treat RIF patients with elevated Th17/Treg ratio: a double-blind, phase II randomized clinical trial. Int Immunopharmacol. 2019;74:105730.
79. Kwak JY, Quilty EA, Gilman-Sachs A, Beaman KD, Beer AE. Beer, intravenous immunoglobulin infusion therapy in women with recurrent spontaneous abortions of immune etiologies, J Reprod Immunol. 1995;28(3):175-88.
80. Abdolmohammadi-Vahid S, Pashazadeh F, Pourmoghaddam Z, Aghebati-Maleki L, Abdollahi-Fard S, Yousefi M. The effectiveness of IVIG therapy in pregnancy and live birth rate of women with recurrent implantation failure (RIF): a systematic review and meta-analysis, J Reprod Immunol. 2019;134-135:28-33.
81. Li J, Chen Y, Liu C, Hu Y, Li L. Intravenous immunoglobulin treatment for repeated IVF/ICSI failure and unexplained infertility: a systematic review and a meta-analysis. Am J Reprod Immunol. 2013;70(6):434-47.

82. Royal College of Obstetricians and Gynaecologists. (2016). The Role of Natural Killer Cells in Human Fertility. Scientific Impact Paper No. 53. [online] Available from https://www.rcog.org.uk/guidance/browse-all-guidance/scientific-impact-papers/the-role-of-natural-killer-cells-in-human-fertility-scientific-impact-paper-no-53/ [Last accessed November, 2022].
83. Yu N, Zhang B, Xu M, Wang S, Liu R, Wu J, et al. Intrauterine administration of autologous peripheral blood mononuclear cells (PBMCs) activated by HCG improves the implantation and pregnancy rates in patients with repeated implantation failure: a prospective randomized study. Am J Reprod Immunol. 2016;76(3):212-6.
84. Li S, Wang J, Cheng Y, Zhou D, Yin T, Xu W, et al. Intrauterine administration of hCG-activated autologous human peripheral blood mononuclear cells (PBMC) promotes live birth rates in frozen/thawed embryo transfer cycles of patients with repeated implantation failure. J Reprod Immunol. 2017;119:15-22.
85. Yakin K, Oktem O, Urman B. Intrauterine administration of peripheral mononuclear cells in recurrent implantation failure: a systematic review and meta-analysis. Sci Rep. 2019;9:1-7.
86. Wu Y, Li L, Liu L, Yang X, Yan P, Yang K. Autologous peripheral blood mononuclear cells intrauterine instillation to improve pregnancy outcomes after recurrent implantation failure: a systematic review and meta-analysis, Arch Gynecol Obstet. 2019;300(5):1445-59.
87. Busnelli A, Somigliana E, Cirillo F, Baggiani A, Levi-Setti PE. Efficacy of therapies and interventions for repeated embryo implantation failure: a systematic review and meta-analysis. Sci Rep. 2021;11(1):1747.
88. Liu Z, Xu H, Kang X, Wang T, He L, Zhao A. Allogenic Lymphocyte Immunotherapy for Unexplained Recurrent Spontaneous Abortion: a Meta- Analysis. Am J Reprod Immunol. 2016;76(6):443-53.
89. Sarno M, Cavalcante MB, Niag M, Pimentel K, Luz I, Figueiredo B. Gestational and perinatal outcomes in recurrent miscarriages couples treated with lymphocyte immunotherapy. Eur J Obstet Gynecol Reprod Biol X. 2019; 3:100036.
90. Alhalabi M, Samawi S, Taha A, Kafri N, Modi S, Khatib A, et al. Prednisolone improves implantation in ICSI patients with high peripheral CD69 + NK Cells. Hum Reprod. 2011;26(suppl1):i219.
91. Lédée N, Prat-Ellenberg L, Petitbarat M, Chevrier L, Simon C, Irani EE, et al. Impact of prednisone in patients with repeated embryo implantation failures: beneficial or deleterious? J Reprod Immunol. 2018;127:11-5.
92. Quenby S, Kalumbi C, Bates M, Farquharson R, Vince G. Prednisolone reduces preconceptual endometrial natural killer cells in women with recurrent miscarriage. Fertil. Steril. 2005;84(4):980-4.
93. Cooper S, Laird SM, Mariee N, Li TC, Metwally M. The effect of prednisolone on endometrial uterine NK cell concentrations and pregnancy outcome in women with reproductive failure. A retrospective cohort study. J Reprod Immunol. 2019;131:1-6.
94. Boomsma CM, Keay SD, Macklon NS. Periimplantation glucocorticoid administration for assisted reproductive technology cycles. Cochrane Database Syst Rev. 2012;(6): CD005996.
95. Demetri GD, Griffin JD. Granulocyte colony-stimulating factor and its receptor. Blood. 1991;78(11):2791-808.
96. Scarpellini F, Klinger FG, Rossi G, Sbracia M. Immuno-histochemical study on the expression of G-CSF, G-CSFR, VEGF, VEGFR-1, Foxp3 in first trimester trophoblast of recurrent pregnancy loss in pregnancies treated with G-CSF and controls. Int J Mol Sci. 2019;21(1):285.
97. Eftekhar M, Naghshineh E, Khani P. Role of granulocyte colony-stimulating factor in human reproduction. J Res Med Sci. 2018;23:7.
98. Li J, Mo S, Chen Y. The effect of G-CSF on infertile women undergoing IVF treatment: a meta-analysis. Syst Biol Reprod Med. 2017;63(4):239-47.
99. Eftekhar M, Hosseinisadat R, Baradaran R, Naghshineh E. Effect of granulocyte colony stimulating factor(G-CSF) on IVF outcomes in infertile women: an RCT. Int J Reprod Biomed. 2016;14(5):341-6.
100. Arefi S, Fazeli E, Esfahani M, Borhani N, Yamini N, Hosseini A, et al. Granulocyte-colony stimulating factor may improve pregnancy outcome in patients with history of unexplained recurrent implantation failure: An RCT. Int J Reprod Biomed. 2018;16(5):299-304.
101. Aleyasin A, Abediasl Z, Nazari A, Sheikh M. Granulocyte colony-stimulating factor in repeated IVF failure, a randomized trial. Reproduction. 2016;151(6):637-42.
102. Obidniak D, Gzgzyan A, Feoktistov A, Niauri D. Randomized controlled trial evaluating efficacy of autologous platelet-rich plasma therapy for patients with recurrent implantation failure. Fertil Steril. 2017;108(3):e370.
103. Nazari L, Salehpour S, Hosseini MS, Hashemi Moghanjoughi P. The effects of autologous platelet-rich plasma in repeated implantation failure: a randomized controlled trial. Hum Fertil (Camb). 2020;23(3):209-13.
104. Tezuka H, Sawada H, Sakoda H, Itoh K, Nishikori M, Amagai T, et al. Suppression of genetic resistance to bone marrow grafts and natural killer activity by administration of fat emulsion. Exp Hematol. 1988;16(7):609-12.
105. Singh N, Davis AA, Kumar S, Kriplani A. The effect of administration of intravenous intralipid on pregnancy outcomes in women with implantation failure after IVF/ICSI with non-donor oocytes: a randomised controlled trial. Eur J Obstet Gynecol Reprod Biol. 2019;240:45-51.
106. Zhou P, Wu H, Lin X, Wang S, Zhang S. The effect of intralipid on pregnancy outcomes in women with previous implantation failure in in vitro fertilization/intracytoplasmic sperm injection cycles: a systematic review and meta-analysis. Eur J Obstet Gynecol Reprod Biol. 2020;252:187-92.
107. Plaçais L, Kolanska K, Kraiem YB, Cohen J, Suner L, Bornes M, et al. Intralipid therapy for unexplained recurrent miscarriage and implantation failure: case-series and literature review. Eur J Obstet Gynecol Reprod Biol. 2020;252:100-04.
108. Fatemi HM, Kasius JC, Timmermans A, van Disseldorp J, Fauser BC, Devroey P, et al. Prevalence of unsuspected uterine cavity abnormalities diagnosed by office hysteroscopy prior to in vitro fertilization. Hum Reprod. 2010;25(8):1959-65.
109. Cenksoy P, Ficicioglu C, Yıldırım G, Yesiladali M. Hysteroscopic findings in women with recurrent IVF failures and the effect of

correction of hysteroscopic findings on subsequent pregnancy rates. Arch Gynecol Obstet. 2013;287(2):357-60.
110. Demirol A, Gurgan T. Effect of treatment of intrauterine pathologies with office hysteroscopy in patients with recurrent IVF failure. Reprod Biomed Online. 2004;8(5):590-4.
111. Rackow BW, Arici A. Fibroids and in-vitro fertilization: which comes first? Curr Opin Obstet Gynecol. 2005;17(3):225-31.
112. Strandell A, Lindhard A, Waldenström U, Thorburn J, Janson PO, Hamberger L. Hydrosalpinx and IVF outcome: a prospective, randomized multicentre trial in Scandinavia on salpingectomy prior to IVF. Hum Reprod. 1999;14(11):2762-9.
113. Kontoravdis A, Makrakis E, Pantos K, Botsis D, Deligeoroglou E, Creatsas G. Proximal tubal occlusion and salpingectomy result in similar improvement in in vitro fertilization outcome in patients with hydrosalpinx. Fertil Steril. 2006;86(6):1642-9.
114. Barash A, Dekel N, Fieldust S, Segal I, Schechtman E, Granot I. Local injury to the endometrium doubles the incidence of successful pregnancies in patients undergoing in vitro fertilization. Fertil Steril. 2003;79(6):1317-22.
115. Siristatidis C, Kreatsa M, Koutlaki N, Galazios G, Pergialiotis V, Papantoniou N. Endometrial injury for RIF patients undergoing IVF/ICSI: a prospective nonrandomized controlled trial. Gynecol Endocrinol. 2017;33(4):297-300.
116. Simon C, Bellver J. Scratching beneath 'the scratching case': systematic reviews and meta-analyses, the back door for evidence-based medicine. Hum Reprod. 2014;29(8):1618-21.
117. Nastri CO, Lensen SF, Gibreel A, Raine-Fenning N, Ferriani RA, Bhattacharya S, et al. Endometrial injury in women undergoing assisted reproductive techniques. Cochrane Database Syst Rev. 2015;(3):Cd009517.
118. Vitagliano A, Di Spiezio Sardo A, Saccone G, Valenti G, Sapia F, Kamath MS, et al. Endometrial scratch injury for women with one or more previous failed embryo transfers: a systematic review and meta-analysis of randomized controlled trials. Fertil Steril. 2018;110(4):687-702.e2.
119. Rubio C, Bellver J, Rodrigo L, Bosch E, Mercader A, Vidal C, et al. Preimplantation genetic screening using fluorescence in situ hybridization in patients with repetitive implantation failure and advanced maternal age: two randomized trials. Fertil Steril. 2013;99(5):1400-7.
120. Hatirnaz S, Ozer A, Hatirnaz E, Atasever M, Başaranoglu S, Kanat-Pektas M, et al. Pre-implantation genetic screening among women experiencing recurrent failure of in vitro fertilization. Int J Gynaecol Obstet. 2017;137(3):314-8.
121. Coulam CB. What is implantation failure?. J Reprod Endoc Infer. 2017;2(1).
122. Teklenburg G, Salker M, Heijnen C, Macklon NS, Brosens JJ. The molecular basis of recurrent pregnancy loss: impaired natural embryo selection. Mol Hum Reprod. 2010;16(12):886-95.
123. Ruiz-Alonso M, Blesa D, Díaz-Gimeno P, Gómez E, Fernández-Sánchez M, Carranza F, et al. The endometrial receptivity array for diagnosis and personalized embryo transfer as a treatment for patients with repeated implantation failure. Fertil Steril. 2013;100(3):818-24.
124. Hashimoto T, Koizumi M, Doshida M, Toya M, Sagara E, Oka N, et al. Efficacy of the endometrial receptivity array for repeated implantation failure in Japan: a retrospective, two-centers study. Reprod Med Biol. 2017;16(3):290-6.
125. Taguchi S, Funabiki M, Hayashi T, Tada Y, Iwaki Y, Karita M., et al. The implantation rate of Japanese infertile patients with repeated implantation failure can be improved by endometrial receptivity array (era) test: A randomized controlled trial. Fertil Steril. 2018;110(4):e90.
126. Lo Monte G, Murisier F, Piva I, Germond M, Marci R. Focus on intracytoplasmic morphologically selected sperm injection (IMSI): a mini-review. Asian J Androl. 2013;15(5):608-15.
127. Caseiro AL, Regalo A, Pereira E, Esteves T, Fernandes F, Carvalho J. Implication of sperm chromosomal abnormalities in recurrent abortion and multiple implantation failure. Reprod Biomed Online. 2015;31(4):481-5.
128. Coughlan C, Clarke H, Cutting R, Saxton J, Waite S, Ledger W, et al. Sperm DNA fragmentation, recurrent implantation failure and recurrent miscarriage. Asian J Androl. 2015;17(4):681-5.
129. Halpern JA, Schlegel P N. Should a couple with failed in vitro fertilization/intracytoplasmic sperm injection and increased sperm DNA fragmentation use testicular sperm for the next cycle? Eur Urol Focus. 2018;4(3):299-300.
130. Romany L, Garrido N, Motato Y, Aparicio B, Remohí J, Meseguer M. Removal of annexin V-positive sperm cells for intracytoplasmic sperm injection in ovum donation cycles does not improve reproductive outcome: a controlled and randomized trial in unselected males. Fertil Steril. 2014;102(6):1567-75.e1.
131. Miller D, Pavitt S, Sharma V, Forbes G, Hooper R, Bhattacharya S, et al. Physiological, hyaluronan-selected intracytoplasmic sperm injection for infertility treatment (HABSelect): a parallel, two-group, randomised trial. Lancet. 2019;393(10170):416-22.
132. Armstrong S, Bhide P, Jordan V, Pacey A, Marjoribanks J, Farquhar C. Time-lapse systems for embryo incubation and assessment in assisted reproduction. Cochrane Database Syst Rev. 2019;5(5):CD011320.
133. Bontekoe S, Heineman MJ, Johnson N, Blake D. Adherence compounds in embryo transfer media for assisted reproductive technologies. Cochrane Database Syst Rev. 2014;2014(2):CD007421.
134. Singh N, Gupta M, Kriplani A, Vanamail P. Role of Embryo Glue as a transfer medium in the outcome of fresh non-donor in-vitro fertilization cycles. J Hum Reprod Sci. 2015;8(4):214-7.
135. Chun S, Seo JE, Rim YJ, Joo JH, Lee YC, Koo YH. Efficacy of hyaluronan-rich transfer medium on implantation and pregnancy rates in fresh and frozen thawed blastocyst transfers in Korean women with previous implantation failure. Obstet Gynecol Sci. 2016;59(3):201-7.
136. Almog B, Levin I, Wagman I, Kapustiansky R, Schwartz T, Mey-Raz N, et al. Interval double transfer improves treatment success in patients with repeated IVF/ET failures. J Assist Reprod Genet. 2008;25(8):353-7.
137. Fang C, Huang R, Li TT, Jia L, Li LL, Liang XY. Day-2 and day-3 sequential transfer improves pregnancy rate in patients with repeated IVF-embryo transfer failure: A retrospective case-control study. Reprod Biomed Online. 2013;26(1):30-5.
138. Niu Z, Chen Q, Sun Y, Feng Y. Long-term pituitary downregulation before frozen embryo transfer could improve pregnancy outcomes in women with adenomyosis. Gynecol Endocrinol. 2013;29(12):1026-30.
139. Tremellen K, Russell P. Adenomyosis is a potential cause of recurrent implantation failure during IVF treatment. Aust N Z J Obstet Gynaecol. 2011;51(3):280-3.

Lifestyle Factors in Infertility

T Shilpa Reddy

INTRODUCTION

Reproduction is considered to be an important biologic event in all living organisms. Over the last five to six decades, there have been reports of deteriorating reproductive health indices from different parts of the world, especially in industrialized/developed countries as a result of modifiable lifestyle factors.[1]

Lifestyle factors refer to the modifiable behavior and ways of life that could influence the general health and wellbeing of individuals including fertility.[2] The role of lifestyle factors in the etiology of infertility has generated a growing interest among researchers. Several authors have provided evidence of an association between lifestyle factors and infertility in both men and women. Age is considered to be an important nonmodifiable risk factor. Smoking, eating of fat-rich diets, alcohol and caffeine consumption, lack of exercise, risky sexual behaviors, drug misuse, anxiety/depression, cellular phones, and radiation are among the list of modifiable lifestyle factors as depicted in **Figure 1**.

Around 20–30% of couples worldwide are infertile as per the WHO with about 50% of infertile women in developing countries.[3] It has been estimated that about one in six couples or approximately 15% of the population in industrially developed countries is affected.[4] Infertile couples suffer both emotional and psychological trauma due to pressure from family members and society. Fortunately, most of the causes of infertility are treatable with major procedures belonging to the assisted reproductive technology (ART) methods. However, the normalization of some modifiable lifestyle factors could restore normal oocyte maturation in women and improve semen quality in the males. The understanding of the various mechanisms whereby modifiable lifestyle behaviors impair fertility in both males and females will go a long way to assist in the management of affected subjects. This chapter seeks to highlight the adverse effects of some lifestyle behaviors and suggests ways to optimize the infertile couple's chances of obtaining conception and live a better quality of life.

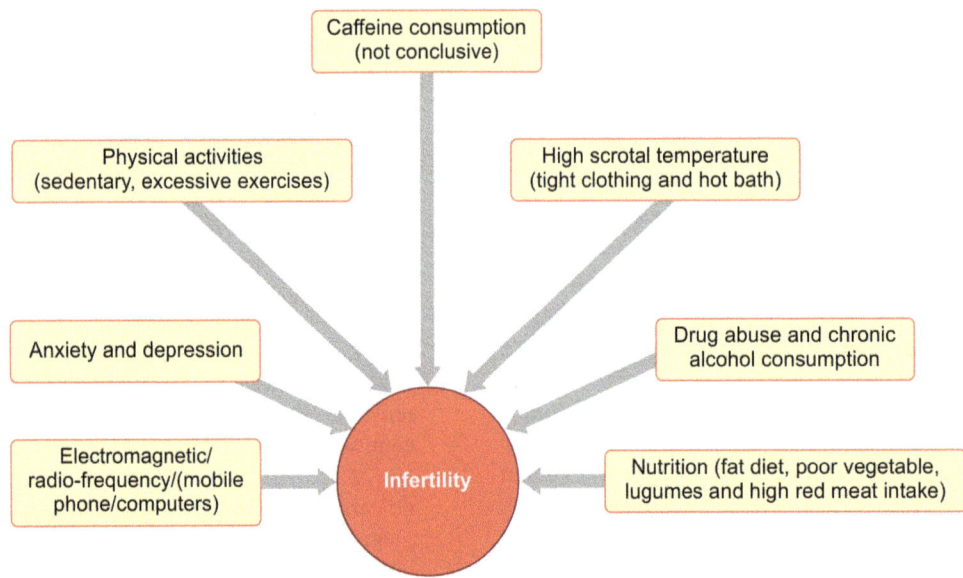

Fig. 1: Modifiable lifestyle factors on fertility.
Source: Emokpae MA, Brown SI. Effects of lifestyle factors on fertility: practical recommendations for modification. Reprod Fertil. 2021 Jan 8; 2(1):R13-R26.

LIFESTYLE FACTORS EFFECTING FERTILITY

Nonmodifiable

Delayed Childbearing/Age of Starting a Family

Age plays a significant effect on human reproduction. Many physiological changes take place in men and women as they grow older.

Aging in men: Although men can produce semen even at an older age, increased paternal age has been reported to be a major determinant for testicular function, sex hormones, sperm quality, sperm deoxyribonucleic acid (DNA) integrity, telomere length, and epigenetic factors.[5] These changes due to aging adversely impact fertility and are known to cause bad reproductive outcomes such as congenital birth defects, fetal death, recurrent abortion. Paternal age has also been linked with autism, schizophrenia, bipolar disorders, and achondroplasia.

The exacerbated effect of ageing on increased DNA fragmentation has been reported to be a contributing factor to the low success rate of ART treatment in infertile couples.

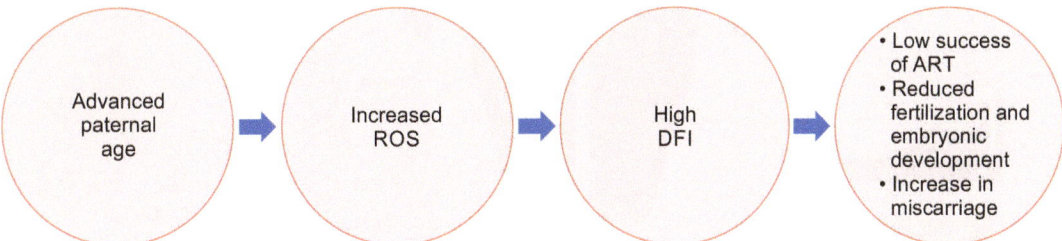

Aging in women: A woman is born with all egg cells she will ever have. They reduce in number and quality over the years and after the age of 35 there is a sharp decline in fertility in females. The incidence of genetic abnormality and spontaneous abortion also increases with maternal age. The biological clock regulating the female reproductive life span has existed to reduce the complications associated with abnormal pregnancy outcomes in advancing age and to save energy for somatic maintenance.

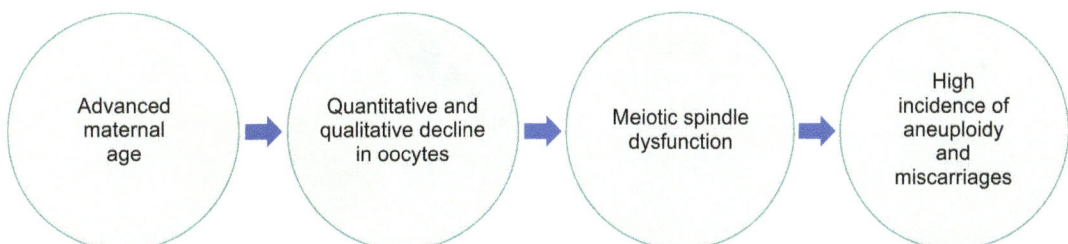

Couples need to understand the biology of aging concerning fertility in both the sex to enable them and healthcare givers to make an informed decision regarding delayed childbearing, age of starting a family, and counseling of those seeking fertility treatments.

Modifiable

Nutritional Factors

Obesity is, however, increasingly common in developing countries due to globalization. The reproductive system is extremely sensitive to influences from the external environment. **Figures 2 and 3** depict the effect of obesity on female and male fertility, respectively.

Anorexia Nervosa/Bulimia and Infertility

The combined prevalence of *bulimia nervosa* and *anorexia nervosa* is approximately 5% among women of reproductive age.[6] Bulimia nervosa is an eating disorder that is characterized by binge eating which is followed by fasting or self-induced vomiting or purging. It is an emotional disorder that makes one have a distorted body image and an obsessive desire to lose weight. Anorexia on the other hand is also an eating disorder that is more of a psychological condition marked by extreme self-starvation due to a distorted body image.

Leptin, a hormone produced by adipocytes, is thought to be an important mediator of the hypothalamic-pituitary-ovarian axis balance. Chronic dietary restriction results in a reduction in body fat, leading to a drop in leptin levels. This is followed by a cascade of events involving several mediators [ghrelin, insulin, peptide YY, corticotropin-releasing hormone (CRH), cortisol, dopamine and opioids]. This results in inhibition of pulsatile gonadotropin-releasing hormone (GnRH) secretion thereby leading to anovulation.

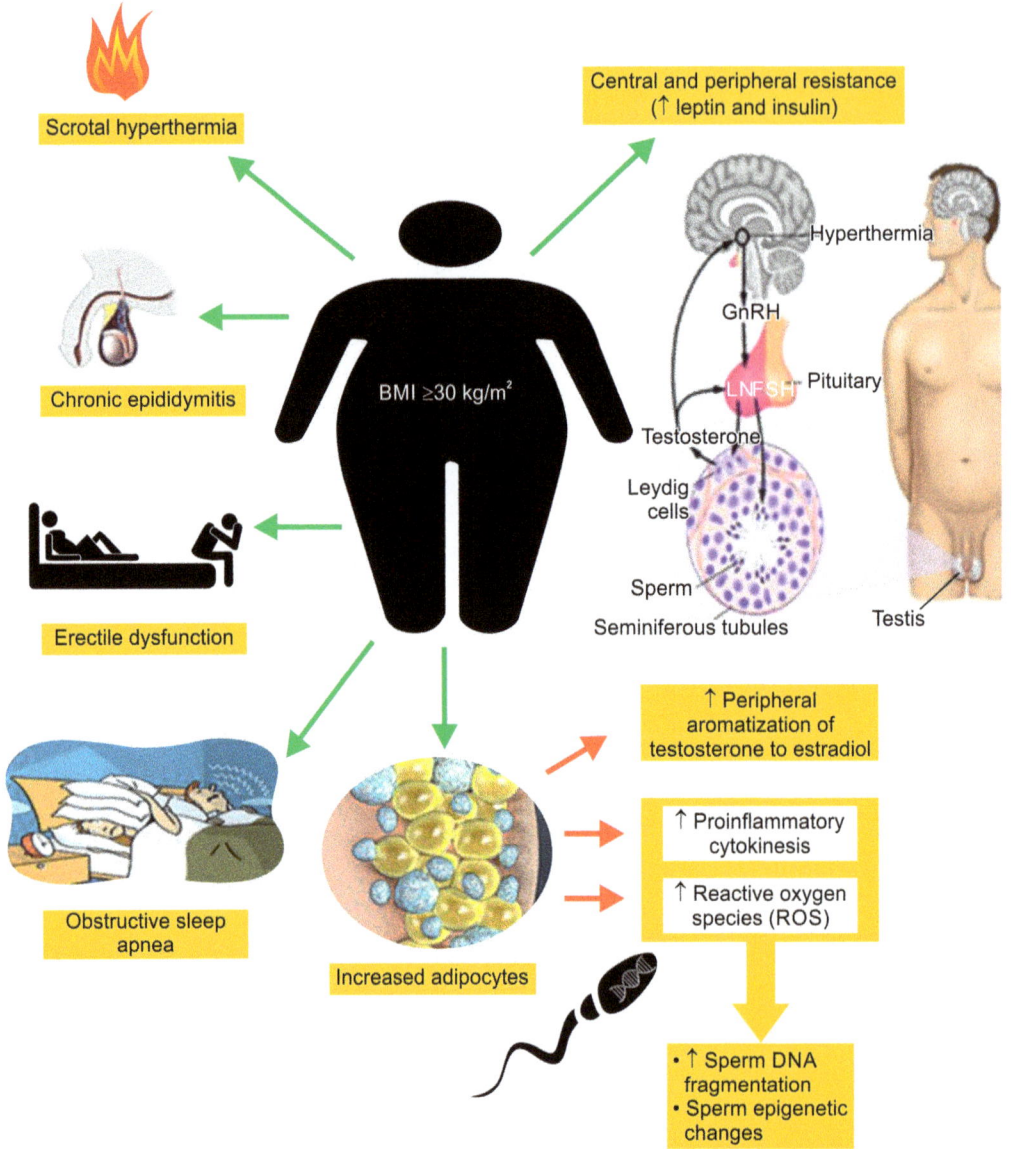

Fig. 2: Obsesity related male infertility.
Source: Abd El Salam, Mohamed. (2018). Obesity, An Enemy of Male Fertility: A Mini Review. Oman Medical Journal. 33. 3-6. 10.5001/omj. 2018.02.

Both disorders suppress ovulation in severely affected women and account for up to 60% of women with anovulatory infertility.[6]

Smoking

In males smoking has been observed to reduce sperm concentration, motility, morphology and also leads to an increased DNA damage. The exact mechanisms underlying the impact of smoking on sperm quality is not completely understood. Tobacco smoke contains several substances such as nicotine, cadmium, lead, superoxide, and hydroxyl radicals that can adversely affect reproductive health. Superoxide and hydroxyl radicals can take part in Fenton reactions to produce hydrogen peroxide and ultimately cause oxidative stress and cause DNA damage. A study that evaluated the levels of DNA fragmentation index (DFI) in infertile smokers and infertile nonsmokers reported a significantly higher ($p <0.001$) DFI (37.66%) among infertile smokers than infertile nonsmokers (19.34%) and controls (14.51%).[7] The study demonstrated the contribution of smoking to infertility. The effect of smoking on sperm quality was reported to be more pronounced in heavy smokers (those who smoke >20 cigarette sticks/day) and moderate smokers (10-20 cigarette sticks/day) than mild smokers (1-10 cigarette sticks/day).[8]

In females, smoking can lead to increased thickness of the *zona pellucida* which makes sperm penetration difficult.[5] Menopause has been reported to occur 1-4 years earlier in smoking women when compared to nonsmoking women. Cigarette contains several harmful constituents that have been detected in the follicular microenvironment of smokers such as cotinine and Cadmium. These constituents

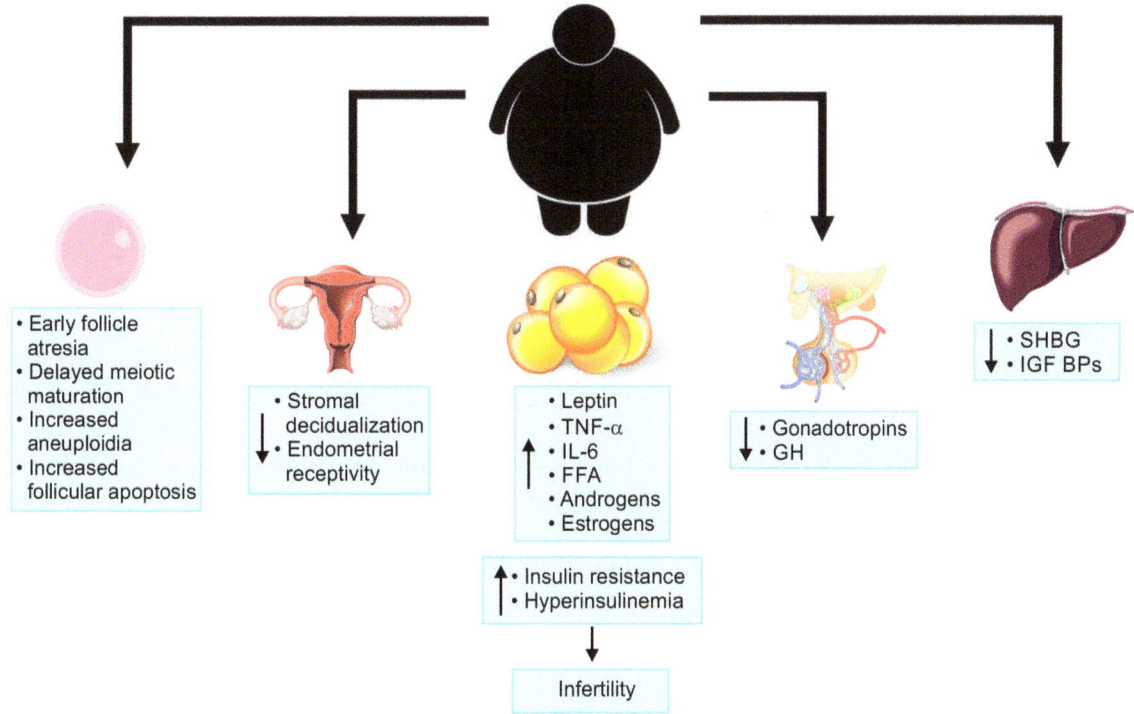

Fig. 3: Obesity related female infertility.
Source: Gambineri, A., Laudisio, D., Marocco, C. et al. Female infertility: which role for obesity? Int J Obes Supp 9, 65–72 (2019).

alter harmone levels in the luteal phase and also effect the developing follicle. Smoking in women significantly decreases the chance of conception by disrupting ovarian function and depleting its reserve.

Alcohol Consumption

The kind of damage done depends on the type, amount, and duration of alcohol consumption. Alcohol depletes many essential nutrients from the body such as vitamin B, zinc, iron, magnesium, calcium, sodium, and potassium, and these vitamins and minerals are needed for most functions including reproduction. There is excess estrogen and decrease in testosterone in all types of alcohol misuse. Alcohol is a known teratogen and its consumption has been reported to decrease fertility.

Caffeine

Regular consumption and abuse of high caffeine energy drinks are increasingly popular. These caffeine-rich energy drinks have been reported to readily pass through biological membranes, get rapidly distributed all over the body and may impair male gonadal development and function. The mechanism by which caffeine impairs fertility is not well understood, and there are conflicting reports on its harmful effects by some authors.[5]

There is no definite amount or safe level of caffeine consumption but about 200 mg is considered moderate for those breastfeeding, pregnant, or trying to conceive.

Physical Exercise

Regular exercise affects all individuals' general health and wellbeing and probably provides some protection from obesity, cardiovascular disease, type 2 diabetes, psychological stress, etc. Exercise increases insulin sensitivity and improves ovarian functioning and may improve the chances of achieving conception.

In obese infertile women, increased physical fitness and psychological wellbeing resulted in significant improvement in ovulation and conception. In contrast, female athletes who engage in excessive exercise and have poor dietary habits are at risk of developing a low body mass index (BMI) which may result in a low estrogen level. This affects the menstrual cycle and ovulation.

Drug Abuse

Drugs such as marijuana, heroin, methamphetamine, and cocaine can easily pass through the placenta to the fetus thereby increasing the risk of low birth weight, birth defects, premature birth, sudden infant death syndrome (SIDS), and changes in physical features of the fetus. Women who use illicit drugs during pregnancy are up to two times more likely to have a stillbirth.[9]

In males, this risky behavior leads to Sexually transmitted infections (STI's) and infertility. The use of methamphetamine and cocaine can lead to erectile dysfunction and delayed orgasm in men who initially may have experienced benefits such as heightened arousal. Chronic use of marijuana decreases testosterone secretion from Leydig cells, spermatogenesis, sperm motility, etc. Marijuana contains "hashish" which also is capable of binding to receptors in a reproductive organ such as the uterus and ductus deferens

Cellular Phones and Radiation

Emerging evidence suggests a detrimental effect of cellular phones on fertility. The numbers of mobile phone users are increasing by the day and several users keep and/or store mobile phones in their trouser pockets. Mobile phone has been suggested as a source of damaging radiation to the male reproductive organs. Increased levels of DFI have been reported in mobile phone users. These gadgets transmit or receive radiofrequency electromagnetic waves that have adverse effects on sperm motility, number, and morphology. Higher serum free testosterone and a lower luteinizing hormone (LH) level were reported among some users of cellular phones than control subjects who do not use cellular phone.[5]

Anxiety and Depression

There is enough scientific evidence to suggest that anxiety and depression could severely affect spermatogenesis, mainly by depressing testosterone secretion. The hypothalamic-pituitary-adrenal (HPA) axis has a direct inhibitory action on the hypothalamic-pituitary-gonadal (HPG) axis and Leydig cells in the testes. The gonadotropin inhibitory hormone (GnIH) also has an inhibitory effect on the HPG axis which results in a fall in the testosterone levels, which causes changes in Sertoli cells and the blood-testis barrier leading to the arrest of spermatogenesis.[10]

Anxiety and depression have an inhibitory effect on the female reproductive system. CRH inhibits hypothalamic GnRH secretion, and glucocorticoids inhibit pituitary LH and ovarian estrogen and progesterone secretion. These are responsible for the "hypothalamic" amenorrhea.

It is recommended that infertile couples desiring conception are encouraged to avoid anxiety and depression and management programs such as periodic relaxation activities are encouraged to improve conception rates.[11]

Myths and Perception

Misconception and belief is very common among infertile couples and families. In a cross sectional study conducted by Akande et al. regarding attitude and willingness of infertile couple toward uptake of ART in Africa, 52% of the respondents held a negative attitude toward the use of ART.[12] As a result, there is usually a delay in the willingness to access treatment because they want to "wait on God" for the natural process of conception.[13] This practice further reduces the chances of hitherto healthy individuals who would have otherwise benefited from the treatment. Therefore individuals have a responsibility to preserve or increase their fertility potential to some degree by modifying their lifestyle behaviors which may improve or hamper their reproductive health. It is important to advocate reproductive health education to create the necessary awareness of the etiologies of infertility and the importance of in vitro fertilization (IVF) treatment as a means of conceiving "natural" babies.

Environmental Pollutants

While there is a vast and controversial literature on this subject, some environmental agents may adversely affect outcomes of reproductive interventions. It would seem prudent to ask all patients for their occupational and environmental exposures to endocrine disrupting chemicals such as bisphenol, phthalates, insecticides, and other potentially dangerous products.

Sexually Transmitted Diseases

It is increasingly evident that bacterial and viral infections of the reproductive tissue can alter immune and inflammatory parameters in such a way as to impede periconceptional events and reduce fertility. The recommendation is that couples should seek advice from their clinical care provider regarding the detection and treatment of any infection of the reproductive tract, remembering that many infections, e.g., chlamydia are widespread in the community and may not necessarily result in signs/symptoms.

PRACTICAL RECOMMENDATIONS TO MODIFY LIFESTYLE BEHAVIORS

Age plays a major role in determining the fertility of both partners. The peak of fecundability is before age 35 years for men and 30 years for women. Infertile couples should access care early after a maximum of 1 year without contraception and 6 months for women above 35 years or those with known factors affecting fertility.[14]

- Couples trying to achieve pregnancy should limit or quit smoking since there appears to be a significant impact of smoking on reproductive outcomes. Also, passive smoking should be avoided.
- Research shows that weight plays a significant role in fertility; therefore, maintaining a healthier weight will help prevent harmonal imbalance thereby improving ovulation and reducing the risk of miscarriage and other complications. Overweight infertile women on treatment are encouraged to reduce weight for effective treatment outcomes.
- It is better to reduce or abstain from alcohol consumption when trying to achieve pregnancy. Caffeine also appears to have a negative effect and should also be consumed with caution.
- Infertile couple should avoid anxiety and emotional stress. They should be encouraged to embark on relaxation programs to reduce other sources of stress threby enhancing fertility. Moderate regular exercise

- enables the release of endorphins which would help in relaxation.
- Nutrition and exercise may impact fertility both in men and hence good nourishment and a balanced diet should be encouraged. Infertile women should consume foods low in saturated fat, red meat, and high in vegetables, legumes, and antioxidants.
- Recreational and prescription drugs have a significant impact on fertility as most of these drugs alter reproductive processes. It is therefore best to avoid all unnecessary medications and recreational drugs.
- Avoiding excessive irradiation by reducing contact with electronic gadgets like mobile phones that emit electromagnetic waves may prevent infertility. It is not possible to eliminate all hazards in the environment, but efforts can be made to reduce them.

CONCLUSION

Most lifestyle factors are theoretically modifiable that can be reversed with strong determination by affected subjects. Public enlightenment by healthcare providers will go a long way in increasing the knowledge and improving awareness amongst the public since most of them are ignorant of the potential conseqences of lifestyle habits on fertility. Counseling of infertile couples may enhance awareness of the risk of unhealthy lifestyle behaviors and facilitate appropriate lifestyle changes that might improve reproductive health.

REFERENCES

1. Kumar S, Thaker R, Verma V, Gor M, Agarwal R, Mishra V. Occupational, environmental exposure and lifestyle factors: declining male reproductive health. J Gynecol Infertil. 2018;1:1-5.
2. Acharya S, Gowda CR. Lifestyle factors associated with infertility in a rural area: a cross-sectional study. Int J Med Sci Public Health. 2017;6:502-6.
3. Ombelet W, Cooke I, Dyer S, Serour G, Devroey P. Infertility and the provision of infertility medical services in developing countries. Hum Reprod Update. 2008;14:605-21.
4. Sharma R, Biedenharn KR, Fedor JM, Agarwal A. Lifestyle factors and reproductive health: taking control of your fertility. Reprod Biol Endocrinol. 2013;11:66.
5. Ilacqua A, Izzo G, Emerenziani GP, Balari C, Aversa A. Lifestyle and fertility: the influence of stress and quality of life on male fertility. Reprod Biol Endocrinol. 2018;16:115.
6. Tabler J, Utz RL, Smith KR, Hanson HA, Geist C. Variations in reproductive outcomes of women with histories of bulimia nervosa, anorexia nervosa or eating disorder not otherwise specified relative to the general population and closest aged sister. Int J Eat Disord. 2018;51:102-11.
7. Wright C, Milne S, Leeson H. Sperm DNA damage caused by oxidative stress: modifiable clinical, lifestyle and nutritional factors in male infertility. Reprod Biomed Online. 2014;28:684-703.
8. Sharma R, Harlev A, Agarwal A, Esteves SC. Cigarette smoking and semen quality: a new meta-analysis examining the effect of the 2010 World Health Organization laboratory methods for the examination of human semen. Eur J Urol. 2016;70:635-45.
9. Forray A. Substance use during pregnancy. F1000Res. 2016;5:F1000 Faculty Rev-887.
10. Hazra R, Upton D, Jimenez M, Desai R, Handelsman DJ, Allan CM. In vivo actions of the Sertoli cell glucocorticoid receptor. Endocrinology. 2014;155:1120-30.
11. Silvestris E, Lovero D, Palmirotta R. Nutrition and female fertility: an independent correlation. Front Endocrinol (Lausanne). 2019;10:346.
12. Akande SO, Dipeolu IO, Ajuwon AJ. Attitude and willingness of infertile Persons towards the uptake of Assisted reproductive technologies in Ibadan, Nigeria. Ann Ib Postgrad Med. 2019;17(1):51-8.
13. Omokanye LO, Olatinwo AO, Durowade KA, Raji ST, Biliaminu SA, Salaudeen GA. Assisted reproduction technology: perceptions among infertile couples in Ilorin, Nigeria. Saudi J Health Sci. 2017;6:14-8.
14. ESHRE Capri Workshop Group. Fertility and ageing. Hum Reprod Update. 2005;11(3):261-76.

Luteal Phase Support—What and Till When

Sandhya Krishnan

INTRODUCTION

Luteal phase support is the time of uncertainty between implantation and the final outcome that is clinical pregnancy where maximum support has to be provided in form of medicine as well as counselling.

LUTEAL PHASE

The luteal phase of the menstrual cycle starts after ovulation and continues up to the next menstruation. The ovarian follicle's remnants after ovulation are called corpus luteum (CL), which produces progesterone, the hormone that causes endometrial proliferation and makes it ready for implantation.[1]

LUTEAL PHASE DEFECT IN IN VITRO FERTILIZATION (FLOWCHARTS 1 AND 2)

The women's pituitary gland is downregulated/desensitized during in vitro fertilization (IVF) treatment to do controlled ovarian stimulation and get mature oocytes.[1,2] Pituitary desensitization and damage to granulosa cells during oocyte retrieval leads to the CL's inability to produce sufficient progesterone resulting in luteal phase defect. This needs to be supported by progesterone—oral, vaginal, or intramuscular routes to get healthy pregnancy and for the continuation of pregnancy till placental formation gets complete. Human chorionic gonadotropin (hCG) can also be used to stimulate progesterone production. Gonadotropin-releasing hormone (GnRH) agonist can be used to restore luteinizing hormone (LH) levels and support the luteal phase naturally.[1]

LUTEAL PHASE SUPPORT IN ASSISTED REPRODUCTION TECHNIQUE

The impairment of progesterone production in assisted reproduction technique (ART) affects the mid to late luteal phase.[3] Consensus favors early luteal support starting on the evening of oocyte retrieval or the day after.[2] This also has the additional advantage of uterus relaxing properties of progesterone which favor embryo transfer by reducing uterine contractions.[3]

WHAT TO GIVE?

Human chorionic gonadotropin or progesterone during the luteal phase may result in higher rates of live birth or ongoing pregnancy than placebo or no treatment.[1,4]

The addition of GnRH agonist to progesterone appears to improve outcomes as well.[5,6] Human chorionic gonadotropin may increase the risk of ovarian hyperstimulation syndrome (OHSS) compared to placebo. The addition of estrogen or the route of progesterone administration does not appear to be associated with improved outcomes.[1,7]

Flowchart 1: Luteal phase defect and increased miscarriage rate.

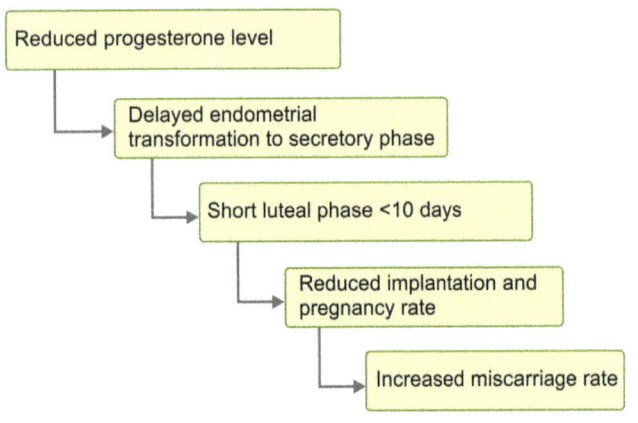

Flowchart 2: increased estradiol and luteal phase defect.

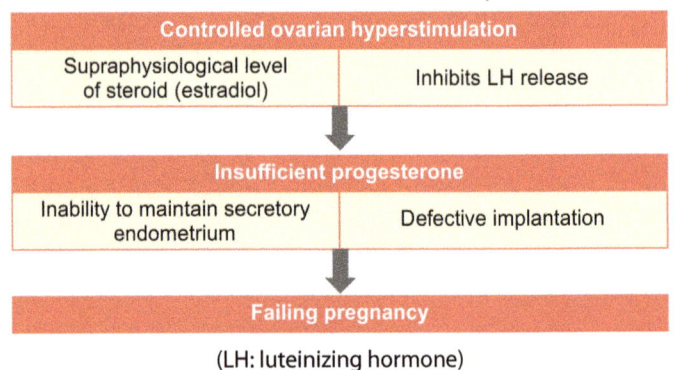

(LH: luteinizing hormone)

ROUTES OF ADMINISTRATION

Different routes of administration of hormones during luteal phase support (LPS) include vaginal, oral, transdermal, and intramuscular **(Flowchart 3)**.[8]

Studies have shown different routes of progesterone administrations to have comparable efficacy with respect to implantation rate, clinical pregnancy, ongoing pregnancy, and livebirth rate. Intramuscular progesterone has shown better pregnancy rates in few studies but with the inconvenience of painful injections. So the choice of progesterone depends on convenience and availability.[10]

WHEN TO START?

- Progesterone is normally started on the day of oocyte retrieval in ART cycles.
- Progesterone administration before oocyte retrieval is associated with premature secretory changes in the endometrium, reducing implantation rates.[11]
- Delaying progesterone administration by 6 days after oocyte retrieval is associated with a 24% reduction in implantation rates.[12]
- No difference was found in pregnancy rates when LPS was started on the day of oocyte retrieval or 24–48 hours after oocyte retrieval.[13,14]
- Common practice is to start progesterone on day of oocyte retrieval.

The questions of when to start luteal supplementation and when to end it are areas that are poorly studied in the literature. Most IVF practitioners arbitrarily start progesterone supplementation after oocyte retrieval and elect to continue it, if the patient is pregnant, until 8–10 weeks of gestation.[11]

Comparison of progesterone alone as luteal support and adding hCG is provided in **Table 1** below.

Luteal phase support with progesterone alone versus progesterone estrogen combination is provided in **Table 2**.

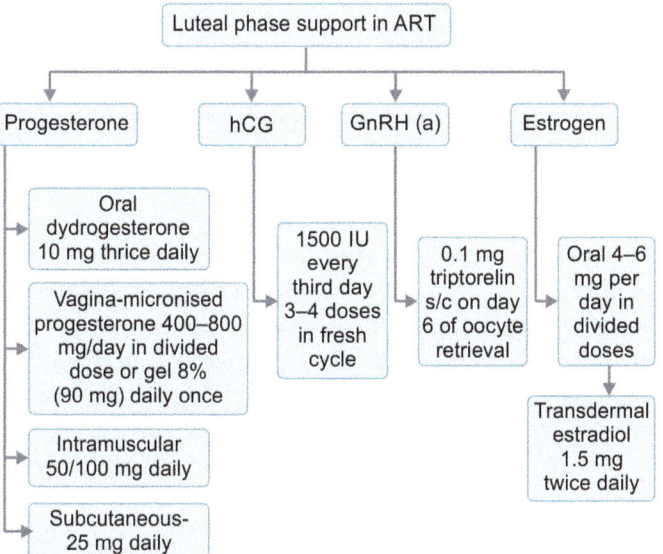

Flowchart 3: Routes and dosage of progesterone administration for LPS in ART.

(ART: assisted reproduction technique; GnRH: gonadotropin-releasing hormone; hCG: human chorionic gonadotropin; LPS: luteal phase support)

TABLE 1: Randomized prospective studies comparing P4 with human chorionic gonadotropin (hCG) ± P4 for luteal phase supplementation.[9]

Trials	Luteal support	Conclusion
Claman (1992); Golan (1993)	hCG vs. IM P4	Higher live birth rate with hCG (not significant)
Araujo (1994); Martinez (2000); Ludwig (2001)	hCG vs. IM P4	No differences in ongoing pregnancy rates
Artini (1995); Martinez (2000); Ludwig (2001)	hCG vs. vaginal P4	No differences in ongoing pregnancy rates
Buvat (1990)	hCG vs. oral P4	Higher pregnancy rate with hCG
Fujimoto (2002)	hCG + IM P4 vs. IM P4	Higher pregnancy rate with the (hCG + IM P4) combination
Mochtar (1996); Ludwig (2001)	hCG þ vaginal P4 vs. vaginal P4	No differences in pregnancy rates

Source: Adapted from Hubayter ZR, Muasher SJ. Luteal supplementation in in vitro fertilization: more questions than answers. Fertil Steril. 2008;89:749-58.

TABLE 2: Randomized prospective studies comparing P4 and E2 with P4 alone.

Trials	Luteal support	Conclusion
Farhi (2000)	E2 + IM P4 vs. IM P4	Higher pregnancy rate with (E2 + IM P4) in women on long gonadotropin-releasing hormone (GnRH) agonist protocol
Lukaszuk (2005)	E2 + vaginal P4 vs. vaginal P4	Higher pregnancy rate with E2 + vaginal P4
Smitz (1993); Lewin (1994); Tay (2003)	E2 þ IM P4 vs. IM P4	No differences in pregnancy rates

DOSAGE

There is limited data regarding optimal dosage of progesterone. Comparative studies did not lead to any conclusion. Commonly used dosage is shown in **Flowchart 1**.

ROLE OF ADJUVANTS IN LUTEAL PHASE SUPPORT

Aspirin

Aspirin is one of the adjuvants used with LPS to increase implantation and pregnancy rates.

Low-dose aspirin by its positive influence on ovarian and endometrial blood flow has been shown to improve folliculogenesis and implantation rates. Aspirin when added is used as 75 mg tablet. Studies have shown different results with the use of aspirin, some showing beneficial effect and while the others are not supporting this. A meta-analysis on aspirin use as luteal support did not support the beneficial role of aspirin on pregnancy rate and delivery rates in ART cycles.[15]

Sildenafil

Vaginal sildenafil has also been shown to be useful in the treatment of women with thin endometrium. Sildenafil citrate, a phosphodiesterase-5 inhibitor, increases the endometrial blood flow by effect on intrinsic vasodilatory effects of nitric oxide. Sildenafil citrate has been used as vaginal suppositories in case of thin endometrium to increase endometrial thickness and vascularity and pregnancy rates. Dose of vaginal sildenafil used varies from 25 to 100 mg vaginally in divided doses, starting from day of ovum pick-up (OPU) or embryo transfer.[16]

Gonadotropin-releasing Hormone Agonist

The GnRH agonist use in luteal phase has been shown to improve implantation and pregnancy rates by acting on GnRH receptors are present in endometrium, CL, and embryo itself. Tesarik et al. showed beneficial effects of GnRH agonist triptorelin in IVF patients given injection triptorelin on luteal day 6 in both agonist and antagonist cycles. Similarly, other studies have shown improved pregnancy rates with luteal phase administration of GnRH agonist. To the contrary, other studies have shown no improvement in pregnancy rates with addition of luteal phase GnRH agonist. Most of studies are done with 0.1 mg of injection triptorelin given 3 days after embryo transfer.[11]

Low-molecular-weight Heparin

Heparin has a proven role in cases of thrombophilia associated repeated implantation failure and recurrent pregnancy loss. Low-molecular-weight heparin (LMWH) has been used empirically in cases of recurrent implantation failure without history of thrombophilias as well.

Mechanism of Action

Heparin has been shown to enhance implantation through interactions with several adhesion molecules, growth factors, cytokines, and enzymes such as matrix metalloproteinase in addition to its antithrombotic effect. Some studies have shown a positive impact of such therapy on implantation while others failed to support this. The dose recommended is 20–40 mg subcutaneous (SC) of LMWH daily.[11,16]

WHEN TO STOP?

Luteal support is given up to 8–10 weeks of pregnancy when the placenta takes over the function of producing hormones.

However, as per the American Society for Reproductive Medicine (ASRM) guidelines, there is no proven benefit of giving progesterone once pregnancy is established.[17]

A recent meta-analysis of six eligible studies and 1,201 randomized subjects concluded there may be no additional benefit of progesterone supplementation beyond the first positive hCG value, showing no difference in live birth, ongoing pregnancy, or miscarriage. Despite these data, most surveyed clinics (72%) continue progesterone until 8 weeks or more of pregnancy and only 15% discontinue progesterone after detection of beta-hCG.[18,19]

As per a few studies, the recommendation is that luteal support is not beneficial after confirmation of pregnancy by ultrasound.[20-22]

LUTEAL SUPPORT IN DONOR CYCLES AND FROZEN THAW CYCLES

In all hormone replacement therapy (HRT) cycles [frozen embryo transfer (FET) cycles], luteal support should be continued till 10–11 weeks of pregnancy, when the luteal placental shift is complete.

In donor egg and FET cycles, LPS consists of both estrogen and progesterone. Normally, estrogen is started in follicular phase and progesterone is added on the day of donor oocyte pick-up in case of donor embryo transfer and 3–5 days prior to embryo transfer in frozen-thawed embryo transfer cycles depending upon stage at which embryo is transferred. Estrogen and progesterone is then continued through luteal phase and till placental take over which normally occurs around 10–11 weeks of pregnancy. Progesterone use by different routes (vaginal or intramuscular) has been shown to have comparable efficacy.

CONCLUSION

- LPS is proven to be necessary for ART.[2]
- LPS is started ideally on the day of oocyte retrieval or a day after.

- Even though documented that LPS can be stopped after the first positive ultrasound or even a positive pregnancy test, many groups continue to prescribe LPS for longer than necessary, in part because this is necessary for HRT cycles in FET as many fear that having two distinct regimens for fresh ART and FET might cause confusion.[2,22,23]

Key Learning Points

- Progesterone production from the CL is critical for natural reproduction and progesterone supplementation seems to be an important aspect of any ART treatment.
- Normally progesterone is started on the day of OPU and embryo transfer done 3 days later in case of eight-cell embryo and 5 days later in case of blastocyst.
- There is limited data regarding the optimal dose of progesterone.
- In routine IVF cases, LPS is continued till β-hCG is checked.[20,21]
- In donor egg IVF, luteal support is continued till placental take over which normally happens around 10–11 weeks.
- In FET cycles where endometrium is artificially prepared with hormones, luteal support is continued till placental takeover (10–11 weeks).
- Effect of addition of estrogen to progesterone for LPS has shown controversial results. Some studies have shown beneficial effect of adding estrogen in long agonist cycles but not in antagonist cycles. However, in FET and donor cycles, estrogen is used for endometrial preparation and continued as luteal support till 10–11 weeks.

REFERENCES

1. van der Linden M, Buckingham K, Farquhar C, Kremer JA, Metwally M. Luteal phase support for assisted reproduction cycles. Cochrane Database Syst Rev. 2015;2015(7):CD009154.
2. Practice Committee of the American Society for Reproductive Medicine. Progesterone supplementation during the luteal phase and in early pregnancy in the treatment of infertility: an educational bulletin. Fertil Steril. 2008;89:789-92.
3. Tryde Schmidt KL, Ziebe S, Popovic B, Lindhard A, Loft A, Nyboe Andersen A. Progesterone supplementation during early gestation after in vitro fertilization has no effect on the delivery rate. Fertil Steril. 2001;75:337-41.
4. Haas J, Kedem A, Machtinger R, Dar S, Hourvitz A, Yerushalmi G, et al. HCG (1500IU) administration on day 3 after oocytes retrieval, following GnRH-agonist trigger for final follicular maturation, results in high sufficient mid luteal progesterone levels—a proof of concept. J Ovarian Res. 2014;7:35.
5. Bar Hava I, Blueshtein M, Ganer Herman H, Omer Y, Ben David G. Gonadotropin-releasing hormone analogue as sole luteal support in antagonist-based assisted reproductive technology cycles. Fertil Steril. 2017;107:130-135.e1.
6. Pirard C, Loumaye E, Laurent P, Wyns C. Contribution to More Patient-Friendly ART Treatment: Efficacy of Continuous Low-Dose GnRH Agonist as the Only Luteal Support—Results of a Prospective, Randomized, Comparative Study. Int J Endocrinol. 2015;2015:727569.
7. Bosch E, Broer S, Griesinger G, Grynberg M, Humaidan P, Kolibianakis E, et al. ESHRE guideline: ovarian stimulation for IVF/ICSI. Hum Reprod Open. 2020;2020:hoaa009.
8. Griesinger G, Blockeel C, Tournaye H. Oral dydrogesterone for luteal phase support in fresh in vitro fertilization cycles: a new standard? Fertil Steril. 2018;109:756-62.
9. Hubayter ZR, Muasher SJ. Luteal supplementation in in vitro fertilization: more questions than answers. Fertil Steril. 2008;89:749-58.
10. Gayet V, Vasilopulos I, de Ziegler D. Luteal-phase support in assisted reproductive technology. In: Weissman A, Howles CM, Shoham Z (Eds). Textbook of Assisted Reproductive Techniques, 5th edition. Florida, United States: CRC Press; 2018. pp. 612-16.
11. Sohn SH, Penzias AS, Emmi AM, Dubey AK, Layman LC, Reindollar RH, et al. Administration of progesterone before oocyte retrieval negatively affects the implantation rate. Fertil Steril. 1999;71:11-4.
12. Williams SC, Oehninger S, Gibbons WE, Muasher SJ. Delaying the initiation of progesterone supplementation results in decreased pregnancy rates following in vitro fertilization: a randomized, prospective study. Fertil Steril. 2001;76:S89.
13. Yanushpolsky E. Luteal Phase Support in In Vitro Fertilization. Semin Reprod Med. 2015;33:118-27.
14. Kaur H. Luteal phase support in assisted reproduction. In: Rao K (Ed). The Infertility Manual, 4th edition. New Delhi: Jaypee Brothers Medical Publishers (P) Ltd.; 2018.
15. Gelbaya TA, Kyrgiou M, Li TC, Stern C, Nardo LG. Low-dose aspirin for in vitro fertilization: a systematic review and meta-analysis. Hum Reprod Update. 2007;13:357-64.
16. Eid ME. Sildenafil improves implantation rate in women with a thin endometrium secondary to the improvement of uterine blood flow; "pilot study". Fertil Steril. 2015;104:e342.
17. Casanova P, Szlit Feldman E, Rey Valzacchi GJ, Blanco LA, Carrere CA, Torno A, et al. The addition of GNRH agonist for luteal phase support in ovum donation cycles. Fertil Steril. 2015;104:e346.
18. Practice Committees of the American Society for Reproductive Medicine and the Society for Reproductive Endocrinology and Infertility. Diagnosis and treatment of luteal phase deficiency: a committee opinion. Fertil Steril. 2021;115:1416-23.
19. Hamdi K, Danaii S, Farzadi L, Abdollahi S, Chalabizadeh A, Sabet SA. The role of heparin in embryo implantation in women with recurrent implantation failure in the cycles of assisted reproductive techniques (without history of thrombophilia). J Family Reprod Health. 2015;9(2):59-64.
20. Griesinger G, Blockeel C, Sukhikh GT, Patki A, Dhorepatil B, Yang D-Z, et al. Oral dydrogesterone versus intravaginal micronized progesterone gel for luteal phase support in IVF: a randomized clinical trial. Hum Reprod. 2018;33:2212-22.
21. Aboulghar MA, Amin YM, Al-Inany HG, Aboulghar MM, Mourad LM, Serour GI, et al. Prospective randomized study comparing luteal phase support for ICSI patients up to the first ultrasound compared with an additional three weeks. Hum Reprod. 2008;23:857-62.
22. Liu XR, Mu HQ, Shi Q, Xiao XQ, Qi HB. The optimal duration of progesterone supplementation in pregnant women after IVF/ICSI: a meta-analysis. Reprod Biol Endocrinol. 2012;10:107.
23. Di Guardo F, Midassi H, Racca A, Tournaye H, De Vos M, Blockeel C. Luteal Phase Support in IVF: Comparison Between Evidence-Based Medicine and Real-Life Practices. Front Endocrinol (Lausanne). 2020;11:500.

Fertility Preservation Techniques

Jasneet Kaur

INTRODUCTION

Fertility preservation (FP) has become a "quality of life" issue and the "standard of care" for cancer survivors and noncancer patients at risk of decreased fertility. Reproductive compromise may occur as a result of treatment with gonadotoxic drugs, radiotherapy (RT), immunological disease or genetic conditions, and also in women, due to advancing age.

Cancer survivorship is steadily increasing due to early detection of cancer and advanced multimodality treatment bringing "quality of life" issues into focus. European and US data suggest a long-term survival in children and adolescents diagnosed with cancer of around 80%.[1] A latest study predicted that amongst the adults in the age group of 20–39 years, 1 in 530 is a childhood cancer survivor.[2] So the need for oncofertility arises due to an increase in cancer survival rates, good obstetric and neonatal outcomes of pregnancy in cancer patients, and possibly no increased risk in cancer progression. FP is also being adopted increasingly for patients on cytotoxic drugs for nonmalignant disorders and genetic issues leading to reduced fertility. The discussion about FP should start early during treatment of patient diagnosed with cancer in reproductive age group as literature suggests a lower level of emotional distress in patients who have an in-depth knowledge regarding their sexual and reproductive health.

Following a multidisciplinary approach and a close collaboration between the oncologists, reproductive medicine specialists, psychologists, and genetic counselors will help patients in decision-making. Use of decision aids, effective FP counseling along with a well-defined referral path may help improve the oncofertility services. Proper documentation and informed consent is vital before starting any FP procedure. The main goal is to preserve fertility but at the same time avoid any complications that might delay the start of chemotherapy (CT)/RT.

This chapter will touch upon the basic aspects of FP and the promising techniques which may well become the future of FP.

EFFECT OF CHEMOTHERAPY AND RADIOTHERAPY ON GONADS

Chemotherapeutic drugs act by interrupting vital cell processes and halting the normal cellular proliferation. Unfortunately, they affect not only the cancer cells but can also be quite disastrous to the metabolically active gonadal cells. Cytotoxic agents produce DNA damage and oxidative stress in the somatic as well as germ cells leading to apoptosis.

Females—Effect of Chemotherapy

Ovarian effects: There is a *reduction in ovarian reserve* which occurs because of apoptosis of the growing follicles and fibrosis of stromal blood vessels. Furthermore, resting follicles are activated and undergo apoptosis, leading to a "burn-out" effect **(Fig. 1)**. The degree of ovarian damage is related to the dose, type of chemotherapeutic agent used, age of the patient, and her baseline ovarian reserve. Gonadotoxicity is greatest with alkylating agents such as cyclophosphamide being responsible for the highest age-adjusted odds ratio of ovarian failure, followed by other

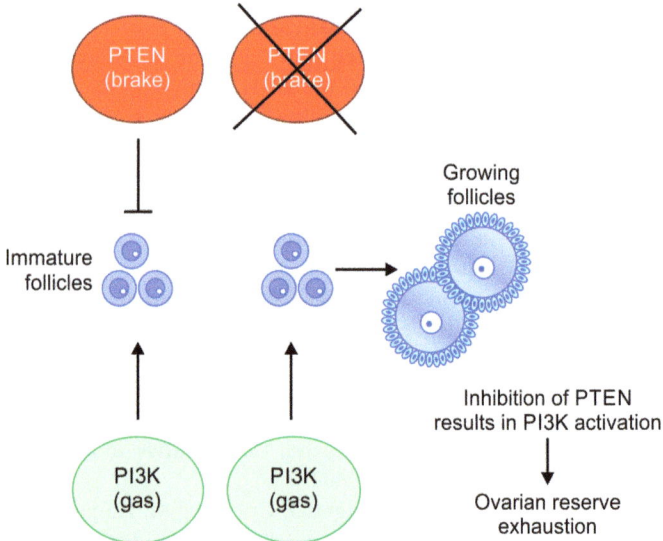

Fig. 1: Burn out phenomenon due to chemotherapy.

TABLE 1: Estimated risk of gonadal dysfunction to cytotoxic drugs.		
High risk	**Medium risk**	**Low risk**
Busulfan	Cisplatin	Vincristine
Chlorambucil	Doxarubicin	Methotrexate
Cyclophosphamide	Carboplatin	Dactinomycin
Dacarbazine		Mercaptapurine
Melphalan		Bleomycin
Nitrogen mustard		Vinblastine
Procarbazine		

Source: Wallace, et al. Lancet Onco. 2005;6:209-18.

TABLE 2: Radiation induced ovarian damage by dose and age.	
Age of treatment (years)	Effective sterilizing dose (Gy): loss of 97.5% of follicles
0	20.3
10	18.4
20	16.5
30	14.3
40	11.3

Source: Rodriguez-Walberg KA, Oktay K. Cancer Treatment Rev. 2012;38:354-61.

drug families.[3] **(Table 1)**. The *prepubertal ovary is less susceptible* to damage by chemotherapeutic agents while older women having a lower ovarian reserve are more susceptible to premature ovarian failure (POF).

The clinical manifestations range from complete amenorrhea to premature menopause and varying degree of infertility.

Effect on oocytes: Most cytotoxic drugs are mutagenic and teratogenic to oocytes exposed during maturation. Persistent unrepaired DNA double-strand breaks (DSBs) initiate apoptotic processes in the oocytes. In humans, the oocyte maturation phase lasts approximately 6 months. It is therefore recommended that conception should be delayed for 6 months after completing gonadotoxic treatments. FP techniques are best carried out prior to CT, however, if a delay is unavoidable then a wait of 6 months after treatment is mandatory. FP should not be performed between treatment cycles.[4] However, the exact safety interval from completion of treatment to oocyte collection for preservation has not yet been established.

Females—Effect of Radiotherapy

Unlike CT, RT affects both the ovary and the uterus.

Ovary and oocytes: Human oocyte is sensitive to radiation, with an estimated median lethal dose (LD_{50}) of <2 gray (Gy). Damage to the ovary by RT is also *dependent on the dose of exposure to RT and the age of the patient* **(Table 2)**. Ovarian failure has been reported in 90% of patients following total body irradiation (TBI) of 10–15.75 Gy and in 97% of females treated with total abdominal irradiation of 20–30 Gy during childhood.[5]

Uterine effect: Uterine growth starts at puberty and is completed almost 7 years post menarche. An increase in uterine blood flow is also seen during puberty. Exposure to radiation leads to reduced vascularity, fibrosis, and hormone-dependent endometrial insufficiency which is responsible for adverse reproductive outcomes such as infertility, miscarriages, and preterm labor. The uterine volume is lower and endometrium atrophies completely if there is direct radiation, more so if the exposure is prepubertal. Radiation doses of *>25 Gy directly to the uterus* in childhood appears to induce irreversible damage.[6]

Males—Effect of Chemotherapy and Radiotherapy

Testis is highly susceptible to the effects of CT and RT throughout life. The prepubertal testis is especially vulnerable as there is a constant turnover of early germ cells and maturation of the Leydig cell pool and other somatic compartments.

Low-dose CT and RT: Can deplete progenitor and differentiating spermatogonia in both the pubertal and adult testis. Clinical effects range from *temporary oligospermia to azoospermia.*

High doses of CT/RT: May lead to all the spermatogonial stem cells undergoing apoptosis or alternatively getting damaged. Sertoli cells are unable to support the spermatogonial stem cells. This may lead to complete depletion of spermatogonial stem cell pool and seminiferous tubules causing *Sertoli cell-only (SCO) syndrome, permanent azoospermia, and sterility.*

Complete Leydig cell failure resulting in androgen insufficiency and requiring testosterone replacement therapy is rare after CT.[7] Majority of males undergo a normal puberty and most produce normal adult levels of testosterone. Partially compensated Leydig cell failure [increased luteinizing hormone (LH) with low normal testosterone levels or exaggerated follicle stimulating hormone (FSH) and LH responses to LH-releasing hormone] and gynecomastia have been reported in patients treated with MOPP (mechlorethamine, vincristine, procarbazine, and prednisone) for Hodgkin disease and after treatment with high dose of cyclophosphamide.[8]

FERTILITY PRESERVATION TECHNIQUES IN FEMALES

Embryo Cryopreservation

Embryo cryopreservation by vitrification is a time-tested technique, however, it requires participation of the husband

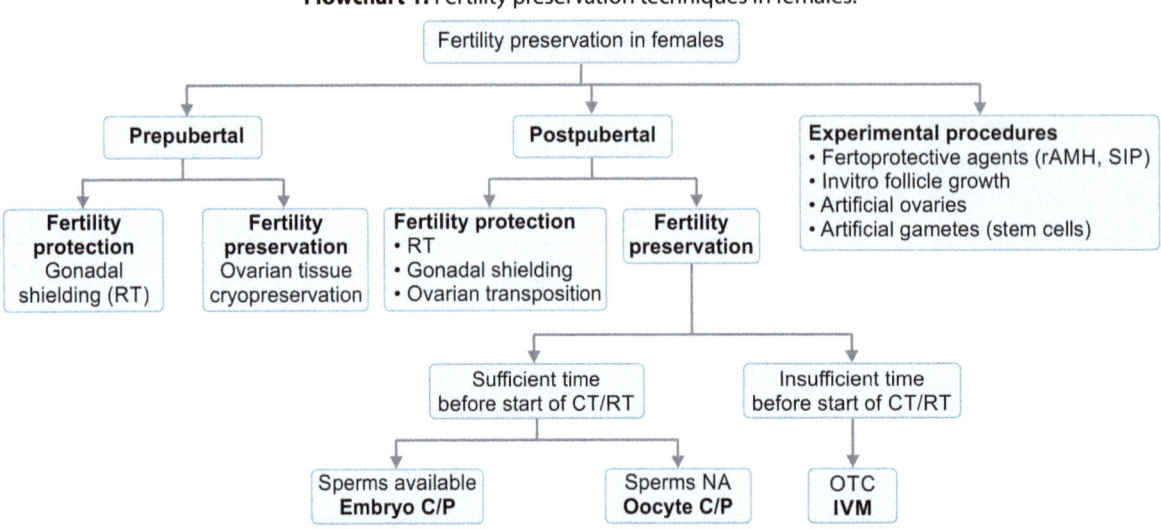

Flowchart 1: Fertility preservation techniques in females.

(SIP: sphingosine-1-phosphate; IVM: in vitro maturation; FP: fertility preservation; OTC: ovarian tissue cryopreservation; CT: chemotherapy; RT: radiotherapy; C/P: cryopreservation; NA: not available)

or partner (**Flowchart 1**). It involves ovarian stimulation (OS) from day 2 of the menstrual cycle (MC) and oocyte retrieval, therefore a period of approximately 12–14 days is required before CT. The desired protocol is the antagonist protocol with a gonadotropin releasing hormone agonist (GnRH-a) trigger for oocyte maturation, as it is shorter and decreases the risk of ovarian hyperstimulation syndrome (OHSS). To avoid delay in CT, a random start protocol has been introduced where OS is started at any time of the MC without affecting the outcome.[9] Literature suggests that age is a vital factor that contributes to a decrease in the number of oocytes recovered in oncological patients, though few studies suggest a preexisting reduced ovarian reserve in patients with BRCA mutations and lymphoma.[10] Women should be informed about the risk of losing reproductive autonomy and possible issues with ownership of stored embryos.

Limitations of the procedure:

- The process of controlled ovarian stimulation (COS) usually takes around 2 weeks which may lead to a delay in starting the cancer treatment (**Figs. 2A to F**).
- High estradiol (E2) levels during COS might have an effect on estrogen-sensitive tumors.
- Reproductive autonomy in future might be affected.
- Repercussions regarding discarding of embryos in case the patient dies before the embryos are used.

Mature Oocyte Cryopreservation

Unlike embryo cryopreservation, oocyte cryopreservation helps maintain the reproductive autonomy in young cancer patients and is now an established technique, no longer considered experimental. Women with a partner should be offered the option to cryopreserve unfertilized oocytes or to split the oocytes to attempt both embryo and oocyte cryopreservation.[11]

Though studies assessing the pregnancy outcomes in cancer patients who undergo oocyte cryopreservation are limited, an oocyte survival rate of 85.2%[12] and a live birth rate of 35% have been reported in oncofertility patients who underwent oocyte cryopreservation. Recently, it is also postulated as an alternative for adolescent females who are peripubertal and premenarchal. Due to paucity of studies at present, it is difficult to decide if cancer patients have comparable outcomes to elective FP or donor oocyte patients.

Ovarian Stimulation for Embryo or Mature Oocyte Cryopreservation

Gonadotropin releasing hormone antagonist protocol with a GnRH-a trigger is preferred as it reduces the duration of stimulation and circumvents the risk of OHSS. At times in cases where there is an urgency to start cancer therapy random start protocols are used without compromising the outcome. Normal follicular growth and development is seen despite the raised progesterone levels in the luteal phase or a spontaneous LH surge which might occur when the initial lead follicle reaches maturity. In luteal halt protocol, administration of GnRH antagonist in the luteal phase induces corpus luteum regression, menses ensues 2–4 days later, and OS is initiated earlier than awaiting spontaneous menses. If the patient with cancer presents in the late follicular phase, OS without GnRH antagonist can be started if the follicle cohort following the lead follicle is smaller than 12 mm and stays smaller than 12 mm before a spontaneous LH surge. After the LH surge, GnRH antagonist is started when the secondary follicle cohort reaches 12 mm to prevent premature secondary LH surge. If however, the

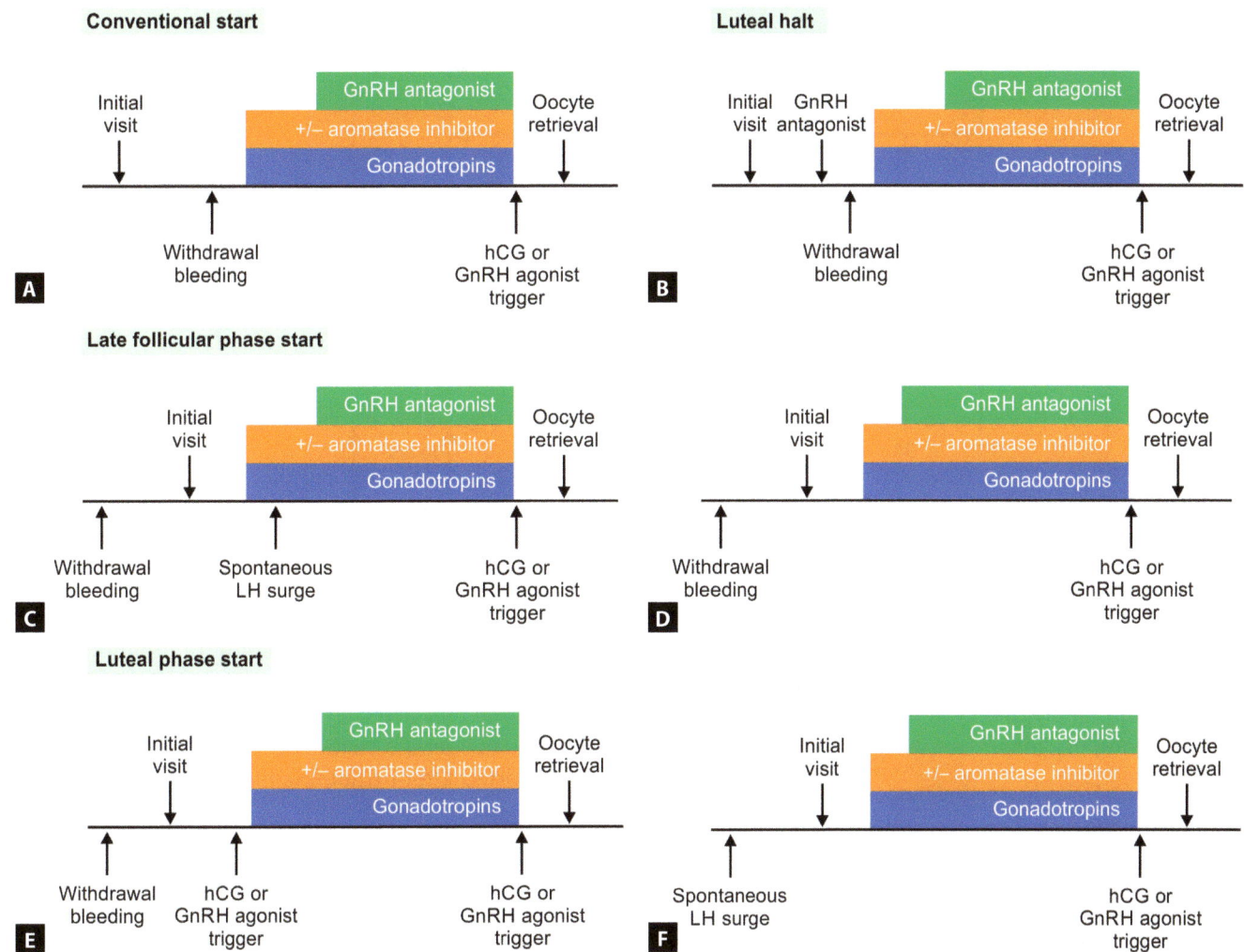

Figs. 2A to F: Controlled ovarian stimulation protocols in patients with cancer.
(Cakmak H, Katz A, Cedars MI, Rosen MP. Effective method for emergency fertility preservation: random-start controlled ovarian stimulation. Fertil Steril 2013 Aug 26.)

follicle cohort following the lead follicle reaches 12 mm before the spontaneous LH surge, pituitary suppression with GnRH antagonist is initiated and continued until triggering final oocyte maturation. If the patient is in the late follicular phase, ovulation can be induced with human chorionic gonadotropin (hCG) or GnRH-a when the dominant follicle reaches 18 mm in diameter and OS is started in 2–3 days in luteal phase. If the patient presents in the luteal phase, OS can be started in the absence of GnRH antagonist and GnRH antagonist administration is initiated later in the cycle, when the follicle cohort reached 12 mm to prevent premature secondary LH surge.[9]

Random-start require higher total gonadotropin dose, but the number of retrieved oocytes and the number of cryopreserved oocytes [9.0 (range 0–24) vs. 10.6 (range 0–40)] and embryos [4.8 (range 0–29) vs. 4.8 (range 0–16)] are similar between the groups. Double stimulation can also be considered for urgent FP cycles.[11]

Suprarphysiological E2 levels achieved during OS have raised concerns in hormone-sensitive cancers. This can be managed effectively by the addition of letrozole, an aromatase inhibitor (AI), along with gonadotropins during OS. It is administered from the start of OS in a dose of 2.5–5 mg daily and continued till after oocyte retrieval, until the E2 levels normalize. Its use does not affect the ovarian response or fertilization rate, though few studies have suggested a lower oocyte maturation rate.[12] Tamoxifen, a selective estrogen receptor modulator (SERM), is used routinely in breast cancer (BC) patients to reduce recurrence. It has also been used during OS in hormone-sensitive BC patients, a follow-up of 10 years has not shown an increase in recurrence rate in these patients[3,13,14] **(Fig. 3)**.

Precautions that need to be taken when performing OS in oncology patients involve using an antagonist protocol, triggering with an agonist, and adding AIs/SERMs such as letrozole and tamoxifen when dealing with hormone-sensitive tumors.[15,16] However, a safe time interval between conclusion of CT/RT and oocyte or embryo cryopreservation has not been found though the European Society of Human Reproduction and Embryology (ESHRE) guidelines

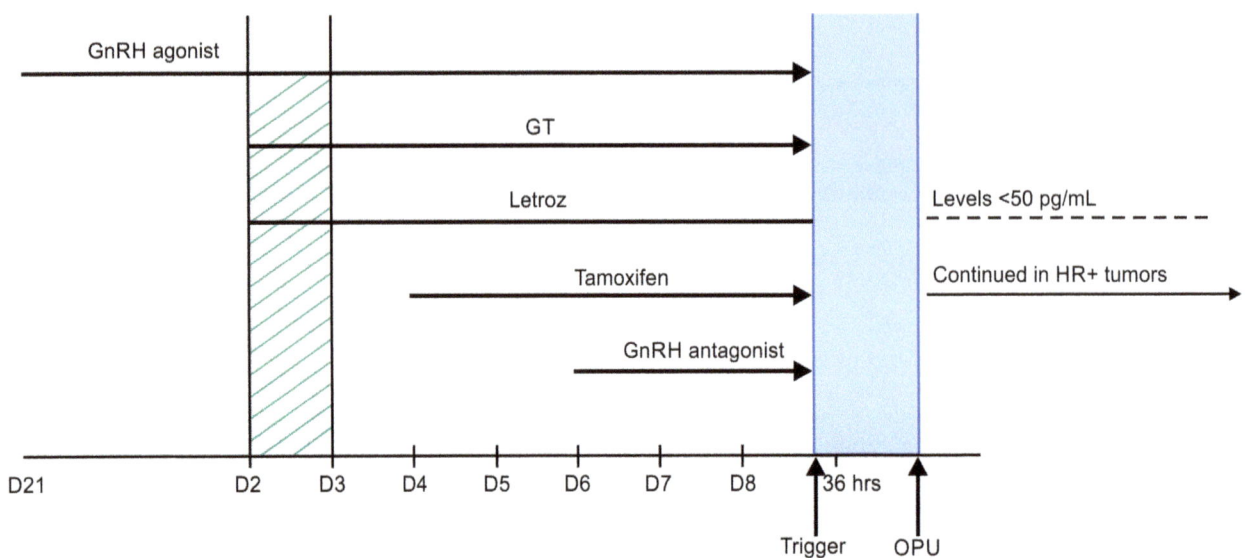

Fig. 3: Controlled ovarian stimulation (COS) strategies for ovarian stimulation (OS) in cancer patients. (OPU: oocyte pickup; D: day; GT: gonadotrophins; E2: estradiol; GnRH: gonadotrophin releasing hormone; HR+: hormone receptor positive)

suggest an interval of at least 1 year following CT and an interval of 2 years if both CT and RT have been administered before attempting pregnancy in order to reduce the risk of pregnancy complications.[11]

Complications: Delay in starting cancer therapy, risk of OHSS, thromboembolic complications, and a theoretic stimulation of estrogen-sensitive cancers always need to be kept in mind and the patient counseled accordingly.

In Vitro Maturation

It has not witnessed universal success as in vitro oocyte maturation is technically challenging. Improved culture techniques have led to better pregnancy rates in appropriately selected patients.[17] Pregnancy rates per embryo transfer vary from 0–36% and spontaneous abortion rate between 17–63%.[18] Studies assessing the health risks of children conceived after in vitro maturation (IVM) have been reassuring. The advantage of IVM is that it can be performed when delay in CT is not possible. Additionally no gonadotropin stimulation is required and therefore can be used in estrogen-sensitive tumors. According to the ESHRE guidelines, IVM is now regarded as an innovative procedure, with better results lately due to the biphasic culture media, though IVM after ex vivo extraction is still considered experimental.[11]

Cryopreservation of Ovarian Tissue

It is the only FP technique available for prepubertal girls. Ovarian cortical tissue which is rich in primordial follicles is removed by laparoscopy or by minilaparotomy and then cryopreserved by either slow freezing or lately by vitrification after tissue preparation. Reimplantation of tissue is done preferentially to the ovary/pelvic cavity (orthotopic), however, heterotopic transplantation (abdominal wall or forearm) can be carried out if required. A live birth rate of 23% has been reported with ovarian tissue cryopreservation (OTC) and the trend is on the rise.[19] Over 130 live births have been reported after orthotopic transplantation of thawed ovarian tissue.

Success of transplantation depends on the patient's age, baseline ovarian reserve, and expertise of the surgeon and cryobiologist performing the procedure. Ovarian function usually resumes between 60–240 days posttransplant and persists for up to 7 years.[20] The first ongoing pregnancy with heterotopic implantation of ovarian tissue has been reported lately by Stern et al. 2013.[21]

Intraoperative aspiration of immature oocytes from ovarian tissue can be followed by IVM and cryopreservation of mature oocytes or embryos which are produced during the process of OTC.[22]

According to ESHRE FP 2020 guidelines, OTC should not be offered in patients with a low ovarian reserve [anti-Müllerian hormone (AMH) <0.5 ng/mL and antral follicle count (AFC) <5], advanced age considering the unfavorable risk/benefit ratio. Current evidence suggests that the efficiency of OTC procedure is questionable above the age of 36 years.[11]

According to American Society for Reproductive Medicine (ASRM) Practice Committee 2019 data on the effectiveness, safety, and reproductive outcomes after OTC are inadequate. However, with the current literature in hand, OTC should be considered an *established* medical procedure with limited effectiveness and should be offered to carefully selected patients.

According to ESHRE FP guidelines, OTC should be considered as an *innovative* technique. OS can be performed immediately after OTC, however, OTC at the time of oocyte pick-up after OS should not be done unless in a research context. Ovarian transposition can also be performed at the same time as OTC in patients who will receive pelvic irradiation.[11]

Since OTC can be technically challenging it should be offered only by clinics with the essential laboratory and surgical expertise.

Advantages:
- No delay in CT
- OS not required
- No increase in E2 levels
- Preserves a greater pool of follicles
- Resumption of ovarian function—avoids negative effects of premature menopause
- Spontaneous pregnancy possible
- Can be done in prepubertal girls
- Can be done in patients unwilling for COS.

Disadvantage and Risks: OTC requires the patient to undergo surgery twice once to take out the tissue and once for transplantation. There is also a risk of tumor reseeding especially for malignancies, such as leukemia, which are systemic in nature. Extensive testing of tissue using immunohistochemistry (IHC), molecular analysis by reverse transcription quantitative polymerase chain reaction (RT-qPCR), histology, and xenografting prior to transplantation improve safety though complete elimination of risk is not possible.[23] On the basis of the available data, the risk of reseeding in various malignancies was predicted as: High risk for leukemia, moderate risk for gastrointestinal cancers, low risk for BC, sarcomas of the bone and connective tissue, gynecological cancers, and Hodgkin's and non-Hodgkin's lymphoma[24] **(Table 3)**. Also carriers of BRCA mutations are at an increased risk and so autologous transplantation is not done in these cases.[25] Only one live birth after autologous transplantation of tissue in a patient with leukemia has been reported in which tissue xenotransplantation was done in a severe combined immunodeficiency (SCID) mouse.[26]

Ovarian Transposition

This is indicated in patients who need local pelvic radiation as transposition keeps the ovaries away from the area of maximal radiation exposure. Post transposition, however, there may be a difficulty in performing transvaginal oocyte retrieval and transabdominal retrieval may be needed in some patients.[27] Since this procedure does not prevent ovarian damage by cytotoxic drugs it *should be avoided if patient has to undergo both CT and RT.*

Uterine Transposition

Ribeiro et al. 2017[28] for the first time reported it in a patient with rectal cancer. In this procedure, they performed laparoscopic transposition of the uterus to the upper abdomen, away from the field of radiation to preserve fertility. After conclusion of RT, rectosigmoidectomy was done and the uterus was repositioned into the pelvis. Patient resumed menses in 2 months and at 18 months uterine and ovarian functions were stated to be normal.

Fertoprotective Adjuvant Therapy

The additional stress and strain of FP procedures could be avoided if drugs were available to protect the gonads against the ill effects of CT. Though there is ongoing research to develop such agents, the only drug available for clinical use so far is the long-acting GnRH-a. It acts as a fertoprotective agent by the following mechanisms:
- Hypogonadotropic state is achieved similar to that seen in the prepubertal ovary.
- Reduced ovarian blood flow due to hypoestrogenic status
- Direct effect on ovary (GnRH receptors are found in ovary)
- Upregulation of antiapoptotic molecules such as sphingosine-1-phosphate (S1P) in the ovary
- Prevention of gonadotoxicity on oogonial stem cells.[29-31]

Gonadotropin releasing hormone agonists are started at least a week prior to CT to reduce damage caused by follicular activation due to its "flare effect", and it should be continued till 2 weeks after completion of therapy. GnRH-a have been shown to reduce the risk of premature ovarian insufficiency in BC patients, but is no replacement to other FP alternatives. They may also help to decrease the heavy bleeding in patients with thrombocytopenia related to CT and stem cell transplantation.

According to ESHRE FP 2020 guidelines, in premenopausal women with BC, GnRH-a during CT can be offered as an option for ovarian function protection only in those cases where other FP options cannot be offered. In malignancies other than BC and in premenopausal patients

TABLE 3: Ovarian metastasis risk according to the type of cancer Sommezer Human reprod update. 2004;10:251-66.

High Risk (>11%)	Moderate Risk (0.2-11%)	Low Risk (<0.2%)
• Leukemia • Neuroblastoma • Burkitt lymphoma	• Breast cancer (stage 4/infiltrating lobular type) • Colon cancer • Adenocarcinoma of cervix • Non Hodgkins lymphoma • Ewings sarcoma	• Breast cancer (stages 1,2/infiltrating ductal type) • Squamous cell carcinoma cervix • Hodgkins lymphoma • Osteogenic carcinoma • Nongenital rhabdomyosarcom • Wilms tumor

with autoimmune diseases receiving cyclophosphamide, GnRH-a should be used only after discussing the uncertainty about its benefits. GnRH-a should not be considered an equivalent or alternative option for FP but can be offered after cryopreservation techniques or when they are not possible.[11]

Special Clinical Conditions

Breast cancer: FP is important in these patients as they invariably receive alkylating agents or long-term hormonal therapy which shortens the reproductive window drastically. Patients with BC have time between surgery and CT to undergo in vitro fertilization (IVF). For patients with hormone receptor positive tumors AIs/SERMs are used to avoid high E2 levels. IVM or ovarian tissue preservation is an alternate option for patients not willing for OS **(Flowchart 2)**.

Hematologic malignancies: Patients with hematologic malignancies (such as leukemias and lymphomas) have an urgent requirement for CT. OTC can be carried out though the risk of surgical complications increases due to abnormal hematological parameters. OTC can also be carried out after the first CT when patient's condition has improved, though it may be less effective. Patients diagnosed with leukemia may benefit by GnRH-a coadministration to manage ovulation and menstrual bleeding during CT.

Children and adolescents: Extreme sensitivity is required when broaching the topic of FP. Postpubertal girls under the age of 18 and peripubertal girls can undergo OS followed by mature oocyte cryopreservation. IVM and OTC are also alternative options. In prepubertal girls OTC is presently the only established technique to cryopreserve gametes.

According to the new Assisted Reproductive Technology (ART) Act 2021 consent/assent (in minors) needs to be taken before for cryopreservation of gametes when offering FP services. The gametes can be cryopreserved for 10 years and even longer after the permission of the national board.

FERTILITY PRESERVATION STRATEGIES IN MALES

Ejaculated Sperm Cryopreservation

Postpubertal males should be offered sperm cryopreservation, preferably before administration of gonadotoxic therapy as it is simple and an established FP technique. Patients need to be counseled about the quality of the cryopreserved sample and potential for future use.[32] In some cases, there may be an impairment in the semen parameters even prior to start of cancer therapy which could be due to the cancer itself, as it might cause disruption of the normal hypothalamic-pituitary-gonadal axis and damage to the germinal epithelium. In some patients who have a difficulty in ejaculation other therapeutic options such as phosphodiesterase type 5 (PDE5) inhibitors, penile vibratory stimulus, or electroejaculation can be considered.[33]

Cryopreservation of Surgically Extracted Sperm

Surgical sperm extraction is an option for men who cannot ejaculate despite trying the abovementioned techniques, or those who are azoospermic.[34] This procedure has been mentioned as "onco-TESE (testicular sperm extraction)" and this may be the only option of viable sperm in some patients **(Flowchart 3)**.

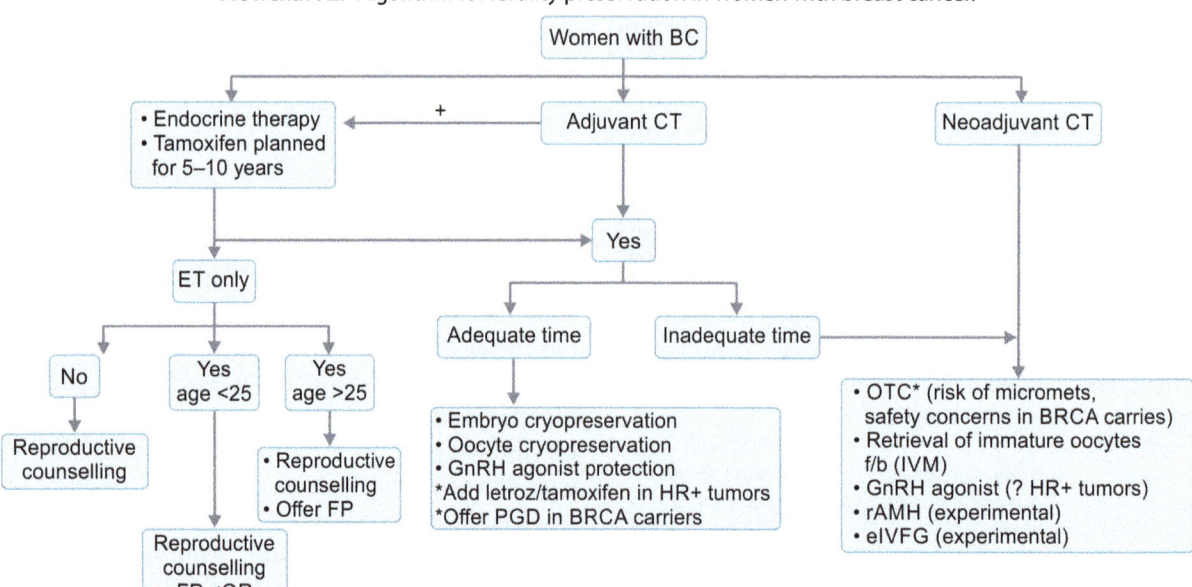

Flowchart 2: Algorithm for fertility preservation in women with breast cancer.

(BC: breast cancer; ET: endocrine therapy; OR: ovarian reserve; CT: chemotherapy; HR+: hormone receptor positive; IVM: in vitro maturation; AMH: anti-mullerian hormone; eIVFG: encapsulated in vitro follicular growth; FB: followed by)

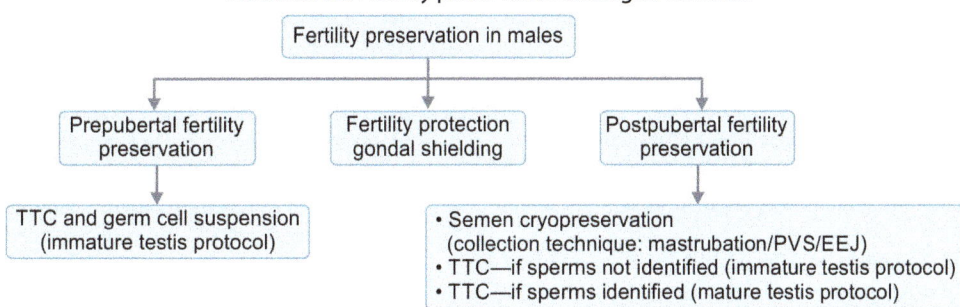

Flowchart 3: Fertility preservation strategies in males.

FUTURE DIRECTIONS

Technologies in the field of reproductive and regenerative medicine are evolving at an incredibly fast pace. Many new fertoprotective agents such as imatinib, S1P, ovarian activation by interrupting the Hippo signaling pathway, in vitro follicular activation, and generation of artificial ovaries may be the future for FP in females. Cryopreservation of immature testicular tissue (ITT) and germ cell suspension can be offered in prepubertal males, but currently regeneration of mature sperm is in the experimental stage. Generation of artificial gametes from stem cells may be the future to help improve oncofertility care, though there have been concerns about methylation pattern of imprinted genes using total in vitro protocol for generation of germ cells.

CONCLUSION

Early detection of cancer and advanced multimodality treatments are improving cancer survivorship and bringing 'quality of life' issues into focus. Fertility preservation (FP) is now the 'standard of care' for cancer survivors. For postpubertal women oocyte and embryo freezing is available and is an established technique. GnRH antagonist protocol with an agonist trigger is employed due to its shorter duration of stimulation and decreased risk of ovarian hyperstimulation syndrome (OHSS). To avoid any delay in Chemotherapy(CT), random start protocols have been introduced in which ovarian stimulation (OS) is started at any day of the menstrual cycle without compromising the outcome. In women where we have an urgency to start CT and in pre-pubertal girls, ovarian tissue freezing can be offered. Success of transplantation depends on the patients age, baseline ovarian reserve and skill of the surgeon and cryobiologist performing the procedure. Postpubertal males can be offered sperm cryopreservation since it is a standardized fertility-preservation method. Surgical sperm extraction is also an alternative approach for some. Many experimental therapies have evolved for follicular growth and generation of gametes from stem cells. At this point they are considered merely experimental and should be carried out only in the context of a research setting.

Key Learning Points

- Fertility preservation has become the standard of care for patients at risk of losing their reproductive potential due to cancer treatment, immunological diseases, or genetic makeup.
- FP techniques can be used separately or together in the same patient to maximize efficiency.
- For postpubertal women oocyte and embryo freezing is available and is an established technique. It needs to be performed before CT and requires a time period of 2 weeks.
- In women where there is an urgency to start CT and in prepubertal girls, ovarian tissue freezing may be offered. OTC requires a double surgery though it has the advantage of allowing for spontaneous conception and restoration of endocrine secretion. As more births are being reported, it has lost the experimental tag in some countries. Screening of tissue for malignant cells before transplantation is of paramount importance.
- Sperm cryopreservation is an established FP technique in postpubertal males and surgical extraction of sperms maybe needed in certain circumstances.
- For the prepubertal males freezing of ITT and germ cell suspension can be offered but currently regeneration of mature sperm is in the experimental stage.
- In the future, IVM of gametes, stem cell therapy, and effective fertoprotective agents may be available to improve oncofertility care.
- A multidisciplinary approach is vital for offering effective FP services.

REFERENCES

1. Hudson MM. Reproductive outcomes for survivors of childhood cancer. Obstet Gynecol. 2010;116(5):1171-83.
2. Ward E, DeSantis C, Robbins A, Kohler B, Jemal A. Childhood and adolescent cancer statistics, 2014. CA Cancer J Clin. 2014;64(2):83-103.
3. Meirow D, Epstein M, Lewis H, Nugent D, Gosden RG. Administration of cyclophosphamide at different stages of follicular maturation in mice: effects on reproductive performance and fetal malformations. Hum Reprod. 2001;16(4):632-7.
4. Su HC, Haunschild C, Chung K, Komrokian S, Boles S, Sammel MD, et al. Prechemotherapy antimullerian hormone, age, and body size predict timing of return of ovarian function in young breast cancer patients. Cancer. 2014;120(23):3691-8.
5. Wallace WH, Thomson AB, Kelsey TW. The radiosensitivity of the human oocyte. Hum Reprod. 2003;18(1):117-21.

6. Wo JY, Viswanathan AN. Impact of radiotherapy on fertility, pregnancy, and neonatal outcomes in female cancer patients. Int J Radiat Oncol Biol Phys. 2009;73:1304-12.
7. Meistrich ML, van Beek MEAB. Radiation Sensitivity of the Human Testis. Adv Radiat Biol. 1990;14:227-68.
8. Mitchell RT, Saunders PTK, Sharpe RM, Kelnar CJH, Wallace WHB. Male fertility and strategies for fertility preservation following childhood cancer treatment. Endocr Dev. 2009; 15:101-34.
9. Cakmak H, Katz A, Cedars MI, Rosen MP. Effective method for emergency fertility preservation: random-start controlled ovarian stimulation. Fertil Steril. 2013;100(6):1673-80.
10. Kim J, Turan V, Oktay K. Long-term Safety of Letrozole and Gonadotropin Stimulation for Fertility Preservation in Women with Breast Cancer. J Clin Endocrinol Metab. 2016;101(4):1364-71.
11. Anderson RA, Amant F, Braat D, D'Angelo A, Chuva de Sousa Lopes SM, Demeestere I, et al; ESHRE Guideline Group on Female Fertility Preservation. ESHRE guideline: Female fertility preservation. Hum Reprod Open. 2020;(4):hoaa052.
12. Cobo A, Garrido N, Pellicer A, Remohí J. Six years' experience in ovum donation using vitrified oocytes: report of cumulative outcomes, impact of storage time, and development of a predictive model for oocyte survival rate. Fertil Steril. 2015;104(6):1426-34.e1-8.
13. Meirow D, Raanani H, Maman E, Paluch-Shimon S, Shapira M, Cohen Y, et al .Tamoxifen co-administration during controlled ovarian hyperstimulation for in vitro fertilization in breast cancer patients increases the safety of fertility-preservation treatment strategies. Fertil Steril. 2014;102(2):488-95.e3.
14. Soleimani R, Heytens E, Darzynkiewicz Z, Oktay K. Mechanisms of chemotherapy-induced human ovarian aging: double strand DNA breaks and microvascular compromise. Aging (Albany NY). 2011;3(8):782-93.
15. Hawkins MM. Pregnancy outcome and offspring after childhood cancer. BMJ. 1994;309(6961):1034.
16. Green DM, Zevon MA, Lowrie G, Seigelstein N, Hall B. Congenital anomalies in children of patients who received chemotherapy for cancer in childhood and adolescence. N Engl J Med. 1991;325(3):141-6.
17. Grynberg M, El Hachem H, de Bantel A, Benard J, le Parco S, Fanchin R. In vitro maturation of oocytes: uncommon indications. Fertil Steril. 2013;99(5):1182-8.
18. Holte TO, Norderhaug IN. In Vitro Maturation of Oocytes within Assisted Reproduction. Oslo, Norway: Knowledge Centre for the Health Services at the Norwegian Institute of Public Health (NIPH); 2007.
19. Van der Ven H, Liebenthron J, Beckmann M, Toth B, Korell M, Krüssel J, et al; FertiPROTEKT network. Ninety-five orthotopic transplantations in 74 women of ovarian tissue after cytotoxic treatment in a fertility preservation network: tissue activity, pregnancy and delivery rates. Hum Reprod. 2016;31(9):2031-41.
20. Kim SS. Assessment of long term endocrine function after ovarian transplantation of frozen-thawed human ovarian tissue to the heterotopic site: 10 year longitudinal follow-up study. J Assist Reprod Genet. 2012;29(6):489-93.
21. Stern CJ, Gook D, Hale LG, Agresta F, Oldham J, Rozen G, et al. First reported clinical pregnancy following heterotopic grafting of cryopreserved ovarian tissue in a woman after a bilateral oophorectomy. Hum Reprod. 2013;28(11):2996-9.
22. Fadini R, Dal Canto M, Mignini Renzini M, Milani R, Fruscio R, Cantù MG, et al. Embryo transfer following in vitro maturation and cryopreservation of oocytes recovered from antral follicles during conservative surgery for ovarian cancer. J Assist Reprod Genet. 2012;29(8):779-81.
23. Masciangelo R, Bosisio C, Donnez J, Amorim CA, Dolmans MM. Safety of ovarian tissue transplantation in patients with borderline ovarian tumors. Hum Reprod. 2017;33(2).
24. Rosendahl M, Andersen MT, Ralfkær E, Kjeldsen L, Andersen MK, Andersen CY. Evidence of residual disease in cryopreserved ovarian cortex from female patients with leukemia. Fertil Steril. 2010;94(6):2186-90.
25. Rodriguez-Wallberg KA, Oktay K. Fertility preservation and pregnancy in women with and without BRCA mutation-positive breast cancer. Oncologist. 2012;17(11):1409-17.
26. Shapira M, Raanani H, Barshack I, Amariglio N, Derech-Haim S, Marciano MN, et al. First delivery in a leukemia survivor after transplantation of cryopreserved ovarian tissue, evaluated for leukemia cells contamination. Fertil Steril. 2018;109(1):48-53.
27. Zinger M, Liu JH, Husseinzadeh N, Thomas MA. Successful surrogate pregnancy after ovarian transposition, pelvic irradiation and hysterectomy. J Reprod Med. 2004;49(7):573-4.
28. Ribeiro R, Rebolho JC, Tsumanuma FK, Brandalize GG, Trippia CH, Saab KA. Uterine transposition: technique and a case report. Fertil Steril. 2017;108(2):320-4.
29. Roness H, Kalich-Philosoph L, Meirow D. Prevention of chemotherapy-induced ovarian damage: possible roles for hormonal and non-hormonal attenuating agents. Hum Reprod Update. 2014;20(5):759-74.
30. Blumenfeld Z, Evron A. Endocrine prevention of chemotherapy-induced ovarian failure. Curr Opin Obstet Gynecol. 2016;28(4):223-9.
31. Lambertini M, Moore HCF, Leonard RCF, Loibl S, Munster P, Bruzzone M, et al. Gonadotropin-Releasing Hormone Agonists During Chemotherapy for Preservation of Ovarian Function and Fertility in Premenopausal Patients with Early Breast Cancer: a Systematic Review and Meta-Analysis of Individual Patient-Level Data. J Clin Oncol. 2018;36(19):1981-90.
32. Meirow D, Schenker JG. Cancer and male infertility. Hum Reprod. 1995;10(8):2017-22.
33. Hallak J, Kolettis PN, Sekhon VS, Thomas AJ Jr, Agarwal A. Sperm cryopreservation in patients with testicular cancer. Urology. 1999;54(5):894-9.
34. Furuhashi K, Ishikawa T, Hashimoto H, Yamada S, Ogata S, Mizusawa Y, et al. Onco-testicular sperm extraction: testicular sperm extraction in azoospermic and very severely oligozoospermic cancer patients. Andrologia. 2013;45(2):107-10.

CHAPTER 34

Third Party Reproduction

Sowmya Dinesh HR

INTRODUCTION

The development of in vitro fertilization (IVF) in 1978 has marked a remarkable milestone in the history of human reproduction and evolution. IVF opened new vistas and possibilities and has affected many institutions in the society.

A revolutionary concept has been the introduction of a "third party", when a couple has not been able to bear a child with conventional assisted reproductive technologies (ARTs).

The three essential elements for reproduction are egg, sperm, and uterus. Even if the couple or intended person has one of those, they could achieve parenthood.

The desire to have their own offspring is so strong that it makes the intended parent(s) cross their cultural, social, and moral beliefs, and legal restrictions. Many times, they do undertake an international or intercontinental journey to realize their dream.

HISTORY

The major milestones in IVF leading to third party reproduction (TPR) have been enumerated in **Table 1**.

TABLE 1: Third party reproduction—milestones.		
Year	Procedure	Credit
1866	Artificial insemination of husband's sperm (AIH)	Dr Marion Sims
1890	Artificial insemination of donor sperm (AID)	Dr Robert L. Dickinson
1978	In vitro fertilization (IVF)	Patrick Steptoe and Robert Edwards
1978	IVF	Dr Subhash Mukhopadhyay
1976	The first formal surrogacy (Gestational with AID)	USA
1984	Egg donation	Trounson et al.
1986	The first gestational surrogacy	USA

Definition

The American Society for Reproductive Medicine (ASRM),[1] defines TPR as the use of eggs, sperm, or embryos that have been donated by a third person (donor) to enable an infertile individual or couple (intended recipient) to become parents.

The person who donates nuclear DNA in the form of sperm, eggs, or embryos, or carries the pregnancy (gestational carrier), or provides a combination of these is called the "third party". The person(s) who will raise the child after birth is/are called "intended parent(s)". A third-party donor can be someone the intended parents know or they may be anonymous.[13]

Types

The types of TPR are as shown in the **Box 1**.

Social Issues

Infertility brings a tremendous pressure on the couple from social and personal realms. Cultural, religious, and personal beliefs influence the extent to which the intending parent(s) utilize the range of services, under the umbrella of IVF. TPR enables couples, who would not have otherwise had a baby, to have treatment confidentially and to get relief from social pressure and stigmata of infertility.

Legal Issues

The laws and regulations governing TPR vary from country to country, while some are very lenient, some completely prohibit such services.

Since the donors or surrogates are mostly paid, there is a complex mixture of money and power between them and the

BOX 1: The types of third party reproduction.
- Egg donation
- Sperm donation
- Embryo donation/adoption
- Surrogacy
- Posthumous reproduction

agencies which procure such services to recipients. In a class-stratified society, usually the donors are underprivileged which can lead to their exploitation.

Also, there is a risk of misunderstanding and confusion in the contract between the donor and recipient, leading to a long-drawn legal battle. Hence, strong and thoughtful laws are needed to govern these special reproductive services.

In India, IVF services were not governed by any law till recently. In 2021, the ART (Regulation) and Surrogacy laws were enacted leading to a lot of reforms in the way such services are provided. In this chapter, TPR is discussed in the context of Indian laws.

Psychological and Ethical Issues

Third party reproduction brings about significant psychosocial issues for all the parties that are directly involved that is the couple/intending woman, gamete donors, and surrogate. Moreover, the partners and children of surrogates are also affected.

Surrogacy has led to a lot of debates, the prime concern being the exploitation and commodification of women and that there could be a significant chance of these women being coerced into agreeing to provide such services. On the other hand, its proponents argue that a woman has the right to make decisions regarding her body and the compensation she receives could change her and her children's lives for better.

There are dilemmas about maintaining the gamete donor's details in secrecy versus the need to reveal it to the child, who might seek the information after reaching adulthood or for some health concerns.

There would be an intense psychological conflict when one must make a choice between being childfree versus accepting another person's gametes or participating in getting the desired offspring.

New Kinship Patterns

Third party reproduction has introduced a bunch of social and personal dilemmas like never before. A child can have three types of mothers: genetic—who gives oocyte, gestational—who raises him in her womb, and social—who raises him after birth. It would also raise concerns as to what is the relationship between women contributing to the birth of a child and whether multiple motherhood is acceptable.

So, the mother who carries her daughter and son-in-law's embryos is the offspring's social mother as well as the genetic grandmother while the offspring is the social sister of the genetic mother. It could get more complex with intergenerational gamete donation as in a mother donating her eggs to her daughter.

With TPR, the scope of motherhood has widened to include same-sex couples with offspring born to a lesbian couple having double legal mothers. The impact of these emerging forms of family among LGBTQ (lesbian, gay, bisexual, transgender, and queer/questioning) couples extends beyond the relationship between the immediate parents and their offspring involving and affecting the generation of grandparents and the wider kin group in several ways.

Primary eligibility criteria to procure TPR services in India are listed in **Table 2**.

Protocol for Providing Third Party Reproduction

Since there are complex sets of ethical, moral, psychological, and personal issues involved in this type of reproduction, the service providers are expected to follow a set of rules and regulations laid down by each country to safeguard the interest of all parties involved. The steps are as shown in **Box 2**. In this chapter, the regulations in Indian context are discussed in detail.

■ EGG DONATION

Egg donation has made a remarkable impact in the lives of many women with poor egg quality and numbers enabling them to achieve motherhood.

TABLE 2: Eligibility for TPR according to Indian ART Act 2021.

Who can solicit these services	*Sperm, egg, and embryo donation* • Married couple • Unmarried or ever married single woman *Surrogacy* • Married Indian/OCI couple • Unmarried or ever married single woman • Not having their own healthy biological/adopted child
What is the age limit	*Sperm, egg, and embryo donation* • Husband: 21–55 years • Wife/intended woman: 21–50 years *Surrogacy* • Husband: 26–55 years • Wife/intended woman: 23–50 years
Identity	• Aadhar card • Marriage certificate for couple

(ART: assisted reproductive technology; OCI: overseas citizen of India; TPR: third party reproduction)

BOX 2: Protocol to be observed while providing third party reproduction.

- Counseling of intended or commissioning couple/woman (IC/W)
- Ascertaining the third-party donor/surrogate (TPD/S)—known or nonidentified
- Counseling of TPD/S
- Screening of IC/W
- Screening of TPD/S
- Consenting of all parties involved
- Legal compliance and clearance
- Provision of assisted reproductive technology (ART) keeping safety and confidentiality of TPD/S in mind

TABLE 3: Indications for donor eggs.

Ovarian dysfunction

Premenopausal	*Postmenopausal*
• Poor ovarian responders • Diminished ovarian reserve • Premature ovarian failure (includes genetic, autoimmune, iatrogenic causes, etc.) • Previous assisted reproductive technology (ART) failure • Resistant ovarian syndrome • Unexplained	• Natural aging • Oncology-related chemoradiotherapy • Surgical ophorectomy • Genetic

Normal ovarian function
- Genetic transmittable disorder in female partner
- Recurrent pregnancy loss with/without recurrent aneuploidy
- Frozen pelvis/severe endometriosis/inaccessible ovaries where oocyte retrieval is difficult/risky
- Same sex couples

BOX 3: Egg donor eligibility criteria [assisted reproductive technology (ART) Act 2021].
- The donor should be
- Between 23 and 35 years of age
- An ever-married woman with a living child of her own
- Altruistic
- Having Aadhar as a proof of identity
- Donating for the first time and hence only once in her lifetime
- Medically and psychologically fit
- Registered and undergo screening at an ART bank

BOX 4: Screening of egg donor—prerequisites.
- The donor should undergo a detailed counseling regarding pros and cons of the intended procedure and to assess her psychological readiness
- Screening for general health and medical fitness
- Screening for infectious diseases: HIV 1 and 2, HBV, HCV, and VDRL

(HBV: hepatitis B virus; HCV: hepatitis C virus; HIV: human immunodeficiency virus; VDRL: venereal disease research laboratory test)

Indications for Donor Eggs

When the ovaries are primarily affected due to age, disease, or have been surgically removed, donor eggs become a viable option. The various indications are listed in **Table 3**.

Types of Egg Donors

The intending couple/woman (IC/W) can procure donor eggs from a known person, or an anonymous person recruited through agencies called ART banks.

In India, only altruistic egg donation is permitted. The USA and many other countries allow commercial egg donation where a donor is compensated financially.

Known or directed donor: Usually, the donor would be a close relative or a friend. When it is a relative, it must be made sure that it would not amount to incest or preferably does not increase the risk of consanguinity. Many a couples advertise in social or print media requesting for an egg donor and procure their own donor.

Anonymous or nonidentified donors: Assisted reproductive technology banks advertise for egg donors and recruit them for ART clinics. Their identity would be kept confidential.

Peer patient donor: In IVF programs, a woman with good number of eggs can donate few of her eggs to a fellow patient who is needing eggs. The recipient will bear part of the cost of IVF for the donor. This is called *egg sharing*. However, an infertile woman is not the ideal donor unless the cause of infertility is purely related to the male.

In India, it is illegal to do egg sharing and all donors must be altruistic, that is they would help the IC/W without any monetary expectations.

Alternatives to Egg Donation

Since there is a huge demand for donor eggs and number of altruistic donors is less leading to long waiting period, the usage of following techniques which utilize the existing reserve in the woman are expected to increase in the coming years.
- Egg/embryo pooling
- In vitro maturation (IVM) of oocytes
- Ovarian rejuvenation using autologous platelet rich plasma (PRP) or bone marrow-derived stem cells (BMSC).

Criteria for Eligibility to Be an Egg Donor

The Indian ART Regulation Act (December, 2021) mandates following eligibility criteria shown in **Box 3**.

Screening of the Egg Donor

The Indian ART (Regulation) Act 2021 lays down the following requisites for screening the donor shown in **Box 4**.

To optimize safety and outcomes for both gamete donors and recipients, the United States Food and Drug Administration (US FDA), American Association of Tissue Banks, US Centers for Disease Control and Prevention (CDC), and ASRM have released a fully comprehensive guideline in 2021.[2]

Food and Drug Administration donor eligibility determination focuses on infectious risk (includes screening for chlamydia, gonorrhea, rapid plasma reagin for syphilis, etc.) while the ASRM guidance also incorporates prenatal optimization, psychoeducational counseling of donors and recipients, and genetic risk assessment including genetic screening for cystic fibrosis, spinal muscular atrophy, and thalassemia, and fragile X syndrome carrier status **(Box 2)**.

Screening of the Recipients

Apart from routine screening as needed for couple/women undergoing IVF, additional screening would depend on the cause of ovarian insufficiency.

TABLE 4: Additional screening for donor egg recipients.

Test/intervention	When to do	Remarks
HSG/SSG/hysteroscopy	Within 2 years of planned IVF	More recent this evaluation, the better
Screen for glucose intolerance	Before scheduling for IVF	–
Karyotype	• High FSH in young women • Abnormal phenotype	High risk if Turner's syndrome
Cardiac risk assessment	Before scheduling for IVF in all women aged >44 years	–
Management by high-risk obstetrics specialist	• Women aged >40 years • Those with additional comorbidities	–

(FSH: follicle stimulating hormone; IVF: in vitro fertilization; HSG: hysterosalpingogram; SSG: sonosalpingogram)

TABLE 5: Recipient and donor cycles management.

Intervention	Donor	Recipient
Fresh transfer		
Synchronization of cycles	With OCPs or luteal progesterone	• With OCP or luteal progesterone • GnRH-a from luteal phase Aim to get periods at least 1–3 days prior to donor
Controlled ovarian stimulation (COS)*[14]	Antagonist protocol (As GnRH-a can be used for trigger and has the least risk of OHSS)	–
Frozen transfer		
Synchronization of cycles	Not needed	
Endometrial preparation	–	Women with functioning ovaries • Natural cycle • Modified natural cycle • Letrozole-induced cycle • Programmed cycle with HRT with/without pituitary downregulation Women with nonfunctioning ovaries • Programmed cycle with HRT

*The protocols for COS, oocyte pick-up in donor, and embryo transfer in the recipient are as per the standard accepted protocols for women with IVF programs with self-oocytes.
(GnRH-a: gonadotropin-releasing hormone agonist; HRT: hormone replacement treatment; OCP: oral contraceptive pills; OHSS: ovarian hyperstimulation syndrome)

In younger women, karyotype is indicated. The women with Turner's syndrome need to be carefully assessed and counseled as mortality in pregnancy is three times higher than control group due to risk of aortic dissection or rupture, hepatic disease, and other endocrine diseases.

American Society for Reproductive Medicine consensus 2012 states that in a woman with Turner's syndrome, *pregnancy is absolutely contraindicated if any cardiac defects on magnetic resonance imaging (MRI), including aorta size index (ASI) >2 cm/m² and pregnancy is relatively contraindicated, even if no cardiovascular defects.*[3]

In women aged >40 years, cardiac function assessment and management with a high-risk obstetrics specialist is important to decrease morbidity during pregnancy.

Additional factors to consider while screening the recipients of donor eggs are shown in **Table 4**.

Recipient and Donor Cycles Management

The recipient and donor cycles management is shown in **Table 5**.

The steps involved in egg donation are as shown in **Flowchart 1**.

Complications of Egg Donation

The various complications of egg donation in both donor and recipient are listed in **Table 6**.

The Impact of Donor Gamete Conception on the Resultant Children

It is difficult to assess how conception through donor gametes affects the resulting children psychologically as very few couples disclose to their children that they were conceived with donor gametes.

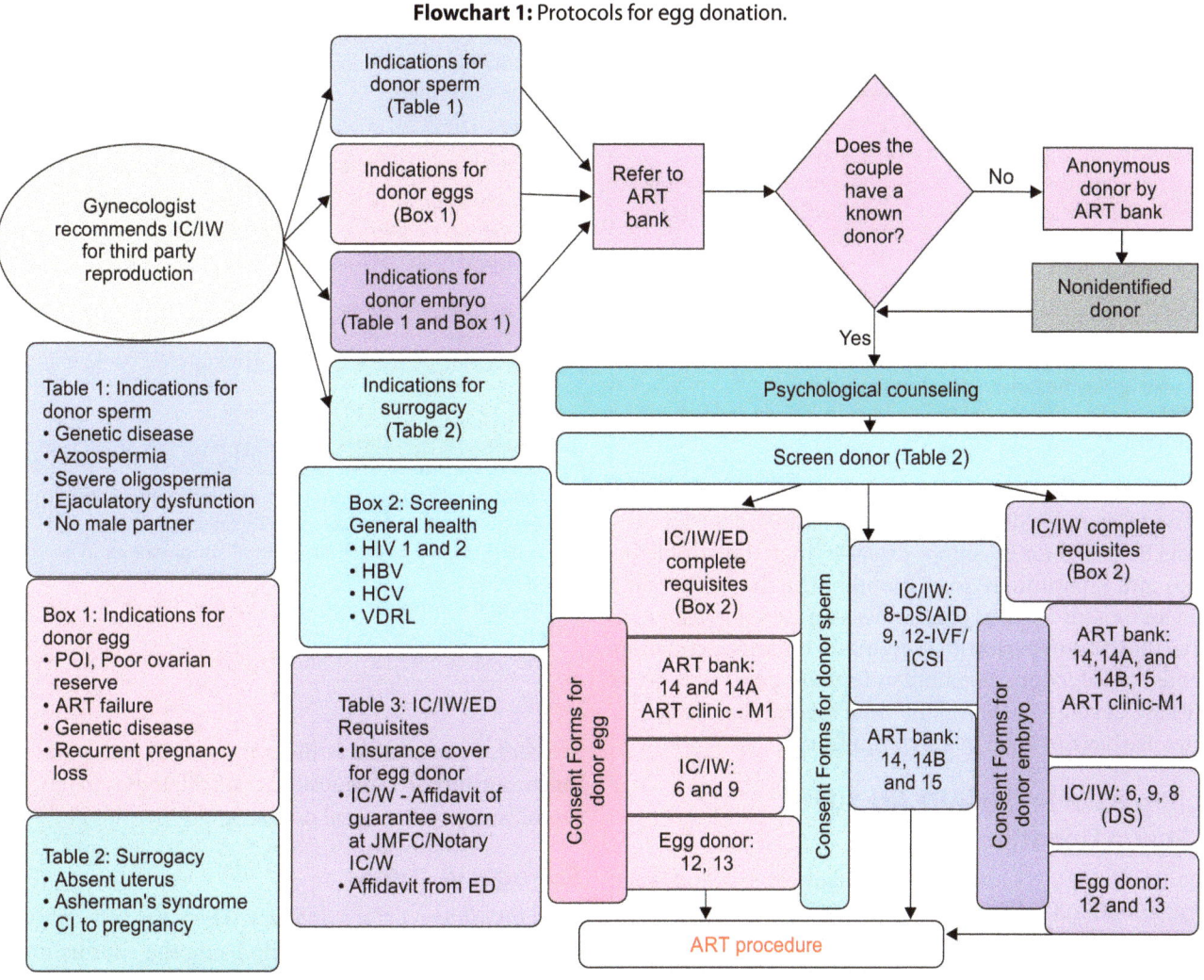

Flowchart 1: Protocols for egg donation.

(AID: artificial insemination of donor sperm; ART: assisted reproductive technology; CI: confidence interval; DS: donor sperm; ED: egg donation; HBV: hepatitis B virus; HCV: hepatitis C virus; HIV: human immunodeficiency virus; IC/W: intended or commissioning couple/woman; ICSI: intracytoplasmic sperm injection; IVF: in vitro fertilization; JMFC: judicial magistrate of first class; POI: premature ovarian insufficiency; VDRL: venereal disease research laboratory)

TABLE 6: Complications specific to egg donation in donors and recipients.

	Donor	Recipient[4]
Short-term	• Ovarian hyperstimulation syndrome (OHSS) • Ovarian torsion • Corpus luteal cyst rupture • Oocyte retrieval related-hemorrhage, injury to internal organs, sepsis, risks due to anesthesia	• Multiple gestation • Preterm birth • Hypertensive disorders • Small for gestation baby • Risk of transmission of infection from donor (remote)
Long-term	• Increased risk of breast, ovarian, and uterine cancers (In women with multiple egg donation cycles) • Risk of infertility • Premature ovarian insufficiency • Psychological disturbance	• Psychological disturbance • Conflicts and dilemmas regarding revealing to the child that he/she was donor-conceived

When electively disclosed by parents, young children showed curiosity and wished to know more about their genetic parent. Adolescents as well showed similar desire more so to know more about themselves. This is in line with adopted children who tend to seek more information about their origin. However, when they learnt later in life, particularly those who found out by accident or under situations like divorce of parents, showed more negative responses including anger toward their social parents and feelings of betrayal and distrust.[5]

SPERM DONATION

Artificial insemination using donor sperms was the first form of TPR which slowly paved way for more advanced methods with the advent of IVF.[15]

The indications for use of donor sperms in either intrauterine insemination (IUI) or as a part of advanced ARTs are shown in **Table 7**.

TABLE 7: Indications for donor sperms.	
Primary defect in sperm quality/quantity	*Normal sperm production*
• Nonobstructive azoospermia • Severe oligozoospermia • Severe teratospermia • Medical and/or surgical procedures (cancer treatments) • Failure to fertilize eggs with intracytoplasmic sperm injection (ICSI)	• Obstructive azoospermia [congenital bilateral absence of vas deference (CBAVD), post vasectomy] • Genetic diseases or anomalies in the male partner • Ejaculatory dysfunction
Other indications: • Severe Rh isoimmunization in female partner • Absence of a male partner (single woman, lesbian couple) • CBAVD	

TABLE 8: Indian assisted reproductive technology (ART) Act mandates for sperm donation.	
The age of the man	21–55 years
Identity	Aadhar card
How many times he can donate	Only once in lifetime
How many could receive gametes from a donor	Only one intended couple/woman
Accessibility to information	ART banks, national registry In exceptional cases to parents/child on a legal order
Source	Through ART banks only

> **BOX 5:** Indications for embryo donation.
> - Menopausal and perimenopausal women with subfertile partner
> - Recurrent in vitro fertilization (IVF) failures
> - Carriers of genetic or chromosomal abnormalities in any/both partners
> - Financial constraints in couple with poor prognosis with self-gametes
> - Untreatable infertility/severe abnormalities in both partners

The FDA and ASRM guidelines recommend that sperm donors be tested for infectious diseases, then the sample be frozen and quarantined for 6 months. The donor is tested again for those infections before releasing the sample for use, so that the window period for covering for the long incubation periods for infections like human immunodeficiency virus (HIV) are covered. However, in India quarantine of sperms before use has not been made compulsory.

Highlights of Indian ART Act 2021 on Sperm Donation

Indian ART Act 2021 mandates the following guidelines for sperm donation **(Table 8)**.

The steps involved in sperm donation are as shown in **Flowchart 1**

■ EMBRYO DONATION

This form of reproduction is chosen by the couple when there are significant compromises in both the partners and the female partner has a normal uterine cavity and endometrium.

Indications

The indications for embryo donation are shown in **Box 5**.

Shifting of Gametes/Embryos

The Assisted Reproductive Technology (Regulation) Act, 2021 mandates that the individuals or couples wishing to transfer their eggs, sperms or embryos from one IVF clinic to another or from India to abroad should follow the protocols as specified in Forms 16 to 20 and could use them only for personal use. The clinics holding the gametes or sperms and the clinics receiving the same shall follow the protocol as per Forms 21 to 24.

■ SURROGACY

In surrogate motherhood, the IC/W take the help of another woman who carries their baby in her uterus till term and delivery. Perhaps this is the type of TPR which has raised maximum number of questions and dilemmas in the ethical, moral, and psychological domains.[16]

Surrogacy—Types

Traditional or partial surrogacy: The surrogate contributes her own eggs and uterus while using the sperms from the male partner of the intended couple which could be done via either IUI or IVF. *It is not permitted in India.*

Gestational or full surrogacy: In gestational surrogacy, the woman is not genetically related to the child and carries the embryo of the intended couple and delivers, legally handing over the baby to the intended or commissioning couple or woman.

Commercial surrogacy: The surrogate receives financial compensation for the service provided. *It is not permitted in India.*

Altruistic surrogacy: The surrogate wishes to carry the embryos of intending parents/woman without any expectation in return. She would mostly be a woman known to the couple like a sister or friend.

Indications for Surrogacy

The various indications are as shown in the **Box 6**.

Eligibility to Become a Surrogate

Known gestational surrogates can be relatives or friends of the intended parents who volunteer to carry a pregnancy for them.

BOX 6: Indications for surrogacy.

Women without a uterus
- Absent [Mullerian agenesis—Mayer-Rokitansky-Küster-Hauser (MRKH) syndrome]
- Absence of a uterus secondary to surgery [fibroids, cancer, severe postpartum hemorrhage (PPH), uterine rupture, etc.]

Women with uterus
- Diseased endometrium (severe Asherman syndrome, endometrial tuberculosis)
- Diseased uterus (severe adenomyosis, multiple myomectomies, etc.)
- Recurrent implantation failure in in vitro fertilization (IVF)
- Recurrent thin endometrium in IVF
- Recurrent miscarriage/adverse obstetric outcomes such as abruption and severe preeclampsia
- Women with a medical contraindication to pregnancy (Eisenmenger syndrome, chronic kidney disease, etc.)

TABLE 9: Eligibility criteria for a surrogate according to Indian Assisted Reproductive Technology (ART) Act 2021.

Age	21–35 years
Married status	An ever-married woman
Medial/psychological status	Healthy and fit as determined by the ART clinic/bank
Parity/children	She should have at least one living child
Intention	Altruistic
How many times	Only once in her lifetime
How many embryo transfers per couple	Maximum of three embryo transfers

Alternatively, surrogates could be sought from an ART bank who would advertise to get interested surrogates to be registered whose identity would be kept confidential.

The eligibility criteria to become a surrogate are shown in **Table 9**.

India in 2021, categorically banned commercial surrogacy and allowed only altruistic interaction between the IC/W and surrogate.

Surrogacy Program—Steps

The steps involved in executing a surrogacy program are shown in **Flowchart 2**.

Requirements for Altruistic Surrogacy in India

As per the Surrogacy Act, 2021 – These are additional requirements other than those shown in **Flowchart 2**.
- The Couple undergoing Surrogacy must have both gametes from the intending couple & donor gametes are not allowed.
- A single woman (widow/divorcee) undergoing Surrogacy must use her own eggs and donor sperms to avail surrogacy procedure.

Lesbian motherhood—reception of partner's oocytes[6]: Different countries have different policies when it comes to surrogacy and in general, TPR. Hence, they have varying permissions in circumstances such as homosexual couple, unmarried couple, and single men wishing to have their own genetically related children.

Recently, a technique of assisted reproduction was developed to assist lesbian women to share biological motherhood of their offspring—the *ROPA* method (in Spanish, *Recepción de Ovocitos de Pareja*; in English reception of partner's oocytes), also known as *lesbian shared motherhood*. One partner provides the oocytes (genetic mother) and the other receives the embryo and carries pregnancy (gestational mother). Extending it further, when both women wish to carry pregnancy, ROPA could be *reciprocal* when both partners play both the roles simultaneously and *reverse* when they switch their roles consequently.

Posthumous reproduction: Posthumous reproduction is defined as birth of a child after death of one of the biological parents. Posthumous gamete procurement is harvesting sperms or eggs from a recently deceased person.

The causes of death would mostly be involving motorcycle accidents, sudden cardiac arrest, cerebrovascular accidents, or cancer. The development of cryopreservation made posthumous is possible.

Cryopreserved gametes/embryos: Indian law gives prominence to the procreative liberty of the gamete-providers, even following the death of one of them.

The ART Act 2021 permits posthumous use of cryopreserved sperms or embryos by the surviving spouse, provided the deceased has given written consent prior to their death.

In the case of minors, it gives provision for the gametes to be handed over to the parent or legal guardian in case of the death as per the previous written consent.

Posthumous sperm or egg retrieval[7,8]: Many studies have shown that sperm quality is favorable when retrieved within 24 hours of death but could be performed within 72 hours. The methods include vasal or epididymal irrigation and excisional procedures after death and electroejaculation could be used in brain-dead men.

In women ovarian stimulation with egg retrieval or ovarian tissue cryopreservation could be performed.

Posthumous gamete retrieval cannot be done on the request of parents or relatives in the absence of a *will* or *advanced directive* by the deceased.

Alternatives to TPR: For couples/women not wishing to go for TPR, the conventional alternatives are either adoption or childfree life. However, there are some newer methods to help such couples to have genetically related children. Since, there is a long waiting list at the ART banks as

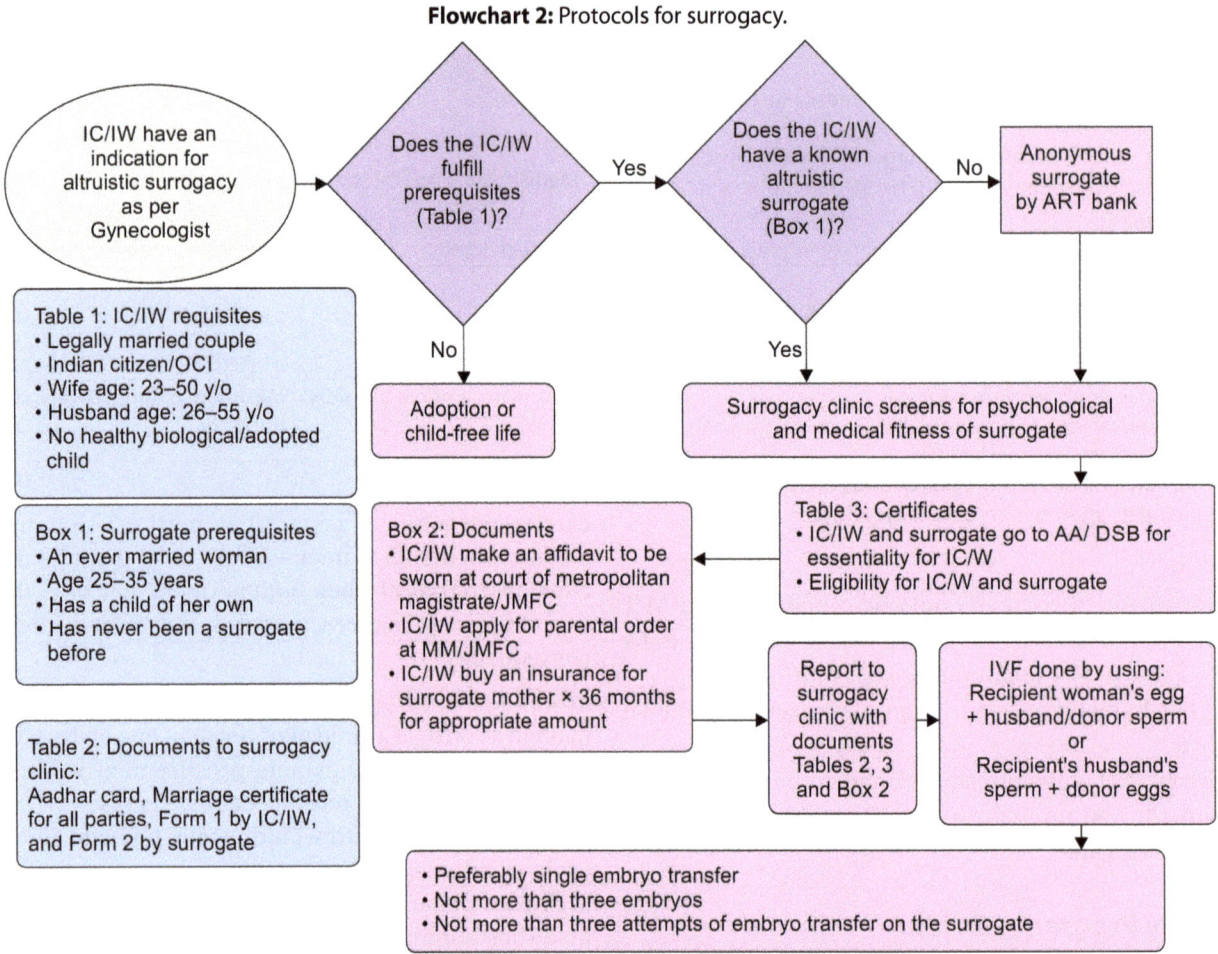

Flowchart 2: Protocols for surrogacy.

(AA: appropriate authority; DSB: district surrogacy board; IC/W: intended or commissioning couple/woman; JMFC: judicial magistrate of first class; MM: metropolitan magistrate; OCI: overseas citizen of India; y/o: years old)

TABLE 10: Newer alternatives to third party reproduction.	
Procedure	**Alternative to**
In vitro gametes through stem cells	Donor egg/sperm
Preimplantation genetic testing	Donor egg/sperm
Ovarian transplantation	Donor egg
Uterine transplantation	Surrogacy
Autologous bone marrow-derived stem cell therapy (BMSC)	Surrogacy

many couples are not able to procure their own or known third party. The newer developments which could offer hope in reducing the need for a third party are listed in **Table 10**.

ADOPTION

Though scientific advances have bypassed many causes of infertility leading to successful conception, there remain many a causes such as nonobstructive azoospermia and absent uterus where there is no solution other than TPR. Also, the treatment may not be in the reach of the affected or the couples might not opt for such services.

The clinician needs to assess the situation with sensitivity and empathy. Notably, during the training period, the fertility specialist lacks much exposure to address the needs of a couple whose only option seems to adopt a child. In such scenarios, it is vital to explore this option with them with transparency and to guide them to the right resources.

In India, the process of adoption is centralized. The Ministry of Women and Child Development oversees this process through Central Adoption Resource Authority (CARA).[9] This statutory body functions as the nodal body for adoption of Indian children and is mandated to monitor and regulate in-country and intercountry adoptions. CARA is designated as the central authority to deal with intercountry adoptions in accordance with the provisions of the Hague Convention on Intercountry Adoption, 1993, ratified by Government of India in 2003.

Central Adoption Resource Authority primarily deals with adoption of orphan, abandoned, and surrendered children through its associated/recognized adoption agencies. The adoption process is governed by rules as described in Adoption Regulations 2022.[10]

CHILDFREE LIFE

Childlessness, also called being childfree, describes the decision not to have children. A person or couple could be childfree by choice or by chance. It could be voluntary when the person chooses not to reproduce for various personal, cultural, or religious reasons. In infertile couples, there is a portion where the treatment has not been successful, or they would not utilize the entire spectrum of fertility treatments as a matter of personal choice or due to financial constraints. Such couples would need additional support and access to resources to make them accept the situation gracefully and lead a productive and fulfilling life. The fertility specialist providing care to such couples has an opportunity to guide them to appropriate support groups to facilitate this process.[11,12]

What Conflicts Could Arise?

Here are some examples:
- A sperm donor may decide later that he wants to parent the child as his own.
- An egg donor may lie about how many times she has donated in the past.
- A gestational carrier may purposefully lie or not disclose relevant medical information that may be important to the health of the pregnancy.
- The intended parents may decide that they plan to divorce prior to the birth of their child when the surrogate is carrying their child and the surrogate wants to deliver the child to a couple with stable marriage.
- The ART bank might not have procured the egg donor the required insurance.
- Not all advocates will be familiar with legal requirements of these ART services and may unknowingly leave out important parts of a TPR contract.
- The clinician in charge may get emotionally involved and bypass legal requirements like providing ART services to a couple without eligibility.

How to Avoid Conflicts?

- *Be informed:*
  - The head of the fertility center providing services should be aware of the legal requirements and make sure every service provider follows them.
  - Everyone involved (physician, intended parents, donors, gestational carriers, agencies, and attorneys) must read the consent forms and contracts in detail.
- *Be transparent:* Everyone involved should be honest and forthcoming about their qualification status and expectations surrounding the arrangement.
- *Express concerns:* If there are any doubts or concerns, it is important to bring these up early in the process.
- *Counsel, consent, and document:* It is vital to provide all the required information to all parties involved through a qualified counselor, take informed consent and to document if there are any additional issues addressed.
- *Follow a protocol:* Having a protocol based on the national guidelines and legal requirements helps not to miss vital steps. A flowchart in the clinic could help the staff involved in this process.
- *Follow the law:* The clinician needs to be empathetic but not emotionally involved while providing care.
- *Use professionals:* It is important that the agency or advocate being used has adequate experience to draft the agreement according to the existing legal requirements.
- *Take a second opinion:* Whenever confronted with a complex scenario, it is important to seek a second opinion from a colleague or an expert in this field and document the same.

Key Learning Points

- Third party reproduction opens vast possibilities for infertile couples. However, as with any situation involving more than one person, conflicts and disputes can arise. The clinician who bridges both the sides should be aware of the consequences of this emotionally charged arrangement.
- So, it is helpful to know what type of conflicts could arise and how to avoid them. ASRM guideline has outlined such good practice tips.[11]

CONCLUSION

Third Party Reproduction has led to a wide spectrum of reproductive choices. The clinician catering to the needs of infertile individuals should cultivate deep empathy to address their special requirements and should be well versed in the laws of the land governing these services. Apart from assisting childless individuals, the all-round wellbeing of gamete donors, surrogates, and the children born as a result remains the core objective of this distinctive category of services.

ACKNOWLEDGMENT

I want to thank to Advocate (Dr) Hitesh Bhatt, MBBS, MD, PGDMLS, LLB for reviewing the legal protocols.

REFERENCES

1. ASRM Information Bulletin. (2006). Third-Party Reproduction. [online] Available from https://www.asrm.org/topics/topics-index/third-party-reproduction/#:~:text=The%20phrase%20%E2%80%9Cthird%2Dparty%20reproduction,intended%20recipient)%20to%20become%20parents [Last accessed December, 2022].
2. Practice Committee of the American Society for Reproductive Medicine and the Practice Committee for the Society for Assisted Reproductive Technology. Guidance regarding gamete and embryo donation. Fertil Steril. 2021; 115(6):1395-410.

3. Practice Committee of American Society For Reproductive Medicine. Increased maternal cardiovascular mortality associated with pregnancy in women with Turner syndrome. Fertil Steril. 2012;97(2):282-4.
4. Jeve YB, Potdar N, Opoku A, Khare M. Donor oocyte conception and pregnancy complications: a systematic review and meta-analysis. BJOG. 2016;123(9):1471-80.
5. Golombok S, Readings J, Blake L, Casey P, Mellish L, Marks A, et al. Children Conceived by Gamete Donation: Psychological Adjustment and Mother-child Relationships at Age 7. J Fam Psychol. 2011;25(2):230-9.
6. Brandão P, de Pinho A, Ceschin N, Sousa-Santos R, Reis-Soares S, Bellver J. ROPA—Lesbian shared in vitro fertilization—Ethical aspects. Eur J Obstet Gynecol Reprod Biol. 2022;272:230-3.
7. Simana S. Creating life after death: should posthumous reproduction be legally permissible without the deceased's prior consent? J Law Biosci. 2018;5(2):329-54.
8. Ahluwalia U, Arora M. Posthumous Reproduction and Its Legal Perspective. Int J Infertil. Fetal Med. 2011;2(1):9-14.
9. Central Adoption Resource Authority—Ministry of Women & Child Development, Government of India. [online] Available from https://cara.nic.in/[Last accessed December, 2022].
10. The Juvenile Justice (Care and Protection of Children) Amendment Act, 2021 stands enforced from 1st September 2022. [online] Available from https://cara.nic.in/PDF/adoption_regulations_2022_2709.PDF [Last accessed December, 2022].
11. Chehreh R, Ozgoli G, Abolmaali K, Nasiri M, Karamelahi Z. Child-Free Lifestyle and the Need for Parenthood and Relationship with Marital Satisfaction among Infertile Couples. Iran J Psychiatry. 2021;16(3):243-9.
12. Resources. The NotMom. Retrieved December 21, 2022, from https://www.thenotmom.com/resources.
13. Reproductivefacts. www.Reproductivefacts. Retrieved December 21, 2022, from https://www.reproductivefacts.org.
14. Patel NH, Esteves SC. Advances in assisted teproductive technology. Jaypee Publishers; 2020.
15. Goldfarb JM (Ed). Third Party Reproduction: a comprehensive guide, 1st edition. Netherlands: Springer New York; 2014.
16. Ryan-Flood R, Payne JG (Eds). Transnationalising Reproduction: Third Party Conception in a Globalised World. (Routledge Studies in the Sociology of Health and Illness), 1st edition. United Kingdom: Taylor & Francis; 2018.

CHAPTER 35

PGT: When and Where to Offer

Abha Majumdar, Bhawani Shekhar

INTRODUCTION

Preimplantation genetic testing (PGT) is a technique that involves testing of in vitro fertilized embryos to identify monogenic disorders, structural chromosomal rearrangements, or aneuploidy.[1]

Since its advent in 1990s, scope of PGT has been expanding. Clinicians should be familiar with its indications, its benefits, and limitations.

TYPES OF PREIMPLANTATION GENETIC TESTING

Preimplantation genetic testing-M for monogenic disorders, PGT-SR for structural rearrangements (both previously known as preimplantation genetic diagnosis or PGD), and PGT-A for aneuploidy (previously known as preimplantation genetic screening or PGS).[2]

Preimplantation genetic testing-M and PGT-SR are mainly indicated in fertile couples carrying an inheritable genetic defect whereas PGT-A is mostly offered to infertile couples undergoing in vitro fertilization (IVF).

Preimplantation Genetic Testing-Monogenic Disorders

- *Single gene disorders*: PGT-M involves testing of single gene disorders for which causative genetic mutation is known. These gene mutations could be recessive or dominant. If two copies of the abnormal gene are required to cause disease, it is an autosomal recessive disorder, but if only one abnormal gene is needed to produce a disease, it is a dominant hereditary condition. Frequent indications for PGT-M include the following:[3]
  - *Autosomal recessive* conditions where both parents are carriers. Hence, the risk of genetic disorder would be in 25% of offspring, 25% would be completely free from the disorder, and the remaining 50% would be carriers such as in cystic fibrosis and hereditary hemoglobinopathies.
  - *Autosomal dominant* conditions where the genetic condition would be transmitted in 50% of offspring and the other 50% would be free of the disease. Examples include Marfan syndrome, osteogenesis imperfecta, neurofibromatosis, and Huntington's disease.
  - *X-linked recessive* conditions mainly manifest as a disease only in males and females are carriers. Examples of X-linked recessive diseases are Duchenne's and Becker's muscular dystrophy, hemophilia, and red/green color blindness.

    Risk calculation: X chromosome from a male is transmitted to daughters, and the Y chromosome is transmitted to sons. If an affected male has children with a healthy wife, none of his male offspring's will be affected; however, all his female offspring will be carriers. If a carrier female has children with a healthy male, there is 50% chance of male offspring being affected, and 50% chance of female offspring being a carrier.[4]
  - *X-linked dominant* inheritance affects both males and females to cause the disease. Affected males can transmit the defective gene to female offspring but not to male offspring. Affected females can transmit the defective gene to 50% of her male offspring and 50% of her female offspring. Examples of X-linked dominant inheritance are Fragile X syndrome, hypophosphatemic rickets, incontinentia pigmenti, and Alport syndrome.
- *Mitochondrial disorders:* Mitochondria contain their own deoxyribonucleic acid (DNA) which consists of 37 genes and is separate from the genes of the cell nucleus. In normal women, all mitochondrial DNA (mt-DNA) copies are identical or homoplasmic. Affected patients usually have mixed (heteroplasmic) mitochondrial genes of mutated and normal ones. There is a threshold level of mutation of mt-DNA that causes mt-DNA disease (60–90%).[5] PGT-M for mitochondrial disorders allows selection of embryos with a pathogenic mt-DNA load below threshold of clinical expression. Mitochondrial

disorders can affect both males and females, but are only passed on by females because all mitochondria in child come from the mother and can appear in every generation. Examples of such diseases are Leber's hereditary optic neuropathy, and Kearns–Sayre syndrome.[6]

- *Human leukocyte antigen (HLA) typing:* Apart from testing for single gene disorders another special indication for PGT-M is HLA typing which is not to prevent disease in the child who is being tested but to treat an affected sibling already born with a hematopoietic disorder. PGT-M is used to select an embryo that is HLA matched with an affected sibling. Hematopoietic stem cells from the bone marrow of this HLA-matched progeny can be used for bone marrow transplantation in the affected sibling.

Preimplantation Genetic Testing-Structural Rearrangements

The PGT-SR involves analyzing the chromosomal constitution of embryos derived from couples carrying a structural chromosomal rearrangement, most commonly a balanced translocation. These couples have a 60% risk of having a progeny with an unbalanced translocation which can lead to failure to achieve a pregnancy, pregnancy loss, or abnormal live birth. In couples with recurrent implantation failure (RIF), recurrent pregnancy loss (RPL), or abnormal progeny, PGT-SR is indicated if either partner carries a balanced translocation (reciprocal or Robertsonian) or rarely certain other chromosomal rearrangements.[7]

- *Reciprocal translocation:* Fragments of two non-homologous chromosomes interchange positions.
- *Robertsonian translocation:* It results due to exchange of arms between two nonhomologous acrocentric chromosomes (chromosomes 13, 14, 15, 21, and 22). The long arms of two nonhomologous acrocentric chromosomes fuse to form one chromosome and the chromosome formed by fusion of two short arms is lost. It can lead to monosomy, trisomy such as trisomy 13 (Patau syndrome), trisomy 21 (Downs syndrome), or uniparental disomy in the progeny.[8,9]
- *Deletion/duplication:* A segment of chromosome is deleted or duplicated.
- *Inversion:* Segment of a chromosome is inverted and reinserted back into the same chromosome.

Most commonly next-generation sequencing technology is used to count chromosome fragments and detect large chromosomal imbalances in embryos. Additional genetic test methods may be necessary for cases involving small chromosomal imbalances that are difficult to diagnose with the usual technologies. Therefore, it is pertinent for the IVF team to ensure that the translocation has been identified by the genetic laboratory, as they need to develop probes to identify the translocated segment of chromosome. All laboratories may not be able to identify smaller segments of lost or added pieces of chromosome.

Preimplantation Genetic Testing-Aneuploidy

The PGT-A involves analysis of chromosome copy number of embryos to rule out aneuploidy. Traditionally, embryo selection was only based on morphological grading. PGT-A is used to detect embryo aneuploidy, thus ensuring euploid embryo transfer. Aim of PGT-A is to increase live birth rates, decrease early pregnancy loss rates, and also reduce time to pregnancy.

After extensively reviewing the evidence, the American Society for Reproductive Medicine (ASRM) published a practice guideline in 2018 concluding that there is insufficient evidence to recommend the routine use of PGT-A in all IVF patients. However, a subset of patients may benefit from PGT-A. These include advanced maternal age (AMA), RIF, RPL, severe male factor (SMF), or centers/patients opting for elective single embryo transfer (eSET).[10]

Advanced Maternal Age

A randomized controlled trial (RCT) including women between 25 and 40 years of age found that PGT-A did not improve pregnancy outcomes among all women. However, in the subgroup of age >35 years there was a significant improvement in pregnancy outcomes.[11] Another RCT found that women between 38 and 41 years of age had significantly higher live birth rates, lower miscarriage rates, and a shorter time to pregnancy with PGT-A.[12]

Recurrent Implantation Failure

There is data that suggests that patients with RIF have higher incidence of chromosomal abnormalities, particularly aneuploidy. However, currently there is insufficient evidence to recommend for or against PGT-A in RIF.[13]

Recurrent Pregnancy Loss

Fair number of first trimester pregnancy losses may be attributed due to aneuploidy, providing plausibility for PGT-A. However, The European Society of Human Reproduction and Embryology (ESHRE) guideline group 2018 states that couples with a history of RPL have a high chance of successfully conceiving naturally and that PGT-A for RPL without a genetic cause is not recommended.[14]

Severe Male Factor

Limited evidence suggests that patients with severe oligozoospermia have a higher incidence of sex chromosomal aneuploidy and may choose to pursue PGT-A.[15]

Elective Single Embryo Transfer (eSET)

The PGT-A may be beneficial in increasing utility of eSET. A 2015 study showed a significant improvement in live birth rate per embryo transfer cycle with eSET along with PGT-A.[16]

PATIENT SELECTION AND COUNSELING

The PGT-A is offered to couples mainly by IVF specialists in cases with high risk of embryo aneuploidy. However, couples requiring PGT-M and PGT-SR are encountered by all obstetricians and gynecologists in their practice. Hence, clinicians should be well versed with all aspects of patient selection for PGT to adequately counsel the patients.

- PGT-M or SR should be applied only when genetic diagnosis is technically possible and there is a high likelihood regarding its reliability. To ensure this, pre-PGT workup is essential in cases of PGT-M and PGT-SR by the genetic laboratory conducting the test.
- Cost involved should be discussed. Cost depends on type of PGT being performed, number of embryos tested and laboratory performing the test. This cost is in addition to the cost of IVF cycles.
- Feasibility of procedure should be discussed in patients with low ovarian reserve. Probability of finding genetically normal embryos increases with number of biopsied embryos. Consecutive IVF cycles or dual stimulation with pooling of embryos can be considered in these couples.
- If there are financial constraints or low ovarian reserve, option of natural conception with prenatal diagnostic testing (chorionic villus sampling/amniocentesis) can be offered to fertile couples instead of PGT-M or SR. However, the procedure associated risk of an added miscarriage (1–2%) may increase the overall risk of abortion in subsequent pregnancy (24–40%) even in the absence of a genetic abnormality in the embryo.[17]
- PGT should not be considered if the woman has serious health concerns due to a genetic disorder for which PGT is desired, as it could lead to medical complications during ovarian stimulation, oocyte retrieval, pregnancy or medical risks at birth. Examples of such situations are cystic fibrosis, sickle cell anemia, and Huntington's disease which could worsen during the above procedures.
- Patient concerns regarding effect of embryo biopsy should be addressed of which most important are the following:
  - *Embryo damage:* Trophectoderm (blastocyst stage biopsy) has very little impact on embryo viability compared to cleavage-stage biopsy. Even though more cells (5–10) are removed in trophectoderm biopsy, it constitutes a very small percentage of embryo mass and these cells do not contribute to formation of fetus. Conversely, cleavage-stage biopsy occurs at a time when cell lineage has not been established and the cell removed could potentially impact embryo and fetal development.[18]
  - *Pregnancy outcomes:* Recent meta-analysis of 15 studies by Zheng et al. showed that PGT pregnancies may be associated with increased risk of low birth weight (LBW), preterm delivery (PTD), and hypertensive disorders of pregnancy (HDP) compared with spontaneously conceived pregnancies. The overall obstetric and neonatal outcomes of PGT pregnancies are comparable with those of IVF/intracytoplasmic sperm injection (ICSI) pregnancies, although PGT pregnancies were associated with a higher risk of HDP.[19]
- Possibility of a misdiagnosis due to false negative or false positive results owing to mosaicism should be explained. Decision regarding transfer of mosaic embryos should also be discussed.[20]

MOSAICISM

- Mosaicism is the presence of two or more cell lines with different sets of chromosome in an embryo. It occurs due to errors in the mitotic cell divisions and various other events which occur during embryo development.
- Incidence of mosaicism appears to be less at the blastocyst stage, possibly because some chromosome errors may be associated with developmental arrest and hence, such embryos do not reach blastocyst stage. This is one of the reasons that most IVF laboratories now culture embryos to the blastocyst stage to select competent embryos for biopsy.
- Incidence of mosaicism in clinical testing of trophectoderm is between 3 and 20% depending upon the type of testing platform used.
- For reporting embryo results, the suggested cut-off point for definition of mosaicism is >20% abnormal cells, so levels <20% should be considered euploid, >80% should be considered aneuploid, and the ones between 20 and 80% should be considered as mosaic.[21]
- Mosaic embryo transfer may be considered in the hope that either the mosaic diagnosis is due to an analytical error, or a mosaic embryo may "self-correct", not be clinically impacted by the presence of some abnormal cells, or fail to implant, or miscarry through natural means.
- The Preimplantation Genetics Diagnosis International Society (PGDIS) position on transfer of mosaic embryos:[22]
  - Embryos showing mosaic euploid/monosomy are preferable to euploid/trisomy, because monosomic embryos (except 45X) are not viable.
  - If a decision is made to transfer mosaic embryos with single chromosome trisomy, one can prioritize selection based on the level of mosaicism and the specific chromosome involved
    - The preferable transfer category consists of mosaic embryos with trisomy for chromosomes 1, 3, 4, 5, 6, 8, 9, 10, 11, 12, 17, 19, 20, 22, X, Y. All these trisomies are nonviable

TABLE 1: Pros and cons of PGT-A.

Pros	Cons
• In patients with advanced age >35 years, it reduces time and number of embryo transfers required to attain a live birth • It reduces miscarriage rates due to high risk of aneuploidy in advanced age patients • It promotes single embryo transfer thus reduces risks associated with multiple gestation • It helps clinician to determine which embryos to transfer on priority • It helps to identify and discard aneuploid embryos. This could reduce the burden of excess cryopreserved embryos	• Does not increase the chance of live birth among women of all age groups • Expensive procedure, in addition to IVF costs • Need for increased resources and hours of labor for the embryology team for each biopsy case • Due to technical challenges, there is a small risk that test results may not reflect true embryo status • Some embryos have a mixture of normal and abnormal cells (mosaicism). This can result in false-positive or false-negative PGT-A result • Sometimes no embryo may be suitable for biopsy or transfer

(IVF: in vitro fertilization; PGT-A: preimplantation genetic testing-aneuploidy)

- Embryos mosaic for trisomies 14 and 15 are of lesser priority as they are associated with uniparental disomy
- Embryos mosaic for trisomies 2, 7, and 16 are of lesser priority as they are associated with intrauterine growth retardation
- Embryos mosaic for trisomies 13, 18, and 21 are of least priority as they are capable of liveborn viability with various abnormalities

- Couples being offered PGT-A should be counseled regarding its pros and cons **(Table 1)**.

ROLE OF PRENATAL DIAGNOSTIC TESTING

Prenatal diagnostic testing in PGT-M or PGT-SR conceived pregnancies by chorionic villus sampling or amniocentesis should be offered to all patients for confirmation of the PGT result. In patients who have undergone PGT-A, noninvasive prenatal testing (NIPT) should be offered. Prenatal diagnostic testing is not recommended for pregnancies conceived after PGT-A unless abnormal findings on 11–14 weeks scan or NIPT indicates high aneuploidy risk. In PGT-A conceived pregnancies with mosaic embryo transfer, prenatal diagnostic testing is mandatory.[23]

THAW, BIOPSY, RECRYOPRESERVE, RETHAW, AND TRANSFER

Patients with previously cryopreserved unbiopsied embryos may want their embryos to be rebiopsied. Reasons for this could be previous miscarriages, disease discovery, or desire to utilize new technology. This would involve thawing embryos for biopsy and testing followed repeat cryopreservation, thawing, and transfer. A study found that while fresh biopsy is preferable, reproductive outcomes are not significantly compromised on surviving euploid embryos after a sequence of thaw, biopsy, revitrification, and rethawing.[24] Another study found that the embryo survival rate was lower after the second thawing (87.5% vs. 98.3% in first thaw). Therefore, many patients may benefit from this approach; however, there may be a reduction in the number of embryos available for transfer.[25]

NONINVASIVE PREIMPLANTATION GENETIC TESTING

To obtain embryonic genetic material for PGT analysis, a biopsy is required which needs the removal of one or more cells. This invasive procedure increases the cost of PGT and there are concerns that embryo viability could be compromised in some cases. The recent discovery of DNA within the blastocoele fluid (BF) of blastocysts and in spent embryo culture media (SCM) has led to the development of noninvasive PGT (niPGT). However, its efficiency has been limited by the technical complications associated with the low quantity and quality of the DNA obtained. Reported levels of concordance between SCM/BF samples and biopsied embryonic cells vary widely. In a recent study, trophectoderm biopsy sample showed no amplification failure and high genotype concordance rate (99.8%) whereas BF samples showed high amplification failure (72.6%) with low genotype concordance (13.3%) and SBM samples showed low amplification failure (10.3%) and a moderate genotype accordance rate of 59.5%. The observed poor accuracy of niPGT (SCM/BF samples) was possibly due to contamination from maternal DNA, a major risk factor for genetic misdiagnosis. Therefore, it is necessary to further develop techniques to discriminate between embryonic and nonembryonic DNA.[26] Further research is needed to understand the mechanisms involved in the release of embryonic DNA and to determine the extent to which this material reflects the true genetic status of the embryo. Currently, the clinical potential of niPGT remains unknown.[27]

CONCLUSION

Preimplantation genetic testing (PGT) has attained significant relevance in current clinical practice. Clinicians should be well versed with its types, indications, advantages and limitations. Detailed counselling is of utmost importance when selecting a patient for PGT. Potential of new technology such as non invasive PGT needs to be explored further **(Table 2)**.

TABLE 2: Summary of types of PGT.

	PGT-A	PGT-M	PGT-SR
Genetic test	Detects aneuploidy	Detects single gene disorders	Detects unbalanced chromosomal rearrangements
Indication	IVF patients (particularly AMA, RIF, RPL, SMF, eSET)	Patients at high risk of having a child with single gene disorder	Patients with chromosomal rearrangements (particularly balanced translocations)
Aim	Reduce time to successful pregnancy	Reduce risk of transmitting a heritable genetic disorder to the progeny	Increase chances of successful pregnancy with a normal/balanced chromosomal constitution
Pre PGT work up by genetic lab	Not required	Extensive pre PGT work up (6–8 weeks) Includes blood samples for mutation analysis of couple and family members	Case review and approval (1–2 days)
Prenatal testing	NIPT	CVS/Amniocentesis	CVS/Amniocentesis

(AMA: advanced maternal age; eSET: elective single embryo transfer; IVF: in vitro fertilization; NIPT: noninvasive prenatal testing; PGT: preimplantation genetic testing; RIF: recurrent implantation failure; RPL: recurrent pregnancy loss; SMF: severe male factor)

Key Learning Points

- Clinical indication and utility for PGT-M and PGT-SR is firmly established. PGT-M is indicated in couples at an increased risk of having a child with a specific single gene disorder. PGT-SR is indicated in couples with a bad obstetric history carrying heritable chromosomal rearrangements, particularly balanced translocations.
- Role of PGT-A in clinical practice remains to be determined. However, a subset of patients, particularly those with AMA of >35 years, has been found to benefit by reducing the number of embryo transfers and time to live birth.
- In couples where PGT-M or PGT-SR are indicated, a pre-PGT workup by the genetic laboratory is essential to determine feasibility of the procedure.
- Financial counseling is a must in these patients, as it is an expensive procedure in addition to the cost of IVF.
- In patients with low ovarian reserve need for multiple IVF cycles for pooling embryos or option of natural conception with prenatal testing should be discussed.
- Small risk of false-positive or false-negative results owing to mosaicism should be explained to patients.
- Prenatal diagnostic testing (chorionic villus sampling/amniocentesis) should be done for confirmation of the PGT-M or PGT-SR result. In patients who have undergone PGT-A, NIPT is recommended.

REFERENCES

1. De Rycke M, Berckmoes V, De Vos A, Van De Voorde S, Verdyck P, Verpoest W, et al. Preimplantation genetic testing: clinical experience of preimplantation genetic testing. Reproduction. 2020;160(5):A45-58.
2. Siermann M, Claesen Z, Pasquier L, Raivio T, Tšuiko O, Vermeesch JR, et al. A systematic review of the views of healthcare professionals on the scope of preimplantation genetic testing 2022;13:1-11.
3. NIH. What are the different ways in which a genetic condition can be inherited? [online] Available from https://ghr.nlm.nih.gov/primer/inheritance/inheritance patterns. [Last accessed February, 2023].
4. Basta M, Pandya AM. Genetics, X linked inheritance. Treasure Island (FL): StatPearls Publishing; 2022.
5. Amato P, Tachibana M, Sparman M, Mitalipov S. Three-parent in vitro fertilization: gene replacement for the prevention of inherited mitochondrial diseases. Fertil Steril. 2014;101:31-5.
6. Genetic Alliance; The New York-Mid Atlantic Consortium for Genetic and Newborn screening services. Understanding Genetics: A New York Mid Atlantic Guide for Patients and Health professionals. Washington (DC): Genetic Alliance; 2009.
7. Scorio R, Tramontano I, Catt J. Preimplantation genetic diagnosis (PGD) and genetic testing for aneuploidy (PGT-A): status and future challenges. Gynecol Endocrinol. 2020;36:6-11.
8. Benn P. Uniparental disomy: Origin, frequency, and clinical significance. Prenat Diagn. 2021;41;564-572.
9. Kleigman RM. Cytogenetics. In: Kleigman RM (Ed). Nelson Textbook of Pediatrics, 21st edition. Philadelphia: Elsevier; 2020.
10. Practice Committees of the American Society for Reproductive Medicine and the Society for Assisted Reproductive technology. The use of preimplantation genetic testing for aneuploidy (PGT-A): a committee opinion. Fertil Steril. 2018;109:429-36.
11. Munne A, Kaplan B, Frattarelli J, Child T, Nakhuda G, Shamma F, et al. Preimplantation genetic testing for aneuploidy versus morphology as selection criteria for single frozen-thawed embryo transfer in good-prognosis patients: a multicenter randomized clinical trial. Fertil Steril. 2019;112:1071-9.
12. Rubio C, Bellver J, Rodrigo L, Castillon G, Guillen A, Vidal C, et al. In vitro fertilization with preimplantation genetic diagnosis for aneuploidies in advanced maternal age: a randomized, controlled study. Fertil Steril. 2017;107:1122-9.
13. Shaulov T, Sierra S, Sylvestre C. Recurrent implantation failure in IVF: A Canadian Fertility and Andrology Society Clinical Practice Guideline. Reprod Biomed Online. 2020;41:819-33.
14. Atik R, Christiansen B, Elson J, Kolte A, Lewis S, Middeldrop S, et al. ESHRE guideline: recurrent pregnancy loss. Hum Reprod Open. 2018;2018:hoy004.
15. Coates A, Hesla JS, Hurliman A, Coate B, Holmes E, Matthews R, et al. Use of suboptimal sperm increases the risk of aneuploidy of the sex chromosomes in preimplantation blastocyst embryos. Fertil Steril. 2015;104:866-72.

16. Ubaldi FM, Capalbo A, Colamaria S, Ferrero S, Maggiulli R, Vajta G, et al. Reduction of multiple pregnancies in the advanced maternal age population after implementation of an elective single embryo transfer policy coupled with enhanced embryo selection: pre- and post-intervention study. Hum Reprod. 2015;30:2097-106.
17. Regan L, Braude PR, Trembath PL. Influence of past reproductive performance on risk of spontaneous abortion. BMJ. 1989;26:541-5.
18. De Vos A, Staessen C, De Rycke M, Verpoest W, Haentjens P, Devroey P, et al. Impact of cleavage-stage embryo biopsy in view of PGD on human blastocyst implantation. Hum Reprod. 2009;24:2988-96.
19. Zheng W, Yang C, Yang S, Sun S, Mu M, Rao M, et al. Obstetric and neonatal outcomes of pregnancies resulting from preimplantation genetic testing: a systematic review and meta-analysis. Hum Reprod Update. 2021;27:989-1012.
20. Carvalho F, Coonen E, Goossens V, Kokkali G. ESHRE PGT Consortium good practice recommendations for the organisation of PGT. Hum Reprod. 2020;2020: hoaa021.
21. Preimplantation genetic testing: ACOG Committee Opinion, Number 799. Obstet Gynecol. 2020;135:e133-7.
22. Preimplantation Genetic Diagnosis International Society. (2016). PGDIS position statement on chromosome mosaicism and preimplantation aneuploidy testing at the blastocyst stage. [online] Available from https://pgdis.org/docs/newsletter_071816.html. [Last accessed February, 2023].
23. Zwingerman R, Langlois S. Committee Opinion no. 406: Prenatal testing after IVF with Preimplantation Genetic testing for Aneuploidy. J Obstet Gynaecol Can. 2020;42:1437-43.
24. Taylor TH, Patrick JL, Gitlin SA, Michael Wilson J, Crain JL, Griffin DK. Outcomes of blastocysts biopsied and vitrified once versus those cryopreserved twice for euploid blastocyst transfer. Reprod Biomed Online. 2014;29:59-64.
25. Liu M, Su Y, Wang WH. Assessment of clinical application of preimplantation genetic screening on cryopreserved human blastocysts. Reprod Biol Endocrinol. 2016;14:16.
26. De Rycke M, Berckmoes V. Preimplantation genetic testing of monogenic disorders. Genes. 2020;11:871.
27. Leaver M, Wells D. Non-invasive preimplantation genetic testing (niPGT): the next revolution in reproductive genetics? Hum Reprod Update. 2020;26:16-42.

Viral Infections and IVF—Hepatitis B, Hepatitis C, and HIV

Sweta Gupta, Sapna Yadav, Rahul Kumar Gupta

INTRODUCTION

In vitro fertilization (IVF) and other assisted reproductive technologies are becoming more popular nowadays. Aside from very well-predictive factors such as the woman's age, the ovarian stimulation protocol, the number and quality of embryos to be transferred, and so on for the success of an infertility treatment, other factors such as contamination or viral infection transmission can all have an impact on the success rates of an IVF treatment.[1]

Hepatitis B, hepatitis C, and human immunodeficiency virus (HIV) are common viral infections that can be found chronically in subfertile patients. They can be found in both males and females. They present particular difficulties at many stages, including evaluation, treatment, pregnancy, and newborns. Current times have changed these critical situations, making it ethically and in terms of preventing infection, possible to increase the probability of having a healthy baby.

The chances of viral infection in reproductive technologies are still a widely discussed topic, particularly for the hepatitis C virus (HCV). It is a major cause of parenterally transmitted viral hepatitis. Besides that, it has been implicated in other modes of transmission, such as sexual and nosocomial infections. Infertility treatment in terms of dealing with widely spread viral infections has sparked debates about the potential risk of infection spreading to noninfected individuals and embryos. It is very apparent that the risk of viral transmission to noninfected individuals is via biological fluids, including blood, body fluids, semen, or follicular fluid. Only the strict use of standard operating procedures (SOPs), along with the proper initial detection and segregation of potentially harmful materials, can reduce or eliminate this risk. Techniques and protocols have been developed to enable andrologists and embryologists to protect patients from such risks, and they should be strictly followed at all the centers.[2]

Screening assists in identifying these infections and allowing us to take adequate infection control with successful treatment. According to the American Society for Reproductive Medicine (ASRM), patients with severe viral infections cannot be denied fertility services ethically if a center has the resources to provide care.[3] However, centers that lack such resources should assist in referring patients to a facility that has the protocols necessary to manage such patients. The recommendations are as follows:[4]

- Reducing viral load in a partner who is infected
- Reducing exposure and susceptibility in a partner who is not infected
- Promoting open discussions with patients about available research findings and risk-reduction strategies to lay the groundwork for explicit consent.

PRECONCEPTION COUNSELING

Couples infected with a sexually transmissible viral infection should be counseled extensively prior to conception about the risks of sexual and vertical transmission of their infections **(Table 1)**. In some cases, the viral infection can be effectively treated to eliminate the risk of transmission during intercourse, whereas in others, it cannot be effectively treated due to an infertility diagnosis such as low sperm counts, blocked fallopian tubes, and so on.[5] As a result, the only way for such patients to conceive is to use assisted reproductive technology (ART).

During infertility treatment, counseling and education about safe sexual practices should be provided and emphasized. If only the male partner is infected, the couple should be educated on the importance of using condoms and strictly following antiviral therapy throughout the fertility process.[6] Serial diagnostic testing of the uninfected partner is recommended throughout the treatment and pregnancy, as well as for both mother and newborn during the first year after birth.[7] Informed consent should be as clear and specific as possible; stating that, despite the use of specific risk-reduction strategies, the risk of transmission cannot be completely eliminated. Such patients should ideally receive comprehensive psychological, medical, and obstetrical care from a multidisciplinary medical team that includes infectious disease experts.[8]

TABLE 1: Risks of sexual and vertical transmission of viral infections.							
Infection	Infection type	Availability of vaccine	Horizontal sexual transmission	Horizontal transmission during assisted reproduction	Inhibition of vertical transmission by CS	Inhibition of vertical transmission by breastfeeding	Prophylaxis in newborn
HIV	Acute/persistent	No	Yes	Yes	Yes	Yes	Yes
HBV	Acute/persistent	Yes	Yes	Yes	Possibly not	Possibly not	Yes
HCV	Acute/persistent	No	Limited	Limited	Possibly not	Possibly not	No

(HBV: hepatitis B virus; HCV: hepatitis C virus; HIV: human immunodeficiency virus)

GENERAL LABORATORY PROTOCOLS

For Treating Infected Personnel

Couples wherein one partner or both partners are infected with viral infections pose a great risk of transmission of the infection to their newborns, laboratory personnel, medical staff, as well as the gametes/embryos of other noninfected patients. This risk of viral transmission can be reduced by:
- Early detection and identification of potentially hazardous materials
- Strict implementation of SOPs.

Preventive Measures for Handling Infected Sample in Laboratory

- *General:*
  - Wear appropriate personal protective equipment such as eye protectors, face masks, gloves, shoe covers, and disposable scrubs
  - Avoid using mouth pipetting
  - Avoid fluid splashing and aerosol exposure
  - Avoid injuries from sharp objects and needle punctures
- *Strict waste management protocols:*
  - Seal test tubes and dustbin lids to prevent aerosol-borne viruses from escaping.
  - Label all the dustbins being used for the disposal of infected waste and instruct the person in charge to take appropriate precautions when disposing of the waste.
  - To avoid aerosol release into the environment, transfer the infected sample into a disposable container and tight cap it before discarding it into a designated dustbin.
  - Clean all workstations thoroughly with 6% hydrogen peroxide, followed by distilled water.
- *Precautions to be followed to prevent cross-contamination:*
  - Label all disposable items and trash cans properly to prevent waste mixing and proper waste disposal.
  - Change micropipette tips, flexipets, transfer pipettes, injection, and holding needles regularly by the end of the case to prevent cross-contamination between infected and noninfected patients.

For Sperm Preparations

Several studies have investigated the effects of assisted reproduction with sperm washing in virally infected couples. The presence of viral particles in the seminal plasma but not in the spermatozoa was found in the semen of HCV positive men. Many studies have shown that the risk of sexual transmission of HCV infection is extremely low. However, because the virus is present in the seminal plasma, there is a possibility of nosocomial contamination, and thus necessary safety precautions should be taken in all ART laboratories.[9] Similarly, proper semen preparation technique is required to separate sperm from seminal plasma, including the HIV virus, in order to obtain an HIV-free fraction with an adequate amount of morphologically normal and progressive motile sperm.

To separate motile sperm free from any viral infections, sperm-wash procedures that included density-gradient centrifugation followed by sperm swim-up are recommended.[10] A quantitative analysis of HIV in sperm before and after washing reveals that >99% of the HIV is removed. Before using the significant proportion of sperm for insemination, it can be tested for the presence of detectable HIV using polymerase chain reaction (PCR)-based techniques.[11]

Similar semen washing techniques have been used to isolate HCV from sperm and may be effective for other viral infections where the large part of the virus is reported free or associated with sperm somatic cells (i.e., white blood cells and epithelial cells).[12]

For Oocyte Retrieval

Ovum pickup (OPU) is a transvaginal ultrasound aspiration method for oocyte retrieval in which an ultrasound probe and needle are inserted into the vagina to identify follicles and retrieve oocytes. The follicular fluid is then examined under a microscope to see if there are any oocyte-cumulus complexes (OCC) present. Patients with viral infections who are undergoing OPU require more care and attention than noninfected patients. It is always preferable to have a separate set of instruments for these patients so that their cases do not interfere with the cases of the other patients. In the absence of a separate facility, however, these cases

TABLE 2: The possibility of viral infections being transmitted to sperm and oocytes, their detection in semen sample and follicular fluid, and the effect of viral infections on the outcomes of fertility treatment.

Infection	Can virus be detected in sperm	Can virus be detected in oocytes	Can virus be detected in placenta	Can virus be detected in breast milk	Impact on assisted reproduction outcomes	
					When husband is infected	When wife is infected
HIV	No	No	No clear evidence is available	Yes	No	Yes
HBV	Yes	Yes	Yes	Yes	No clear evidence is available	No
HCV	Possibly not	Possibly not	Possibly not	Possibly not	No clear evidence is available	No clear evidence is available

(HBV: hepatitis B virus; HCV: hepatitis C virus; HIV: human immunodeficiency virus)

can be managed in an IVF laboratory by scheduling their procedure at the end of the daily workflow to isolate the patients in time and cross contamination.

It is also suggested that viruses may be present in follicular fluid and attach to OCC; therefore, trimming and washing of OCC in culture media is advised to dilute the viral titer.[1] To further reduce viral titer, complete denudation of oocytes and only insemination with intracytoplasmic sperm injection (ICSI) over IVF is recommended. After insemination, wash the oocytes in culture media again and transfer them to a new culture dish with fresh media. The discarding of follicular fluid in a container and capping it tightly post-OPU is also recommended. Finally, disinfect the workstations using 6% hydrogen peroxide before cleaning with distilled water.

Based on the available evidence, **Table 2** summarizes the possibility of viral infections being transmitted to sperm and oocytes, their detection in semen sample and follicular fluid, and the effect of viral infections on the outcomes of fertility treatment in these patients.

Embryo Culture and Cryopreservation

To isolate patients in space, gametes and embryos should be cultured in separate incubators or incubator chambers. The number of embryos to be transferred is chosen at the time of embryo transfer only with the vision of avoiding multiple pregnancies, a complicated delivery, or both. In such cases, a single embryo transfer is recommended as an option. Depending on the virus [hepatitis B virus (HBV), HCV, and HIV], frozen embryos, and gametes should be stored in separate cryopreservation tanks, or they can be stored in the same cryotanks if a leak proof system, such as heat-sealed high security vitrification straws, is used.

Virus Specific Management

Following are the virus-specific recommendations.

Recommendations Related to Hepatitis B Virus

Hepatitis B: Following recommendations need to be kept in consideration while treating a HBV positive patient[13] and are summarized in **Flowchart 1**:

- Partners of HBV positive individuals should be vaccinated.
- Barrier contraception should be used until the completion of the HBV vaccination protocol.
- Staff providing the service of assisted reproduction should be vaccinated against HBV.[14]
- All patients with an active or chronic HBV infection must be reviewed by an infectious disease specialist before initiating any infertility treatment.
- Commencement of infertility treatment in HBV positive patients should be a joint decision of patient, their partner, the fertility doctor, and the infectious disease specialist. In the case of the female testing positive for HBV, the possibility of viral vertical transmission, the availability of vaccination during pregnancy and newborn prophylaxis should also be discussed.
- Men testing positive for HBV should be informed that no current semen preparation technique can select HBV deoxyribonucleic acid (DNA)-free spermatozoa for use during their treatment.
- Semen processing using density gradient method followed by swim-up method is recommended in men testing positive for HBV.
- Based on the current evidence, HBV DNA testing on seminal fluid or sperm is not recommended.
- Cesarean delivery is not recommended on the basis of maternal HBV-positivity alone.[15]
- Breastfeeding is probably not contraindicated in women testing positive for HBV.[15]
- All neonates born to HBV-positive couples should be vaccinated.
- Administration of hepatitis B immunoglobulin (HBIG) in addition to vaccination is recommended for children born to mothers testing positive for HBV. HBIG administration should follow local or national guidelines.

Recommendations Related to Hepatitis C Virus

The overall global prevalence of HCV infection in 2015 was 1%, with the highest estimated prevalence in the Eastern Mediterranean region (2.3%), followed by the European

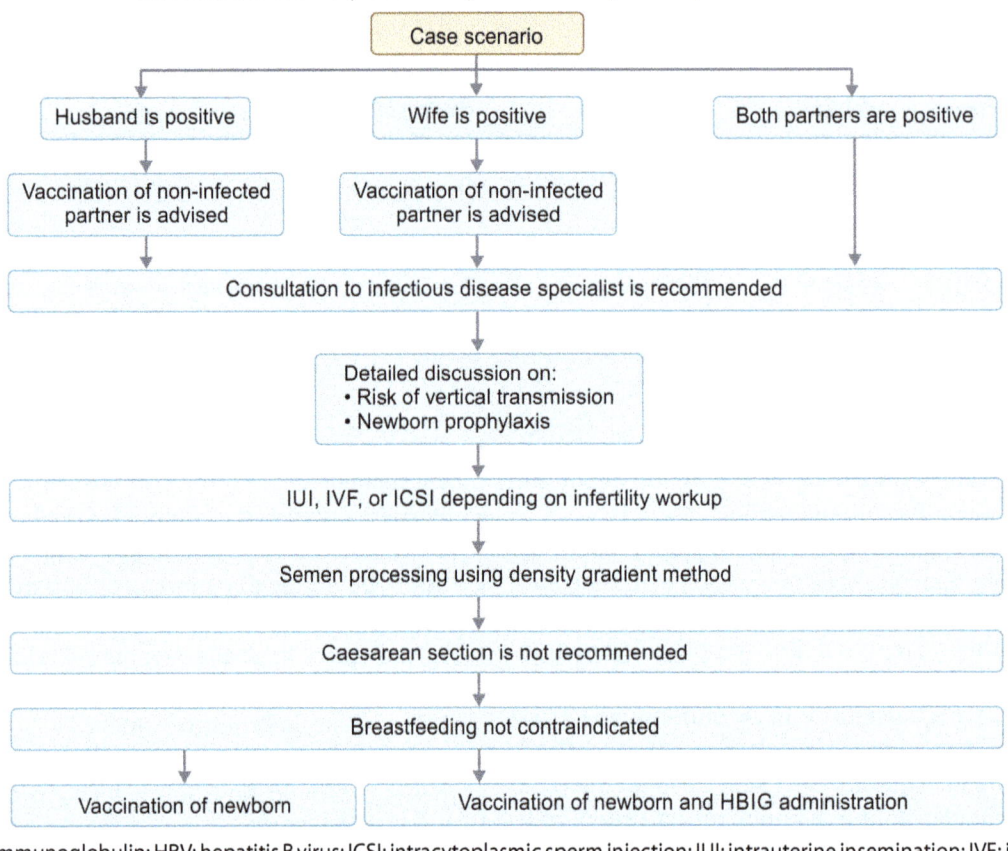

Flowchart 1: Summary of infertility treatment in patients positive with HBV.

(HBIG: hepatitis B immunoglobulin; HBV: hepatitis B virus; ICSI: intracytoplasmic sperm injection; IUI: intrauterine insemination; IVF: in vitro fertilization)

region (1.5%), the African region (1.0%), the region of the Americas and Western Pacific region (both 0.7%) and the South-East Asian region with the lowest estimated prevalence (0.5%).[16]

Hepatitis C virus testing is mandatory according to the European Tissues and Cells Directive as a preventative measure to reduce the risks of transmission to partners and offspring. Following recommendations need to be kept in consideration while treating a HCV positive patient[13] and are summarized in **Flowchart 2**:

- In a monogamous heterosexual relationship of >12 months, there is no indication for the use of barrier contraceptives to reduce the risk of HCV transmission in a serodiscordant infected couple.
- No studies have reported a HCV ribonucleic acid (RNA) serum threshold below which horizontal transmission does not occur.
- No publications could be identified where maternal HCV viral load was measured before pregnancy to avoid vertical transmission.
- All patients with an active or chronic HCV infection must be reviewed by an infectious disease specialist before initiating any infertility treatment.
- Good practice points (GPP) commencing with infertility treatments in patients positive for HCV should be a joint decision between the patient, their partner, the fertility doctor, and the infectious disease specialist. In the case of the female testing positive for HCV, the possibility of viral vertical transmission should be discussed prior to the treatment.
- From the perspective of horizontal and vertical transmission, there is currently not enough evidence to recommend one technique [intrauterine insemination (IUI)/IVF/ICSI] over another in patients infected with hepatitis C. Therefore, the cause of infertility should dictate the specific technique (IUI/IVF/ICSI) used in couples where one or both partners test positive for HCV.
- Women testing positive for HCV should be informed that assisted reproduction does not eliminate the risk of vertical transmission.
- There are contradictory results evaluating effects of male HCV infection on infertility treatments outcomes. Although the fertilization rate has been reported significantly lower in couples with HCV-RNA positive men, other studies report that HCV infection does not affect the IVF-ICSI cycle outcomes in these couples.
- There are contradictory results evaluating effects of female HCV infection on infertility treatments outcomes. Although some studies report significantly reduced implantation rates, higher cycle cancellations, and higher follicle-stimulating hormone (FSH) use in HCV positive women, other report no significant differences.

Flowchart 2: Summary of infertility treatment in patient positive with hepatitis C virus (HCV).

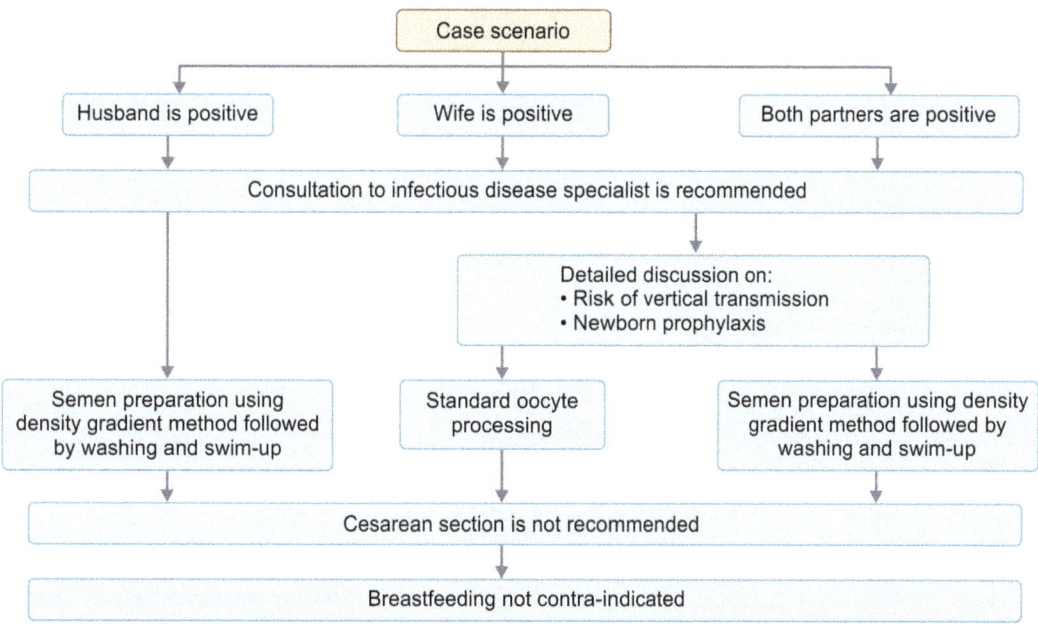

- Good laboratory practice regarding semen processing should be applied irrespective of whether only the male or both partners are testing positive for HCV.
- High plasma HCV viral load is likely to be predictive of the presence of HCV RNA in semen. Strong evidence for the correlation of HCV viral load between serum and semen is currently lacking.
- Cesarean delivery is not recommended on the basis of maternal HCV positivity alone.[17]
- Breastfeeding is not contraindicated in women testing positive for HCV.[17]

Recommendations Related to Human Immunodeficiency Virus

Human immunodeficiency virus infection has become a manageable chronic health condition, enabling people with HIV to lead long and healthy lives. In 2019, 68% of adults and 53% of children living with HIV globally were receiving lifelong antiretroviral therapy. HIV testing is mandatory according to the European Tissues and Cells Directive as a preventative measure to reduce the risks of transmission to partners and offspring.[18]

Following recommendations need to be kept in consideration while treating a HIV positive patient[13] and the process of decision making while treating these patients are summarized in **Flowchart 3**:

- HIV-1-serodiscordant couples should be informed that there is a risk of sexual transmission of the virus to the unaffected partner. To reduce this risk, couples must be advised to use barrier contraception and seek active therapy to reduce viral load.
- In individuals testing positive for HIV-1, antiretroviral therapy can suppress viral replication. These patients should remain on antiretroviral therapy and providing undetectable viral loads in serum can be achieved and sustained, the risk of horizontal transmission through unprotected intercourse is minimal in the absence of other sexually transmitted diseases.
- Commencing of infertility treatment in patients positive for HIV-1 or 2 should be a joint decision between the patient, their partner, the fertility doctor, and the infectious disease specialist.
- All patients testing positive for HIV, wishing to have a child should be counseled about the risk of horizontal and vertical transmission. In the case of the male testing positive for HIV, antiretroviral therapy can reduce the viral load in blood and semen to undetectable levels, allowing the possibility of natural conception. Reproductive counseling should include fertility and antiretroviral covariates.
- In the case of the female testing positive for HIV-1 or 2, and even with undetectable viremia, the possibility of viral vertical transmission should be discussed prior to the treatment.
- HIV infection status is not a reason to deny treatment. The cause of infertility should dictate the specific technique (IUI/IVF/ICSI) used in couples where one or both partners test positive for HIV.
- Serodiscordant couples with a male partner testing positive for HIV-1 should be informed that the efficacy of ART is not impacted compared to HIV-seronegative couples.
- Serodiscordant couples with a female partner testing positive for HIV should be informed that the efficacy of IVF/ICSI could be reduced compared to HIV-seronegative couples.

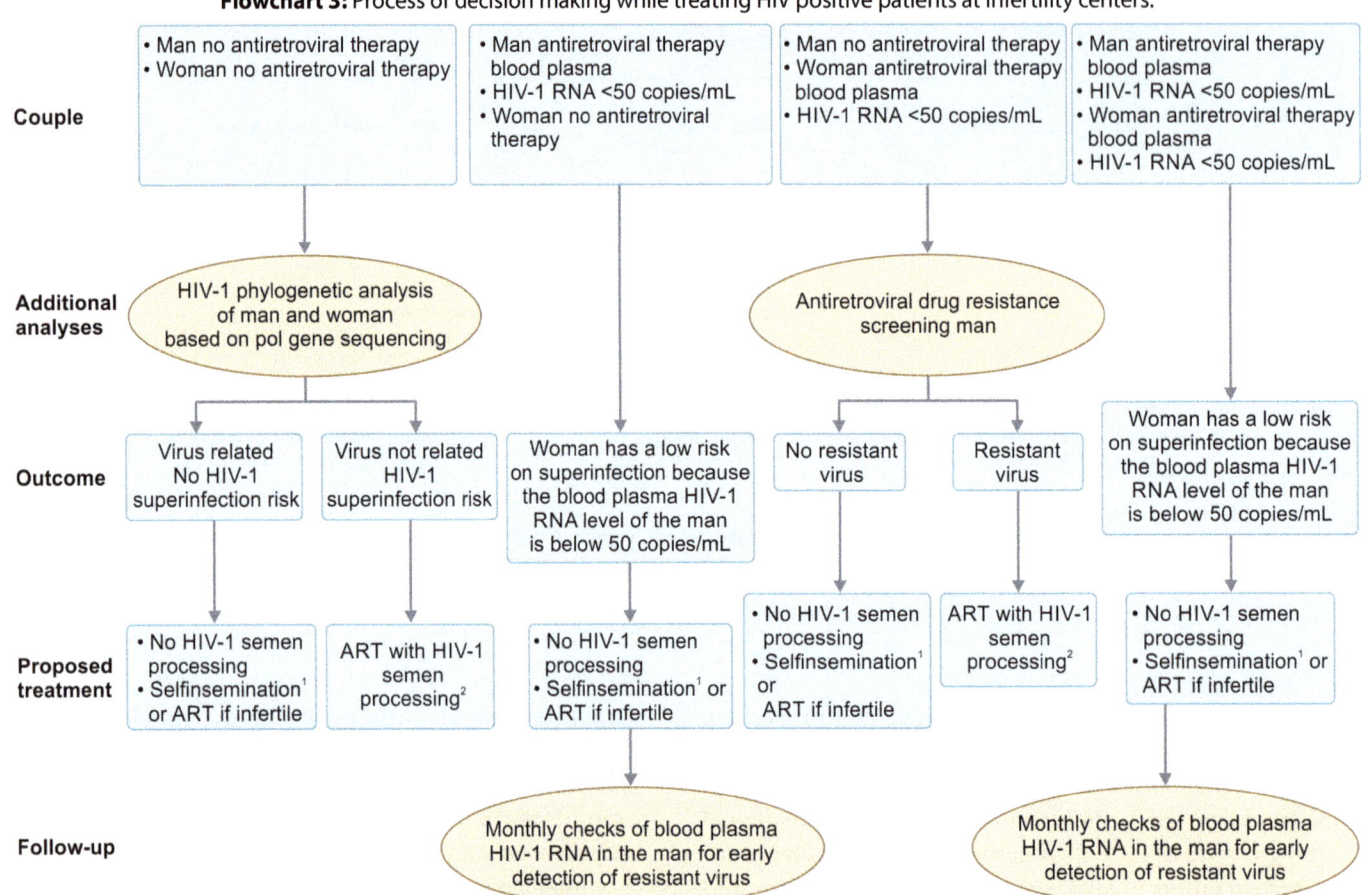

Flowchart 3: Process of decision making while treating HIV positive patients at infertility centers.

1. For all couples the formal advice is selfinsemination instant of unprotected intercourse to prevent HIV-1 superinfection of the male parter.
2. HIV semen processing is desired in case of discordant HIV-1 strains, in the presence of proven resistant virus in the male partner or when blood plasma HIV-1 RNA levels are detectable under antiretroviral therapy in the male partner

(ART: assisted reproductive technology; HIV: human immunodeficiency virus; RNA: ribonucleic acid)

Transmission of Viral Infections to Newborn

A woman is subjected to viral infections during childbirth, which can be forwarded vertically to the newborn. A few of these viruses cause clinically significant harm to the newborn after vertical transmission, whereas others, even when transmitted vertically, are rarely clinically significant. These viral infections can infect a newborn through the uterus (congenital), during labor (perinatal), or after birth (postnatal). The implications of this viral transmission from infected mother to fetus can result in intrauterine death, abortion, preterm birth, and other pregnancy complications.

The viral infection can be transmitted intrauterine either by the umbilical vessels or after the infection of the maternal and fetal limbs and consequent infection of the amniotic fluid. Perinatal transmission, on the contrary hand, can be due to prolonged rupture of membranes, which can result in contamination of amniotic fluid, placenta, umbilical cord, or fetal membranes via an ascending route while postnatal infections are primarily transmitted by breastfeeding. Viral infections such as hepatitis B and C and HIV are transmitted vertically to the child. Studies state that around 30–50% of HIV transmission from mother to the child is due to breastfeeding and in remaining cases it is intrauterine, mostly during the third trimester of the pregnancy or during labor.[19] Similarly, the vertical transmission of HBV infection from positive mother with both hepatitis B surface antigen (HBsAg) and hepatitis B e antigen (HBeAg) to child is 70–90% which can be reduced to 10–30% when mother is HBeAg negative[20] while the chances of HCV transmission from infected mother to child is 5%.[21] However, the exact cause of transmission is still unknown but few studies have suggested that viral transmission can occur both intrauterine or during labor.

In recent years, prophylactic initiatives have been adopted to reduce the risk of viral infection transmission from mother to child. In the case of HIV, administration of antiretroviral drugs during pregnancy, cesarean delivery, and the utilization of powdered milk to feed the newborn are recommended instead of breastfeeding, which can help in reducing the risk of transmission by up to 70%.[22] Moreover, since the introduction of highly active antiretroviral therapy (HAART), the probability of vertical transmission of HIV has

Flowcharts 4A and B: Transmission of HBV infection from mother to offspring.

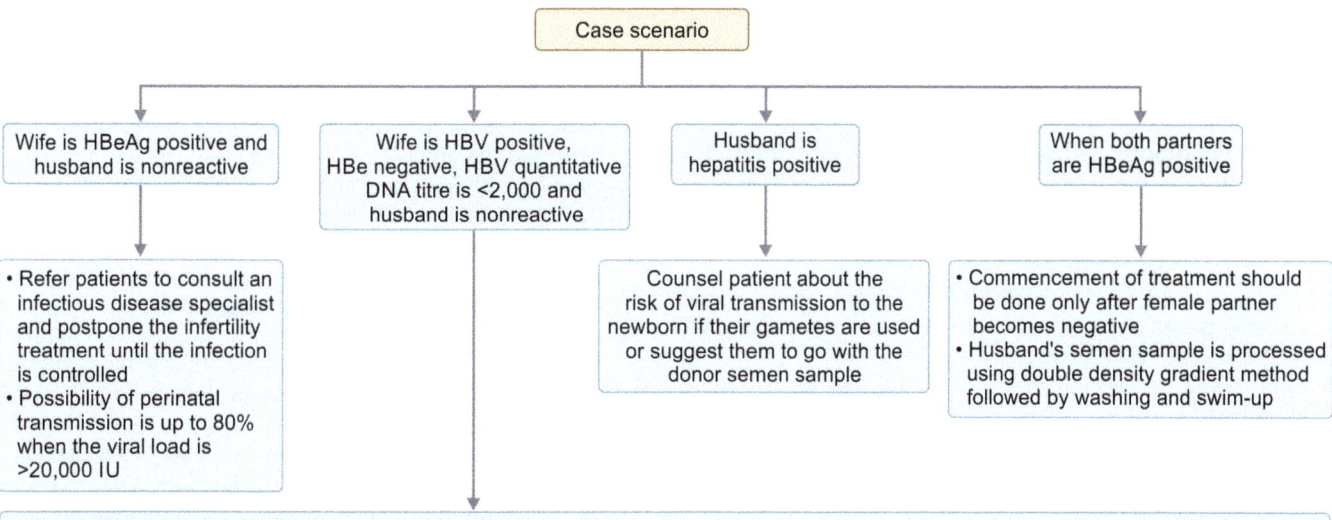

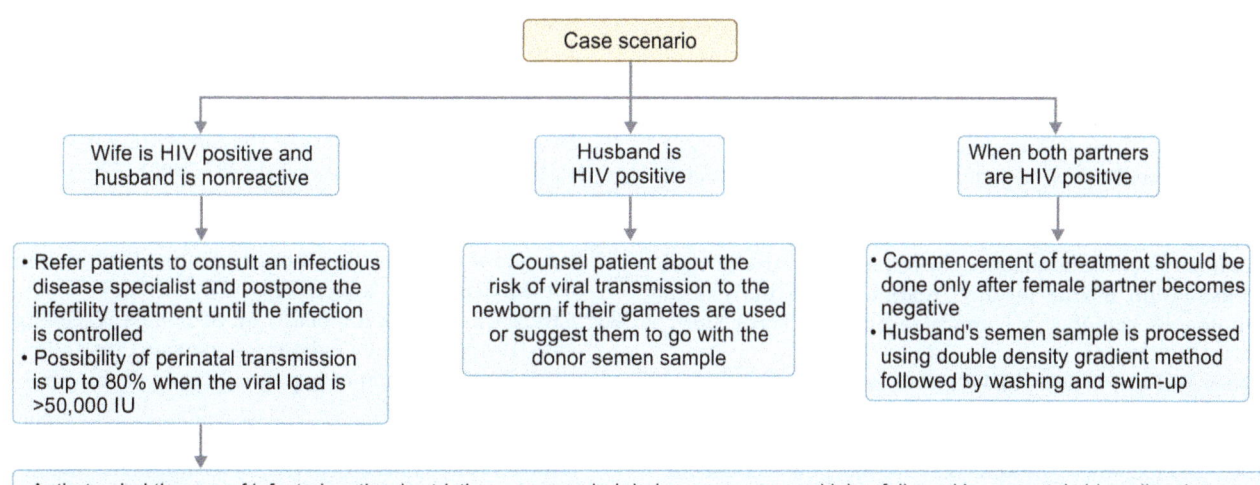

(DNA: deoxyribonucleic acid; HBeAg: hepatitis B e antigen; HBV: hepatitis B virus; HIV: human immunodeficiency virus)

been reduced to current levels.[23] On the other hand, active and passive vaccination of newborns can collectively help in reducing perinatal HBV transmission by up to 90–95%, whereas only active vaccination can reduce transmission by up to 70–90%.[24] In the case of perinatal HCV transmission, a combination of interferon-α and ribavirin has proven to eliminate the infection in 50% of cases, as no other approaches are currently available to prevent perinatal transmission.[25] Detailed process is summarized in **Flowcharts 4A and B**.

CONCLUSION

It is strongly advised that if the center has the necessary resources to provide care, individuals with chronic viral infections, including HIV, should not be denied fertility services. It is also appropriate to refer to a center with such capabilities. There is strong evidence to support the recommendation that antiretroviral drugs be used to reduce HIV viremia in the HIV-infected partner. Sperm-washing methods could be used to further reduce viral load during insemination via IUI, IVF, or ICSI. Separate culturing conditions and storage in different cryotanks can help to reduce the risk of cross-contamination to laboratory personnel as well as other patient cases.

Key Learning Points

- All patients seeking ART treatments should be screened for HIV, HCV, and HBV viral infections.
- Appropriate counseling and informed consents are very important.
- Individualization as per the case etiology for subfertility with multidisciplinary input for viral infection is required.
- Viral load of infection needs to be assessed and minimized with adequate treatment and prevention measures.
- SOPs should be written and validated by infection control and hygiene committee of the hospital.
- Management needs to be planned after careful evaluation.

REFERENCES

1. Steyaert SR, Leroux Roels GG, Dhont M. Infections in IVF: review and guidelines. Hum Reprod Update. 2000;6(5):432-41.
2. Abou-Setta AM. Transmission risk of hepatitis C virus via semen during assisted reproduction: how real is it? Hum Reprod. 2004;19(12):2711-7.
3. Ethics Committee of the American Society for Reproductive Medicine. Human immunodeficiency virus (HIV) and infertility treatment: a committee opinion. Fertil Steril. 2015;104:e1-8.
4. Practice Committee of American Society for Reproductive Medicine. Recommendations for reducing the risk of viral transmission during fertility treatment with the use of autologous gametes: a committee opinion. Fertil Steril. 2020;114:1158-64.
5. Vause TD, Jones L, Evans M, Wilkie V, Leader A. Preconception health awareness in infertility patients. J Obstet Gynaecol Can. 2009;31(8):717-20.
6. Chandranipapongse W, Koren G. Preconception counseling for preventable risks. Can Fam Physician. 2013;59(7):737-9.
7. Lu MC, Kotelchuck M, Culhane JF, Hobel CJ, Klerman LV, Thorp JM Jr. Preconception care between pregnancies: the content of internatal care. Matern Child Health J. 2006; 10 (Suppl 5):S107-22.
8. Nekuei N, Nasr-Esfahani MH, Kazemi A. Preconception Counseling in Couples Undergoing Fertility Treatment. Int J Fertil Steril. 2012;6:79-86.
9. Savasi V, Oneta M, Parrilla B, Cetin I. Should HCV discordant couples with a seropositive male partner be treated with assisted reproduction techniques (ART)? Eur J Obstet Gynecol Reprod Biol. 2013 Apr;167(2):181-4. doi: 10.1016/j.ejogrb.2012.12.012. Epub 2013 Jan 11. PMID: 23317917.
10. Marina S, Marina F, Alcolea R, Expósito R, Huguet J, Nadal J, et al. Human immunodeficiency virus type 1–serodiscordant couples can bear healthy children after undergoing intrauterine insemination. Fertil Steril. 1998;70(1):35-9.
11. Politch JA, Xu C, Tucker L, Anderson DJ. Separation of human immunodeficiency virus type 1 from motile sperm by the double tube gradient method vs. other methods. Fertil Steril. 2004;81:440-7.
12. Pasquier C, Daudin M, Righi L, Berges L, Thauvin L, Berrebi A, et al. Sperm washing and virus nucleic acid detection to reduce HIV and hepatitis C virus transmission in serodiscordant couples wishing to have children. AIDS. 2000;14:2093-9.
13. European Society of Human Reproduction and Embryology. Medically assisted reproduction in patients with a viral infection or disease. Strombeek-Bever: European Society of Human Reproduction and Embryology; 2021.
14. Lemon SM, Alter MJ. Viral hepatitis. In: Holmes KK, Mardh PA, Sparling PF, Lemon SM, Stamm WE, Piot P, Wasserheit JN (Eds). Sexually transmitted diseases, 3rd edition. New York: McGraw-Hill; 1999:361-84.
15. Mast EE, Weinbaum CM, Fiore AE, Alter MJ, Bell BP, Finelli L, et al. A comprehensive strategy to eliminate hepatitis B virus transmission in the United States. Recommendations of the Advisory Committee on Immunization Practices (ACIP) part II: Immunization of adults. MMWR Recomm Rep. 2006; 55(RR-16):1-25.
16. Petruzziello A, Marigliano S, Loquercio G, Cozzolino A, Cacciapuoti C. Global epidemiology of hepatitis C virus infection: An up-date of the distribution and circulation of hepatitis C virus genotypes. World J Gastroenterol. 2016; 22(34):7824-40.
17. AASLD-IDSA HCV Guidance Panel. Hepatitis C guidance 2018 update: AASLD-IDSA recommendations for testing, managing, and treating hepatitis C virus infection. Clin Infect Dis. 2018;67:1477-92.
18. Deeks SG, Lewin SR, Havlir DV. The end of AIDS: HIV infection as a chronic disease. Lancet. 2013;382(9903):1525-33.
19. Nduati R, John G, Mbori-Ngacha D, Richardson B, Overbaugh J, Mwatha A, et al. Effect of breastfeeding and formula feeding on HIV-2 transmission. 1: a randomized clinical trial. JAMA. 2000;283:1167-74.
20. Sevens CE, Neurath RA, Beasly RP, Szmuness W. HBeAg and anti-HBe detection by radioimmunoassay. Correlation with vertical transmission of hepatitis B virus in Taiwan. J Med Virol. 1979;3:237-41.
21. Thomas SL, Newell ML, Peckham CS, Ades AE, Hall AJ. A review of hepatitis C virus (HCV) vertical transmission: risks of transmission to infants born to mothers with and without HCV viraemia or human immunodeficiency virus infection. Int J Epidemiol. 1998;27:108-17.
22. Connor EM, Sperling RS, Gelber R, Kiselev P, Scott G, O'Sullivan MJ, et al. Reduction of maternal-infant transmission of human immunodeficiency virus type 1 with zidovudine treatment. Pediatric AIDS Clinical Trials Group Protocol 076 study group. N Engl J Med. 1994;331:1173-80.
23. European Collaborative Study. Mother-to-child transmission of HIV infection in the era of highly active antiretroviral therapy. Clin Infect Dis. 2005;40:458-65.
24. Shepard CW, Simard EP, Finelli L, Fiore AF, Bell BP. Hepatitis B virus infection: epidemiology and vaccination. Epidemiol Rev. 2006;28:112-25.
25. Wirth S, Lang T, Gehring S, Gerner P. Recombinant alfa-interferon plus ribavirin therapy in children and adolescents with chronic hepatitis C. Hepatology. 2002;36(5):1280-4.

Index

Page numbers followed by *b* refer to box, *f* refer to figure, *fc* refer to flowchart, and *t* refer to table.

A

Abdominal bulge 78
Abdominal distension 86
Abdominal mass, suprapubic 61
Abdominal pain 25, 78
    mild 170, 176
Abdominal ultrasonography 25
Abortion, post spontaneous 90
Abruptio placentae, recurrent 231
Abscesses 70
Achondroplasia 251
Acid tyrode 241
Acid-fast bacilli 87
Acinetobacterium 192
Acquired uterine anomalies 240
Adenoma, recurrence of 59
Adenomyomectomy, techniques of 17*t*
Adenomyosis 13, 15, 114, 116, 221
    diffuse 114
    effects of 115
    hysteroscopic features of 17*b*
    management of 115*fc*
    ultrasound of 114
Adhesion
    barriers 96
    lesser risk of 12
    location of 92
Adnexa
    complete rotation of 185
    partial rotation of 185
Adnexal pathology 73
Adnexal torsion
    evaluation 186
    investigations 186
    pathophysiology 185
Adolescent congenital hypogonadotropic hypogonadism 68
Adrenal androgen production 22
Adrenal gland 44, 44*fc*
Adrenal hyperplasia
    classification of congenital 44, 44*fc*
    congenital 24, 25, 44, 46
Adrenal hypoplasia congenita 67
Adrenal hypothesis 118
Adrenal tumors, functional 25
Adrenarche, premature 25, 26
Adrenocorticotropic hormone 65
Agents, injectable 135
Agonist protocols 163*t*
Alcohol
    consumption 253
    limit 228
Alpha-hydroxylase 226
    deficiency 40
Alprostadil 218
Altruistic surrogacy 274
    requirements for 275
Ambiguous genitalia 33, 44
Amenorrhea 33, 56, 61, 62*fc*, 78, 97, 261
    causes of 62*f*, 63, 65*fc*
    ovarian causes of 63, 64*f*
    primary 42*f*, 61, 61*fc*
    secondary 61, 62, 74
    work-up of secondary 64*fc*
Amniotic fluid, contamination of 290
Anabolic steroids 4
Analgesia 12
Androgen
    major 131
    secreting tumors 61
    source of 131
    testing 236
Androgen action
    classification of disorders of 41*fc*
    disorders of 41
Androgen insensitivity syndrome 35, 41, 63, 64
    partial 41, 46
    spectrum of presentation of 41
Androgen synthesis 35
    disorders of 40
Androgenization, signs of 215
Androstenedione 41
Anejaculation 217
Aneuploidy 35
Aneurysms 70
Anorexia nervosa 251
    prevalence of 251
Anovulatory infertility, second-line therapy for 127
Antagonist cycles 128
Antagonist protocol 164*t*, 166*f*
    mild 166*f*
Antagonist regimen 142*f*
Antagonist stimulation protocol, mild 163
Antenatal care 94
Antiandrogen therapy 133
Antiapoptotic molecules, upregulation of 265
Antibiotic therapy 96, 243
    use of 96
Antiestrogens 168
Antigen–antibody interaction 57
Anti-inflammatory agents 219
Anti-Müllerian hormone 1, 35, 46, 69, 119, 161, 168, 172, 241, 266
Antinuclear antibody 231
    testing 234
Antiphospholipid antibody 231, 233, 235
    syndrome 240
Antiphospholipid syndrome 236
Antiretroviral therapy 128
    highly active 290
Antisperm antibody testing 6
Antituberculosis treatment 87
Antral follicle count 161, 168
Anxiety 254
Aortic dissection 38
Apareunia 78
Arcuate nucleus, dorsal portion of 54
Aromatase 226
    inhibitors 137
Arousal disorders 220
Array comparative genomic hybridization 45, 233, 234
Artificial cycle 197
    with suppression 201, 203
    without suppression 199, 203
Artificial reproductive technique 144
Asherman's syndrome 63, 89, 89*f*, 92*t*, 94*fc*, 194
    classification 92, 93*t*
    clinical features 90
    diagnosis 90
    management 93
Aspirin 168, 174, 192, 258
Assisted conception rates 108
Assisted reproduction technique 239, 256, 266, 285
Assisted reproductive technology 17, 37, 50, 106, 108, 112, 115, 172, 196, 219, 270, 273, 290
    Act 271*b*, 274*t*, 275*t*
    cycle 144
    emergence of 239
    methods 250
Asthenozoospermia 5, 157
Atopic dermatitis 221
Atrophic epithelial mono-layer 89
Atrophic uterine remnant 81*f*
Audiometry 38
Autoimmune 226
Autologous bone marrow stem cell transplant 96
Autosomal recessive disorder 40, 44
Axillary hair 61
Azoospermia 5, 72, 207, 207*f*, 208*f*, 208*t*, 261
    classification system of 207, 207*b*
    etiology of 207*b*
    incidence of 207
    management of 210, 210*fc*, 211*f*
    obstructive 207, 211, 211*t*
    permanent 261
    work-up of 207
Azoospermic factor 209

B

Bacterial growth 222
Bacteroidetes 192
Bardet–Biedl–Moon syndrome 67
Bariatric surgery, indications of 128
Barker's hypothesis 118
Barrier contraception 287
Bartholin and paraurethral gland palpation 224
Basal estradiol 161
Beta-human chorionic gonadotropin 186, 198*f*

Bilateral tubal
  block 9f
  spill 11f
Bilateral tubes 10f
Biopsy 87
Biphasic basal body temperature 3
Bipolar disorders 251
Bipolar resectoscope 113
Birth defects 253
Bladder neck closure 216
Blastocyst transfer 241
Bleeding, regular withdrawal 129
Bleomycin 261
Blind vagina 43f
Blindness
  green color 279
  red color 279
Blood 285
  mononuclear cells, peripheral 242
  pressure 208
  tests 173
Blood sugar
  fasting 86
  levels 196
Body fluids 285
Body mass index 2, 61, 161, 168, 172, 215, 227, 239, 253
Bone
  densitometry 71
  health management 229
  marrow-derived stem cell transplant, administration of 96
  mineral density 40
Breast 42f
  cancer 266, 266fc
    patient 229
  development 61, 73
  examination 2
Breastfeeding 287
Bromocriptine 58
Bulimia nervosa, prevalence of 251
Burn out phenomenon 260f
Busulfan 261

C

Cabergoline 58, 175
Caffeine 253
Cancer 263
  survivorship 260
  type of 265t
Carboplatin 261
Carboxymethylcellulose 96
Cardiac magnetic resonance scan 37
Cardiovascular health management 229
Cardiovascular system 208
Cell sorting, magnetic activated 154, 155f
Cellular phones and radiation 254
Central adoption resource authority 276
Central nervous system 24, 63, 65fc, 70, 216
Central precocious puberty 23-25
Cervical
  agenesis 81
  cerclage 236, 236t
  insufficiency 236
  integrity 233
  motion tenderness 186
  pathology 221
  secretions 2

Cervix 77, 82f, 86
Cesarean delivery 287
CHARGE syndrome 67
Chemical stimulators mediated sperm selection 157, 158f
Chemotherapeutic drugs 260
Chemotherapy 260f, 262, 266
  effect of 260, 261
Childhood cancer survivor 260
Chlamydia 192
  antibody test 8, 11
Chlorambucil 261
Choanal atresia 67
Chromopertubation 8, 10
Chromosomal abnormalities 36f
Chromosomal aneuploidies 241
Chromosomal microarray analysis 45
Chromosomal sex 43
Chromosome analysis, indications for 36
Cisplatin 261
Citalopram 218
Clinical pregnancy rate 168
Clitoral atrophy 222
Clitoral hypertrophy, degrees of 47
Clitoral pathology 221
Clitoroplasty 47
Cloacal exstrophy 35
Clomiphene citrate 136, 163, 190
  mechanism of action of 136fc
Clomipramine 218
Coagulation 17
Coenzyme Q10 168
Cognitive, stage of 21
Cogwheel appearance 87
Colloid infusion-plasma expanders 175
Coloboma 67
Combined hormonal contraceptive pills 228
Combined oral contraceptive pills 73, 124
Comparative genomic hybridization 233
Complete androgen insensitivity syndrome 46
Complete blood count 71, 86, 176
Conception karyotyping, products of 233
Conception, products of 233
Congenital anomalies 222
Congenital hypogonadotropic hypogonadism 67
Congenital sensorineural deafness 67
Contraceptive vaginal
  patch 133
  rings 133
Contralateral ovary 42
Conventional testicular sperm extraction 211, 212
Corifollitropin alfa 163, 166f
Coronavirus disease-2019 196
Corpus luteum 256
Corticotropin-releasing hormone 251
Cortisol 41, 251
Couple, counseling of 196
Craniopharyngioma 70
C-reactive protein levels 186
Cryomyolysis 114
Cryptomenorrhea 61
Cryptorchidism 4
Cryptozoospermia 207
Cumulative pregnancy rates 74
Cushing's syndrome 25, 30

Cycle cancelation 161, 175
Cyclic adenosine monophosphate 175
  selective inhibitor of 192
Cyclophosphamide 261
  high dose of 261
CYP17A1 gene 40
Cystic fibrosis 210
  transmembrane regulator mutation 5
Cystoscopy 219
Cytokine polymorphism 236
Cytomegalovirus 226
Cytotoxic drugs 261t

D

Dacarbazine 261
Dactinomycin 261
Dapoxetine 218
Deep infiltrating disease 99
Deeper digital palpation 224
Dehydroepiandrosterone 24, 25, 41, 120, 168
  sulfate 41, 46, 64, 120
Delayed puberty 27, 67
  treatment of 29
De-novo mutations 41
Density gradient 148f
  centrifugation 148, 149f
  method 148
Deoxyribonucleic acid 1, 235, 287, 291
  integrity of 5
  percentages of 144
Depression 254
Desire disorders 220
Diabetes mellitus, type 2 129
Diethylstilbestrol 78, 79
Dihydrotestosterone 46, 48
Direct swim-up 146, 146f
Directly observed treatment short-course 88
Distal tubal block 17
Distension media, types of 14t
Diverticulitis 187
Donor cycles 258
  management 272, 272t
Donor egg
  indications for 271, 271t
  recipients, additional screening for 272t
Donor gamete conception 272
Donor oocyte 229
Donor sperm 273
  artificial insemination of 273
  indications for 274t
Dopamine 54, 251
  agonist 175
Double flap technique 17
Double stimulation 163
  protocol 166f
Doxarubicin 261
Drug
  abuse 253
  and medications, use of recreational 5
Dual hypothalamic regulation 54
Duchenne's and Becker's muscular dystrophy 279
Dyslipidemia 128
Dysmenorrhea 114
  severe 83
Dyspareunia 2, 78, 220, 222, 224
  causes of 223t

classification of 220, 221*t*, 222*t*
etiology 220
management 222
oocytes 229
ovarian tissue 229
signs 222
symptoms 222

E

Ear abnormalities 67
Early follicular phase 167
Eating disorders 63
Ecosprin 192
Eflornithine 133
Egg
   quality 241
   recipients, screening of 271
   use of 269
Egg donation 269, 270, 273
   complications of 272
   protocols for 273*fc*
Egg donor 277
   eligibility criteria 271*b*
   screening of 271
   types of 271
Ejaculated sperm cryopreservation 266
Ejaculation
   by prostatic massage, stimulation of 219
   delayed 217
   retrograde 216, 219
Ejaculatory duct
   obstruction 208
   transurethral resection of 208-210
Ejaculatory dysfunction 215, 216
   diagnosis of 217*fc*
Electrocardiogram 177*f*
Electroejaculation 219
Electromyography 216
Electrophoretic method 153
Electrosurgical vaporization 113
Elevated intracranial pressure,
      symptom of 25
Elevated thyroid-stimulating
      hormone 50, 170
Embryo
   adoption 269
   cryopreservation 261, 287
   culture 287
      media, spent 282
   damage 281
   donation 269, 274, 274*b*
      indications 274
   freezing 197
   mosaic 282
   ovarian stimulation for 262
   pooling 196
   synchronization of 197
   transfer 196, 204, 239, 256, 258
      elective single 280, 283
      sequential 244
   transfer cycles 190
      frozen-thawed 258
   use of 269
Embryology 77
Emotional distress, lower level of 260
Endocrine
   abnormalities 241

evaluation 25
therapy 266
Endogenous gonadotropins, release of 161
Endometrial aspirate 87
Endometrial biopsy 4, 13
Endometrial carcinoma, increased risk
      for 129
Endometrial cavity
   normal 10*f*
   outlining 92
Endometrial coring 194*f*
Endometrial hyperplasia 73
Endometrial injury 243
Endometrial mesenchymal cells,
      proliferation of 96
Endometrial pattern 191
Endometrial polyps 13, 15, 241
Endometrial preparation protocols 205
Endometrial proliferation, causes of 256
Endometrial receptivity
   analysis 196
   array 191
   assay 244
Endometrial scratching 96, 237
Endometrial shedding 89
Endometrial stromal cells, proliferation of 96
Endometrial thickness 181, 190, 191, 241
   measurement of 181
Endometrial tissue 236
Endometrial vascularization 191
Endometrioma 100*b*
Endometriosis 16, 99, 99*fc*, 100*b*, 104*b*, 104*t*,
      105, 105*b*, 106, 107*f*, 221, 222
   fertility index 103*f*, 106
   management of 99, 103
      pain with 104
   pain with 105
   stage of 100, 107*fc*
   work-up of 99
Endometriotic excision 17
Endometritis
   chronic 13, 15, 16*b*, 192
   role of antibiotics of 194
Endometrium 10*f*, 89, 92*f*, 257, 258
   causes 190
      of thin 190*fc*
   functional 81*f*
   management of thin 190
   normal 191*f*
   synchronization of 197
   thin 191*fc*, 192*f*
   treatment 192
      of thin 193*fc*
Endoscopic surgery 19
Endoscopic techniques 87
Enzyme deficiencies 226
Ependymal sperm aspiration,
      microscopic 211, 212
Epidermal growth factor 194
Epididymis 4
Erectile dysfunction 56, 215, 218
   management of 216*fc*
Erection, medicated urethral system for 216
Erythrocyte sedimentation rate 29, 86, 191
Escherichia coli 192
Estradiol 41, 51, 175, 264
   levels 22
   serum concentrations of 25

Estrogen 258, 259
   component 228
   replacement, duration of 200
   treatment 73
Estrogenization, loss of 67
Ethambutol 87
European tissues 288
Euthyroid 51
Euthyroidism 51
Exercise 255
   regular 228
Exogenous progesterone 74
   initiation 201
Exosomes therapy 229
External genitalia 61
   development 42

F

Facial hair, excessive 42*f*
Fallopian tube 8*f*, 77, 185, 187
   distended 87
Female external genitalia 43*f*
Female genital
   mutilation 222
   system 77*f*
   tract 86
   tuberculosis 86, 222, 223
      drug sensitive 88*t*
Female orgasm disorders 220
Female reproductive tract 77
Female sexual dysfunction 220
Ferriman and Gallway score, modified 121*f*
Ferriman-Gallwey
   chart, modified 132*f*
   score, modified 131
Fertility 37*t*, 96, 109, 115
   evaluation 123
   expert 1
   female 55*f*
   male 56*f*
   natural 37
   options for 48, 228
   preservation 196, 262
      strategies 266, 267*fc*
      techniques 260, 261, 262*fc*
   treatment 287*t*
Fertilization rates, impaired 51
Fertoprotective adjuvant therapy 265
Fetal cystic hygroma 36
Fibroids 108
   classification of 108
   diagnosis of 108
   effects of 109
   management of 112, 112*fc*
   with infertility, management of 111
Filtration techniques 149
   advantages 149
   disadvantages 149
Fluid
   management 177*b*
   overload 13
Fluorescence in situ hybridization 233
Fluoxetine 218
Focal adenomyosis 114
Follicle-stimulating hormone 1, 2*f*, 22, 24, 25,
      46, 62-65, 71, 74, 119, 120*f*, 135, 136,
      139-142, 161, 172, 207, 209, 210,
      215, 216, 261, 272
   higher 288
   receptor, mutated 170

Follicular early cessation protocol 162
Follicular fluid 285
Folliculogenesis 73, 258
Foods to eat 125
Fragile X mental retardation gene 1 227
Fragile X premutation 230
    carrier screening 227
Franulocyte colony-stimulating factor 193
Free triiodothyronine levels 50
Freeze-all cycles 196*b*
Freeze-all protocol 128*f*
Frozen embryo transfer 115, 128, 168, 196, 203*t*, 204, 241, 242
    cycles 258
        monitoring of 200
    endometrial preparation for 196
    indications for 196
    modified natural cycle, types of 197*fc*
    planning 197
    protocols 197
    timing 200
Frozen thaw cycles 258
Frozen transfer 272
Fundoscopic examination 25
Fungal culture 224
Fungal growth 222

G

Galactorrhea 2, 56, 61
Galactose-1-phosphate uridylyltransferase 226
Galactosemia 226
Gametes and embryos, vital portal for transport of 8
Ganirelix 141
Gender dissatisfaction 35
Gender dysphoria 35
General illness 61
Genetic analysis 209
Genetic syndromes 226
Genetic testing 5, 45, 70, 227
Genexpert 87
Genital abnormalities 67
Genital infections, evidence of 4
Genital mutilation 221
Genital outflow tract 61
    obstruction 62*fc*, 63
Genital pituitary hormone deficiency 67
Genital surgeries 45
Genital tract, chronic infectious disease of female 86
Genital tuberculosis 18*t*, 19*fc*, 90
    clinical features of female 86, 86*b*
    diagnosis of female 86
    management of 19*fc*
Genitalia, degree of internal 42
Genitopelvic pain 220
Genitourinary function 229
Genome of mycobacterium, rapid sequencing of entire 87
Gestational surrogacy 274
Ghrelin 251
Glass bead filtration 150
Glass wool filtration 150*f*
Glucocorticoids 175, 237
    levels of 41

Glyceryl trinitrate 168
Glycine 113
Gonadal dysfunction 261*t*
Gonadal dysgenesis 40*fc*, 61
    mixed 40
    partial 40
    pure 40
Gonadal estrogen production 22
Gonadectomy 40, 48
    bilateral 47
Gonadoblastoma, risk of developing 43
Gonadotoxic drugs, treatment with 260
Gonadotoxic therapy, administration of 266
Gonadotoxicity, prevention of 265
Gonadotropin 22, 126, 142, 175, 212, 264
    choice of 139
    dose of 142
    inhibitory hormone 254
    injectable 139
    release of 67
    therapy 72, 73
    treatment 73
    use of 128
Gonadotropin-dependent precocious puberty 24, 25
    treatment of 26
Gonadotropin-independent precocious puberty 24, 25
Gonadotropin-only protocols 139
Gonadotropin-releasing hormone 54, 56, 62, 71, 74, 104, 106, 118, 136, 163, 167, 178, 223, 257, 264
    agonist 112, 128, 133, 144, 164*f*, 172, 175, 244, 256, 258, 265
        long protocol 115
    analogs, role of 141
    antagonist 141, 262
        premenstrual 161
    deficiency 67
    inhibition of pulsatile 251
    neuronal migration 68
    receptor synthesis 68
    therapy 72, 212
Gonadotropin-stimulation, monitoring during 141
Gonads 44, 260
Gordon Holmes syndrome 68
Granulocyte colony-stimulating factor 193, 204, 237, 241, 242
Granulomas 70
Granulosa cells, aspiration of 175
Growth disorders in adolescent age 29
Growth factor, transforming 194
Growth failure, severe 30
Growth hormone 48, 65, 168, 193
Growth retardation 67
Guideline development group 100, 104
Gynecological history 2
Gynecomastia 5, 261

H

Hair, abnormal pigmentation of 67
Headache 61
Heart
    defect 67
        left-sided congenital 36
    disease, worsening of 216
    rate 176

Hematocrit 176
Hematologic malignancies 266
Hematometrocolpos 84
Hemivagina, obstructed 79
Hemoglobin 233
Hemophilia 279
Hemorrhage, internal 185
Heparin 242, 258
Hepatitis B 285, 287
    E antigen 290, 291
    immunoglobulin 288
        administration of 287
    virus 271, 273, 286-288, 291
        transmission 291
Hepatitis C 285
    virus 271, 273, 285-287
        testing 288
Hepatotoxicity 87
Hereditary thrombophilias 240
Hermaphroditism, true 42
Hirsutism 2, 61, 121, 131, 132*f*
    diagnosis 131
    differential diagnosis for 131, 132*t*
    evaluation of 131
    incidence 131
    laser therapy in 134
    management of 131, 132
    mild 134
    patient-important 134
    red flags of 131
Hodgkin's disease 261
Homocysteine levels 236
Hormonal assay 227
Hormonal evaluation 5
Hormone
    administration of 257
    medication 29
    replacement treatment 228, 228*t*
    sensitive cancer 228
    supraphysiological doses of 73
    therapy 37, 37*fc*, 48, 65, 70*t*, 73, 212
Hormone replacement therapy 192
    cycles 258
    regimen 73
Human albumin 175
Human chorionic gonadotropin 71, 74, 126, 139-142, 161, 163, 167, 172, 175, 178, 182, 193, 199*f*, 204, 212, 227, 256, 257, 257*t*
    trigger 174
Human immunodeficiency virus 86, 271, 273, 285-287, 290, 291
Human leukocyte antigen 231
    typing 280
Human menopausal gonadotropin 71, 73, 74, 139-142, 163
Huntington's disease 279
Hyaluronic acid 96
    binding 153
        physiological method of 153, 153*f*
Hybrid leiomyomas 109
Hybrid myomas 110*f*, 113
Hydrops 36
Hydrosalpinges 243
Hydrosalpinx 17, 87, 241
    management of 18*fc*
Hydroxyethyl starch 175
Hydroxylase, deficiency of 44

Hydroxyprogesterone 41, 46
Hymen, imperforate 222
Hyperandrogenemia, manifestation of 131
Hyperandrogenism 120
    biochemical markers of 120*t*
    evaluation of 131
    signs of 131
    symptoms of 61
Hypercortisolism 30
Hypergonadotropic hypogonadism 28, 29, 37
Hyperpigmentation 67
Hyperprolactinemia 54, 58*t*, 59
    causes of 55, 55*f*
    effects of 55, 55*f*, 56*f*
    evaluation of 56
    management 57
    medical management of 58*fc*
    microadenoma-associated 57
    surgical management of 58*fc*
Hypertension 229
Hyperthyroidism 51
    infertile women with 51
Hypogonadism 67, 68
    anabolic steroid-induced 213
    primary 5, 207
    secondary 5
    signs of 215
Hypogonadotropic hypogonadal
    female, management of 72
    male, management of 67, 70
Hypogonadotropic hypogonadism 29, 55, 67, 69, 71, 207, 210
    adult-onset 68
    causes of 27
    clinical condition of 67
    differential diagnoses 68
    etiological types of 67*fc*
Hypogonadotropic state 265
Hypo-osmotic swelling 157*f*
    test, modified 156
Hypoplasia 70
Hypothalamic amenorrhea 63
Hypothalamic gonadotropin-releasing hormone 67
    pulsatile secretion of 22
Hypothalamic neurons 54
Hypothalamic-pituitary-adrenal axis 67, 254
    normal 266
Hypothalamus, suprachiasmatic nucleus of 55
Hypothyroidism 50, 51
    primary 59
Hysterography 89
Hysterolaparoscopy 100*b*
    procedure 13
Hysterosalpingo-contrast sonography 3*f*, 4, 8, 10, 10*f*, 109
Hysterosalpingogram 9*f*, 13, 79, 107, 272
    normal 8*f*
Hysterosalpingography 3, 3*f*, 4*f*, 8, 63, 87, 91, 92*f*, 93*t*, 94, 223
Hysteroscope
    flexible 13
    parts of 12, 13*f*
    types of 13*t*
Hysteroscopic adhesiolysis 95*f*, 96, 97, 194
Hysteroscopic morcellator 113
Hysteroscopic myomectomy 16*t*, 116
    methods of 16

Hysteroscopic surgery 93
Hysteroscopy 4, 13, 63, 78, 87, 92, 93*t*, 109, 112, 191, 192
    indications of 13*t*
    usage of 12, 13

I

Idiopathic hirsutism 134
Idiopathic hyperprolactinemia 55
Idiopathic infertilit 50
Idiopathic short stature 30
    severe 36
Immotile spermatozoa 157
Immunological disease 260
Immunotherapy 242
Implantation failure, repeated 204
In vitro activation 229
In vitro fertilization 51, 71, 105, 107, 124, 144, 161, 163, 167, 175, 178, 186, 196, 200, 204, 210, 234-236, 242, 254, 256, 272, 282, 285, 288
    cycles 111, 168*t*
    development of 269
    planning 40
    treatment 256
        regimens 174
In vitro follicular growth, encapsulated 266
In vitro maturation 174, 262, 264
Indian ART Act 270*t*, 274
Infections 240
Infertile couple 51, 108, 158, 250, 254
Infertility 18*fc*, 33, 37, 54, 67, 78, 114, 115*fc*, 251, 253
    causes of 1, 8, 99, 108
    degree of 261
    duration of 4
    etiology of 2, 2*f*, 19*fc*
    female 51, 253*f*
    indications of 1
    lifestyle factors in 250, 251
    male 51
    management of 17, 74*f*, 105*fc*, 112, 112*fc*, 125
    obesity related male 252*f*
    treatment of 71, 73
    tubal evaluation for 8*fc*
    unexplained 6, 13
    with endometriosis, management of 105
    work-up of 1, 1*t*
Innovative molecular tests 45
Insemination 287
Insulin 251
    hypothesis 118
    resistance, signs of 131
    sensitizers 174
    sensitizing agents 137
Insulin-like growth factor 65
    binding protein 138
Intercourse, timed 126
Interferon gamma release assay 86
Intermenstrual bleeding 114
Intracellular cyclic adenosine monophosphate levels 157
Intracervical adhesions 89
Intracytoplasmic morphologically selected sperm injection 152*f*

Intracytoplasmic sperm injection 51, 151, 163, 210, 287, 288
    bypass 144
    cycles 111, 161
    treatment 192
Intralipids 243
Intramural extension, degree of 15
Intramural fibroids 108
    distorting 109
Intramuscular progesterone 175, 257
Intraovarian renin-angiotensin system, activation of 171
Intrauterine adhesions 16*b*, 63, 89, 91*f*, 95*f*, 97
    causes of 16*b*
    classification of 16*t*
    hysteroscopic appearance of 92*f*
    management of 16*b*
Intrauterine androgens, abnormal levels of 44
Intrauterine anomalies 243
Intrauterine device 94, 221
    malfunction of 222
Intrauterine fetal deaths, recurrent 231
Intrauterine insemination 71, 74, 105, 106*b*, 107, 108, 112, 126, 145, 210, 288
    processing techniques, use of effective 144
    ovulation induction protocols for 135
Intrauterine synechiae 13, 15
Intravaginal ejaculation latency time, basis of 216
Intravenous calcium gluconate 175
Intravenous immunoglobulin 237, 242
In-vitro fertilization 48
Ipsilateral renal anomaly syndrome 79, 82
Iris, abnormal pigmentation of 67
Isoniazid 87
Isosorbide monohydrate 168
Isothermal amplification, loop-mediated 87

K

KAL1 gene 68
Kallmann's syndrome 67, 210
Karyotype testing, indication of 45
Kearns–Sayre syndrome 280
Ketoconazole 175
Klinefelter's phenotype 5
Klinefelter's syndrome 38, 38*fc*, 47*fc*, 209

L

Laparoscope, parts of 12*f*, 12*t*
Laparoscopic chromopertubation 11*f*
Laparoscopic entry techniques 14*fc*
Laparoscopic myomectomy, robotic-assisted 114
Laparoscopic ovarian drilling 124, 127
    indications of 128
Laparoscopic uterosacral nerve ablation 223
Laparoscopy 4, 8, 10, 113
    diagnostic 87
    instruments for 12
Laser, types of 134
Lasmar's classification 16*t*
Lasmar's STEPW preoperative classification 113*t*
Leber's hereditary optic neuropathy 280

Leiomyoma 13, 108, 221
    classification of 109*t*
Leptin 251
Lesser blood loss 12
Letrozole 137, 163, 167, 168
Leukocyte antigen antibodies,
    anti-human 236
Leydig cell 254
    failure 261
Lifestyle behaviors, modify 254
Lifestyle factors 250
Lifestyle modifications 125, 215
Lignocaine, topical 218
Lipid profile 38, 215
Live birth rate 168
Liver function test 29, 71, 86, 176
Long follicular
    agonist protocol 162
    gonadotropin-releasing hormone agonist
        protocol 164*f*
Lower abdominal pain 86
    acute onset of 186
Lower luteinizing hormone level 254
Low-molecular-weight heparin 233, 258
Luteal agonist protocol, long 162
Luteal antagonist administration 175
Luteal estradiol 161
Luteal phase
    agonist 194
    defect 256, 256*fc*
    support, role of 258
Luteinizing hormone 1, 2*f*, 35, 46, 62, 64, 67,
        74, 118, 119, 120*f*, 127, 136, 164, 192,
        198*f*, 204, 210, 215, 216, 242, 256
    increased 261
    induction of 55
    kit, positive 3
    levels 22, 256
        restore 256
    premature 161
    testing 236
Luteofollicular transition 139*f*
Luteoplacental transition 74
Lymphocyte
    immunization therapy 237
    immunotherapy 243

M

Macroadenoma 57, 70
Macroprolactinemia 55, 56, 57*fc*
Malaria 226
Mannitol 175
Mantoux test 86
Marfan's syndrome 279
Marijuana contains 254
Maternal age, advanced 283
Matrix metalloproteinase 258
Mayer-Rokitansky-Küster-Hauser
    syndrome 46, 63, 64, 222
McCune-Albright syndrome, treatment of 26
Mechlorethamine 261
Medical illness, chronic 61
Medroxyprogesterone 163
Menopause, premature 261
Menorrhagia 114
Menstrual cycle 240
    irregular 121

    luteal phase of 256
    time in 167
Menstrual disorders 86
Menstrual early cessation agonist protocol
    162, 165*f*
Menstrual history 2, 61
Menstrual pathway, normal 62*f*
Menstrual pattern 93
Menstruation, absence of 61
Mental disorders, statistical manual of 220
Mental retardation 68
Mercaptapurine 261
Metabolic disorder 123
Metabolic syndrome 128
Metformin 168, 174
    mechanism of action of 138
Methotrexate 261
    management 180
Metroplasty 82*f*
Metrorrhagia 114
Microadenoma 57
Microcode flare agonist protocol 162
Microfluidic channels 156
Microprolactinoma 55
Midluteal progesterone measurement 3
Migraine 229
Migration sedimentation 147, 147*f*
Mimicking estradiol levels 73
Minimally invasive surgery 12
    role of 12
Miscarriage 197
    age-related risk of 232*t*
    increased risk of 108
Misconception 254
Mitochondrial activation 229
Mitochondrial disorders 279
Mitochondrial genes, mixed 279
Monofollicular cycles 142
Monogenic disorders 279
Monopolar resectoscope 113
Mosaicism 281
Motile sperm
    organelle morphology examination 152*f*
    selection of 157
Müllerian agenesis 63, 80
Müllerian anomalies 13, 15, 78*t*, 243
    complex 84
    hysteroscopic features of 17*t*
    management of 77, 79, 79*fc*
Müllerian duct 15
    anomalies 77
        classification 77
    derivatives
        embryogenesis of 77*f*
        embryological development of 77
Müllerian structures, well-formed 44
Multidisciplinary team 229
Multifollicular cycles 142
Multifollicular development 142
Multiple dense adhesions 93
Multiple pregnancies 161
    lower risk of 137
Mumps 226
Muscular dystrophy 67
Musculoskeletal conditions 221
Mutation 41
Mycobacterium
    bovis 18, 86
    tuberculosis 18, 86, 90

Mycoplasma 192
Myolysis 114
Myomas, role of 240
Myomectomy 13, 112
    indications of 111

N

National TB Elimination Program 88
Natural cycle
    modified 198, 198*f*, 203
    transferred in 197
    true 197
Natural killer cell 236
Neodymium-doped yttrium aluminum
    garnet 133
Neonatal congenital hypogonadotropic
    hypogonadism 68
Nerve conduction velocity 216
Nervous system, peripheral 216
Neuritis, peripheral 87
Neurobiological causes 216
Neurofibromatosis 279
Newer molecular methods 87
Next-generation sequencing 45, 233
    platform 68
    technology 87
Nifedipine 168
Nimodipine 168
Nitric oxide 192, 258
Nitrogen mustard 261
Nocturnal penile tumescence 215
Nocturnal sperm emissions 219
Nonapoptotic spermatozoa 154
Non-classical congenital adrenal hyperplasia
    48, 120
Noninvasive preimplantation genetic
    testing 282
Noninvasive prenatal testing 282, 283
Noninvasive tests 191
Nonmalignant disorders, cytotoxic drugs for
    260
Nonobstructive azoospermia 209, 211, 212
    evaluation of 210*fc*
Nonsteroidal anti-inflammatory drugs 79,
    95, 104
Nosocomial infections 285
Nuclear receptors 87
Nucleic acid amplification,
    cartridge-based 87
Nucleotide polymorphism, single 233
Nutrition 255
Nutritional factors 251

O

Obesity 68, 253*f*
Obstetric history 2
Ocular lens assembly 12
Ocular toxicity 87
Olfactory placode aplasia 70
Oligoasthenospermia, severe 5
Oligoasthenoteratozoospermia 5
Oligomenorrhea 56
Oligospermia 5, 261
Oligozoospermia 157
Oocyte 261, 270
    cryopreservation, mature 262, 266

cumulus complexes 286
    effect on 261
    pickup 264
    retrieval 200f, 286
Oogonial stem cells 265
Oophoropexy 188
Opioids 251
Oral agents 135
Oral contraceptive pill 65, 129, 104, 133
    pretreatment 161
    third-generation 133
Oral estradiol 72
Oral glucose tolerance test 137
Oral ovulation induction agents 138
Oral ovulogens 125
Oral prednisolone 243
Orgasm disorder 220
Osada's triple-flap technique 17
Osmotic diuretic 175
Osteogenesis imperfecta 279
Ostium, atresia of internal 93
Ovarian cyst 186
    functional 25
    ruptured 187
Ovarian drilling 135
Ovarian dysfunction 271
Ovarian effects 260
Ovarian endometrioma 17b, 100
Ovarian endometriosis 17
Ovarian enlargement, unilateral 186
Ovarian failure
    following chemotherapy 63
    premature 190
Ovarian function
    normal 271
    resumption of 265
Ovarian hyperstimulation
    controlled 112, 161, 163
    rates 142
Ovarian hyperstimulation syndrome 163, 164, 170, 171-173, 173t, 175-177, 177f, 178, 196
    classification of 170
    clinical features of 171
    complications of 172, 173b
    management of 170, 176fc, 177
    pathogenesis of 172f
    pathophysiology of 171, 171f
    predicting 171
    prevention of 161, 172
    risk of 74, 256
    severity of 171t
    types of 170, 170t
Ovarian hypothesis 118
Ovarian implants, morphology of 100
Ovarian insufficiency, primary 61, 94
Ovarian metastasis risk 265t
Ovarian reserve 266
    diminished 50
    hormonal tests for 2
    reduction in 260
    tests of 2, 236
Ovarian stimulation 174, 197, 264
    controlled 162f, 167, 264
    effects of 51f
    iatrogenic complication of 170
    protocol, controlled 136fc, 161, 263f

Ovarian tissue cryopreservation 48, 262, 264
Ovarian torsion
    clinical features 186
    diagnosis of 185
    differential diagnosis 187
    management of 185, 187
    risk factors for 186
Ovarian transposition 265
Ovarian tumors 186
Ovary 86, 185, 261
    support system of 185f
Overt hypogonadism 56
Overt thyroid dysfunction 51
Ovotestes 42
    bilateral 42
Ovulation induction
    agent, second-line 126
    indications of 135
    methods of 135
    prerequisite for 135
Ovulatory cycles 204fc
Ovulatory dysfunction 120, 121
    categories of 3f
    tests for 3, 122t
Ovulatory response rates 74
Ovum donation 196
Ovum pick-up 197, 258, 286

P

Pain
    adjunctive treatment of 105b
    cyclical 61
    management for 104fc
        medical 104t
        surgical 104b
Painful ejaculation 219
Painful injections 257
Parasite 226
Parental aneuploidies 241
Parental genetic analysis 233
Paroxetine 218
Partner's oocytes, reception of 275
Pelvic
    adhesions 221
    examinations 2
    floor muscle spasm 220
    infections 222
    inflammatory disease 8, 168, 187, 221-223
    organ prolapse 221
    pain 114, 220
        chronic 86
    tuberculosis 86
    ultrasonography 25
Penetration disorder 220
Penile Doppler clubbed 215
Penile vibratory stimulation 219, 266
Pentoxifylline 157, 168, 193
    compound 157
    use of 157
Peptide YY 251
Percutaneous ependymal sperm aspiration 211, 212
Percutaneous sperm aspiration 219
Perimenopausal women 200
Perinatal morbidity 128
Perineal muscles 216
Peritoneal endometriosis 16, 17b
    types of 17t

Peritoneal implants, morphology of 100
Peritoneal lesions 99
Peritoneal pathology 8
Persistent hypogonadism 29
Pharmacological therapy, first-line 129
Phenotypic females 33
Phenotypic males 33
Phosphodiesterase-5 218
    inhibitor 215, 258, 266
Photoepilation, sources of 134
Physical exercise 253
Physiological intracytoplasmic sperm injection 235, 236
Pituitary adenoma 63
Placenta express thyroid peroxidase 50
Platelet-derived growth factor 194
Platelet-rich plasma 94, 193, 242, 243
    intraovarian infusion of 229
Pleasurable sensation 216
Polycarbophil-based gel 224
Polycystic ovarian morphology 120, 122, 172
Polycystic ovarian syndrome 13, 46, 50, 55, 61, 64, 118, 119, 131, 135-137, 161, 168, 227, 233
    diagnosis of 120, 173
    etiopathogenesis of 119fc
    management of 118
    pathophysiology of 118
    related infertility 124, 125
Polycystic ovary 62, 122f
Polydactyly 68
Polyglandular autoimmune syndrome 226
Polymerase chain reaction 87, 234, 286
Polyp
    hysteroscopic appearance of 15b
    management of 15b
Polypectomy 13
Postcoital cervical mucus test 4
Postcoital testing 6
Postejaculate urinalysis 209
Postepididymal obstruction 211
Posthumous reproduction 269, 275
Posthumous sperm 275
Postsurgery, monitoring 211
Potential reproductive options 80
Pouch of Douglas 186
Precocious puberty 23
    classification of 23
    evaluation of 24, 25
    incomplete 24
    peripheral 24
    treatment of 25
Preconception counseling 285
Prednisone 261
Pregnancy 37, 96, 229
    complications 290
    ectopic 180, 187
    high-risk 229
    hypertensive disorders of 231
    intrauterine 180
    loss 232fc
        recurrent preterm 231
        type of 90
    management, multidisciplinary approach in 229
    medical termination of 79
    nonviable 180
    test, positive 181, 259
    viable 180

Pregnancy of unknown location 180, 182
   classification of 180
   clinical features 181
   diagnosis 181
   differential diagnosis 181
   management of 182
Pregnant women, management for 59
Preimplantation genetic
   diagnosis 233
   screening 242, 244
Preimplantation genetic testing 196, 234, 279, 282, 283
   aneuploidy 163, 280, 282
   types of 279, 283*t*
Pre-in vitro fertilization treatment 106*fc*
   role of 106
Premature ejaculation 216, 218
   evaluation of 218*fc*
   management of 218*fc*
   pharmacotherapy for 218*t*
Premature ovarian insufficiency 50, 226, 227, 229, 230
   causes 226
   management of 226
   prevalence 226
   risk factors 226
   sequelae 228, 228*f*
   terminology 226
Prenatal diagnostic testing, role of 282
Prepubertal ovary 261
Priapism 216
Prilocaine 218
Procarbazine 261
Progesterone 41, 73, 129, 161, 182, 256-259
   administration 257
     delaying 257
     different routes of 257
      routes and dosage of 257*fc*
   luteal phase support with 257
   micronized 228
   optimal dosage of 258
   primed ovarian stimulation 128, 163, 167*f*
   production 259
     impairment of 256
   receptor membrane component variants 226
   role of 236
   supplementation 242
     benefit of 258
   support 242
   type of 202
Progestin medication 29
Prolactin 55, 56, 58, 62
   disorders 61
   inhibitory factors 54
   measurement, prerequisites for 56
   neuroregulation 54*f*
   releasing factor 54
   secretion 55
     regulation of 54
Prolactinomas 55
Prostaglandin E1 analog 216
Prostate-specific antigen 71
Protein-rich fluid, massive transudation of 171
Proximal tubal block
   causes of 18*fc*
   management of 18*fc*

Pseudoprecocious precocious puberty 24
Psychosexual development 34, 35*fc*
Psychosexual health 33
Psychosexual therapy 215
Psychotropic agent 59
Pubarche, premature 26
Pubertal development, evaluation of delayed 28
Pubertal events 22
Pubertal milestones, sequence of 22
Puberty 21, 73
   absent 33
   disorders of 21
   induction of 37, 70, 70*t*
Pubic hair development 61
Pudendal nerve, regulated by 216
Pulmonary tuberculosis, secondary to 86
Pulse
   amplitude increases 55
   frequency 55
   generator 55
Pyelonephritis 187
Pyrazinamide 87
Pyridoxine 87

Q

Quality of life 220, 260

R

Radial artery-resistance index 191
Radiation therapy 63
Radiofrequency ablation 114
Radiotherapy 260, 262
   effect of 261
Rathke pouch cysts 70
Recipient cycles management 272, 272*t*
Reciprocal translocation 280
Recombinant follicle-stimulating hormone 71
Reconstruction surgery
   decision for 211
   type of 211
Reconstructive surgery 211
   advantages of 211
Recreational drugs 255
Rectal examination 215
Rectovaginal septum, palpation of 224
Recurrent implantation failure 239-241, 245, 280, 283
   management of 241, 242*f*
   pathology of 240
   risk factors for 239, 239*t*
Recurrent miscarriage 231, 233*fc*, 236
   risk factors for 231, 232*t*
Recurrent pregnancy loss 78, 89, 231, 234, 234*fc*, 235-237, 258, 280, 283
   diagnosis of 231
   evaluation of 233
Relcovaptan 175
Renal agenesis, unilateral 209
Renal function test 86, 176
Reproductive hormones 69
Reproductive maturation, maintenance of 70*t*
Reproductive technologies 285
Ribonucleic acid 290
Rifampicin 87

Rigid hysteroscope 13
Ringer lactate 177
Robert's uterus, obstructed 83
Robertsonian translocation 280

S

Saline
   infusion sonography 4*f*, 63, 109, 109*f*
   slide preparation, diagnosis 224
   sonography 4
   sonosalpingogram 9*f*
Salpingo-oophorectomy 188
Salvage reproductive potential 229
Schistosoma 90
Schizophrenia 251
Scoliosis 38
Scrotalization 44
Segmentation strategy 177*f*
Seizures 25
Semen 285
   analysis 5
     abnormalities in 5
   culture 5
   deposition of 216
   parameters, abnormal 5
   processing 287
   sample 5
   volume, normal 210*fc*
Seminiferous 56
Sephadex columns 150
Septate vagina 82*f*
Septoplasty 13
Septum, partial 84
Serial diagnostic testing 285
Serotonin reuptake inhibitor, selective 218
Sertoli cell-only syndrome 261
Sertraline 218
Serum
   anti-müllerian hormone 2
   CA-125 86, 181
   concentrations 41
   estradiol 192
   human chorionic gonadotropin 181, 182
Serum progesterone 181, 182
   levels
     increased 41
     measurement of 181
Sex chromosome 35, 38
Sex development
   differences of 33, 46
   disorders of 35
Sex hormone-binding globulin 120, 133, 138
   increased levels of 51
Sex hormones, management with 29
Sex-steroid
   deficiency shunting 40
   hormones, doses of 74
Sexual abuse 222
Sexual activity 47
Sexual characteristics, secondary 48, 70
Sexual development
   crucial, stage of secondary 31
   disorders of 33, 35
   type of abnormal 33
Sexual differentiation
   classification of abnormal 35*t*
   normal 34, 34*fc*

Sexual dysfunction 215
    causes of 215
    evidence of 4
Sexual function 229
Sexual health inventory 215, 216
Sexual history 2
Sexual infections 285
Sexual maturation, complete 29
Sexual maturity 26
Sexual organs, secondary 61
Sexual pain disorder 220
Sexual transmission of viral infections,
    risks of 286t
Sexuality, expression of 220
Sexually transmitted
    diseases 4, 254
    infections 219, 253
Sharma's ascending colonic adhesion 87
Sharma's blue python sign 87
Sharma's compartmentalization sign 87
Sharma's hanging gallbladder sign 87
Sharma's kissing fallopian tubes sign 87
Sharma's parachute sign 87
Sharma's sigmoid colonic adhesive band 87
Short luteal phase 56
Short stature 29
Sildenafil 168, 215, 218, 258
    citrate 192, 258
Single gene
    defect testing 5
    disorders 279
    variants 227
Singular dense adhesion 93
Skin, abnormal pigmentation of 67
Smoking 232, 239, 252
Social issues 269
Sonohysterography 4
Sonohysterosalpingography 8, 9, 78
Sonosalpingogram 272
Sorbitol 113
Sperm
    birefringence 153, 153f, 158
    concentration 5
    donation 269, 273, 274t
    donor 277
    found 207
    membrane 154
    morphology 51, 158
    number, total 5
    parameters, evaluation of 5
    preparations 286
    sorting technologies 158
    transport, impairment of 115
    use of 269
Sperm deoxyribonucleic acid
    fragmentation 5, 234
    integrity 251
Sperm retrieval techniques 211t
    advantages of 212t
    disadvantages of 212t
Sperm selection 145, 151, 153
    laser-assisted 157, 157f
    magnetic activated 244
    microfluidics based 155, 156f
Spermatogenesis 210, 254
Spermatozoa 219
    free 287
    quality of 144

Spermicide free condoms 219
Sphingosine-1-phosphate 262, 265
Spontaneous ovarian hyperstimulation
    syndrome 170, 170t
Spontaneous pregnancy possible 265
Standard operating procedures, use of 285
Standard sperm selection techniques 157
Staphylococcus spp 192
Stem cell 193, 229
    platelet-rich plasma 193
    treatment 96
Step-down protocol 139f
Sterility 261
Sterilization, permanent 133
Steroidogenesis 44, 44fc
    pathway 40
Stimulated cycle 199, 199f, 203
Stimulated ovaries 186
Stimulation protocols 139
Stimulation, types of response to 161
Streptococcus spp 192
Streptomycin 88
Stress 5, 232
Strict waste management protocols 286
Stromal cells, installation of 96
Stromal edema 185
Subclinical hypothyroidism 50
Subfertility 78
Submucosal fibroids 15, 108, 109, 109f
    hysteroscopic features of 15b
Submucosus leiomyomas 109
Submucous fibroid 110, 110f, 113f, 116
    classification of 108, 108t
Submucous myoma 113t
    multiple 113
    removal of 61
Subserosal fibroids, multiple 110f
Substance abuse 2
Sudden infant death syndrome 253
Supraphysiological E2 levels 263
Supraphysiological estradiol levels 161
Surgery, principles of 17b
Surgical sperm retrieval 210
    methods 219
    techniques 211
Surgically extracted sperm, cryopreservation
    of 266
Surrogacy 115, 269, 270, 274
    commercial 274
    cycles 196
    indications for 274, 275b
    partial 274
    program 275
    protocols for 276fc
    traditional 274
    types 274
Swim-up technique 145f
Swyer syndrome 40, 63
Sympathetic nervous system 216

T

Tadalafil 215, 218
Tall stature 30
Tamoxifen 137, 168
Tanner scale 22f
Telomere length 251
Teratozoospermia 5

Terminal hair 121
Testes 42
Testicular azoospermia 212
Testicular biopsy 6
    role of diagnostic 210
Testicular development, disorders of 35
Testicular extraction 219
Testicular failure, primary 207
Testicular sperm
    cryopreserved 212
    extraction 48
        microsurgical 210-212
Testis, bilateral 4
Testosterone 4, 25, 168
    enanthate 70
    gel 70
    patch 70
    production 210
    replacement therapy 39, 71
    secretion 254
    supplementation 39
    undecanoate 70
Thelarche, premature 27
Theophylline 157
Third party reproduction 269, 269t, 276t
    protocol for providing 270
    types of 269
Thrombophilia 233
    history of 258
Thyroid
    autoantibodies 227
    autoimmunity 50, 51f
    disease, history of 2
    disorders 50, 51, 52fc
        management of 51
        prevalence of 51
    disturbances, symptoms of 61
    dysfunction 51
    examination 61
    fertility 50
    function 196
        ovarian stimulation on 50, 51
        tests 25
    hormone 51
        replacement 59
        treatment 29
    peroxidase antibodies 50
    stimulating hormone 1, 2f, 3, 58, 63-65, 69,
        215, 227, 241
Thyrotropin-releasing hormone 54, 55
Thyroxine-binding globulin 50
Torsion
    chronic 187
    early-stage of 186
Total body irradiation 261
Tramadol 218
Transdermal estradiol 72
Transdermal testosterone 70
Transglutaminase antibodies 38
Transmembrane migration 147, 147f
Transplanted mesenchymal stem cells 193
Transrectal ultrasonography 217
Transthoracic echocardiogram 37
Transvaginal color Doppler 181
Transvaginal scan 4f, 114
Transvaginal sonography 180, 191, 196
Transvaginal ultrasonography 4
Transvaginal ultrasound 9

Transverse vaginal septum 84
Triggering factor 171
Trocars, primary 12
Trophoblastic human chorionic
　　　　gonadotropin 170
Tubal cannulation 13
Tubal evaluation methods 8
Tubal factor 17
　　infertility, assessment of 8
　　tests of 3, 3*f*
Tubal mucosal thickening 87
Tuberculosis 18, 190, 208, 221, 223, 226
Tubo-ovarian
　　abscess 187
　　relationship play 8
Tumor 70
　　necrosis factor 243
Turner mosaic syndrome 229
Turner's syndrome 35, 36, 36*f*, 37, 37*fc*,
　　　　38*t*, 48, 63, 226, 229
　　clinical characteristics of 36*f*
　　management of 37
　　mode of delivery in 38

U

Ultrasonography 69, 91*f*, 191, 198*f*, 199*f*, 204,
　　　　223, 233, 236
Ultrasound 91, 100
Umbilical cord 290
Ureaplasma 192
Urethra
　　increasing pressure of posterior 216
　　posterior 216
Urinary tract infection 221, 223
Urine
　　analysis, routine 219
　　pregnancy test 94, 126
Urogenital examination 215
Urogenital sinus 44
Uterine
　　anomalies, management of 78
　　cavity 82*f*, 90, 96, 109
　　curettage 182
　　effect 261
　　factor, tests for 4, 4*f*
　　microbiota 192
　　sepsis 61
　　size 2
　　structural malformations 234*fc*
　　transposition 265

Uterine artery 185
　　embolization 114
　　pulsatility index 191
Uterine fibroids 108, 116
　　hysteroscopic features of 15
Uterocervical characteristics 15
Utero-ovarian ligament 185
Uterus 9*f*, 77
　　arcuate 17
　　assessment of 15
　　bicornuate 17, 82, 82*f*
　　complete septate 83*f*
　　didelphys 82, 82*f*
　　hysteroscopic assessment of 15*b*
　　normal 15*t*
　　septate 17, 82, 83*f*
　　unicornuate 17, 81, 81*f*

V

Vacuum constriction devices 216
Vagina 77, 86
Vaginal atresia 35
Vaginal atrophy 222
Vaginal delivery 229
Vaginal dilatation 47
Vaginal discharge, abnormal 86
Vaginal dryness 220
Vaginal lubricants, water-based 224
Vaginal pH test 224
Vaginal secretions 2
Vaginal septum 222
　　longitudinal 79, 83, 83*f*
Vaginal sildenafil 258
Vaginismus 220
Vaginitis 220, 223
Vaginoplasty 47
Vaporization 17
Vaporizing electrodes 113
Vardenafil 218
Varicella 226
Varicocele 5, 212
　　treatment 212
Vas deferens
　　absence of 208
　　bilateral 4
　　congenital bilateral absence of 208-210
Vascular endothelial growth factor 171,
　　　　172, 176
Vasoactive angiogenic factors 176
Vasoactive intestinal peptide 54
Vasodilators 168

Vasoepididymostomy 210
Vasovasostomy 210
Venereal disease research laboratory test 271
Venous blood flow, impairment of 185
Venous thromboembolism 229
Veress needle 12, 14*fc*
　　parts of 13*f*
　　proper positioning of 14*b*
Vestibulitis 221
Vhromosomal abnormalities 38
Viable nonmotile spermatozoa,
　　　　selection of 156
Vinblastine 261
Viral hepatitis, transmitted 285
Viral infection 285, 287*t*
　　chances of 285
　　effect of 287*t*
　　transmission of 290
　　risk of 290
Virilization, severe 47
Virilizing congenital adrenal hyperplasia 44
Virus specific management 287
Vitamin E 193
Vulva 86
Vulvodynia 220, 223

W

Waardenburg syndrome 67
Whirlpool sign 187, 187*f*
Whole-genome sequencing 45, 233

X

X chromosome 41, 279
　　deletions 226
　　disorders 226
　　structural rearrangement of 35
X syndrome, triple 226
X trisomy 230
X-linked dominant inheritance 279
X-linked recessive diseases 279

Y

Y chromosome 279
　　microdeletion 5
　　microdeletion tests 209

Z

Zeta potential method 154, 154*f*
Ziehl–Neelsen staining 87

www.ingramcontent.com/pod-product-compliance
Ingram Content Group UK Ltd.
Pitfield, Milton Keynes, MK11 3LW, UK
UKHW051315150425
457399UK00006B/4